# PRINCIPLES OF PATHOLOGY
# FOR DENTAL STUDENTS

J. B. WALTER, *T.D.*,
M.D., M.R.C.P., F.R.C.Path.
*Department of Pathology, Banting Institute, University of Toronto,
and Departments of Medicine and Pathology, Toronto General
Hospital, Toronto, Canada*

MARGARET C. HAMILTON
F.D.S.R.C.S.(ENG.)
*Department of Dental Health, University of Birmingham, England*

M. S. ISRAEL
M.B., M.R.C.P., M.R.C.Path., D.C.P.
*Department of Pathology, Institute of Basic Medical Sciences,
Royal College of Surgeons of England, and
Lewisham Group Laboratory, London*

# Principles of Pathology for Dental Students

## THIRD EDITION

J. B. WALTER
MARGARET C. HAMILTON
M. S. ISRAEL

CHURCHILL LIVINGSTONE
Edinburgh London & New York
1974

CHURCHILL LIVINGSTONE
Medical Division of Longman Group Limited

Distributed in the United States of America by
Longman Inc., 19 West 44th Street, New York, N.Y.
10036 and by associated companies, branches and
representatives throughout the world.

First Edition 1967
Reprinted 1969
Second Edition 1971
Third Edition 1974
Reprinted 1976
Reprinted 1978
Reprinted 1979

ISBN 0 443 01093 5

Library of Congress Catalog Card Number
73-84619

Printed in Hong Kong by
Wilture Enterprises (International) Ltd

# PREFACE

The student who embarks on a career in dentistry must achieve within a period of five years sufficient skill to recognize, diagnose correctly, and treat the diseases which occur in the oral cavity. He must acquire much theoretical knowledge as well as become adept in many complicated practical procedures. This knowledge should be based on sound general principles, and the first part of this book is intended to cover the principles of general pathology in a manner suited to the particular needs of the dentist.

The dental surgeon must treat not only diseases of the oral cavity but also people—each patient as an individual with problems which may not be confined to the mouth. Dental treatment must be related to other diseases in so far as these may modify the treatment and necessitate certain precautions. Nowhere is this more evident than in a patient with heart disease. Although the dentist need not be medically qualified, he should have sufficient insight into common diseases to enable him to appreciate his patient's general condition and thereby cooperate effectively with his medical colleagues. The latter part of this book is designed to cover the basic principles of the pathology pertaining to some of the special systems. Of necessity this coverage is brief but it is intended to be adequate, so that when time and opportunity arise the dentist will be able to consult specialized texts without the feeling that he is venturing into foreign fields.

When studying pathology for the first time, the student meets many new words and concepts; these we have endeavoured to define when they are first introduced so that learning may proceed by a series of progressive steps. We have appended a list of references to each chapter in the hope of fostering the spirit of inquiry in our students. For it may be stated as an axiom that those who wish to learn consult a book, but those who seek to understand consult a library. From this vantage point they may proceed alone by planned experimentation and careful observation.

Two years have elapsed since the second edition, and, although no dramatic advances have been made in medicine during this period, many sections have required modification. The section on immunology has undergone considerable change—in particular, the nature of the cell-mediated response and the lymphokines. Amyloid is now believed to be a component of immunoglobulin, and the section on its pathogenesis has therefore been rewritten. Other subjects which have been modified or introduced for the first time include cell-membrane structure, the Y chromosome dot, biosynthesis of collagen, serum enzymes in myocardial infarction and liver disease, the mediators of acute inflammation (in particular the role of prostaglandins and complement), verrucous carcinoma, angiosarcoma, Kaposi's sarcoma, carcinoma of the colon, melanoma of the skin, carcinoid tumours of the gastrointestinal tract, the classification of the lymphomata, the action of RNA-containing oncogenic viruses and the role of reverse transcriptase, malignant hyperpyrexia, kwashiorkor, the hyperviscosity syndrome, cryoglobulinaemia, enzyme defects as a cause of haemolytic anaemia, and the lipoproteins. In addition, a chapter on diseases of the skin has been added, for a number of these conditions also affect the mucosa of the mouth, and their presence may first be noted by the dental surgeon.

J. B. W., Toronto, Canada
M. C. H., Birmingham, England
M. S. I., London, England

# ACKNOWLEDGEMENTS

Many of the gross specimens illustrated are photographs of preparations in the Wellcome Museum of the Royal College of Surgeons of England, and these are acknowledged with each corresponding caption. We thank the President and Council of the Royal College of Surgeons of England for permission to use them.

We owe special thanks to those who have given us unpublished photographs or who have permitted us to utilize or modify their published material: Brookes, W. S., Fig. 20.1; Bywaters, E. G. L., Fig. 33.8; Cohen, A. S., Fig. 25.4; Crick, F. H. C., Fig. 2.11; Cullen, J. B., Fig. 30.2; David, J. R., Fig. 13.2; Dixon, J. F., Fig. 13.1; Epstein, M. A., Figs. 2.4 and 2.8; Foster, T. D., Fig. 33.1; Gladstone, G. P., Fig. 13.1; Hoggins, G. S., Figs. 20.3 and 35.1; Horne, R. W., Figs. 16.1, 16.2, and 16.3; Kavanau, J. L., Fig. 2.5; Kemp, N. H., Figs. 2.14 and 3.4; Killey, H. C., Fig. 33.2; le Beux, Y., Figs. 2.6 and 2.7; Levene, C. I., Fig. 2.17; Lewin, P. K. and Conen, P. E., Fig. 2.15; Miles, A. A., Fig. 5.2; Miyai, K., Figs. 2.10, 4.3, and 4.4; Nirenberg, M. W., Fig. 2.12; Sheward, J. D., Fig. 18.2; Smallwood, W. C., Fig. 3.5; Thompson, J. S. and M. W., Fig. 2.13; Thomson, A. D., Fig. 33.6; Waldenström, J., 25.1; and Warner, J. R., Fig. 2.12.

J. B. W., M. C. H., and M. S. I.

# CONTENTS

*Chapter 1*

# INTRODUCTION

In the practice of medicine it is soon apparent that the majority of patients who seek help do so because of some abnormality which is causing them distress. Often such *symptoms* can be dispelled by simple remedies—quite often by time and reassurance. Much of medicine is an art which its practitioners, whether doctors, dentists, nurses, or physiotherapists must learn. Nevertheless, there have always been individuals who were not content simply to observe disease and the effects of empirical time-honoured remedies upon it. They have attempted to describe and record the abnormalities in their patients in an objective manner; by introducing measurements they initiated the science which is called pathology.

*Disease* itself is as difficult to define as is the normal, from which it is a departure. As generally used, the term disease is employed to describe a state in which there is a sufficient departure from the normal for signs or symptoms to be produced. The variations from the normal are called *lesions*, and although generally structural in nature, the term may also be used to describe functional abnormalities, for example *biochemical lesions* (p. 44). The cause of the disease is called its *aetiology* and the development of the lesions its *pathogenesis*. Although aetiology and pathogenesis are generally described as separate entities, in practice it is often difficult to distinguish between them. Indeed, the aetiology of one era may become part of the pathogenesis of the next. An example will suffice. A patient takes a large dose of strychnine, develops convulsions, and dies. Clearly the aetiology of the disease is administration of strychnine. However, a closer consideration may reveal that the drug was self-administered during a phase of depression. The suicidal administration of strychnine would then be part of the pathogenesis of the fatal disease depression.

Although this instance may appear to be an exaggeration of the difficulty in delineating the cause of a disease, many other examples will be encountered. The great advances in bacteriology which started at the end of the nineteenth century fostered the concept that each disease had a single cause. To state that a boil is always caused by the *Staphylococcus pyogenes* is true, but nevertheless this is an incomplete statement. It is known that patients with diabetes mellitus are prone to develop recurrent boils. Which is the cause of the boils, the staphylococcus or the diabetes? Present doctrine would still favour the organism, but the diabetes would be labelled a major predisposing factor. Multiple causes are probably much more common than we think. The doctrine of one cause for one disease has certainly failed to be a profitable concept in the search for the aetiology of many common diseases such as cancer, arteriosclerosis, emphysema, chronic bronchitis, and dental caries.

An attempt to avoid the difficulty in defining disease has been the introduction of the term *syndrome*. This is a condition in which there occurs a defined collection of lesions, signs, or symptoms which are not necessarily always caused by the same agent. Thus Mikulicz's syndrome is defined as bilateral painless enlargement of the lacrimal and salivary glands from whatever cause. It may be found in leukaemia, but frequently the cause is unknown and it is then said to be *idiopathic*. Clearly the diseases in which the cause is not known are difficult to distinguish from syndromes. Indeed, the two terms are frequently used quite indiscriminately and interchangeably.

*Pathology* is thus the scientific study of disease. It describes the cause, course, and termination of disease, and the nature of its lesions. In almost all diseases the lesions are of varying nature, and may be morphological, chemical, or functional. Anything which can be measured is within the domain of pathology. The height of the blood pressure, the rate of the heart, and the temperature of the patient are all valid measurements, which if accurately recorded are as scientific as are measurements of the size of a muscle fibre on a section or the amount of fat in a liver.

All good clinicians are thus practising pathologists, and it is for this reason that pathology is such an important part of the curriculum for both dental and medical students.

# Chapter 2

# NORMAL STRUCTURE

## THE CELL

### Introduction

The body is composed of innumerable cells which are bound together by a variable amount of intercellular material. Each cell is enclosed by an outer limiting membrane, the *cell* or *plasma membrane*, and contains a nucleus which is bounded by the *nuclear membrane*.

Development from the fertilized ovum is accomplished by two processes:

1. *Division*, whereby more cells are produced.

2. *Maturation*, or *differentiation*, whereby cells develop specific structures which enable them to perform specialized functions, e.g. contraction in the case of muscle fibres. Some highly specialized cells, e.g. neurones, lose their ability to divide as they become differentiated, but others do not, e.g. liver cells. What is lost during the process of maturation is the ability to differentiate along other lines. While the fertilized ovum is *totipotent*, i.e. capable of producing all the tissues of the body, its cellular progeny are not all alike and do not have this ability. Both cytoplasmic and nuclear factors are probably involved in differentiation, but the nature of this process, which may be regarded as a type of ageing, is not understood.

The cells of the body show a considerable diversity of structure and function, and each is in fact remarkably independent. Each receives a supply of oxygen and foodstuff from the blood stream with which it must produce its own structural components and secretions, and from which it must release the energy required for mechanical, chemical, or electrical work. It is therefore not surprising that all cells are built upon a similar basic plan.

The number of chemical reactions known to occur inside the cell is so great that it would be difficult to understand how these could proceed in a structure as simple as the cell appears to be under the light microscope. The electron microscope has changed all this—from a barren wilderness, the internal structure of the cell is now seen to resemble a large industrial city with its factories, warehouses, streets, power-stations, etc. (Fig. 2.1 and Fig. 2.6).

### Functions of the Plasma Membrane[1, 2]

### Motility[3]

Examination of living cells reveals that the plasma membrane is not a rigid structure, but is in constant motion. This motility is particularly well developed in certain cells, and permits them to move bodily through the tissues. The white blood cells—polymorphonuclear leucocytes, lymphocytes, and monocytes—behave in this way. The undulating surface of the macrophage is particularly characteristic. Folds of the membrane have been observed to entrap a droplet of fluid by a process known as *pinocytosis*.

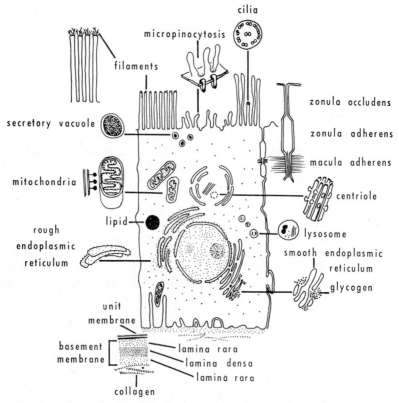

Fɪɢ. 2.1. Diagrammatic representation of a hypothetical composite cell, with
some organelles shown around it at a higher magnification. The free
surface of the cell has projecting microvilli, which on the left are arranged
regularly to form a brush border. In the centre, the villi are irregular,
and micropinocytotic vacuole formation is depicted. On the right cilia are
shown. The cell adjoins its neighbours with some interdigitation of their
plasma membranes; one junctional complex is shown. The nucleus contains
one nucleolus, and is surrounded by a double-layered membrane. Between the
nucleus and the free border is the cell centre, or centrosome, surrounded by
sacs of the Golgi apparatus. There are two centrioles lying at right angles to
each other. The base of the cell rests on a basement membrane which at high
magnification has three components; the plasma membrane, like other membranes in the cell, has a trilaminar structure. Ribosomes are scattered free
in the cell cytoplasm, and are also attached to the rough endoplasmic reticulum and the outer nuclear envelope.

(*Drawn by Margot Mackay, Department of Art as Applied to Medicine,
University of Toronto*)

## Phagocytosis

Apart from locomotion, the surface movement of monocytes and polymorphonuclear leucocytes produces another effect. By pushing out projections, or *pseudopodia*, around particles, they are able to surround and
finally engulf them. This process of ingestion is called *phagocytosis*.

## Cell Recognition

In addition, the cell membrane contains specific substances (antigens) by which the body is able to recognize its own cells and tolerate them. Cells from another individual are regarded as aliens, and are attacked (p. 168).

## Cell Adhesiveness

The cell membrane is concerned with adhesiveness, which is a factor that induces cells of like constitution to stick together. If the cells of an embryo are separated from each other and are then allowed to come together again, they aggregate to form organs and tissues. This affinity which cells have for their own kind must be an important mechanism in the development and maintenance of the architecture of multicellular animals. But not all cells behave in this manner. The cells of the blood do not exhibit adhesiveness, nor to some extent do cancer cells, for they are able to infiltrate freely into the surrounding tissues.

## Cell Growth[4, 5]

The mitotic activity in epidermis is greatly increased in an area of skin adjacent to a wound. The increased production of cells continues until epidermal cells from one side of the wound meet those migrating from the other side. Contact of like cells with like then inhibits cell division; the phenomenon is called *contact inhibition* (p. 108). It appears to be a function of the cell membrane. Malignant transformation, infection of a cell by a virus, and treatment with proteolytic enzymes all appear to alter the cell membrane and release cells from this inhibition.

## Exchange Surface Activity

The cell membrane acts as an exchange surface across which the cell constituents interchange with those of the extracellular fluids. In this way it acts as a chemical barrier as well as a mechanical one. Cells are rich in $K^+$, $Mg^{++}$, and phosphate ions as well as proteins, while the extracellular fluids contain $Na^+$, $Cl^-$, and bicarbonate ions and very little protein. The integrity of the plasma membrane is an important factor in maintaining this special chemical composition of the cell substance. The cell membrane is able to exclude $Na^+$ ions and thereby allow $K^+$ ions to accumulate within the cell. This is sometimes spoken of as the *sodium pump*, and is a mechanism which requires energy. Ionic calcium is required for normal cell membrane permeability, but its role is obscure.

The free surface of some cells is covered by short finger-like processes, or *microvilli*, which appear to be concerned with absorption. On light microscopy they produce the appearance of a brush border seen for example on the intestinal epithelium, a surface where absorption is very necessary (p. 418).

## Membrane Structure in Relation to Function

Electron microscopy has shown an intact membrane some 7·5 nm* in

* 1 mm = 1 000 $\mu$m. 1 $\mu$m = 1 000 nm. The Ångström unit (Å) is a tenth of 1 nm, and is no longer used in measurement.

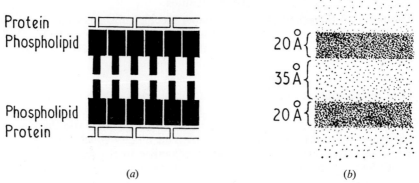

*(a)*            *(b)*

FIG. 2.2. The unit membrane is composed of two electron-dense laminae separated by a third clear zone *(b)*. The chemical structure shown in *(a)* is compatible with this appearance.

width, which at high magnification of suitably prepared material can be resolved into two electron-dense laminae with an intervening clear space. This trilaminar structure is known as a *unit membrane*, and it appears to have no pores such as have been postulated to explain the observed permeability of the cell membrane.[6]

In *micropinocytosis* small invaginations of the cell membrane become nipped off to form vesicles. In this way small quantities of fluid may be imbibed by a process which resembles pinocytosis but on a small scale. The formation of micropinocytotic vesicles on one surface of a cell and their discharge from another surface is one postulated mechanism whereby substances may cross a cellular barrier, e.g. blood-vessel endothelium. The process is known as *cytopempsis*.[7]

Studies on the rate of diffusion of small molecules across the cell membrane led Pappenheimer to conclude that it contained small pores.[6] No such

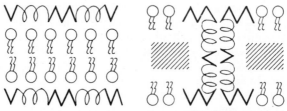

FIG. 2.3. Two diagrams to illustrate the possible structure of the cell membrane. *(a)* A modification of the Davson–Danielli–Robertson unit membrane. The outer layers are depicted as composed of protein, either helical, or random coil which is shown as straight lines forming W or M. The lipid molecules are in the centre of the membrane with their polar heads, shown as circles, pointing outwards. *(b)* The membrane as suggested by Lenard and Singer. The central cross-hatched areas is assumed to be occupied by relatively non-polar constituents (hydrophobic amino-acid residues or lipids) and single polypeptide chains are drawn to traverse the entire membrane.

*(After Lenard, J. and Singer, S. J. (1966), Proc. N.Y. Acad. Sci.* **56**, 1824.)

static pores have been seen, but it is conceivable that the formation of a micro-pinocytotic vesicle and subsequent diffusion of its contents or fusion with other membranes in the cytoplasm of the cell constitute the equivalent *functional pore.*

There is considerable evidence that the cell membrane is not homogeneous. Its nature is complex, and although many chemical structural arrangements have been postulated, none is entirely satisfactory. It is generally believed that

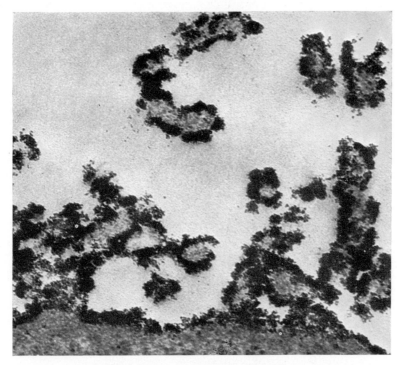

FIG. 2.4. Detail of the plasma membrane of a HeLa cell with much surface activity in the form of profuse filamentous microvilli. After staining for enzymes splitting adenosine triphosphate, dense reaction-product has been deposited with close precision at the cell membrane, indicating that the enzymes are localized there, presumably for the supply of energy require-ments. × 55 000.

(*Electron micrograph provided by Dr. M. A. Epstein and Dr. S. J. Holt*)

a lipid-protein combination is the basis of its structure, and one concept of the cell membrane is that of a bimolecular lipid leaflet as suggested by Davson and Danielli, The two layers of lipid molecules have their polar (hydrophilic) ends turned outwards, and are covered by protein (Fig 2.2(a)). This concept fits well with the observed electron microscopic appearance of an approximately 7·5 nm thick trilaminated membrane as described by Robertson. It is now agreed that this arrangement is physically unsound and other alternative models must be considered. Fig. 2.3 depicts that proposed by Lenard and Singer,[8] in which both protein and lipid molecules reach the surface. Furthermore, a pore lined by polypeptide chains is proposed, although there is no evidence bearing on this point. Rigid structures, such as those depicted in Fig. 2.2, fail to account for the observed activity of the membrane, which is by no means a static structure. It is constantly changing in shape, and change indicates the performance of work. The presence of ATPase at the cell surface (Fig. 2.4) supports the concept that energy is released at the cell membrane. A model which allows for this is that proposed

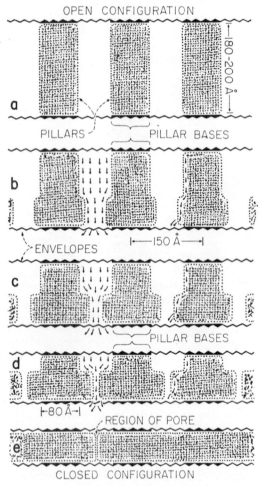

Fig. 2.5. A diagrammatic cross-sectional representation of the plasma membrane. The protein envelope is depicted as zig-zag lines and between them are pillars of lipid, each with a base (heavy zig-zag lines). The pillars are widely separated when the membrane is in the open position (*a*). As the pillars collapse (*b, c, d*), fluid in the pores is pumped in the direction of the arrows. In the closed position fluid is pumped in the direction of the arrows. In the closed position some of the pores may remain (*e*—left-hand end), or else fusion of the pillars takes place and the membrane structure is then very similar to that depicted in Fig. 2.2. (*From: Kavanau, J. L.* (1963). Nature (Lond.) **198**, 525.)

by Kavanau.[9] The membrane is pictured as having pillars of lipid covered by protein (Fig. 2.5). Between the bases of the lipid pillars are pores, which are large in the open and small in the closed configuration. This concept of cell membrane structure allows for ready change in membrane shape and in its permeability. The amoeboid movement of the polymorphs and the changed permeability of the plasma membrane of a neurone when an impulse passes are more readily explained than by the static structure depicted in Fig. 2.2. The technique of surface replication electron microscopy has indicated that this structure of cell membrane may indeed exist.[10]

It should be noted that the membrane in the closed configuration clearly approximates to the structure of Davson and Danielli. The "normal" appearance of the membrane as seen in routine electron microscopy may indeed be an artefact if the membrane readily adopts the closed configuration when subjected to fixation.[8]

An interesting feature of the red-cell envelope is the ability with which influenza viruses attach themselves to it. The relationship between the two is quantitative, and it seems probable that viruses attach themselves to specific areas on the cell surface. These hypothetical areas which are presumably dependent upon particular chemical groupings are known as *cell* or *surface receptors*. It is likely that many substances, e.g. drugs, toxins, etc., act in a similar manner by becoming fixed on to specific receptors. If the receptor units of the membrane are capable of rotation, a substance attached to an external receptor could enter the cell quite readily.

The cell-receptor concept harmonizes well with the concept of active transport of chemicals across the cell membrane. Thus amino acids are actively transported across membranes in the gut (for absorption) and in the renal tubules (for reabsorption). A failure in a transport system can result in disease: for example, in cystinuria the kidney cannot reabsorb cystine, lysine, ornithine, or arginine—amino acids which share a common transport system. The disease was one of the original group of "inborn errors of metabolism" studied by Garrod, and is characterized by the formation of cystine renal stones.

Another interesting application of the receptor concept is the supposition that many hormones react with specific receptors on their target cells. The interaction activates an enzyme adenyl cyclase which, in the presence of magnesium ions, leads to the formation of adenosine 3′,5′-cyclic monophosphate, or *cyclic AMP*.[11] This substance triggers a sequence of events specific for that cell and leads to its response associated with the hormone. Cyclic AMP is therefore a *second messenger*.

In summary, the structure of the plasma membrane is very complex and contains lipid and protein. It can consume energy and change its shape in response to stimuli. Its protein molecules are heterogeneous, some being responsible for the receptor sites, others for antigenicity, enzyme activity, etc.

### The Cytoplasm

The cytoplasm is that part of the protoplasm not included in the nucleus, and electron microscopy has revealed that its structure is very complex indeed. It is subdivided into many compartments by membranes which

closely resemble the plasma membrane in structure. The most extensive
subdivision is effected by the *endoplasmic reticulum*, but the cytoplasm
contains many membrane-bound structures, or *organelles*—mitochondria,
lysosomes, etc. (Fig. 2.6).

## Endoplasmic Reticulum

This consists of a series of membranes which are formed into an inter-
communicating series of tubes, vesicles, and cisterns (Fig. 2.1 and Fig. 2.7).
It is in these spaces that the secretion of some glands first appears. Situated
on the outer surface of the endoplasmic reticulum there are granules, about
15 nm in diameter, which are rich in *ribonucleic acid (RNA)*. These are called
*ribosomes*, and give the endoplasmic reticulum a rough appearance. Similar

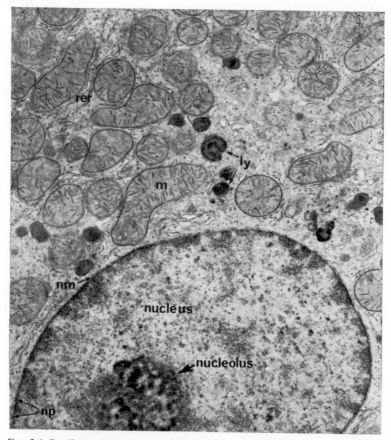

Fig. 2.6. Rat liver cell showing the main features of a cell as revealed by electron-
microscopy. The nucleus is bounded by the nuclear membrane (nm) in which
there is a nuclear pore (np). A nucleolus is present in the part of the nucleus
which is included. In the cytoplasm there are mitochondria (m) with cristae,
lysosomes (ly), and rough endoplasmic reticulum (rer). The tissue was fixed in
osmic acid and embedded in epon-araldite mixture. × 17 300.

(*Photograph supplied by Dr. Y. le Beux*)

granules lie free in the cytoplasm and are not attached to the endoplasmic reticulum. The ribosomes play a very important part in cellular metabolism because it is in relation to them that *protein synthesis* occurs (p. 17). When the ribosomes are lying free the protein is for the cell's own internal requirements. Protein for export is synthetized in relation to the endoplasmic reticulum.

The endoplasmic reticulum and its associated ribosomal granules cannot be distinguished in the "paraffin" sections used in routine pathology. The RNA content, however, is distinguishable by its blue staining (*basophilia*) with haematoxylin—the latter, being a basic substance, combines with acids, e.g. the nucleic acids. It follows that the cytoplasm of cells actively engaged in protein synthesis appears blue or mauve in haematoxylin and eosin stained (H. & E.) sections. Plasma cells are an excellent example of this. RNA stains red with pyronin (see p. 143). The endoplasmic reticulum and its associated granules is called the *ergastoplasm*.

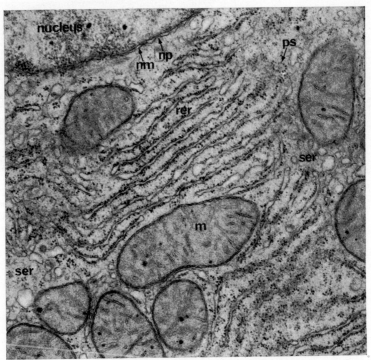

FIG. 2.7. Rat liver cell. The double-layered nuclear membrane (nm) and nuclear pores (np) are well shown. The endoplasmic reticulum has two components, rough (rer) with its attached ribosomes forming parallel arrays, and smooth (ser) seen lower down in the section without ribosomes. Note the group of ribosomes (ps) apparently lying free in the cytoplasm; this probably corresponds to a polysome. The mitochondria (m) are bounded by a double membrane, the inner component of which is folded on itself to produce the cristae. The dense aggregates in the cytoplasm are composed of glycogen. The tissue was fixed in osmic acid and embedded in epon-araldite mixture. Lead hydroxide stain. × 41 250.    (*Photograph supplied by Dr. Y. le Beux*)

In some cells the endoplasmic reticulum also forms a complex lattice of tubules which has no attached ribosomes and therefore appears *smooth*. The smooth and rough elements of the endoplasmic reticulum are continuous with each other, with the outer lamina of the nuclear membrane, and perhaps also with the plasma membrane.

## Golgi Apparatus

The *Golgi apparatus* consists of a series of flattened sacs and small vesicles, much smaller than those of the endoplasmic reticulum. They usually surround the *centrosome*, a clear area near the centre of the cell and which contains one or more *centrioles*. The Golgi apparatus is best developed in glandular cells, and is usually situated close to the nucleus on the side nearest the lumen. It is believed that in exocrine glands, such as the pancreas and the salivary glands, secretion is formed in the endoplasmic reticulum, collects in the

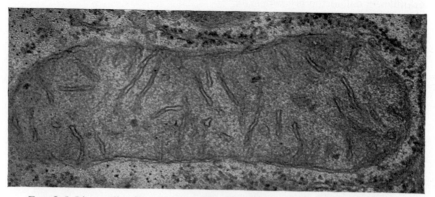

FIG. 2..8 Liver cell mitochondrion. The organelle is surrounded by an outer membrane with a second, inner membrane close within it; the inner membrane is folded into shelf-like cristae which protrude into the interior. ×52 000.                    (*Photograph supplied by Dr. M. A. Epstein*)

Golgi apparatus, and that the vesicles so formed are then discharged on to the surface.

## Centriole

The centriole is a cylindrical body about 15 nm long, which divides into two immediately before mitosis, and is concerned with the orientation of the spindle (p. 22).

## Mitochondria[12, 13]

These rod-shaped bodies have a smooth outer limiting membrane and an inner, electron-dense membrane which is folded into incomplete septa, or *cristae*, that subdivide the mitochondria into compartments (Fig. 2.7 and Fig. 2.8).

This complex structure of the mitochondria is a reflection of their function. They contain all the enzymes of the Krebs cycle and of the terminal electron transport system (cytochrome system). The *Krebs cycle* is a system whereby products of carbohydrate, fat, and protein metabolism are oxidized to produce energy (Fig. 2.9). The latter is stored in the form of the high energy bonds of adenosine triphosphate (ATP), and is utilized whenever the cell performs any kind of work. The mitochondria are the power-stations of the cell, and are among the first structures to be affected when adverse conditions prevail. Mitochondria are capable of enlargement, and replicate by transverse division. Mitochondrial DNA may play a role in this process (see p. 22).

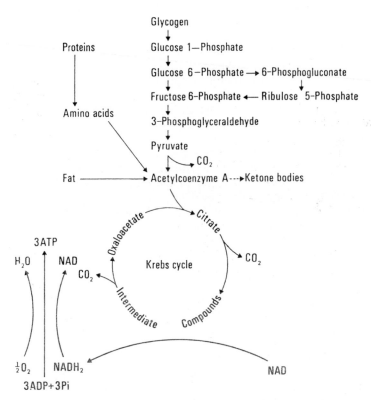

FIG. 2.9. Outline of the metabolic pathways concerned in energy production. Products of protein, fat, and carbohydrate metabolism are fed into the Krebs cycle *via* acetylcoenzyme A. Several enzymic reactions of the Krebs cycle involve the reduction of NAD to $NADH_2$. Reoxidation of $NADH_2$ by the cytochrome system is coupled with phosphorylation of ADP to ATP, viz. The hexose monophosphate shunt shown on the right is an alternative pathway. An aerobic process, it is of importance in the metabolism of red cells. Defects of glucose 6-phosphate dehydrogenase, which converts glucose 6-phosphate to 6-phosphogluconate, result in haemolytic anaemia (see p. 346).

$$NADH_2 + \tfrac{1}{2}O_2 + 3ADP + 3Pi \rightarrow NAD + H_2O + 3ATP.$$

*Key:* NAD— Nicotinamide adenine dinucleotide. $NADH_2$— Dihydronicotinamide adenine dinucleotide. Pi—Inorganic phosphate. ADP— Adenosine diphosphate. ATP— Adenosine triphosphate.

**Lysosomes** [14, 15]

These are rounded membrane-bound bodies described by de Duve in 1955, which contain the lytic* enzymes that are active at a low pH, i.e. acid phosphatase and the proteolytic enzymes previously grouped under the term *cathepsins* (Fig. 2.6). In the polymorphonuclear leucocytes lysosomes are easily visible as the characteristic granules, and these are undoubtedly concerned in the digestion of phagocytosed particles. After cell death the lysosomal enzymes are probably responsible for the cell's digestion and ultimate dissolution. They also play a part as mediators of acute inflammation, and their release from polymorphs can cause local tissue damage. This is particularly prominent in immune-complex reactions (see p. 163). Whether the potentially damaging enzymes of the lysosomes can be released in the living cell is less certain. However, it does seem likely that they are involved in the removal of redundant cells during embryonic development and following some forms of cell injury. Hydrocortisone is said to stabilize the lysosomal membrane, and this may explain how it protects cells against damage.[16, 17]

Particles ingested by the cell appear as membrane-bound bodies, and are called *phagosomes*. These acquire digestive enzymes and may then be regarded as a type of lysosome. Sometimes phagosomes contain recognizable cell components, e.g. mitochondria; evidently as parts of a cell wear out or are damaged, they are removed by digestion.[18] Such bodies are called *cytolysomes*, or *autophagocytic vacuoles*. Lipofuscin and other undigested material may remain to form yet another type of lysosome. Various names have been applied—residual body, dense body, etc. (Fig. 2.10).

The concept of the lysosome is therefore in part biochemical and in part morphological. It is a membrane-bound structure containing lytic enzymes, and its morphology varies according to whether it is inactive (primary lysosome) or is actively engaged in digesting material, either of endogenous or exogenous origin.

**Microtubules and Microfilaments**

High-resolution electron microscopy has revealed that most cells contain fibrillar material which is composed of either thin filaments or tubules. Their composition, structure, and function probably vary from one cell type to another and only a brief description will be given here.

*Microtubules.* These are tubular structures 20–27 nm in diameter. Their centres are composed of material of low electron density, and they therefore appear as hollow tubes. The outer dense wall is actually composed of approximately thirteen longitudinal filamentous subunits with a distance of 5·5–6 nm between them. In some cells, e.g. diatoms, the microtubules appear to give the cell rigidity, acting as a cytoskeleton, and they may be responsible for the relatively fixed shape of some cells, e.g. blood platelets. The transport of material within the cytoplasm is another suggested function. The filaments of the spindle at mitosis are composed of microtubules.

* Lyse—to render soluble.

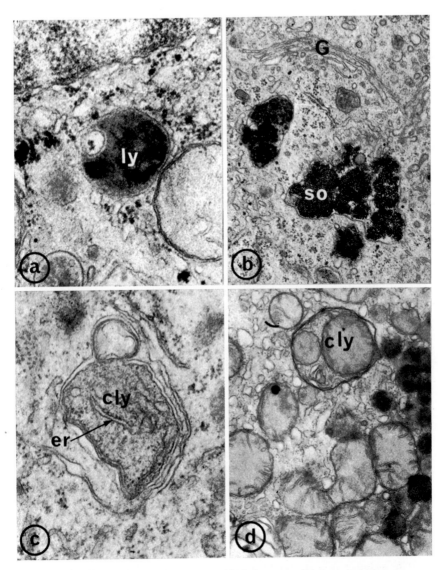

FIG. 2..10 Various types of lysosome. (*a*) A lysosome (ly) in a normal parenchymal liver cell. Lead hydroxide. × 43 750. (*b*) Membrane-bound structures
containing ferritin granules. These are sometimes called siderosomes (so).
G—Golgi apparatus. Lead hydroxide. × 22 400. (*c*) A cytolysome (cly)
in a normal rat hepatocyte containing small fragments of the rough-surfaced
endoplasmic reticulum (er). Lead hydroxide. × 46 200. (*d*) A cytolysome
(cly) containing structures which are probably degraded mitochondria.
Lead hydroxide. × 17 900. (*Photographs supplied by Dr. Katsumi Miyai*)

*Microfilaments.* Most cells also contain filaments about 5 nm in diameter. Bundles of these converging on a macula adherens, or desmosome (Fig. 2.1), are known as tonofibrils on light microscopy.

Other cytoplasmic components include glycogen granules, fat globules, etc. Some cells contain specialized structures, e.g. myofibrils in muscle and granules in eosinophils. Furthermore, as the resolution of the electron microscope is being increased, so further structures are being described. In many instances their function is not known, but there is little doubt that in due course the ultrastructure of cells will turn out to be very complex—as complex indeed as life itself.

## The Nucleus

Situated within the cell and enclosed by a membrane is the *nucleus,* an important structure because it contains, in chemical form, the coded information which is handed down from one cell to its progeny and from one generation to the next. The chemical which performs this vital function is a nucleoprotein consisting of a histone combined with *deoxyribonucleic acid* (DNA). The acidic components of the nuclear material, since they combine with basic dyes like haematoxylin, are responsible for the basophilia with H. & E. The basophilic material in the nucleus is often called *chromatin,* a name coined before the discovery of DNA.

### Chemical Structure of DNA

Much work has been done on the chemical structure of DNA. It is a polymer of high molecular weight (6–10 million) composed of a long chain of monounits, or nucleotides (Base–Deoxyribose sugar–Phosphate). The deoxyribose molecules are linked together by a phosphate, and a base is attached to each sugar (Fig. 2.11.). The common bases are either purines (adenine and guanine) or pyrimidines (thymine and cytosine). As a result of x-ray diffraction studies, Watson and Crick[19] proposed a structure which fits remarkably well with our concept of DNA as a self-reduplicating genetic material. They postulated that the molecule is composed of two polynucleotide chains spiralled around a common axis. The bases are directed towards the axis, and the two chains are linked by hydrogen bonds between a purine and a pyrimidine. They showed that only adenine could pair with thymine, and guanine with cytosine.

### Role of the Nucleic Acids as Genetic Material[20-23]

It is believed that the DNA in the nucleus contains genetic information which is passed *via* RNA into the cytoplasm, where it is utilized in the manufacture of proteins (often enzymes) of exact composition. The word *gene* is used to describe the hypothetical unit of heredity for any single characteristic. Genes are present in the DNA, and are an expression of its contained genetic information.

The order of the bases in DNA constitutes the genetic code, a sequence of three bases corresponding to a single amino acid. A type of RNA (*messenger RNA,* or mRNA) is made in the nucleus in the presence of DNA-dependent RNA polymerase. The process is called *transcription,* and the mRNA is

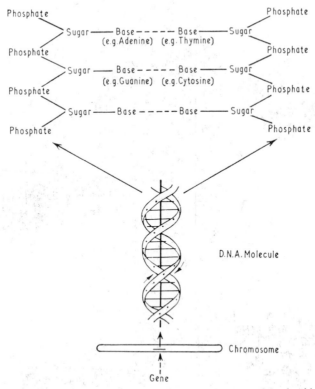

FIG. 2.11. Suggested chemical structure of DNA. The two polynucleotide chains are united by their bases, the order of which constitutes the genetic code. (*After Watson, J. D. and Crick, F. H. C.* (1953). Nature, (Lond.) **171.** 737).

modelled on one of the polynucleotide chains of DNA which acts as a template. The base sequence of the RNA is thus complementary to that of DNA, i.e. cytosine corresponds with guanine, etc. This mRNA passes into the cytoplasm and becomes associated with a group of ribosomes (*a polysome*). Here protein synthesis occurs. Each triplet, or *codon*, of the RNA base order is responsible for one amino acid.* As the ribosomes "read along" the RNA molecule, successive amino acids are added to an ever increasing polypeptide chain. In this way a protein of exact composition is built up; secondary and tertiary structure are presumably a consequence of this. The actual addition of each amino acid is effected by another type of RNA (*transfer RNA*, or tRNA), a separate form of which exists for each of the amino acids. The process is complex and is described as *translation*, for the code of the DNA finally appears legible in the form of a polypeptide chain (Fig. 2.12).

Thus the genetic code of DNA consists of codons which determine the insertion of particular amino acids in the peptide chain. The sequence of the

* With 4 bases, 64 triplets are possible, but as only about 20 amino acids have to be coded, some duplication occurs. The code is therefore said to be degenerate. Thus UUU and UUC both correspond to phenylalanine. The actual order of the three bases in each triplet is not known. It is thought that the code is universal, i.e. the same for all organisms.

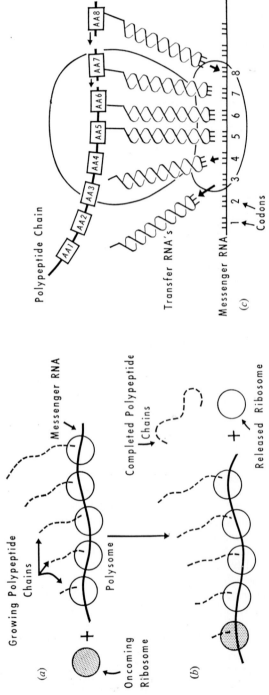

FIG. 2.12. Schematic model of protein synthesis. In (a) and (b) a long single-stranded molecule of messenger RNA (mRNA) is seen associated with a group of ribosomes to form a polysome. As each ribosome moves along the mRNA, an ever-growing polypeptide chain is produced. In (c) a single ribosome is depicted as a combination of two particles of unequal size. The sequence of bases of the mRNA forms triplets, or codons, which for the sake of clarity are drawn as groups of three upright lines. Each molecule of transfer RNA (tRNA) is composed of a long thread bent on itself to form a helical structure. At one end of the molecule there is a particular amino acid (AA1, AA2, etc.), and at the other end, where it is bent on itself, there are three unpaired bases which form an anticodon. Each codon of the mRNA is "recognized" by a corresponding anticodon of a tRNA. In this way specific amino acids are added to the polypeptide chain in a specific linear sequence determined by the mRNA which is itself modelled on the nuclear DNA.

(Drawn by the Department of Art as applied to Medicine, University of Toronto, after Warner, J. R. and Soeiro, R. (1967) New Engl. J. Med., **276**, 613, and Nirenberg, M. W. (1965). In "The Living Cell". San Francisco and London : Freeman.)

codons is colinear with the sequence of amino acids. The codons responsible for a whole peptide chain form a group called a *cistron*. It is believed that a number of cistrons are grouped together to form a larger unit, the *operon*,[24] which is described below. The actual code has been investigated by various means. Synthetic polyribonucleotides have been prepared and can act as mRNA in cell-free preparations containing ribosomes, suitable substrates, and a source of energy. Thus a polynucleotide containing uridine only (poly U) leads to the formation of phenylalanine. Hence the code for this amino acid is UUU.

**Control of Gene Action.** It is evident that each nucleated cell of the body contains the necessary information for the manufacture of every protein of which the body is composed. That they do not do so all the time is evidence that there is some very adequate control mechanism. Thus erythroid cells manufacture haemoglobin, plasma cells immunoglobulin, etc. Nevertheless, it

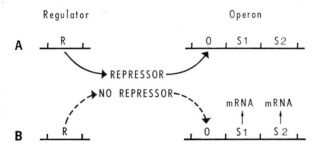

FIG. 2.13. The regulator-operator hypothesis.

A. The regulator gene (R) forms a repressor substance which acts through the cytoplasm to repress the operator gene (O). When O is thus inhibited, the structural genes (S1 and S2) in its operon cannot form mRNA.

B. If the regulator gene cannot form repressor substance, or if the repressor does not reach the operator gene, the operator is *derepressed* and S1 and S2 are then able to produce mRNA.

(*Diagram redrawn from Fig. 3.10 in Thompson, J. S. and Thompson, M. W. (1966). "Genetics in Medicine". Philadelphia and London: Saunders. The hypothesis is that of Jacob, F. and Monod, J. (1961). J. molec. Biol., 3, 318*).

is not surprising that under abnormal circumstances cells produce substances which are alien to their accustomed products. This occurs in metaplasia, and an extreme example is the secretion by certain cancer cells of hormones which normally are produced only in the very specialized cells of the endocrine glands (p. 249).

The control of gene action is poorly understood, but is being actively investigated at the present time. Some genes lead to the production of proteins which are enzymes, or which are used in the metabolism of the cell. These are termed *structural genes*. In certain bacteria it has been found that a group of genes are closely linked, and either function together or are completely repressed, i.e. no mRNA is produced. The mechanism of control is also under genetic influence, and Fig. 2.13 illustrates a scheme of this based on that proposed by Jacob and Monod.[25, 26] Each group of genes, or *operon*, is controlled by a closely associated gene called the *operator gene*. This itself is regulated by another gene, the *regulator gene*, which through its own mRNA leads to the production in the cytoplasm of a protein (*repressor substance*) which suppresses the operator gene. The regulator gene may itself be inhibited, and in that event the operator is derepressed and the genes of the operon are allowed to act; mRNA is produced and protein synthesis proceeds (Fig. 2.13). The complexity of the subject is apparent when it is appreciated that in every cell, every gene is under continuous control and so regulated that the requirements of the body are met. This applies not only during adult life but also during the complex process of development. The ovum provides an excellent example of how protein synthesis can be inhibited, only to be switched on suddenly by the event of fertilization.

It should be noted that each resting somatic cell nucleus contains a constant amount of nucleic acid. This is termed the 2c amount (see below). Certain exceptions are found. In the liver some cells contain a greater amount of DNA (e.g. 3c), while in tumours even greater amounts may be found. The phenomenon is known as *polyploidy*.

**Chromosomes**

The DNA molecules are not lying free in the nuclear sap, but are contained in long threads called *chromosomes*. Each resting somatic cell contains a definite number of chromosomes, the *diploid*, or 2n, number. This corresponds to a definite amount of DNA, the 2c amount. In humans the diploid number is 46, and of these 23 are derived from each parent. Two chromosomes are related specifically to sex, and these are called the *sex chromosomes*. One is considerably larger than the other and is called an X chromosome, while the smaller one is called a Y chromosome. Females have two X chromosomes whereas males have an X and a Y chromosome. The remaining 22 pairs are identical in appearance in both sexes and are called *autosomes*.

During the period between cell division (interphase) the chromosomes are present in the nucleus as long drawn-out threads. These are not visible as such using the light microscope, but in some areas along the thread there is sufficient coiling for the condensation of material to render these areas recognizable as chromatin dots of the nucleus. Such chromatin (*heterochromatin*) appears as areas of deep staining, and is thought to represent regions of the chromosomes which are condensed and relatively inert metabolically. The remainder of the nucleus is lightly stained, and the dispersed chromatin material (*euchromatin*) is in an active form. It follows that the actual morphology of the nucleus varies considerably from one cell to another, and that an assessment of function can be made from nuclear structure. In active cells, e.g. neurones, the nucleus is vesicular and very little heterochromatin is present. Heterochromatin is more abundant in epithelial cells and gives the nucleus a stippled appearance. In inactive cells, e.g. small lymphocytes, late normoblasts, and spermatozoa, the heterochromatin occupies most of the nucleus which therefore appears deeply basophilic. In the mature plasma cells the heterochromatin is disposed close to the nuclear membrane in clumps to produce the cartwheel, or clock-face appearance so typical of this cell (Fig. 10.1).

Some cells which are very large, e.g. the osteoclasts of the bone marrow.

contain many nuclei and are called *multinucleate giant cells*. Some of the RNA component of the nucleus may appear as a separate structure called the *nucleolus*. This is particularly prominent in cells which are actively metabolizing—e.g. cancer cells.

**The Barr Body.** A feature which has assumed great importance is a discrete mass of chromatin, first noted by Murray Barr in the nerve cells of the cat. He noted that this was present in the cells of the female but not in those of the male. It is therefore called the *sex chromatin*, or *Barr body*.[27] It is easily demonstrated in the human by examining suitably stained cells scraped from the buccal mucosa, and appears as a demilune on the nuclear membrane (Fig. 2.14). The Barr body is derived from a single X chromosome, and the number of Barr bodies seen in a cell is one less than the number of X chromosomes present. One X chromosome in each nucleus behaves like the autosomes. It becomes uncoiled between each cell division and therefore is not seen. If another X chromosome is present it remains inactive and appears as a Barr body.[28, 29] It follows that the normal male, having only one X chromosome, is chromatin negative while the normal female is chromatin positive, i.e. has sex chromatin.

**The Y Body.**[30] The Y chromosome selectively takes up the dye quinacrine hydrochloride ("atebrin"), which has the property of fluorescing strongly under ultraviolet light. If a smear of buccal mucosal scraping or peripheral blood is stained with the dye, a bright fluorescent dot in the nucleus indicates the presence of a Y chromosome (Fig. 2.15).

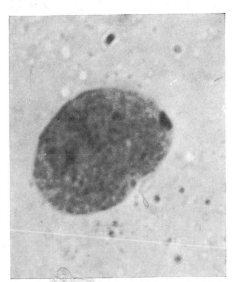

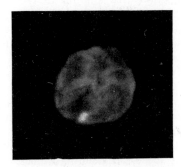

FIG. 2.15. The fluorescent Y chromosome. Blood smears were air-dried, fixed in methanol, and after staining in 0·5 per cent quinacrine dihydrochloride (atebrine) and washing, were examined in ultraviolet light. The Y chromosome shows a characteristic point of fluorescence in the nucleus of a cell of the blood from a normal male. (*Photograph supplied by Dr. Peter K. Lewin. From Lewin, P. K. and Conen, P. E. (1971), Nature, 233, 334.*)

FIG. 2.14. The Barr body. Nucleus of a cell from buccal mucosal smear of a female, showing the sex chromatin mass on the nuclear membrane. Stained by acetic orcein.

(*Photograph supplied by Dr. Nigel H. Kemp*)

## Cytoplasmic DNA

The presence of DNA in the cytoplasm is now well established. Some is present in the mitochondria, and appears to direct protein synthesis *via* specific tRNA. Many other forms of cytoplasmic DNA are known, and have been most extensively studied in bacteria. Some can act as infectious agents (e.g. bacteriophage), or may replicate in unison with cell division and therefore act as cytoplasmic genetic material. These agents are called *episomes*, or *plasmids*, and their presence can greatly alter the function of a cell.[31,32] Thus the production of toxin by the diphtheria bacillus is related to the presence of one of these agents, as is also the development of antibiotic resistance. Their role in mammalian cells is at present speculative, but it may well be related to the inheritance of certain diseases, virus infections (for instance slow viruses), and the development of cancer.

**Individual Chromosome Identification.** New staining techniques involving Giemsa stain and also quinacrine mustard in conjunction with ultraviolet microscopy have revealed that the chromosomes have a characteristic banded appearance. Many individual chromosomes can now be identified and abnormalities in them detected[33].

## CELL DIVISION

### Mitosis

Before cell division occurs it is believed that the DNA molecules split, and that each half acts as a template for the manufacture of another half. In this way the amount of DNA is doubled. The chromosomes divide and become double structures, or *chromatids*, joined closely together at this stage. These strands become coiled along their whole length; in this way they become shortened, thickened, and therefore visible. The cell has now entered the first phase of mitosis—the *prophase*. Meanwhile in the centrosome the two centrioles develop fibrils, and move away from each other; each looks like a star, or *aster* (Fig. 2.16).

The nucleoli and nuclear membrane next disappear, and the cell enters the *metaphase*. By this time the centrioles are at opposite poles of the cell, and their fibrils enter the nuclear region, where the split chromosomes become arranged along an equatorial plate which bisects the cell. The fibrils are attached to the chromosomes, and in this way the *spindle* is formed.

During the next phase, *anaphase*, each set of chromatids, now called chromosomes, is pulled by the fibrils of the spindle to either pole of the cell. The final stage (*telophase*) involves division of the cytoplasm of the cells, and the reconstitution of the nuclear membrane of each daughter cell. The cell now enters the $G_1$ period, which is terminated in due course by the onset of DNA synthesis. The synthetic period is followed by a second, or $G_2$ period, which is short and is terminated by the next mitosis.

It can be readily understood how during mitosis each chromosome reduplicates itself exactly, and the two daughter cells contain an identical quota of nuclear material. Each DNA molecule is also reduplicated exactly. Should an error occur during mitosis such that an abnormal gene is produced, the process is called a *somatic mutation*. Presumably this is related to an abnormal sequence of the bases in the DNA molecule.

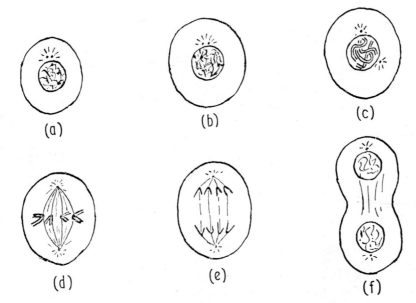

FIG. 2.16. The stages of mitosis.

(a) The resting cell. (b) Prior to mitosis the cell enlarges. There is a build-up of DNA and the nucleus now contains the 4c amount. (c) Prophase. The individual chromosomes become visible—for the sake of clarity only four are shown, but it should be remembered that the normal human cell contains 46 (the 2n number). Each chromosome has already split into two chromatids. (d) Metaphase. The chromosomes are arranged along the equatorial plate, and the spindle is fully formed. (e) Anaphase. The chromatids, now called chromosomes, move apart. (f) Telophase. The daughter nuclei reform, and the cytoplasm divides to produce two new cells each with the 2c amount of DNA corresponding to the normal number of chromosomes (2n number).

## Meiosis

In the testis and ovary the process of cell division is more complex, and is called *meiosis*. The process results in cells which contain only half the number of chromosomes (the n, or *haploid*, number, i.e. 23 in man), and half the amount of DNA. These cells develop into gametes, either sperms or ova. With fertilization the diploid number of chromosomes, 46, is restored. It sometimes happens that during meiosis a pair of chromosomes fail to separate, and both are drawn into the one daughter cell. This is called *non-disjunction*. Sometimes fragments of a chromosome are lost (*deletion*), or become attached to another chromosome (*translocation*). If these abnormal gametes are fertilized, it is evident that an abnormal offspring may result. This is considered in Chapter 3.

### Arrangement of Cells

The majority of cells in the human body do not occur separately, but are grouped together to form tissues. Traditionally, two main types of cells are distinguished—those of the epithelia and those of the connective tissues.

### Epithelial Cells

Epithelial cells cover surfaces, e.g. the skin, or line cavities, e.g. the mouth, and in these situations they are essentially protective in function. Covering epithelium may also perform a secretory function; the respiratory epithelium, for instance, secretes mucus.

In addition to covering extensive surfaces, the secretory type of epithelial cell may be arranged to form glands. These may be simple, like the mucous glands of the colon, or more elaborate, like those of the breast and salivary glands. A feature common to all epithelial cells is that they are closely contiguous to one another. This is evident on light microscopy, and even under the electron microscope these cells appear to be separated by only a thin layer of low electron density, about 15 nm in width.

### Connective Tissue Cells

Connective tissue cells are the other type of cell present in the body. They are usually separated widely from each other by a gelatinous material (*ground substance*) in which are embedded fibres (usually *collagenous*). This type of connective tissue, typified by bone, cartilage, tendon, and fibrous tissue, is primarily supportive in function. Other connective tissue cells have been endowed with specialized cytoplasm, e.g. for contraction (muscle fibres), conduction (nerve cells), phagocytosis (monocytes), and oxygen carriage (red cells).*

It is generally assumed that connective tissue contains primitive multi-potential cells which when suitably stimulated can differentiate into reticulo-endothelial cells, haematopoietic cells, and probably other connective tissue cells as well. These *stem cells* are poorly defined morphologically, and indeed may differ in appearance in different organs. In the bone marrow they may resemble small lymphocytes. In the lymphoreticular tissues they are difficult to distinguish from *reticulum cells*, which form the reticulin-fibre framework of such tissues as spleen and lymph nodes—tissues where stem cells are believed to be plentiful.

The division of the cells of the body into two groups is convenient for some purposes, as will be seen when the classification of tumours is described. Nevertheless, the division is arbitrary and in some ways unsatisfactory. Thus, the flattened cells which line the blood vessels are usually considered to be connective tissue, although they are, in fact, performing a covering function. The same may be said of the mesothelial cells lining the pleura and peritoneum, and those of the synovium.

### The Reticulo-Endothelial System

Among the most important cells of the connective tissue are those that constitute the reticulo-endothelial (RE) system. This system of cells is widely scattered throughout the body, and all share in common an ability to phagocytose coarse particles and to abstract highly diluted dyes from the blood. As these cells are the main phagocytes (scavengers) of the body, they

* Some authorities prefer to restrict the connective tissues to bone, cartilage, etc., and regard the specialized elements as belonging to separate systems, e.g. haematopoietic, nervous, etc.

play a part in many of the pathological processes mentioned later. The RE cells are closely associated with lymphocytes, and they are sometimes considered together as the *lymphoreticular system*.

There are two groups of RE cells:

(*a*) Fixed—these comprise the cells that line the sinuses of certain organs, notably the liver, spleen, bone marrow, and lymph nodes (*sinus-lining*, or *littoral cells*), and also the resting *histiocytes* that lie in the various connective tissues of the body; those in the central nervous system are called *microglia*.

(*b*) Mobile or wandering—these are the blood *monocytes*.

When there is a local pathological process in a tissue, such as infection or haemorrhage, RE cells migrate to the area, become phagocytic, and are then called *macrophages*. They are mobilized both from the blood monocytes and the local histiocytes. It should be noted that the other phagocytic cells of the body, the neutrophil granulocytes of the blood, are not included in the RE system, because they cannot perform the same type of phagocytosis as has been defined for the RE system. The name reticulo-endothelial system derives from the situation of the sinus-lining cells of liver, spleen, etc. which are found in close relationship to the reticulin framework of the organs (p. 26), and which superficially resemble flattened endothelial cells, such as are found in the blood vessels. As the cells differ from vascular endothelial cells and reticulum cells both morphologically and functionally, the name reticulo-endothelial is unfortunate and has been deprecated. An alternate name for this highly phagocytic cell system, the *mononuclear phagocytic system*, has therefore been suggested.[34]

Apart from their essential function of phagocytosis of organisms and debris (Chapters 5, 7, and 10), these cells also play an important part in the immune response (Chapter 11), and in the breakdown of ageing red cells (Chapter 26). They become distended with abnormal lipids in the lipidoses (Chapter 33).

## THE INTERCELLULAR SPACE

### The Ground Substance[35]

The ground substance varies in consistency from an amorphous gel forming the translucent material of hyaline cartilage to the glairy fluid found in the synovial joint cavities. It is in the molecular meshes of the ground substance that the extracellular interstitial fluid is contained. This extracellular interstitial fluid constitutes about one third of the total body water, and lies between the blood vessels and the cells. It contains various electrolytes in a concentration similar to that of the plasma and also small uncharged solute material, such as oxygen, $CO_2$, glucose, and urea, which is conveyed either for cellular metabolism or for excretion. In addition the ground substance contains:

*Glycoproteins.*[36] These are proteins which contain a firmly-bound moiety of carbohydrate. They stain red with the PAS* method.

* *The Periodic Acid-Schiff Reaction.* When periodic acid is applied to a section many carbohydrate components are oxidized to aldehydes. Aldehydes produce a red colour with Schiff's reagent (a solution of basic fuchsin decolorized by sulphurous acid). Therefore if Schiff's reagent is applied to a treated section, the parts containing carbohydrate are stained red. The PAS reaction is useful for the demonstration of glycogen, ground substance, and epithelial mucus.

*Mucoproteins* are loose combinations of protein with acid mucopoly-saccharides. The latter have attracted much attention: they consist of polymers of hexose sugars, some of which possess amino groups, e.g. hexosamines like D-glucosamine and D-galactosamine. The amino groups are presumably responsible in part for the mucoid properties of the polymers. Meyer[37, 38] has subdivided the acid mucopolysaccharides as listed below. The alternative names in brackets are those proposed by Jeanloz.[39]

*Non-sulphated Group*
Hyaluronic acid
Chondroitin
In these the acid grouping is due to uronic acid, e.g. glucuronic acid.
*Sulphated Group*
Chondroitin sulphate A (chondroitin 4-sulphate)
Chondroitin sulphate B (dermatan sulphate)
Chondroitin sulphate C (chondroitin 6-sulphate)
Heparitin sulphate (heparan sulphate)
Keratosulphate (keratan sulphate)

The physical (e.g. optical) and presumably chemical properties of each connective tissue depend upon the nature of the ground substance as well as upon the physical arrangement of the fibres themselves. For example, keratosulphate forms 50 per cent of the total acid mucopolysaccharide in the cornea, but is present only in small quantities in osteoid. It is generally agreed that fibroblasts (and osteoblasts) form acid mucopolysaccharides.

## Collagen[35,40]

Collagen constitutes about one third of the body's protein; it forms a scaffold in all tissues and is the chief component of fascia, dermis (including gingiva), cornea, dentine, and tendon, and gives these structures tensile strength. Isotope studies indicate that although much of the body's collagen is metabolically stable, some of it is rapidly synthetized and degraded; the excretion of hydroxyproline in the urine gives some indication of the amount of collagen which is being degraded. Thus the excretion is high in hyper-parathyroidism. Collagen comprises almost 90 per cent of the organic matrix of bone, and its particular composition is adapted for the deposition of the bone salts.

The collagen of connective tissue is synthetized by fibroblasts or similar cells such as are found in tendon, cornea, bone, and cartilage. An exception to this is the collagen component of basement membrane, which is formed by the adjacent epithelial or endothelial cells and differs in several respects from other collagens. Indeed, as more research is carried out on the composition of collagen, it is evident that many forms exist and it is misleading to talk of collagen as if it were a single entity of fixed composition and structure.

**Light Microscopic Appearance of Collagen.** The first formed collagen consists of fine branching fibres called *reticulin*. These are demonstrated by silver impregnation methods. In many organs of the body collagen formation stops at this stage, and the reticulin forms a scaffold for the parenchyma (e.g. liver, spleen, and lymph nodes). In the connective tissues proper the fibres become further enlarged, and then are called *collagen fibres*. They lose their affinity for silver, but readily take up eosin, or aniline blue combined with phosphotungstic acid (Mallory's stain). They also stain red with picrofuchsin (Van Gieson's stain).

**Electron Microscopic Appearance of Collagen.** The electron microscope reveals that the collagen and reticulin *fibres* are made up of *fibrils*, which show a cross banding with a periodicity of about 64 nm (Fig. 2.17). It is thought that these fibrils are made up of tropocollagen molecules each of which is about 280 nm long and 1·4 nm wide. It was at first thought that the molecules

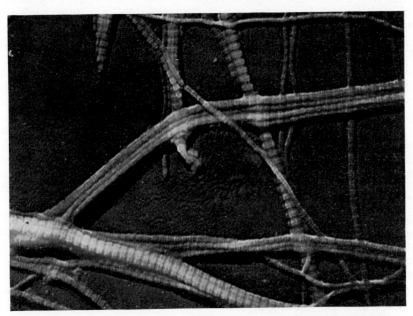

FIG. 2.17. Teased preparation of collagen from the *tendo achilles*. The specimen has been shadowed to accentuate the characteristic 64nm banding. The process involves the throwing of a vaporized heavy metal such as palladium or gold on to the specimen at a small angle. Now that ultra-thin sections can be cut, this technique is not often used. × 34,000.

*(Photograph supplied by Dr. C. I. Levene)*

were joined together with a quarter-length overlap with their lateral neighbours. It is now known that there is a gap of about 41 nm between the head of one molecule and the tail of the next as shown in Fig. 2.19. In osteoid tissue these gaps serve as a nidus for the deposition of bone salts. The thickness of the collagen fibrils varies from tissue to tissue. In cartilage they measure 15–25 nm, while in tendon they reach 130 nm in thickness. It is evident that different lateral arrangements of the tropocollagen could form fibrils with different periodicity, and such have in fact been found to exist.

**Solubility of Collagen.** Adult fully-matured collagen is very insoluble, and only denaturation by strong acids or heat can render it soluble. The final product is then gelatin. In young collagen a fraction can be extracted by cold neutral buffers. This probably contains tropocollagen, and on warming the solution, typical banded fibrils are reformed. An additional fraction can be extracted by dilute acid solutions, and this component persists as maturation proceeds. Ultimately the collagen becomes insoluble due to the increasing numbers of cross-linkages which are formed (p. 30).

**Chemical Composition of Collagen.** Collagen has a characteristic x-ray diffraction pattern, and from this its structure has been surmised. The basic unit of collagen is called tropocollagen, a molecule 280 nm long and 1·4 nm wide, with a molecular weight of about 340 000. Tropocollagen consists of three polypeptide chains; two are identical and called $\alpha_1$ chains, while the third is different and called an $\alpha_2$ chain. A third type of chain has been found in cartilage, and probably others exist. The nomenclature of the polypeptide polymers is confusing. A single polypeptide chain is called an $\alpha$ chain, dimers are called $\beta$ chains, while tropocollagen with three polypeptides is the $\gamma$ chain. Each of these polypeptide chains is coiled, and the three molecules are wound around a common axis like a three stranded rope. It is thus a coiled coil!

Each polypeptide chain consists of about 1 000 amino-acid residues and has a molecular weight of about 95 000. It is coiled to form a helix in which, unlike the usual protein $\alpha$-helix, there are no hydrogen bonds between adjacent amino acids on the same chain. Each helix is stabilized by hydrogen bonds with adjacent polypeptide chains. Throughout most of the chain every third amino acid is glycine, and a common sequence is glycine—proline—hydroxyproline. Collagen is indeed characterized by its high content of glycine (33 per cent) and proline and hydroxyproline which together constitute about 22 per cent. Hydroxyproline is an amino acid which is not found to any great extent in other proteins, and an estimation of its amount in hydrolysates of tissue may therefore be used to measure the amount of collagen present. It is also noteworthy that collagen contains hydroxylysine, and it is to this amino acid that carbohydrate is attached (either galactose or glucogalactose).

**Biosynthesis of Collagen.** The primary polypeptide chains are formed in the rough endoplasmic reticulum under the influence of specific mRNA. The three polypeptide chains are probably formed simultaneously and immediately unite to form a triple helix. The molecule first formed is called protocollagen; it differs from tropocollagen in not containing hydroxyproline, hydroxylysine, or glycosylated hydroxylysine. The next step in the formation of collagen is the *hydroxylation of proline and lysine*; for this specific enzymes, free oxygen, and *ascorbic acid* are required.

Thus hydroxyproline and hydroxylysine in collagen are formed in the polypeptide chains by hydroxylation of the parent amino acids. They are not directly encoded by specific mRNA, and this raises another problem. What factors determine which proline or lysine is hydroxylated? No definite answer can be given, but it is not surprising that the degree of hydroxylation varies somewhat from one collagen to another even within the same individual.

**Glycosylation of Hydroxylysine.** Glycosylation occurs at some of the hydroxylysine residues; to some of these sites glucose is further added to the

galactose. It has been postulated that in diabetes mellitus excessive glycosylation could lead to the deposition of an abnormal collagen in the basement
membrane.

**Formation of Tropocollagen.** The manner by which the three polypeptide
chains are formed simultaneously and united is not known. There is some
evidence that the first formed polypeptide chains have an extension at the
amino terminal end (see p. 30), and that this contains cysteine. Hence
disulphide bonds could be formed, and initiate the formation of the triple
helix. This sulphur-containing component probably persists until the tropo-

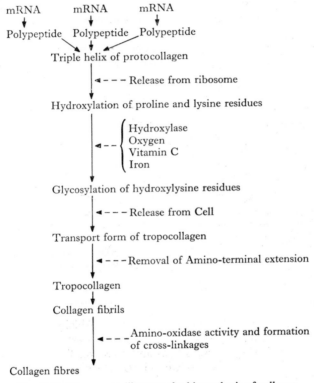

FIG. 2.18. Diagram to illustrate the biosynthesis of collagen.

collagen molecules finally polymerize into mature collagen. These findings
help to explain why sulphur-containing amino acids are necessary for
normal wound healing (p. 112).

**Extrusion of Collagen from the Cell.** Tropocollagen is released from the
ribosomes into the cisternae of the endoplasmic reticulum. It may then leave
the cell *via* the Golgi apparatus as does secretion in exocrine glands, or else
pass by a more direct route. A failure in hydroxylation or glycosylation
inhibits this extrusion. Protein synthesis is not immediately inhibited, but the
defective collagen is not extruded, and extracellular deposition therefore
ceases. This occurs in scurvy.

**Extracellular Incorporation of Tropocollagen into Collagen Fibrils.** Newly synthetized collagen consists of a molecule larger than tropocollagen, due to the presence of the cysteine-containing extension. This is called *procollagen*, or *transport form*. When the extension is removed, aggregation occurs. Fibres are formed by the lateral alignment of the molecules with a quarter overlap as shown in Fig. 2.19. This quarter-stagger arrangement presents problems if one tries to construct a three-dimensional model with match-sticks. Perhaps four or five polymer chains are arranged so that in cross-section they form a square or pentagon. In this way there is limitation of the points of contact between the chains. Whatever the precise arrangement, the carbohydrate content of the collagen and the mucopolysaccharide composition of the ground substance seem to play a part in the determination of the size of the fibres produced.

**Cross-linkage of Fibrils to Form Fibres.**  The fibrils which are formed when tropocollagen aggregates have little strength. It is by the formation of

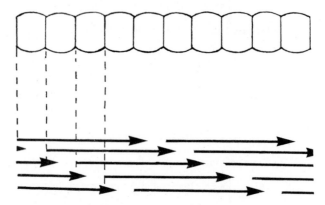

FIG. 2.19. Diagram to illustrate how the lateral arrangement of fibrils, depicted as arrows, results in the formation of a banded collagen fibre.

cross-linkages that tensile strength is produced. Aldehyde groups are produced under the catalytic action of an amineoxidase. These groups form cross-linkages, but the process is slow, and it can readily be understood that tensile strength of collagen in a wound can steadily increase over several months (p. 107).

The first-formed collagen fibres are coated with much ground substance and it is in this that silver is deposited with suitable staining techniques. The maturation of collagen and the formation of cross-linkages has been suggested as a possible mechanism of tooth eruption[41].

### Elastic Fibres

The elastic fibres of the aorta and its large branches, the ligamentum nuchae, lung, etc., appear very different from collagen on light microscopy; they stain *deep red with eosin, dark brown with orcein,* and *black with the resorcinol fuchsin stain of Weigert.* Early electron-microscopic studies of elastic fibres showed them to be amorphous and quite unlike collagen. More recent investigations have shown that elastic tissue consists of two components: one is the microfibril and the other is a homogeneous material of variable electron density. The microfibrils are obvious during the formation of elastic, but with ageing are more difficult to detect. Elastic tissue is very resistant to digestion by acids and alkalis, but is readily attacked by the enzyme elastase produced by some organisms.

Chemically it is thought to consist of a protein, *elastin*, with polysaccharide. Although some authorities regard elastic fibres as being derived from collagen, most maintain that this is unlikely in view of the great difference in amino-acid composition between elastin and collagen. Elastin contains two amino acids, desmosine and isodesmosine, which are thought to be important in forming the cross-linkages which give to elastic tissue the resilience which is its characteristic physical property.[42] With age there is an increase in the content of desmosine and isodesmosine, and this is accompanied by a loss of resilience.[43] Calcification of elastic fibres is another feature of the ageing process; it also occurs in metastatic calcification (see p. 447).

Elastic fibres are formed by the activity of smooth muscle cells in some situations, e.g. in the aortic wall and in atheromatous plaques. In other tissues, cells which resemble fibroblasts appear to be involved. No specific "elastoblasts" have been identified. There is little doubt that new elastic fibres can be formed in adult life. Thus degeneration of elastic tissue is sometimes accompanied by new elastic fibre formation, so as to give an appearance of fraying or reduplication.

## References

1. DALTON, A. J. and HAGUENAU, F. (1968). Edrs., "The Membranes", 223 pp. New York and London: Academic Press.
2. KORN, E. D. (1969). *Fed. Proc.*, **28**, 6.
3. Various Authors (1961). *Exp. Cell Res.* Supp. 8. "Cell Movement and Cell Contact."
4. BURGER, M. M. and NOONAN, K. D. (1970). *Nature (Lond.)*, **228**, 512.
5. Leading Article (1970). *Lancet*, **2**, 1294.
6. PAPPENHEIMER, J. R. (1953). *Physiol. Rev.*, **33**, 387.
7. MOORE, D. H. and RUSKA, H. (1957). *J. biophys. biochem. Cytol.*, **3**, 457.
8. LENARD, J. and SINGER, S. J. (1968). *J. cell Biol.*, **37**, 117.
9. KAVANAU, J. L. (1963). *Nature (Lond.)*, **198**, 525.
10. KAVANAU, J. L. (1966). *Fed. Proc.*, **25**, 1096.
11. Leading Article (1970). *Lancet*, **2**, 1119.
12. LEHNINGER, A. L. (1964). "The Mitochondrion", 263 pp. New York and Amsterdam: W. A. Benjamin Inc.
13. PARSONS, D. F. (1963). *Science*, **140**, 985.
14. Various Authors (1966). *Proc. roy Soc. Med.*, **59**, 867.
15. DINGLE, J. T. and FELL, H. B. (1969). Edrs., "Lysosomes in Biology and Pathology", Vol. 1, 543 pp., Vol. 2, 668 pp., Amsterdam and London: North Holland Publishing Co.
16. WEISSMANN, G. and FELL, H. (1962), *J. exp. Med.*, **116**, 365.
17. WEISSMANN, G. and THOMAS, L. (1962), *J. exp. Med.*, **116**, 433.
18. GLINSMANN, W. H. and ERICSSON, J. L. E. (1966). *Lab. Invest.*, **15**, 762.
19. WATSON, J. D. and CRICK, F. H. C. (1953). *Nature (Lond.)*, **171**, 737.
20. Various Authors (1965). *Brit. med. Bull.*, **21**, 183.

21. PENMAN, S. (1967). *New Engl. J. Med.*, **276**, 502.
22. WARNER, J. R. and SOEIRO, R. (1967). *New Engl. J. Med.*, **276**, 563, 613 and 675.
23. YČAS, M. (1969). "The Biological Code", 360 pp., Amsterdam and London: North Holland Publishing Co.
24. STENT, G. S. (1964). *Science*, **144**, 816.
25. MONOD, J. and JACOB, F. (1961). *Cold Spring Harbor Symp. Quant. Biol.*, **26**, 389.
26. JACOB, F. and MONOD, J. (1961). *J. Molec. Biol.*, **3**, 318.
27. BARR, M. L. and BERTRAM, E. G. (1949). *Nature (Lond.)*, **163**, 676.
28. LYON, M. F. (1961). *Nature (Lond.)*, **190**, 372.
29. LYON, M. F. (1963). *Genet. Res.*, **4**, 93.
30. LEWIN, P. K. and CONEN, P. E. (1971). *Nature (London)*, **233**, 334.
31. Ciba Foundation Symposium (1969). "Bacterial Episomes and Plasmids", ed. by Wolstenholme, G. E. W. and O'Connor, M., 268 pp, London: Churchill.
32. PREER, J. R. (1971). "Extra-chromosomal Inheritance: Hereditary Symbionts, Mitochondria, Chloroplasts". In "Annual Review of Genetics", Vol. 5, p. 361, ed. by Roman, H. L., Pao Alta: Annual Reviews Inc.
33. Editorial (1971). *New. Engl. J. Med.*, **285**, 1482.
34. VAN FURTH, R., *et al.* (1972). *Bull. Wld Hlth Org.*, **46**, 845.
35. WAGNER, B. M. and SMITH, D. E. (1967). Edrs., "The Connective Tissue", 408 pp. Baltimore: Williams and Wilkins.
36. SPIRO, R. G. (1963). *New Engl. J. Med.*, **269**, 566 and 616.
37. MEYER, K. (1959). In "Wound Healing and Tissue Repair", p. 25, ed. Patterson, W. B. Chicago: University of Chicago Press.
38. MEYER, K. *et al.* (1956), *Biochem, biophys. Acta (Amst.)*, **21**, 506.
39. JEANLOZ, R. W. (1960). *Arthritis Rheum.*, **3**, 233.
40. GRANT, M. E. and PROCKOP, D. J. (1972). *New Engl. J. Med.*, **286**, 194, 242, and 291.
41. THOMAS, N. R. (1965). *J. Dent. Res.*, **44**, 1159.
42. PARTRIDGE, S. M., ELSDEN, D. F. and THOMAS, J. (1963). *Nature (Lond.)*, **197**, 1297 and **200**, 651.
43. MILLER, E. J., MARTIN, G. R. and PIEZ, K. A. (1964). *Biochem. biophys. Res. Commun.*, **17**, 248.

*Chapter 3*

# THE CAUSE OF DISEASE

The abnormalities in structure or function which are the hallmark of disease are due to the effects of an interplay between two basic factors—these are the *inherited genetic constitution* of the individual on the one hand and the *environment* on the other.

## INHERITED GENETIC CONSTITUTION

### Introduction

Traditionally much of pathology is concerned with the effects of adverse factors such as heat, trauma, and bacteria acting on a normal individual. Many diseases are regarded as being caused by particular agents—thus tuberculosis may be said to be caused by the tubercle bacillus. Such a one-sided approach to medicine is no longer tenable. If a hundred people were to be exposed to a particular dose of tubercle bacilli, only a few would develop the disease. No two people are the same, nor do they react in exactly the same way. Each individual is different, and the difference is thought to lie in the coded information (or genetic material) which is handed down to him from his parents. This information is very precise, and is capable of exact analysis. Today we think of inheritance in terms of the structure of the DNA molecule and the sequence of its bases. However, the science of inheritance is not new; it started a century ago when the Austrian monk Gregor Mendel, by observing the mode of inheritance of particular characteristics in the garden pea, noted that the characteristics behaved as if they were determined by units which were passed unchanged from one generation to the next. To these units the name *genes* was given, and it is postulated that a pair of them is present in every somatic cell. Each gene is situated at a specific site, or *locus*, on one of a pair of chromosomes, and the genes forming a pair are called *alleles*, or *allelomorphs*. If they are alike the individual is called a *homozygote* for that particular gene, while if dissimilar he is a *heterozygote*. The genetic makeup of an individual is called his *genotype*, and the effects which these genes produce is the *phenotype*.

### The Mode of Inheritance[1,2,3]

In order to explain Mendelian inheritance several assumptions have been made:

(1) Genes occur in pairs.
(2) One gene of each pair is received from each parent.
(3) Genes remain unchanged through many generations.

(4) Some genes may be considered as dominant and some as recessive. A *dominant gene* produces its effect both in the heterozygote and in the homozygote. *Recessive genes,* on the other hand, produce their effects only in the homozygous condition. Genes which occupy an intermediate position are described later. Sometimes a particular locus can be occupied by one of many possible genes. A simple example of this type is illustrated below in respect of the ABO blood groups.

**Dominant Genes.** The pattern of inheritance of a dominant gene may be illustrated by reference to the ABO blood group. The allelic genes concerned occupy one locus, and may be *A, B,* or *O.*

A homozygous individual who has two *A* genes (genotype *AA*) has in his red cells the blood group substance A (phenotype group A). Likewise the heterozygote *AO* is also phenotypically blood group A, because the *A* gene is dominant and the *O* is recessive. The *B* gene, like *A*, is dominant, and both are described as *co-dominants.* The possible blood groups in this system are shown below*:

| Genotype | Phenotype |
|----------|-----------|
| *AA* | A |
| *AO* | A |
| *OO* | O |
| *BB* | B |
| *BO* | B |
| *AB* | AB |

Thus the six gentotypes produce only four recognizable blood groups. The occurrence of two or more genetically different classes of individuals with

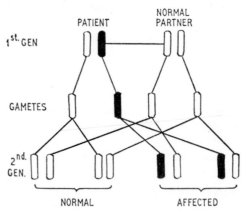

FIG. 3.1. Diagram illustrating the transmission of a disease inherited as a dominant factor. One pair of chromosomes is shown for each individual, the black chromosome being the one carrying the defective gene. It will be seen that half the children of an affected patient are themselves diseased.

* It will be appreciated that the ABO blood group is much more complex than is described in this book.

respect to a single trait is known as *polymorphism*\*.[4] The blood groups provide an excellent example, but many others are also known. Thus there are genetically determined variants of many of the plasma proteins.

Some diseases are inherited as dominant characteristics, e.g. achondroplasia and dentinogenesis imperfecta. The mode of inheritance is shown in Fig. 3.1, and it should be noted that:

(1) The disease appears in every generation, or else it dies out. The occasional instance of poor penetrance (p. 37) and the occurrence of a new mutant provide exceptions to this rule. If the disease greatly reduces the breeding potential of the sufferer, it follows that most cases encountered will be sporadic and due to new mutations.

(2) Unaffected members do not pass on the disease (but see penetrance, p. 37).

(3) The affected members are usually heterozygous, and if the breeding partner is normal, the chances of his offspring being affected are 50 per cent.

(4) Males and females are equally liable to be affected.

**Recessive Genes.** Diseases inherited as recessive characters are frequently severe, and reduce the breeding chances of the sufferer, e.g. galactosaemia (p. 38) and xeroderma pigmentosum (p. 275). The birth of an abnormal individual is often the first indication that an abnormal gene is present in the

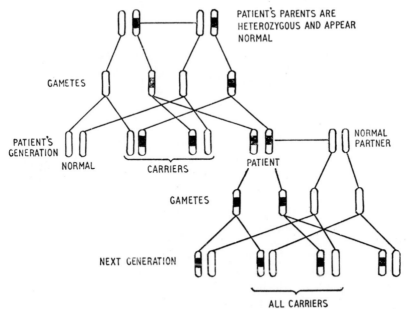

Fig. 3.2. Diagram to illustrate the transmission of a disease inherited as a recessive factor. It will be seen that the patient's parents are both unaffected heterozygotes, and that all his children are likewise carriers.

\* The frequency should be greater than one per cent, since very rare traits can arise by mutation and their occurrence in a population does not constitute polymorphism.

family. Fig. 3.2 shows the mode of transmission, and it can be seen that both parents of the affected individual are themselves heterozygous carriers. Most individuals are heterozygous for several harmful genes, and since some members of one family are likely to have the same recessive gene, the dangers of close interbreeding are apparent.

**Sex-linked Genes.** A gene is said to be sex-linked when it is localized on an X or Y chromosome. Usually the gene is recessive, and is situated on the X chromosome. The bleeding diseases haemophilia and Christmas disease

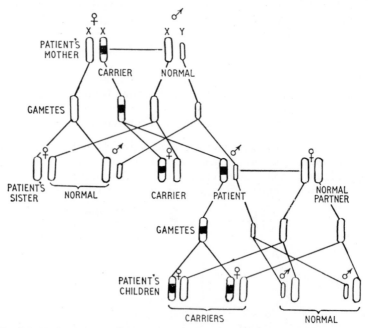

FIG. 3.3. Mode of transmission of a disease like haemophilia, which is inherited as a sex-linked recessive factor. The abnormal gene is situated on the X chromosome, and therefore produces its effect in the male but not in the female except in the rare event of her being homozygous. All the patient's daughters are carriers, but all his sons are normal.

are inherited in this way (Fig. 3.3). Female heterozygotes are protected by the normal gene on their other X chromosome; half the carrier's sons, however, have the disease.

**Intermediate Inheritance.** When the heterozygote differs from either homozygote, the inheritance is described as intermediate. A good example is sickle-cell disease, in which the heterozygote has the sickle-cell trait and differs both from the normal individual and the patient with sickle-cell disease (see below).

**Concept of Expressivity.** So far genes have been considered as behaving either as dominant or recessive. In fact the position is much more complex.[5] A gene may produce a severe disease in one individual but only a minor deformity in another. The concept of *expressivity* has been introduced to explain this. If a gene which usually produces a severe effect is found to cause a minor one in a particular individual, it is said to show poor expressivity. In some instances it produces no detectable effect at all, and a dominant trait may then miss a generation. This is an example of *reduced penetrance*, a term used when some individuals with the appropriate genotype fail to express it. Another complication is the failure of a trait, in other respects behaving as a dominant, to be manifest in one sex. This is called *sex limitation*. Baldness is said to behave in this way since it affects males much more frequently than females.

**Multifactorial or Polygenic Inheritance,** Multifactorial inheritance, where several genes each influence one particular function, is a further complication. Variation in stature is an example of this. With some diseases the mode of inheritance defies exact analysis.

### Molecular Diseases

With the discovery of chromosomes and DNA, it was not unnatural that attempts should be made to equate genes with segments of the DNA molecule. This translation of the mysterious gene action into concrete chemical terms was first achieved successfully with a group of diseases in man known as the *haemoglobinopathies*, in which an abnormal form of haemoglobin is manufactured.

Many other diseases are now known in which the body synthetizes an abnormal form of protein, either a structural protein or an enzyme. These diseases are grouped together as the *molecular diseases*.[1,2]

**Haemoglobinopathies.** The globin of the molecule haemoglobin is a protein of known amino-acid sequence. In certain individuals, usually of African stock, the haemoglobin contains an abnormal globin in which valine replaces the usual glutamic acid in one of the peptide chains in the globin molecule. Presumably this is due to an error in one codon of the DNA molecule. Homozygous individuals manufacture the abnormal haemoglobin Hb-S, and this has the effect of rendering their red blood cells liable to become distorted to a sickle shape at low oxygen tensions. They are more easily removed from the circulation and destroyed, with the result that the patients become severely ill with *sickle-cell anaemia*. Heterozygous individuals suffer from a mild anaemia, and are said to have the *sickle-cell trait*. Their red cells contain both normal adult haemoglobin Hb-A and Hb-S. It might be wondered why the sickle-cell gene, being so harmful, should not have killed off all its carriers and died out. It appears that those with the trait, although at a slight disadvantage in a temperate climate, are at a distinct advantage in the tropics, because they have greater resistance to malaria than do normal individuals. Through natural selection this apparently harmful gene has become widely distributed in tropical climates and has reached a high frequency. The haemoglobin molecule has been the object of intense study, and over 150 variants are now known. This is an example of the *genetic heterogeneity*[6] in the population, and other instances are noted below in respect of certain enzymes.

**Other Molecular Diseases.** Sometimes a particular protein is completely absent, and this is most noticeable when the protein concerned can easily be detected. Thus in the rare analbuminaemia the plasma lacks albumin. Commonly the gene product is an enzyme, and an abnormal gene gives rise to a protein with defective enzymatic activity. As examples there are at least 26 known variants of glucose 6-phosphate dehydrogenase deficiency and three of galactosaemia.[6] This particular subdivision of the molecular diseases falls into the group of genetically determined biochemical defects, or **inborn errors of metabolism,**[7,8] a term coined by Archibald Garrod over 50 years ago.[9] These are uncommon diseases, but they point a finger in the direction which should be followed by those who would unravel the mode of gene action. As noted by William Harvey over 300 years ago, "nature is nowhere accustomed more openly to display her secret mysteries than in cases where she shows traces of her workings apart from the beaten path".*

A representative example of such a disease is *galactosaemia.*[10] Babies with this defect lack an enzyme which converts galactose to glucose. The galactose, or its metabolites, derived from the lactose in milk, accumulates in the blood and interferes with the development of the brain, the eye, and the liver. Mental defect, cataracts, and cirrhosis of the liver are the results of this simple biochemical defect. Many similar examples are known; often they result in mental deficiency. They can be ameliorated by avoiding the particular substance in the diet—for instance, in galactosaemia, by avoiding lactose and galactose. The ethics of condemning a child to a lifelong artificial diet might, however, be questioned.

Many biochemical genetic variants have been discovered. Some result in severe disease, while in other instances they are of no importance save for their anthropological interest. Deficiency or abnormality of an enzyme may induce in the individual an intolerance to a particular drug. For example, those who have a defective *pseudocholinesterase*[11] are very susceptible to the drug suxamethonium used in anaesthesia. This drug is used to produce relaxation or paralysis of muscles, and is inactivated by the enzyme pseudocholinesterase. Patients with this enzyme defect are unable to metabolize the drug quickly, and if given it, are liable to develop prolonged paralysis with cessation of breathing and death. Enzyme-deficient red cells are considered on page 346.

### Disease Associated with Genetic Constitution[1]

In spite of the great advances in biochemical genetics, there are many diseases in which the mechanisms involved are not understood. They appear to be more common in certain families, and are spoken of as *familial diseases,* but their occurrence and distribution cannot be predicted. High blood pressure, obesity, and heart disease seem to fall into this group.

Sometimes particular characteristics are associated with certain diseases, though they themselves are not the obvious cause. The association of a particular disease with race, e.g. diabetes mellitus and Gaucher's disease in Jews, or with sex, e.g. goitres in women and cancer of the lung in men, is an example of this. In addition, innate immunity to infection (see p. 154) is an inherited characteristic, and so is the inherited liability to develop hyper-

* "The Works of William Harvey, M.D." translated by Robert Willis, p. 616, Sydenham Society, London, 1847. (Cited by Garrod, A. E., 1928, *Lancet,* **1,** 1055).

sensitivity (p. 162). The association of blood groups with disease has also been recognized: cancer of the stomach is more frequent in group-A subjects, while duodenal ulceration is more common in those of group O. We are quite ignorant of the mechanisms involved, but undoubtedly this type of association was noted by the great clinicians of the past, who often referred to a characteristic disease diathesis.

## Diseases Associated with Gross Chromosomal Abnormalities[2, 12]

As mentioned on p. 20, man has 46 chromosomes in each cell, of which two are sex chromosomes and the remainder autosomes. Certain individuals have been found to have more than 46 chromosomes, while others have less. Finally, abnormalities in the shape or form of individual chromosomes have also been noted. These abnormalities may be considered under two headings:

(i) *alteration in number of chromosomes*
(ii) *alteration in structure of chromosomes.*

Although the finding of a chromosomal abnormality is regarded as uncommon, it is now apparent that those cases detected in post-natal life represent only the residue of a much larger group of abnormal zygotes. About half the spontaneous abortions in the first three months of pregnancy have chromosomal anomalies, one of the commonest being triploidy (the cells having 69 chromosomes). About 30 per cent of zygotes are aborted spontaneously, and gross genetic errors are clearly a major cause.

### Alteration in Number of Chromosomes

**Additional Chromosomes.** The commonest example is where there is one extra chromosome.

*Trisomy.* The presence of three chromosomes of a kind instead of two is called trisomy. An example is Down's syndrome (trisomy 21, or mongolism) in which a child is born with three of the 21 chromosome.[13, 14] (Fig. 3.4). Usually the total number of chromosomes is 47, and the karyotype is recorded as 47, XX, 21+ (or 47, XY, 21+ according to the child's sex). In occasional cases the additional 21 chromosomes is translocated to the 15 chromosome, so that the total number is 46. This *translocation mongolism* is important because the chromosomal defect is frequently present in one of the parents without producing clinical effects. In these circumstances the chromosomal defect is transmitted to many of the offspring.

The characteristic features of Down's syndrome, the mongoloid features and mental defect, are all too familiar,[15] since such children are produced with an incidence of approximately 1 in every 600 live births (Fig. 3.5).

Several other syndromes are recognized in which other autosomes are trisomic, but they are rare.

The presence of additional sex chromosomes is not uncommon.[16] Certain individuals are found to have an extra X. Some are apparent males, have the genetic constitution 47, XXY, and their cells are chromatin positive. They have small testes which fail to develop at puberty, there is little facial hair, they may have a female type of breast development (*gynaecomastia*), and are sterile. These features become evident at puberty, and the condition

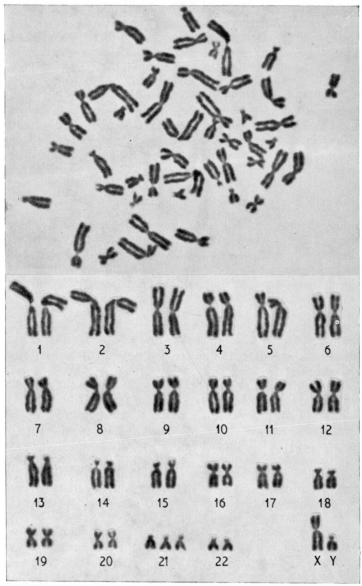

FIG. 3.4. Down's syndrome in a human male. Above are shown the chromosomes of a somatic cell at metaphase, and below these chromosomes are arranged as a karyotype. The latter demonstrates the 22 pairs of autosomes, numbered according to the Denver system of classification, and the two sex chromosomes XY of the male. Note that there are 47 chromosomes due to an extra chromosome No. 21.　　　*(Photograph supplied by Dr. Nigel H. Kemp)*

is known as *Klinefelter's syndrome*.[16] Another group of patients are the *superfemales*, 47, XXX, who are females having an extra X.

In the 47, *XYY syndrome* there is normal male development, but some individuals are abnormally tall and exhibit a criminally aggressive temperament.

**Reduction in Number of Chromosomes.** The loss of an autosome appears to be incompatible with postuterine life. In those cases where such a state has been described, a small chromosome is involved, and it seems likely that

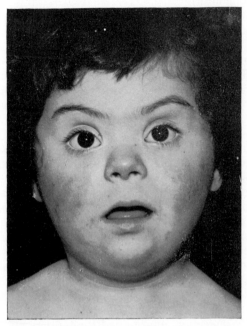

Fig. 3.5. Down's syndrome. Note the oval, slanting palpebral fissures with the prominent epicanthic folds at the inner aspects of both upper eyelids. It is this appearance that is reminiscent of the Mongolian race, and has given rise to the name mongolism. Other typical features are the short nose with depressed bridge, the large tongue, and the rounded lower jaw.

*(Photograph supplied by Dr. W. C. Smallwood)*

the chromosome is in fact present but has become attached to another chromosome (i.e. it has been translocated).

The sex chromosomes appear to be less vital, and deletion of one is compatible with life. About 1 in every 3 000 births produces a female with 45 chromosomes, having the normal number of autosomes but with only one X. This 45, X, or *ovarian dysgenesis syndrome*,[17] becomes obvious at adolescence, when ovulation and menstruation fail to occur. Such individuals are short, stunted, and sterile. When accompanied by two or more of a number of somatic abnormalities, e.g. webbing of the neck, a shield-like chest with widely-spaced nipples, short fourth metacarpal bone, coarctation of the aorta, or hypoplastic nails, the eponym *Turner's syndrome* is applied. Their cells are chromatin negative, since only one X is present.

### Abnormalities of Chromosome Structure

Many abnormalities in the size or shape of chromosomes have been described. These will not be considered in detail. Sometimes a portion of a chromosome is deleted, and the remaining portions join together to form a *ring chromosome*. Translocation results in abnormal chromosomes (see translocation mongolism).

Although certain syndromes, many of them very uncommon, are now recognized as being accompanied by chromosomal abnormality, the actual pathogenesis is obscure. So far only one acquired disease has been found to have any consistent chromosomal abnormality. This is *chronic myeloid leukaemia*, in which the abnormal white blood cells lack one arm of the 22 chromosome (the *Philadelphia chromosome*).[18] Again the significance of this is not understood, but the deletion is a useful diagnostic observation.

### Environmental Factors Causing Disease

Much of human pathology is concerned with those diseases which are acquired in postnatal life as a result of the action of external factors. The effects of physical and chemical agents, living organisms, and dietary deficiencies are the common causes of these *acquired diseases*. It must not be forgotten, however, that the developing fetus is also sensitive to enviromental influences—in some instances much more so than is the adult. Intrauterine events may produce defects which are present at birth (*congenital*), but which are not inherited, since no genetic mechanism is involved. Some congenital lesions of acquired aetiology may copy abnormalities of genetic cause; these are therefore called *phenocopies*. For example, the condition of small brain (microcephaly) may be inherited, or may result from intrauterine irradiation, or infection with toxoplasmosis. The other causes of congenital defects—infection, ionizing radiation, drugs, etc.—are considered in greater detail in Chapter 20.

A final point deserves consideration: hereditary diseases may be congenital, e.g. achondroplasia, but they may also appear later on in life, e.g. polyposis coli (p. 275). The time of onset of a disease gives no indication as to whether the cause is environmental or genetic.

### General Reading

THOMPSON, J. S. and THOMPSON, M. W. (1966). "Genetics in Medicine", 300 pp. Philadelphia and London: Saunders. A very clear and useful introduction to the subject.
CARTER, C. O. (1969). *Lancet*, **1**, 1014, 1041, 1087, 1139, 1203, 1252 and 1303. A series entitled "An ABC of Medical Genetics".

### References

1. Various Authors (1963). Symposium on Genetics. *Amer. J. Med.*, **34**, 583–746.
2. Various Authors (1961). Human Genetics. *Brit. med. Bull.*, **17**, 177–259, and (1969). New Aspects of Human Genetics, **25**, 1–114.

3. FRASER, G. R. (1966). *Brit. med. J.*, **2**, 345, 397 and 453.
4. TOWNES, P. L. (1969). *Med. Clinics of N. America*, **53**, 886.
5. RENDEL, J. M. (1962). *J. theor. Biol.*, **2**, 296.
6. CHILDS, B. and DER KALOUSTIAN, V. M. (1968). *New Engl. J. Med.*, 279, 1205 and 1267.
7. STANBURY, J. B., WYNGAARDEN, J. B. and FREDRICKSON, D. S. (1972). "The Metabolic Basis of Inherited Disease", New York, Toronto and London: McGraw-Hill. 3rd ed. It should be consulted for details concerning any inherited disease.
8. MILNE, M. D. (1966). *Proc. roy. Soc. Med.*, **59**, 1157.
9. CHILDS, B. (1970). *New Engl. J. Med.*, **282**, 71.
10. SMETANA, H. F. and OLEN, E. (1962). *Amer. J. clin. Path.*, **38**, 3.
11. LEHMANN, H. and LIDDELL, J. (1964). In "Progress in Medical Genetics", Vol 3. p. 75, ed. by Steinberg, A. G. and Bearn, A. G. New York: Grune & Stratton.
12. COURT BROWN, W. M. (1962). In "The Scientific Basis of Medicine Annual Reviews", p. 109. London: Athlone Press.
13. LEJEUNE, J. (1964). In "Progress in Medical Genetics", p. 144, *loc. cit.*
14. PENROSE, L. S. and SMITH, G. F. (1966). "Down's Anomaly", 218 pp. London: Churchill.
15. COHEN, M. M. and WINER, R. A. (1965), *J. dent. Res.*, **44**, 197.
16. MILLER, O. J. (1964). *Amer. J. Obst. A Gynec.*, **90**, 1078.
17. JONES, H. W., FERGUSON-SMITH, M. A. and HELLER, R. H. (1963). *Amer. J. Obst. & Gynec.*, **87**, 578.
18. LEADING ARTICLE (1970). *Brit. Med. J.*, 3, 419.

*Chapter 4*

# CELL AND TISSUE DAMAGE

## CELL DAMAGE

Since the tissues of the body are all ultimately derived from a single cell, the fertilized ovum, it is reasonable to assume that all the complex functions of the body and all the intricacies of disease will ultimately be explicable in terms of the function and disorders of individual cells. The concept of *pathology as a cellular study* stems from the invention of the compound microscope by Van Leeuwenhoek in the seventeenth century, and blossomed in the nineteenth century with its application to disease by the German school of pathology headed by Virchow. Recent advances in technology have extended this approach. Electron microscopy, with its resolution several hundred times greater than that of the light microscope, has enabled pathology to enter a subcellular phase. The damaged cells in disease can now be described at a subcellular, or even a molecular, level. This study has been augmented by applying chemistry to the examination of cells, using the techniques of *histochemistry*. A simple example of this is the identification of haemosiderin, an iron-containing pigment which occurs in the tissues after haemorrhage. If acid is added to a section of tissue, haemosiderin granules release $Fe^{+++}$ ions, and these are detected by the addition of potassium ferrocyanide. The intense colour of Prussian blue indicates the previous location of the haemosiderin. Analogous methods are available for the identification of glycogen, polysaccharides, nucleic acids, and many enzymes.

Chemists have, however, exerted a quite different influence on the study of disease by adopting another approach. Instead of concentrating on the individual cell or its organelles, they have turned their attention to specific chemical reactions. Thus, in respect of the metabolism of galactose, all cells may be regarded as one. One important feature in the metabolism of galactose is the enzyme galactose 1-phosphate uridyl transferase, which converts galactose 1-phosphate to glucose 1-phosphate. Deficiency of this enzyme produces the disease *galactosaemia*, which can therefore be explained without recourse to a microscope or the study of individual cells. This second approach to pathology has been of immense value both in the delineation of disease processes and in the treatment of individual patients. Ultimately this broad concept of biochemical disorder must be reduced to a cellular level. In some instances this has already happened, and it is convenient therefore to consider first those examples of cellular damage caused by lesions of known chemical mechanism.

### Biochemical Lesions

The concept of a biochemical lesion was first put forward by Rudolph Peters,[1,2,3] and was based upon the observation that pigeons subjected to a

44

thiamine-deficient diet developed severe neurological symptoms (e.g. convulsions) and died. In spite of the severity of the disease no abnormality could be found by histological examination of the brain. The cells looked normal, but they were not functioning correctly. Peters found that thiamine was one of the factors necessary for the conversion of pyruvate to acetylcoenzyme A (Fig. 2.8). This substance is the fuel, derived from glucose, protein, and fat metabolism, with which the Krebs cycle is fed. Hence in thiamine deficiency Krebs cycle activity is reduced, and with it so also is energy production. Nerve cells, with their high metabolic requirements, are among the first to be affected, and this explains the nervous manifestations of thiamine deficiency. It should be noted that although pyruvate accumulates in the brain and in the blood, it is an effect of the biochemical lesion and not the cause of the symptoms. In other biochemical lesions the unused metabolite does produce a harmful effect. For example, in galactosaemia galactose 1-phosphate accumulates and interferes with other essential metabolic processes. There is no shortage of glucose 1-phosphate, since this can be derived from sources other than galactose.

There are relatively few examples of biochemical lesions in which the detailed changes are known. Certain poisons act by blocking a particular metabolic pathway, and there are the group of inborn errors of metabolism in which a specific enzyme is defective or absent (p. 38). Nevertheless, it is presumed that many bacterial toxins and other damaging agents act in this way. The chemical lesions which they induce are not known, and only the morphological changes in the affected cells are visible. These changes, if severe or prolonged, are liable to lead to the death of the cell—for this reason the changes are generally classified as degenerative, and the group of conditions is spoken of as the *degenerations*.

## The Degenerations

The various morphological types of cellular degeneration may result from the cells being submitted to a wide variety of adverse circumstances which may be either internal or external events. These may be summarized:

**Causes**

**Internal events**    *genetic error*—enzyme defects.
*deprivation of essential chemicals*—e.g. hormones, vitamins, choline, oxygen, etc., *loss of blood supply*.
*hypersensitivity*.

**External agents**    *physical*—heat, cold, trauma, radiation.
*chemical*—poisons, lack of oxygen.
*microbial*—toxins, e.g. diphtheria; microbial invasion.

The names attached to the degenerative processes in the cells are mainly descriptive; while some are appropriate, others are frankly misleading. Two main groups are described. Firstly, there is a group associated with an *excessive accumulation of water* in the cell: these are *cloudy swelling, vacuolar degeneration*, and *hydropic degeneration*. Secondly, there is *fatty change*,

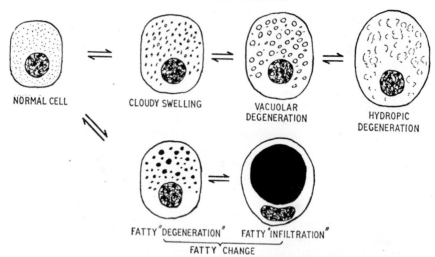

NORMAL CELL          CLOUDY SWELLING          VACUOLAR
DEGENERATION          HYDROPIC
DEGENERATION

FATTY "DEGENERATION"     FATTY "INFILTRATION"
FATTY CHANGE

Fig. 4.1. Diagram to illustrate the cellular changes which are generally described as the "degenerations". A damaged cell may exhibit progressive waterlogging and pass through the stages of cloudy swelling, vacuolar degeneration, and hydropic degeneration. Alternatively, fat may accumulate, first as fine droplets, but as the condition advances, a large globule is formed.

which in the past has been subdivided into fatty degeneration and fatty infiltration (Fig. 4.1).

### Changes Associated with Accumulation of Water

**Cloudy Swelling.** This is generally described in specialized cells, e.g. those of the heart, liver, and kidney. The affected organ is swollen, and its cut surface bulges. It has a grey, parboiled appearance, and the consistency is soft. Microscopically the cells are swollen and the cytoplasm is granular. From being a common descriptive term, cloudy swelling has now largely fallen into disuse. This is partly because the changes are ill-defined, and partly because they are very easily confused with those of autolysis which take place after death[4] (p. 52).

**Vacuolar Degeneration.** The naked-eye appearances described as typical of cloudy swelling are sometimes associated with swollen cells containing vacuoles rather than granules. This is vacuolar degeneration, and its causes and distribution are similar to those of cloudy swelling.

**Hydropic Degeneration.** The cells show great swelling (ballooning) due to an accumulation of fluid. This is the most severe form of this group of degenerative changes, and, although it is reversible, the affected cells frequently rupture and die. Examples of this are to be seen in the liver cells in acute virus hepatitis and in the basal cells of the epidermis in lupus erythematosus.

### Changes Associated with the Accumulation of Fat[5]

An accumulation of excess stainable fat is a frequent finding in parenchymal cells; it is especially common in the liver, and its causes are the same as those of cloudy swelling. In this organ alcohol, carbon tetrachloride, and phosphorus are particularly liable to cause such a change. A fatty liver is enlarged, and is soft in consistency. On section its cut surface bulges and appears greasy. Its colour is pale and in severe cases yellow.

Fatty change is common in the kidneys, where it produces pallor and swelling of the cortex.

An accumulation of fat in the heart muscle, as in severe anaemia, produces yellow flecks on the endocardial surface ("tabby-cat heart").

Microscopically the cells are swollen and contain small droplets of neutral

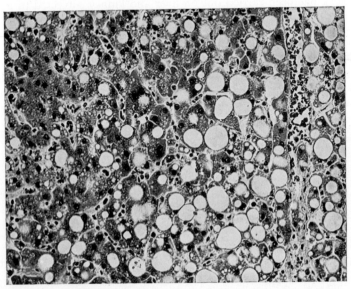

Fig. 4.2. Fatty change of liver. Many of the liver cells are distended with fat globules to the extent that their nuclei are pushed to the cell wall. In others the fat is present as small droplets in the cytoplasm. × 170.

fat (glycerol triesters). In the liver the fat accumulation may proceed until the cell contains one large vacuole of fat and its appearance bears some resemblance to a normal fat cell (Fig. 4.2).

### Nature of the Changes[6,7]

It is often assumed that the cellular changes of cloudy swelling or hydropic degeneration are the same regardless of the organ affected, be it liver, kidney, or islet of Langerhans. Such is not the case. Using the electron microscope, it has been possible to probe more deeply into the nature of these changes. Whereas the light microscope can give a vague impression of intracellular events and detect the changes when they are severe enough to affect the cell as a whole, electron microscopy can reveal which parts of the cell are affected and indicate the sequence of events and metabolic changes which are occurring. The structure of the cell now appears more complex than did the anatomy of the whole body a hundred years ago. Just as "coma" ceased to be an intellectually satisfying ultimate diagnosis when specific conditions affecting the brain were recognized, so cloudy swelling is equally unsatisfactory now that organelles are known to exist. The first steps in the recognition of the cell's response to injury have been taken, and cellular pathology promises to become as complex as organ pathology. At this stage one must expect newly described lesions to prove as useful—and at times as misleading—as were those used initially in organ pathology.

It is not easy to give a clear generalized account of the cell's response to injury, since relatively few cell-types have been investigated to any extent. Most work has been carried out on liver and kidney subjected to a variety of chemical poisons, e.g. carbon tetrachloride, ethionine, barbiturates, ethanol, etc. Some of the changes in the cell's components will be described:

## Nuclear Changes

A variety of nuclear changes have been described in poisoned cells. One of the earliest is clumping of the chromatin along the nuclear membrane and around the nucleolus (Fig. 4.3). The nucleoli show loss of their granular

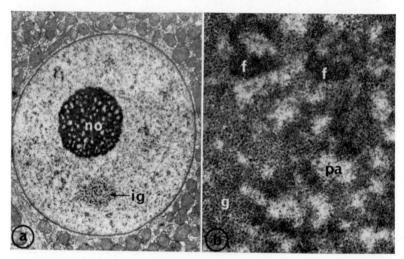

FIG. 4.3. Nucleolar structure of the hepatocyte. (*a*) shows the nucleus of a rat hepatocyte of an animal given ethionine. The nucleolus (no) is large, deeply staining, and shows the nucleolonema as a dense network enclosing spaces of low opacity called the pars amorpha. ig—interchromatin granules. Uranyl acetate. × 7 500. (*b*) is a higher magnification of a nucleolus similar to that shown in (*a*). The fibrillar (f) and granular (g) components are seen, and together surround clear spaces—the pars amorpha (pa). Lead hydroxide. × 45 000.      (*Photographs supplied by Dr. Katsumi Miyai*)

component, and the fibrillar material is sometimes dispersed into separate fragments. Nucleoli are therefore smaller but more numerous. The loss of granular material may indicate impaired synthesis of ribosomal material and messenger RNA. Reduced RNA synthesis is found in damaged cells,[8] and this is reflected in the cytoplasm as reduced protein synthesis. It should be stressed that by light microscopy nuclear changes are not obvious or characteristic in cells showing degeneration.

## Cytoplasmic Changes

These may be considered under five headings:

**Evidence of Increased Cell Function.** Cellular components may proliferate or reorganize in a manner which suggests a state of *hyperfunction*. In response to certain poisons the smooth endoplasmic reticulum becomes more abundant and forms complex whorls or gyrations (Fig. 4.4); this is regarded as an adaptive mechanism and indicates an attempt to increase the cell's ability

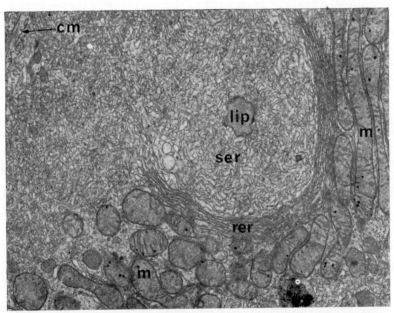

FIG. 4.4. Advanced proliferation of the smooth endoplasmic reticulum (ser) in the periphery of a rat hepatocyte following ethionine administration. The proliferated vesicles of the agranular reticulum are tightly packed and well demarcated from the rough endoplasmic reticulum (rer), which can be identified by the ribosomes studded on the membranes. Mitochondria (m) are elongated. cm—cell membrane; lip—lipid droplet. Lead hydroxide. × 15 750.                           (*Photograph supplied by Dr. Katsumi Miyai*)

to detoxify the substance. Likewise free ribosomes, rough endoplasmic reticulum, and the Golgi apparatus may proliferate; the number of lysosomes may increase, and mitochondria become more abundant, enlarge, and exhibit an increase in their internal complexity. Evidently the cell's metabolism is increased, for protein synthesis, ATP production, and catabolic activity may all be stimulated as may sometimes glycogen synthesis.

Micropinocytotic activity may increase, and this results in the appearance of numerous vacuoles in the cytoplasm.

**Evidence of Decreased Function.** Cellular components may become less numerous and show evidence of *hypofunction*. In damaged liver cells the rough endoplasmic reticulum shows dilatation of its sacs and loss of attached ribosomes. Polysomes are reduced in number. These changes are particularly associated with hydropic degeneration, and indicate *impaired protein synthesis*.

Mitochondrial changes are frequent. These organelles may show swelling and a loss of cristae. An increase in calcium content and the formation of concentric laminated whorls in the matrix have also been described. Impaired function results in reduced oxidative phosphorylation, and ATP production is reduced. Since this substance forms the main immediately available source of energy for cellular metabolism, it is not surprising that many cell functions are impaired. Thus ATP is required for the operation of the mechanism, or pump, regulating the concentration of ions in the cell. The sodium pump is impeded, and sodium and water accumulate in the cell, which in this way becomes progressively enlarged and waterlogged. The electrolytes can pass freely across the cell membrane, but the proteins within the cell cannot escape. When the sodium pump breaks down, there is therefore a *tendency* for the cell to become hypertonic. This is counteracted by the entry of water into the cell which thereupon swells. The breakdown of proteins into smaller molecules may further increase this tendency to hypertonicity. This may not be the complete explanation, but there is little doubt that changes in membrane permeability are an outstanding feature of cells undergoing degeneration.[7] Mitochondrial swelling is commonly found in cells showing cloudy swelling.

**Evidence of Altered Function.** Changes may occur which indicate that the cell has acquired a new function; thus the endothelial cells of the glomerular tuft can become actively phagocytic for fibrin.

**Abnormal Accumulation of Substances in the Cell.** Lipid is an example, and is described later.

**Degenerative Changes.** Localized areas of the cell may appear to become degenerate, and the term *focal cytoplasmic degeneration* has been applied. Sometimes cytoplasmic components, e.g. endoplasmic reticulum and mitochondria, are seen within vacuoles containing lysosomal enzymes. These are called *autophagocytic vacuoles*, *autophagosomes*, or *cytolysomes*, and an increase in their number is an indication of cell injury.[9] Sometimes an area of cytoplasm degenerates and is actually cast off: damaged renal tubular cells can show loss of the brush border, which together with an area of the underlying cytoplasm is desquamated into the lumen. Such changes have been called necrosis of part of a cell.

It should be appreciated that these various changed indicating hyperfunction, hypofunction, altered function, and focal degeneration can all occur within a single cell either simultaneously or sequentially. A damaged cell is not an inactive cell, and its reaction to injury may end in recovery. Parts injured beyond recovery are lysed or extruded, and the remaining structures reform the lost components. The cell may return to normal but some alterations may persist. Thus the retention of an abnormal function is seen in metaplasia and perhaps also neoplasia. The reaction of damaged cells is a highly complex and varied affair, but so far as routine human pathology is concerned it is rarely possible to obtain tissue fresh enough to detect these intracellular events even if time and equipment were available.

Not all the changes described above occur under any single circumstance. Cells subjected to adverse conditions show a complex reaction: some changes may be regarded as degenerative, while others are adaptive. A liver cell showing cloudy swelling due to carbon tetrachloride poisoning would therefore not be expected to show the same changes as one infected with a virus, or a kidney cell damaged by hypoxia.

## Nature of Fatty Change[5,10]

Electron microscopy has revealed that many normal cells contain small droplets of lipid, but these are not visible on light microscopy. An obvious exception to this is the adult fat cell. The excess fat which appears in damaged cells is generally considered to originate from outside the cell.[11] The evidence for this is that if a normal animal is poisoned with phosphorus it develops acute hepatic damage with severe fatty change. If, however, the animal is starved so that its depot fat is severely depleted, poisoning causes cell damage without fatty change. The neutral fat droplets are evidently derived from the fat depots and not by a hypothetical process of *phanerosis*, which is the conversion of phospholipid constituents into visible neutral fat.

Depot fat is composed mostly of neutral fat, and when it is mobilized it is transported in the blood as free fatty acid bound to albumin. This is removed by tissues and utilized for metabolic purposes. If the cells are damaged by hypoxia, poisoned, etc., their metabolic activity is impaired and the fat normally brought to them is inadequately utilized; it accumulates as droplets which are at first small, but later fuse into larger globules.

In the past the appearance of fine droplets was labelled *fatty degeneration*, while cells showing a large globule were said to show *fatty infiltration*. In both conditions the cells contain excess fat which is derived from the fat depots.[11] Clearly the pathogenesis is the same, and to avoid confusion both these terms have now been dropped, and *fatty change*, or *fatty metamorphosis*, substituted. It should not be confused with the accumulation of true fat cells in the tissues such as commonly occurs in the heart and pancreas of obese people. Similar local deposits of fat are also sometimes found accompanying chronic inflammation (p. 129) and following atrophy, e.g. of lymph nodes and thymus. These conditions are sometimes called fatty infiltration, but confusion is most easily avoided if the term *adiposity* is used. *Interstitial fatty infiltration* is an alternative name, but it must be clearly understood that the condition bears no relationship to the lesion depicted in Fig. 4.2, in which the excess neutral fat is in parenchymal cells.

**Fatty Change in the Liver due to Inadequate Diet.** The liver occupies a central position in fat metabolism. Non-esterified fatty acid derived from the adipose tissue is brought to it, metabolized, e.g. by conversion into phospholipids such as lecithin (phosphatidyl choline), and finally passed into the blood in the form of lipoproteins. If because of an indequate diet there is a deficiency of choline, conversion cannot take place and neutral fat accumulates in the cells. This mechanism is the most probable cause of the fatty liver seen in the chronic alcoholic and in people who live on the verge of starvation, as in some parts of Asia and Africa.

## Cell Death and Necrosis[12,13]

Cell death is difficult to define in precise terms, but in practice may be regarded as having occurred whenever a cell is incapable of further division or of continuing its normal synthetic functions.

The appearance of the dead cells varies according to the cause of the injury. If the cells are killed suddenly as the result of physical or chemical trauma, initially they show no changes other than those directly attributable to the agent concerned, e.g. disruption in electrical injuries, effects of freezing, burning, etc.

Cells less severely damaged, e.g. by poisons, may develop biochemical lesions which first result in changes previously described as degenerative, e.g. cloudy swelling and fatty change. It will be recalled that the changes detectable by light microscopy are cytoplasmic, and in themselves do not indicate cell death.

In the dead cell respiration ceases, but glycolysis proceeds for a while and results in the production of lactic acid and therefore a drop in the pH. The synthetic activities of the cell stop, but the lytic destructive enzymes continue their work. These enzymes derived from lysosomes are most active at a low pH, and include a wide range of proteases, lipases, esterases, deoxyribonuclease, ribonuclease, etc. The cell undergoes a process of *self-digestion*, or *autolysis*, and within a few hours shows certain morphological changes (see below) by which cell death can be recognized. This is called *necrosis*[14,15] and it may be defined as the *circumscribed death of cells or tissues with structural evidence of their death*. Necrosis and cell death are therefore not synonymous.

The microscopic changes of necrosis that occur affect the whole cell. The *cytoplasm* becomes homogeneous and often brightly eosinophilic; these early autolytic changes may resemble those seen in the degenerative lesions of living cells. Following cell death, however, the nucleus also shows autolytic changes, and it is these which are to be regarded as pathognomonic (absolutely diagnostic) of necrosis.

**Nuclear Changes of Necrosis.** The nucleus becomes smaller, while the chromatin loses its fine reticular pattern, becomes clumped, and stains intensely. This is termed *pyknosis*. The pyknotic nucleus either breaks up into fragments (*karyorrhexis*), or becomes indistinct as the nuclear material is digested (*karyolysis*).

### Diagnosis of Necrosis by Biochemical Means

A diagnosis of the occurrence of necrosis is frequently of great clinical importance. When areas of heart muscle, pancreas, liver, or brain are dying the patient's life is often in jeopardy. As necrosis occurs, various soluble substances, e.g. enzymes, diffuse out of the cells and are absorbed into the blood stream, and their detection is an aid to clinical diagnosis. Some examples may be cited. A raised level of creatine phosphokinase (CPK) is found after skeletal-muscle necrosis, and is also elevated in some types of myopathy[16] (see also p. 319). Serum glutamate oxaloacetate transaminase (SGOT), hydroxybutyrate dehydrogenase (HBD), CPK, and lactate dehydrogenase (LHD) are all raised after myocardial infarction. Increased serum glutamate pyruvate transaminase (SGPT) and LDH are found after liver-cell necrosis.[17] Some enzymes can be separated into separate fractions by electrophoresis. In the case of LDH these *isoenzymes* are of different origin: LDH 1 and LDH 2 are released from heart muscle, while LDH 5 is of hepatic origin.

## Types of Necrosis

**Coagulative Necrosis.** Necrotic tissue usually becomes firm and slightly swollen. It seems likely that the proteins are denatured.[18] This process involves an unfolding of the three-dimensional arrangement of the molecule without necessarily changing its empirical formula. This causes the tissue to become opaque and firm, as does the white of an egg on boiling. It also becomes more reactive chemically, and side-chains previously saturated become exposed and are available for binding. This explains why the tissue initially binds dyes, e.g. eosin, more avidly than does normal tissue. Thus an increased eosinophilia of heart muscle fibres is a useful *post-mortem* indication of a recent myocardial infarct, and the magnitude of hypoxic brain damage can be judged by the extent and degree of the eosinophilia of the cortical neurones in patients who have died shortly after an episode of cerebral ischaemia, e.g. following cardiac arrest. The increased binding capacity of necrotic tissue might also be a factor in causing the calcification. This is called *dystrophic calcification*, and is important because the deposits of calcium salts show up on x-ray examination and are sometimes of value in diagnosis. Many examples will be met in later sections of this book and only a few will be mentioned here. Calcification of a degenerate *pineal gland* may show up on a radiograph of the skull, and its displacement may help in recognizing an expanding brain lesion. The *caseous material* of tuberculous lesions often calcifies and so also do the degenerate lesions of large arteries in *atherosclerosis*. Dystrophic calcification should not be confused with metastatic calcification, which occurs in normal tissues (p. 447).

A common cause of necrosis is sudden deprivation of the blood supply to a part. This is called *infarction*, and is quite common in the heart and kidney when their supplying arteries are occluded. These infarcts show the typical changes of coagulative necrosis. Microscopically, in addition to the nuclear changes, another feature is noteworthy: the general architecture of the tissue is still recognizable, even though its constituent cells are all dead. This is therefore called *structured necrosis*. In other examples of coagulative necrosis microscopic examination of the dead tissue fails to reveal any structure—this is *structureless necrosis*. The caseous necrosis of tuberculosis is an example of this (p. 192).

Necrosis in certain tissues presents special features. In adipose tissue fat is liberated from the damaged cells, and is phagocytosed by macrophages. These cells, distended with fat, are called *foam cells*. Deposition of cholesterol crystals, giant-cell formation, and fibrosis complete the microscopic picture of *traumatic fat necrosis* (Fig. 4.5). The condition may resemble tuberculosis histologically, and is seen in the breast following injury. Another type of fat necrosis occurs in the peritoneum whenever lipase escapes from the pancreas, as after its injury or inflammation (acute pancreatitis). Necrosis of collagen is described on p. 57.

**Colliquative Necrosis.** This is necrosis with softening, and rarely occurs as a primary event except in infarcts of the brain. Liquefaction is seen as a secondary event in suppuration (p. 70), and following caseation (p. 192).

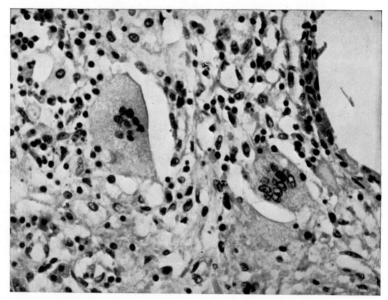

Fig. 4.5. Traumatic fat necrosis of breast. The adipose tissue cells have an opaque, granular cytoplasm due to the breakdown of neutral fat and the production of fatty acid. Two large foreign-body giant cells with a foamy, fat-filled cytoplasm are present. × 330.

### Further Changes in Necrotic Tissue

Necrotic tissue usually excites an *acute inflammatory reaction* followed by a phase of *healing* (Fig. 4.6): these events are considered in later chapters. An occasional complication is gangrene.

### Gangrene

Sometimes the dead tissue is invaded by saprophytic protein-splitting anaerobic bacteria, which cause its decomposition with the production of hydrogen sulphide and other foul-smelling substances. There is blackening of the area due to the formation of iron sulphide from the iron of decomposed haemoglobin. This *necrosis with superadded putrefaction* is called *gangrene*, an old clinical term which was applied to any black, foul-smelling area in continuity with the living.

**Clostridial Gangrene.** The putrefactive bacteria are usually the clostridia of intestinal origin, and therefore necrosis of the bowel is often followed by gangrene. These putrefactive bacteria are of little importance in themselves, because they live on dead tissue and do not invade or harm the living tissue; nevertheless, gangrenous lesions always contain other bacteria which can cause further tissue destruction. It follows that gangrene is a very serious condition, and *unless treated expeditiously is fatal.*

*Gangrene of the Limbs.* This is usually seen in the legs following arterial obstruction (p. 385). It is particularly common in diabetic patients. The limb becomes swollen and black ("wet gangrene"), and in addition to the putrefactive bacteria there are also pathogenic organisms present, which invade the adjacent living tissue. Gangrene of this type therefore steadily spreads.

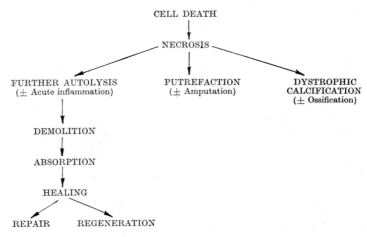

FIG. 4.6. The sequelae of cell death.

If the blood supply to a limb is *slowly* obstructed, the tips of the digits become black and necrotic, and at the same time undergo desiccation. This greatly impedes bacterial growth, and infection with pathogenic organisms is not a feature. The condition slowly extends until a point is reached where the blood supply to the tissue is adequate. A line of demarcation develops, and the dead tissue is discarded by a process of spontaneous amputation. This condition is called *"dry gangrene"*, but since the amount of putrefaction is minimal, the term is somewhat of a misnomer. The process is in fact mummification of an infarcted portion of a limb.

**Gangrene due to Other Organisms.** Some putrefactive bacteria are also pathogenic, e.g. certain strains of anaerobic streptococci (p. 180) and members of the family *Bacteroidaceae.*[19-21] The latter includes the well-known member *Fusobacterium fusiforme,* which is often found in the company of *Borrelia vincenti* ("Vincent's organisms").[22]

The putrefactive organisms mentioned are frequently associated with the common type of ulcerative gingivitis (Vincent's infection, or "trench mouth".) It affects the free gingiva and the interdental papillæ, and may be either acute or run a chronic relapsing course. A more severe gangrenous lesion which affects the soft tissues of the face, and may involve the bone is called *cancrum oris*, or *noma*, and occurs in malnourished debilitated children following an infectious disease like measles.[23] Extensive tissue destruction occurs. Fortunately this condition is almost unknown, at least in civilized communities.

*Gangrene of the lung* may complicate the inhalation of a piece of tooth following extraction performed under general anaesthesia. It is also due to organism of the family *Bacteroidaceae*.

## Damage to Connective Tissue

### Abnormalities of Collagen

The information regarding the appearance and composition of collagen under pathological conditions is contradictory, confusing, and inadequate. In organs where collagen development is incomplete (i.e. where it remains at the reticulin stage), the fibres may mature to form histological collagen. This process is seen in the lymph nodes, the lung, and the spleen. It is one mechanism whereby these organs undergo *fibrosis*, i.e. an increase in their content of fibrous tissue.

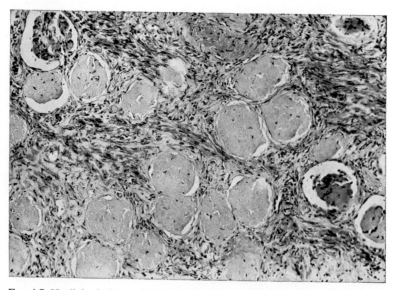

Fig. 4.7. Hyalinized glomerular tufts. Most of the glomeruli have been converted into dense, solid masses of hyalinized material, virtually devoid of cellular components. The section is from a case of chronic pyelonephritis. × 65.

**Hyalinization.** The term hyaline is used in a purely descriptive capacity—it literally means glassy and is employed to describe any homogeneous eosinophilic material. Necrotic cells may take on this appearance, and under particular circumstances they have by tradition been described as hyalinized. Sometimes homogeneous areas in cells have been called hyaline. Thus eosinophilic areas in degenerating liver cells in the alcoholic patient have been called "alcoholic hyaline".

Hyaline can also be used to describe extracellular material, and it is in relation to the connective tissues that the term is most commonly used. In collagen, with the passage of time, the fibres appear to fuse together to form a glassy, eosinophilic material. This hyalinization is very common in fibrous tissue which has been laid down as a replacement for lost parenchyma. Therefore it is very common in scars of any type (Fig. 4.7) and in chronic inflammatory lesions. Hyaline material is also seen in the intima of small blood vessels ("vascular hyaline"); it is a normal ageing process in the spleen, but in other organs, especially the kidneys, it is associated with hypertension. Amyloid may also be described as hyaline material (p. 322).

**Necrosis of Collagen.** When connective tissue is damaged, its associated fibrocytes undergo necrosis and its fibres appear to degenerate. They break up, and are removed in the course of an inflammatory reaction. This necrosis of collagen differs from hyalinization in several important respects.

(a) Hyaline material is extremely stable. Necrotic collagen, on the other hand, is either removed or organized.

(b) Hyalinized collagen retains the staining characteristics of normal collagen. Necrotic collagen, on the other hand, stains brightly with eosin and in fact takes on many of the staining characteristics of fibrin, e.g. it is PAS positive. The term *fibrinoid necrosis* is therefore often used. Fibrinoid necrosis is seen in the *walls of small blood vessels* in a variety of conditions: malignant hypertension (p. 366), the Arthus phenomenon (p. 163), and the generalized Shwartzman reaction (p. 92). The necrotic material may be degenerating collagen, damaged muscle, fibrin, or antigen-antibody complexes. Fibrinoid necrosis, like hyalinization, describes a particular microscopic appearance and does not imply a single morphological change or aetiological agent.

Fibrinoid necrosis occurs in collagen following severe injury, e.g. burning and exposure to ionizing radiation, and is also a feature of some collagen diseases (p. 172). It is particularly prominent in rheumatoid arthritis, and the fibrinoid material, which appears to be altered collagen, excites a chronic inflammatory reaction. The necrosis is sometimes called necrobiosis, but this is unfortunate because this same term is also used to describe the physiological death of cells (p. 229). Necrobiosis is a word best avoided.

**Changes in Elastic Tissue.** An increase in the number of fibres which stain black with orcein like elastic is a common finding in the dermis, and is a reaction to prolonged exposure to the ultraviolet light of sunshine. While there is little doubt that new elastic fibres can be formed in the adult, in *elastosis* of the skin the fibres are probably altered or damaged collagen.

### Changes in the Ground Substance

Sometimes the connective tissue shows an excessive accumulation of ground substance, which appears as a basophilic pool of structureless material. This overhydration of the ground substance is sometimes a physiological event and appears to be under hormonal control: thus the colourful swelling of the sexual skin of the baboon is in large part due to this change. However, sometimes the associated connective tissue fibres undergo degeneration, and the condition is called *myxomatous degeneration*. A good example of this is seen in the aorta, where owing to the resulting weakness in the vessel its wall may rupture with dramatic effects (p. 376).

There is a group of genetically determined diseases involving an abnormality in the metabolism of mucopolysaccharide (*the mucopolysaccharidoses*). They are usually accompanied by skeletal deformities. The best known member of this uncommon group of diseases is *Hurler's syndrome*, which because of the grotesque appearance of the head is also known as *gargoylism*. Specialized texts should be consulted for details.[24]

In this chapter some of the effects of cellular damage have been considered Local injury is usually the prelude to inflammation and healing, and these are described in the chapters that follow. They are all local events, but it must not be forgotten that any injury, except the most trivial, is accompanied by a generalized response. This is considered in Chapter 22. Injury initiates changes which involve the whole individual, and it is a mistake to think of the reaction to injury solely in terms of local cellular degeneration or necrosis. Likewise at a clinical level, not only must the injuries be treated, but also the patient.

## References

1. GAVRILESCU, N. and PETERS, R. A. (1931). *Biochem. J.*, **25**, 1397 and 2150.
2. PETERS, R. A. (1951). *Proc. roy. Soc. B*, **139**, 143.
3. PETERS, R. A. (1963). "Biochemical Lesions and Lethal Synthesis". Oxford: Pergamon Press.
4. TRUMP, B. F., GOLDBLATT, P. J. and STOWELL, R. E. (1965). *Lab. Invest.*, **14**, 343.
5. LOMBARDI, B. and RECKNAGEL, R. O. (1962). *Amer. J. Path.*, **40**, 571.
6. TRUMP, B. F. and ERICSSON, J. L. E. (1965). In "The Inflammatory Process", p. 35, edrs. Zweifach, B. W., Grant, L. and McCluskey, R. T. New York and London: Academic Press.
7. MAGEE, P. N. (1966). *Lab. Invest.*, **15**, 111.
8. VILLA-TREVINO, S., SHULL, K. H. and FARBER, E. (1966). *J. biol. Chem.*, **241**, 4670.
9. SWIFT, H. and HRUBAN, Z. (1964). *Fed. Proc.*, **23**, 1026.
10. FARBER, E., LOMBARDI, B. and CASTILLO, A. E. (1963). *Lab. Invest.*, **12**, 873.
11. DIBLE, J. H. and GERRARD, W. W. (1938). *J. Path. Bact.*, **46**, 77.
12. KING, D. W. *et al.* (1959). *Amer. J. Path.*, **35**, 369, 575, 835 and 1067.
13. DIXON, K. C. (1967). *Proc. roy. Soc. Med.*, **60**, 271.
14. BESSIS, M. (1964). In "Cellular Injury", A Ciba Foundation Symposium, p. 287, ed. de Reuck, A. V. S. and Knight, J. London: Churchill.
15. MAJNO, G. LA GUTTUTA, M. and THOMPSON, T. E., (1960). *Virchow Arch. Path. Anat.*, **333**, 421.
16. ROSALKI, S. B. (1970). *J. Clin. Path.*, **24**, Supplement (*Asso. Clin. Path.*), **4**, 60.
17. WIEME, R. J. and DEMEULENAERE, L. (1970). *J. Clin. Path.*, **24**, Supplement (*Asso. Clin. Path.*), **4**, 51.
18. MAJNO, G. (1964) In "Cellular Injury", p. 87, *loc. cit.*
19. OMATA, R. R. and BRAUNBERG, R. C. (1960). *J. Bact.*, **80**, 737.
20. BAIRD-PARKER, A. C. (1960). *J. gen. Microbiol.*, **22**, 458.
21. MACDONALD, J. B. (1962). *Ann. roy. Coll. Surg. Engl.*, **31**, 361.

22. LINENBERG, W. B., SCHMITT, J. and L. HARPOLE, H. J. (1961). *Oral Surg.*, **14,** 1138.
23. SNIJMAN, P. C. (1966). *Brit. J. oral Surg.*, **4,** 106.
24. McKUSICK, V. A. (1966). "Heritable Disorders of Connective Tissue", 3rd ed., St. Louis: Mosby.

*Chapter 5*

# THE ACUTE INFLAMMATORY REACTION

Acute inflammation is one of the fundamental reactions of the body to injury, and although its pathogenesis is complex, the main features of the response are relatively simple and familiar to anyone who has ever experienced a boil. The area is *red, swollen, warmer* than the surrounding skin, and is *painful*. These four, *rubor, tumor, calor,* and *dolor,* are the *cardinal signs of inflammation* as described by Celsus (first century A.D.). Loss of function has been added subsequently but its origin is obscure. To attribute it to Galen is to perpetuate a misconception which has been handed down by many authors. Its Latin version *functio laesa* gives this origin an air of respectability but not truth.[1]

The suffix -itis is used to denote an inflammatory lesion, e.g. appendicitis or pulpitis. Unfortunately tradition sometimes demands that this rule be broken —e.g. osteitis fibrosa cystica is not an inflammatory lesion.

## Causes of Acute Inflammation

Since the inflammatory reaction is a response to injury, its causes are those of cell damage. These may be enumerated briefly:

*Physical Agents.* Trauma, e.g. mechanical injury such as cutting and crushing, heat, cold, and ionizing radiation.

*Chemical Agents.* There are innumerable chemicals which injure cells. Many, like corrosive acids, alkalis, and phenol, are fairly non-specific in their action, while others affect particular cells, e.g. mercuric chloride causes renal tubular necrosis.

*Deprivation of Blood Supply.* Infarction is described in Chapter 27.

*Living Organisms.* Inflammation is often a feature of infection.

*Antigen-antibody Reactions.* Damage mediated by sensitizing immunoglobulins, immune complexes, and sensitized lymphocytes is described in Chapter 13.

## The Vascular Response

*Hyperaemia.* Changes in the blood vessels are the most obvious manifestation of acute inflammation. Following trauma there may be an initial constriction of the blood vessels, but this is soon followed by a prolonged period of vasodilatation. It affects the arterioles, so that more blood passes into the area. Tissues near the skin surface are normally cooler than the arterial blood which supplies them, and, as the blood flow increases, so the area becomes warmer. This explains the *calor* of inflammation. The first result of arteriolar dilatation is that the blood flows by the most direct route to the veins through the *central,* or *thoroughfare, channels.* Subsequent opening of the precapillary sphincters allows blood to pass into the capillary bed, and vessels which were temporarily shut down become functional. The inflamed part therefore appears to contain an increased number of vessels, in addition, their calibre is increased. The whole area shows *hyperaemia*, i.e. it contains more blood and appears red (*rubor*). If incised it bleeds profusely.

Inflammation can be studied by examining fixed sections of tissue, but it is in the living animal that a truer picture of its ever-changing manifestations can be appreciated. Cohnheim based much of his classical description of inflammation on his observations on the tongue of the frog.[2] The mesentery of the rat and the rabbit ear-chamber (p. 104) can also be used. Using these methods *changes in the blood flow* are particularly prominent.

**Changes in Blood Flow.**[3] In the arterioles of normal tissue the blood flow is so fast that the individual cells cannot be identified other than by the use of high-speed photography. In the venules the flow is considerably slower but it is still difficult to identify individual cells. However, they can be seen to travel in the central, or axial, part of the stream and leave a clear, cell-free *plasmatic zone* adjacent to the endothelium. In acutely inflamed tissue the velocity of the blood increases at first, but it soon diminishes. *Stasis* ensues, and coincidentally the clear plasmatic zone becomes occupied by innumerable colourless, glistening white blood cells. This is called *margination of the white cells*, and very soon the endothelium becomes covered, or *pavemented*, by them. This phenomenon is very characteristic of acute inflammation, and is due to changes in the vascular endothelium—the cells become swollen and *sticky*. White cells which strike the endothelium by chance, instead of bouncing off and passing on their way, are dragged back and retained. The white cells, for the most part polymorphs, soon push pseudopodia between adjacent endothelial cells, penetrate the basement membrane, and emerge on the external surface of the venule. This remarkable process is called *emigration of the white cells*, and eventually large numbers of them accumulate in the extravascular space. The gap in the vessel wall closes up behind the emigrating white cells; a few red cells may, however, be forced out passively by the hydrostatic pressure of the blood. This is called *diapedesis of the red cells*, and must be distinguished from frank haemorrhage due to destruction of the vessel wall.

**The Inflammatory Exudate**[3]

The most important feature of acute inflammation is the formation of the *inflammatory exudate*. This is a collection of fluid in the extravascular tissues and consists of:

*The fluid exudate*

*The cellular exudate*

*The Fluid Exudate.* The really crucial factor in the formation of an inflammatory exudate is an *increased permeability of the vessel walls to plasma proteins*. If trypan blue is injected intravenously into an animal (a "blued animal"), the dye becomes bound to the plasma albumin and does not readily leave the circulation. When an inflammatory response is elicited, the tagged albumin can be seen to pass into the inflamed area as the exudate forms.

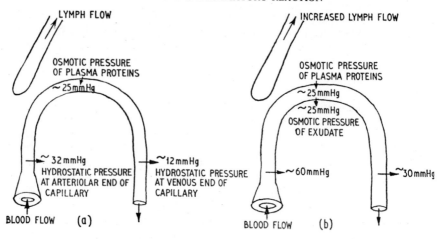

Fɪɢ. 5.1. Fluid exchange between blood and tissue spaces:
(a) under normal conditions,
(b) in acute inflammation.

This experimental method is often used to demonstrate an increase in permeability to plasma proteins. A similar type of labelling may be done with radioactive iodine. In experimentally produced acute inflammation, it has been found that exudation of fluid occurs in two phases. An early transient phase is followed after a latent interval by a prolonged second phase. Fig. 5.2).

*Mechanism of Formation of the Fluid Exudate.* As is described in detail in

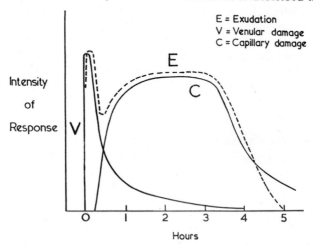

Fɪɢ. 5.2. Multiphase vascular response to mild thermal injury (54° for 40 min.) in rat cremaster muscle.

From Miles, A. A. (1966) in "Wound Healing", ed. by Illingworth, C. p. 9, Fig. 4. London: Churchill.

Chapter 24, the exchange of fluid between the blood vessel lumen and the interstitial tissues is related to the hydrostatic blood pressure within the vessel which drives the fluid out, and the plasma osmotic pressure which draws it into the blood vessel (Fig. 5.1). The effective osmotic pressure is due to the plasma proteins which are too large to pass through the vessel walls. Smaller molecules exchange with ease. In acute inflammation four mechanisms operate to cause excess fluid to leave the blood vessels and form the interstitial exudate.

1. There is an *increased vascular permeability* to plasma proteins. In this way the restraining colloidal osmotic pressure of the plasma is removed, and the hydrostatic pressure is free to drive a protein-rich fluid into the tissues. An exudate has virtually the same protein composition as plasma.

2. There is an *increase in the capillary blood pressure* due to arteriolar dilatation.

3. There is *breakdown of large-molecule tissue proteins* into many small, osmotically-active fragments.

4. There is an *increase in the fluidity of the tissue ground substance*. This has the effect of allowing exudate to diffuse more readily, thereby preventing an immediate rise in tissue tension. A rise in tissue tension is probably the important limiting factor in stopping the accumulation of tissue fluids both under normal conditions and those of acute inflammation. For this reason inflammatory oedema is a prominent feature of inflammation involving, or adjacent to, very lax tissues such as the eyelids and the scrotum. Swelling is not a feature of an infection involving a tissue under tension such as the pulp of a finger.

Since by far the most important factor leading to the formation of the fluid exudate is the increase in vascular permeability, it is not surprising that this has been intensively studied. Two phases of exudation occur after many kinds of injury.[4] The *immediate phase* is obvious in a minute or so and is over within an hour. Then follows a *delayed phase*, which may itself have several components, and this lasts for many hours. In mild thermal injury to the rat cremaster muscle, the immediate phase is accompanied by venular damage while the delayed response is related to capillary damage[5] (see Fig. 5.3). However, in turpentine injury to the rat pleura, both phases are due to venular damage and there is an additional capillary component to the delayed phase.[6] With severe damage the various phases so overlap each other that only one prolonged phase is apparent. The precise response therefore depends upon the tissue involved, the irritant used, and the species of animal. There is evidence that the two phases are mediated by different agents, and this is described later in the section on chemical mediators.

**Vascular Permeability in Normal Tissues.**[7] Normally the walls of the capillaries and venules are freely permeable to water and electrolytes but not to proteins and other large molecules. Rapid exchange takes place between intravascular and extravascular water, and in fact about 70 per cent of the water in the blood crosses the vessel wall every minute and is replaced by water from the interstitial space. The mechanism whereby this exchange takes place has been much debated. In most tissues the barriers which must be considered are:

1. The endothelial cell with its attenuated extensions.

2. The basement membrane, which forms a complete sheath.

3. Pericytes, which form a discontinuous outer coat together with connective tissue fibres.

The following possibilities have been suggested:

*Direct Transport through the Cell by Simple Diffusion.* The lipid (and presumably waterproof) nature of the cell membrane has led many authorities to regard this as an unlikely mechanism.

*Transport across the Endothelial Cell by Cytopempsis* (p. 8). This process does probably take place, but it seems unlikely that it could explain the large volume of fluid which is known to leave the vessels. Furthermore, the vesicles formed by micropinocytosis would be expected to contain protein, but the fluid which escapes from the blood vessels has a low plasma protein content.

*Passage through Pores in the Endothelial Cells.* Pores are present in the sinusoids of the liver; in certain other sites, e.g. kidney and intestine, there are fenestrations which are covered by a very thin membrane. In other areas no pores or fenestrations can be seen on electron microscopy.

*Passage through Spaces between the Endothelial Cells.* The thick cement lines seen in silver-nitrate preparations of endothelium seem to be an artefact, for on electron microscopy the endothelial cells closely adjoin each other and the gap between them is about 15 nm wide. Junctional complexes are present, and in the zonula adherens (Fig. 2.1) the central fused membrane is about 4 nm thick. Pappenheimer and his associates have calculated that the properties of the normal vessel wall could be explained by the presence of circular pores with a radius of about 3 nm or slits about 3·7 nm wide.[8] As noted above, no such pores have been seen in the endothelial cells, but it is possible that the junctions between the cells could act as pores or slits.

The relative importance of these possible methods of transport is not clear at the present time.

A final consideration concerns the basement membrane, for all substances leaving or entering the vessel must cross it. The membrane appears to have no holes nor does it seem to be a barrier to the passage of water or electrolytes. Cells, large particles, and perhaps the plasma proteins are held back and their passage delayed.

**Vascular Permeability in Inflamed Tissue.** Examination of the endothelial cells of capillaries in acutely inflamed tissues has revealed several changes—increase in the number and size of the micropinocytotic vesicles, blebs under the luminal cell membrane, and projections or spikes arising from the membrane. The changes are, however, inconstant and seem inadequate to explain the great increase in vascular permeability. On the other hand, it has been shown that when 5-hydroxytryptamine or histamine is applied to rat cremaster muscle important changes occur in the venules. Gaps (0·1–0·4 $\mu$m in diameter) appear in the endothelial lining due to the separation of adjacent endothelial cells.[9, 10]

If the animal is first given an intravenous injection of mercuric sulphide suspension, the particles, which are 10–15 nm in diameter, are found to be situated between the endothelial cell and the basement membrane. It appears therefore that in acute inflammation the gap between endothelial cells widens, thereby allowing plasma to reach the basement membrane and escape to the extravascular spaces. The particles of mercuric sulphide being unable to penetrate the intact basement membrane accumulate between it and the endothelial cell (Fig. 5.3)

Similar results are obtained if Indian ink is used and trauma applied to produce an acute inflammation.[11-13] Thus, both the early exudation of acute inflammation and the application of histamine are associated with a separation of the endothelial cells and an escape of plasma. Whether other

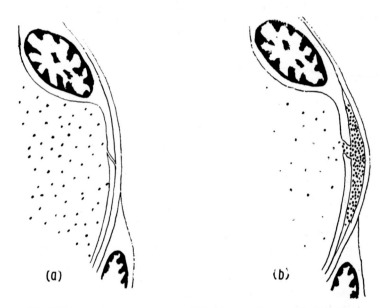

(a)                                        (b)

FIG. 5.3. Diagrammatic representation of the changes in a venule following the intravenous injection of a suspension of mercuric sulphide (particle size 10–15 nm).

(a) Shows the wall of normal venule with the particles distributed in the plasma.

(b) After the local application of histamine. The appearances suggest that the plasma has leaked through the gap between the endothelial cells, and that the basement membrane has held back the particles but allowed the fluid exudate to pass through.

changes occur, for instance in the basement membrane, and whether the second phase of exudation is associated with other features, is not yet clear.

As plasma escapes from the vessels, the plasmatic zone becomes reduced in size. This zone has great functional importance, for the viscosity of plasma is much lower than that of whole blood, and therefore the peripheral resistance is lower than it would be if the blood components were intimately mixed. In inflammation the lubricating action of this zone is impaired or lost, and the blood stream slows. This is the explanation of the *stasis* of inflammation, and it may be so marked that thrombosis sometimes supervenes. This may cause further tissue damage.

*Function of the Fluid Exudate.* All the constituents of the plasma are poured into the area of inflammation. These include natural antibacterial substances, like complement, as well as specific antibodies. Drugs and anti-biotics, if present in the plasma, will also appear in the exudate. The importance of the early administration of therapeutic agents is obvious when it is remembered that they are merely carried to the inflamed area in the exudate, and are in no way concentrated there. The fluid of the exudate (*inflammatory oedema*) has the effect of diluting any irritant substance causing the inflammation. The fibrinogen in it is converted into fibrin by the action of tissue thromboplastin (p. 355) and a *fibrin clot* forms.

*This fibrin has three main functions*:

1. It forms a *union between severed tissues*, as in a cut.
2. It may form a *barrier against bacterial invasion* (p. 95).
3. It aids phagocytosis (p. 68).

The exudate accounts for the remaining cardinal signs of inflammation. It causes swelling (*tumor*), and the increased tissue tension is an important factor in the causation of pain (*dolor*), which is particularly severe in tissues that cannot swell readily, e.g. the pulp space of a finger, the pulp of a tooth (where pain is the only symptom), and the medullary cavity of a bone. Pain limits activity, and this explains the loss of function.

### The Cellular Exudate

The emigration of the white cells and their accumulation in the extra-vascular space has already been described (p. 61). These cells accumulate at the same time as the fluid exudate forms; they constitute the cellular component of the exudate (Fig. 5.4). At first the majority of the cells are poly-morphonuclear leucocytes, but there is also an admixture of monocytes. Within a few days the polymorphs undergo necrosis but the mononuclears remain. It therefore follows that *the cellular exudate changes from poly-morphonuclear initially to mononuclear at a later stage.*

*Mechanism of Formation of the Cellular Exudate.* The stimulus which impels the white cells to force their way through the vascular wall and move to the area of tissue damage is generally thought to be the attraction of some chemical substance. Such directional movement in response to a chemical gradient is well known in biology, and is called *chemotaxis*.[14] The *Boyden chamber*[15] has facilitated the study of the possible mediators. Polymorphs are placed in the upper of a double tissue-culture chamber; the chambers are separated by a membrane of 3 $\mu$m pore size. Test substances are placed in the lower chamber, and the number of cells migrating to the lower side of the filter is a measure of the chemotactic effect.

Both neutrophil polymorphs and monocytes have been shown to be attracted *in vitro* to a number of agents; these include starch and certain bacteria. Antigen-antibody complexes and dead tissue are chemotactic, but only if complement is activated. The activated trimolecular complex C$\overline{567}$ and the anaphylatoxins C3a and C5a are also chemotactic agents. The kinins and nucleic-acid derivatives have also been claimed as chemotactic agents.

Until recently it has been thought that all agents which attracted polymorphs also attracted monocytes, and that a differential chemotactic response was not therefore the explanation of the changing cell population seen in inflammation. It is now known that this is an oversimplification. The reaction of antigen with IgE has been claimed to release a chemotactic factor for eosinophils, cells which are prominent in certain allergic inflammations (p. 162) and parasitic infections.[16] Furthermore sensitized lymphocytes (p. 140) when acted upon by specific antigen release a number of factors called *lymphokines*.[17] These have a chemotactic effect on polymorphs, eosinophils, and monocytes, but it is not certain whether these factors are separate entities (see p. 140).

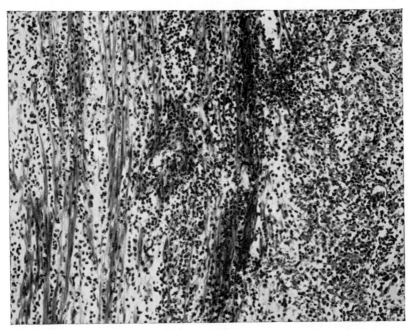

FIG. 5.4. Acute inflammation of the muscular coat of the appendix. There is a very heavy infiltration of polymorphs throughout the wall of the appendix, which has undergone disintegration. × 120.

Lymphocytes are found in certain inflammations, particularly virus infections and acute dermatitis; the mechanism of their accumulation is not known, for no definite chemotactic agents have been found that affect these cells. Nevertheless, lymphocytes can release lymphokines which have many actions relating to the inflammatory response.

**Changes in the Lymphatics.** The small lymphatics of a tissue form a blind-ended system of vessels, which closely resemble the vascular capillaries except that a basement membrane is incomplete or absent and their walls are permeable to proteins. One of their main functions is to allow any plasma protein which has escaped from the blood vessels to drain away and ultimately reach the blood stream again. In acute inflammation the lymph vessels are held widely open, the permeability of the wall is increased, and the flow of fluid, containing excess protein, is augmented.

### Function of the Cellular Exudate

### Phagocytosis

*Polymorphonuclear Leucocytes.* The major function of these cells is phagocytosis. They ingest foreign particles as well as bacteria. Phagocytosis is aided by two mechanisms:

1. *Opsonins.*[18] These are proteins present in the plasma which coat organisms and cause them to be more easily phagocytosed. It is believed that they cover up noxious surface antigens. Two types are recognized:

(a) *Non-specific opsonins,* which are present in all normal individuals.

(b) *Immune opsonins,* which are a type of antibacterial antibody, and are therefore specific for each organism. It follows that phagocytosis is more marked in the individual who has been immunized against the particular infecting organism.

2. *Surface Phagocytosis.*[19] Phagocytes can ingest organisms even in the absence of opsonins, if a suitable framework is provided in which they can trap the organism. Fibrin provides such a surface, and the process is called surface phagocytosis.

Polymorphs which have ingested particles show degranulation. The digestive lysosomal enzymes of the granules are poured into the phagocytic vesicles in which the organisms are contained. The polymorphs release *pyrogen,* and this is probably a factor in the pathogenesis of fever which often accompanies acute inflammation.[20] The manner whereby organisms are destroyed is considered in Chapter 7.

**Macrophages.**[21] These cells are highly phagocytic, and as with the polymorphs, their ingestion of virulent organisms is aided by opsonin. A pyrogen is also released. Macrophages play a part in the initiation of the immune response, probably by processing the antigen. In turn their activity as effector cells is modified and stimulated by lymphokines released by sensitized lymphocytes.

The functions of the eosinophil are not known. The lymphocyte is a key cell in the immune response; this is considered in later chapters.

### Local Sequelae of Acute Inflammation

The changes which follow the formation of an acute inflammatory exudate depend upon two major factors (Fig. 5.5):

(1) The amount of tissue damage sustained.

(2) Whether or not the causative agent remains.

Assuming that the causative agent is removed or destroyed, the initial polymorphonuclear exudate is replaced by a mononuclear one. Their appearance heralds the onset of the demolition phase. The mononuclear cells are phagocytic, and regardless of their origin are called *macrophages.*

*Origin of Macrophages.* The macrophages which accumulate in areas sub-

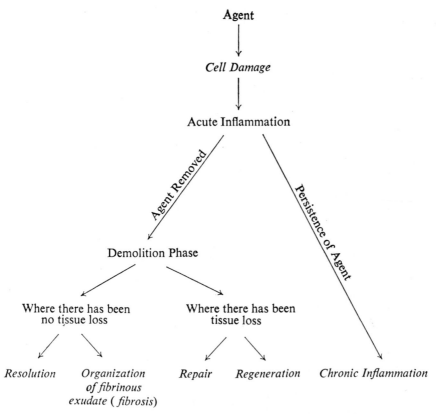

FIG. 5.5. The sequence of events following tissue damage.

jected to injury in lower forms of life appear to be derived from histiocytes, which are resting tissue representatives of the RE system. In mammals tissue histiocytes may also perform a similar function, but the current evidence suggests that the majority of macrophages present in the stage of demolition are the progeny of monocytes that emigrated from the blood stream.

Monocytes originate in the bone marrow where they have a generation time of about 24 hours. They circulate in the blood for one to three days and then randomly leave the circulation to become tissue macrophages.[21] In inflammation they accumulate selectively, presumably in response to chemotaxis. Labelling experiments indicate that monocytes can divide and assume the morphology of histiocytes and macrophages.[22] Reports that lymphocytes can change into macrophages may be misleading. The cellular events in small experimental wounds in human skin have been studied by placing glass cover-slips over the wound and examining the cells adhering to the glass.[23] All stages in the transformation of small lymphocytes to macrophages have been described, but it seems unlikely that the cells described as small lymphocytes are the same as those present in the blood and thoracic-duct lymph. Lymphocytes do not readily adhere to glass, and it may well be that the small cells observed in these experiments are derived from monocytes.

## Demolition Phase

Macrophages engulf fibrin, red cells, degenerate polymorphs, bacteria, etc., and thereby perform a scavenger function. They therefore contain a variety of intracellular structures—fat, haemosiderin, cholesterol, and foreign material. Sometimes they fuse together to form giant cells. If the macrophages ingest large quantities of fat they become swollen and are called *foam cells*.

## Resolution

In acutely inflamed tissue in which cellular damage has been relatively slight, the cellular and tissue changes are reversible, and necrosis does not occur. The demolition phase results in the removal of the exudate, and the organ returns to normal. To this process the term *resolution* is applied, and one of the best examples is found in lobar pneumonia (p. 404). *Resolution thus means the complete return to normal following acute inflammation.*

It should be noted that while demolition is proceeding there is a reversed flow of exudate back into the blood vessels. Most of the exudate, however, is carried away by the lymphatics.

Sometimes removal of the exudate appears to be delayed, and then the fibrin is invaded by granulation tissue. In this way fibrous adhesions, e.g. pleural and peritoneal, are produced.

## Suppuration

When the noxious agent produces much necrosis, resolution is impossible and the process frequently proceeds to *suppuration*. This is typical of pyogenic infection, e.g. boils, but can also occur when the agent is a chemical substance, e.g. turpentine.

The first reaction is circumscribed necrosis accompanied by a profuse polymorph infiltration. The agent kills many of these leucocytes—which are often called "pus cells". The necrotic material undergoes softening by virtue of the proteolytic enzymes released from the granules (lysosomes) of the dead leucocytes as well as through the autolysis mediated by the tissue's own lysosomal enzymes. The resulting creamy fluid material is called *pus*, and is contained within a cavity to form an *abscess*. This is lined by a *pyogenic membrane*, which at this stage consists of inflamed and necrotic tissue with much fibrinous exudate and polymorphs. This soon undergoes organization into granulation tissue.

The pus itself is made up of:

(a) *Leucocytes*, some of which are dead.
(b) *Other components of the inflammatory exudate*—oedema fluid and fibrin.
(c) *Organisms*, many of which are living and can therefore be cultured; if the pus is chemically induced it is sterile.
(d) *Tissue debris*, e.g. nucleic acids and lipids.

The pus tends to track in the line of least resistance until a free surface is reached. Then the abscess bursts and discharges its contents spontaneously—

in clinical practice this is usually anticipated by surgical drainage. An abscess when drained heals by granulation tissue, but sometimes chronic inflammation ensues.

If, as occasionally happens, the abscess is not drained but remains isolated, or sequestrated, in the tissues, its walls become further organized and converted into dense fibrous tissue and the pus undergoes thickening, or *inspissation*, as its fluid component is gradually absorbed. In due course it develops a porridge-like consistency, and may eventually become *calcified*.

When an acute suppurative inflammation involves an epithelial surface, the covering is destroyed, and an *ulcer** is formed. The floor is composed of necrotic tissue and acute inflammatory exudate; this layer of dead tissue forms the *slough*, and is at first adherent because the dead material has not been liquefied. Eventually, however, the slough becomes detached, and the ulcer heals by the processes of repair and regeneration, as described in Chapters 8 and 9.

### Chronic Inflammation

The other sequel of acute inflammation is progression to a state of chronic inflammation in which the inflammatory and healing processes proceed side by side. This is described in Chapter 10.

### Conclusion

Inflammation may be defined as *the reaction of the vascular and supporting elements of a tissue to injury, provided the injury has not been so severe as to destroy the area, and results in the formation of a protein-rich exudate.* Acute inflammation is thus essentially a vascular phenomenon, and cannot occur in an avascular tissue like the cornea or cartilage. The reaction is usually beneficial, but this is not necessarily so under all conditions. The inflammatory cells may themselves spread infection (see tuberculosis, p. 192) and the inflammatory oedema may, in a situation like the larynx, actually endanger life. The relationship between inflammation and infection is further considered in Chapter 7.

The term *subacute inflammation* is used by some authorities; it appears to mean a mild acute inflammation, but since no exact definition is possible, there seems no good reason for retaining the term.

### The Chemical Mediators of Acute Inflammation[3, 4, 24, 25]

The apparent uniformity of the inflammatory response irrespective of its cause has led many investigators to presume that the changes are mediated by chemical agents which are formed when tissue is damaged, rather than being caused directly by the damage itself. The search for these mediators has a practical as well as a theoretical objective. If they could be identified, antagonistic drugs might be designed and administered to prevent or modify the acute inflammatory response.

* An *ulcer* is a localized defect of a covering or lining epithelium. Occasionally the term is applied to a similar defect of mesothelium or endothelium e.g. atheromatous ulcer (p. 374). Dead tissue still adherent to the floor of an ulcer is called a *slough*.

## Histamine

Thomas Lewis under the influence of Henry Dale suggested that *histamine* was an important mediator of the vascular component of acute inflammation. The basis of this view was the demonstration that both trauma and histamine produced an identical *triple response* when applied to human skin.[26]

**The Triple Response.** *The Red Line.* Shortly after stroking the skin firmly, or after the injection of histamine, a red line develops. It is sharply demarcated, and can be shown to be due to capillary dilatation.

*The Flare.* After a further period of 15–30 seconds a flare appears in the area surrounding the red line. This is due to arteriolar dilatation.

*The Weal.* A weal, or swelling, develops on the site of the red line, and is due to an exudation of fluid through the altered vascular wall.

There is now considerable evidence that the liberation of histamine is responsible for the increase in vascular permeability and vasodilatation which occur during the early phase of acute inflammation, and also in allergic states of immediate type (e.g. hay-fever, see p. 161). Antihistamine drugs have proved to be of some value in inhibiting this aspect of acute inflammation. 5-Hydroxytryptamine (5-HT) is a chemical mediator in the rat, but is unimportant in man. The more important and prolonged *second phase* of increased vascular permeability appears to be mediated by other substances.

## Polypeptides: The Kinins[27]

The name kinin is applied to a group of vasoactive polypeptides which can be formed in plasma by the action of proteolytic enzymes. The most important of these in the blood is *kallikrein* which exists as a precursor (see Fig. 5.7). Another enzyme, *plasmin*, can also form kinin from kininogen, but the action is slow. Plasmin can act in another way by activating prekallikrein. The kinin formed in blood is *bradykinin*, a nonapeptide, so called because it causes a slow contraction of guinea-pig small intestinal muscle *in vitro*. Other kinin-forming enzymes are known. One is present in the pancreas, and its release in pancreatic necrosis contributes to the shock seen in this condition. Similar enzymes are present in salivary gland, saliva, and snake venom. They probably play a part in the regulation of the blood flow through the salivary glands.

The kinins cause an increase in vascular permeability and swelling of the endothelial cells; they are chemotactic to white cells and cause pain.[28] Their effect on vascular permeability is the most striking, and it is believed that they are important mediators of the early exudative phase of acute inflammation.

## The Kinin-forming enzymes

Normal plasma can generate a kinin-forming enzyme (*kallikrein*) from a precursor called *prekallikrein*. The exact manner by which this occurs is controversial, but it is probable that there is a *prekallikrein activator*. This appears to be a derivative of the Hageman factor (Factor XII), which is formed by surface activation and also by the action of plasmin (Fig. 5.7). It has been proposed that normal plasma contains a pro-permeability factor

(Pro-Pf/dil) which can be activated *in vitro* by diluting plasma with saline in a glass tube, presumably by the activation of Factor XII to Factor XIIa. The active permeability factor was called the *globulin permeability factor*, or *Pf/dil*, and thought to act directly on the blood vessels. This seems unlikely, and it has been proposed that Pf/dil in fact activates kallikreinogen as shown in Fig. 5.6. Nevertheless, Pf/dil has never been isolated in a chemically pure form and it may well be that it represents a mixture of kinin-forming agents including plasmin, Factor XII, etc. Fig. 5.7 depicts the present situation insofar as it is understood. It will be seen that activation of Factor XII plays a vital role in initiating blood clotting, plasmin formation, and kinin

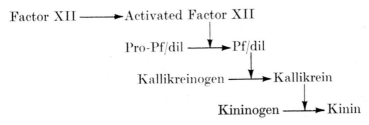

Fig. 5.6.  Possible role of Pf/dil in the formation of kinin.

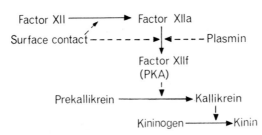

Fig. 5.7.  Series of proposed reactions involved in the *in-vivo* generation of kinin. Activation of Factor XII is presented as a key action.

PKA = Prekallikrein activator.

generation. Nevertheless, patients with Factor XII deficiency show remarkably little disturbance in these various functions. Other pathways must therefore be important.

A number of inhibitors of kallikrein are known; one is an $\alpha_2$-macroglobulin, another is $\alpha_1$-trypsin inhibitor, while a third is Cl-esterase inhibitor (p. 153). It is of interest that patients who are deficient in Cl-esterase inhibitor are prone to develop attacks of angio-oedema, and this may affect the larynx and lead to death (p. 325). The complement system may be more intimately involved, for activated components (C2a and C4a) have kinin-like properties.

In summary, it is believed that kinin formation occurs following injury, and that this is an important aspect of the pathogenesis of the early phase of acute inflammation. Tissues become refractory to the prolonged action of kinins as they do also to histamine. Neither is therefore the mediator of the prolonged second phase of increased vascular permeability.

### Biologically Active Cleavage Products of Complement

Activation of the complement system leads to the formation of anaphyla-toxin, which causes the release of histamine from mast cells. C5a is the classical anaphylatoxin, but C3a has a similar action. Chemotactic components, e.g. C567, are released and have been identified in experimental myocardial infarcts in rats. The alternate pathway for the activation of complement explains how complement could act in the non-immune animal as well as in one with specific antibodies. The actual role of these factors is unknown.[29]

### Biologically Active Components of Polymorphs

Although inflammation can occur in the absence of polymorphs, these cells can release vasoactive compounds which may play a part in the inflammatory reaction. Amongst these are certain cationic (basic) proteins, SRS-A, and lysosomal enzymes. The lysosomal enzymes are liberated when the cells die, but a more selective release occurs when polymorphs phagocytose antigen-antibody complexes.[30,31] The enzymes can activate kallikrein, and therefore act as mediators. In addition, they can lead to local tissue destruction. This is an important mechanism in the pathogenesis of the Shwartzman phenomenon and in immune-complex reactions.

**Prostaglandins.**[32] The prostaglandins are a group of long-chain fatty acids which were first identified in human semen. They are highly active pharmacological agents which cause vasodilatation and smooth-muscle contraction. It has been suggested that they act as mediators in various situations: in the brain, in the uterus during parturition, in the gut, and in the skin during inflammation. When injected into the skin they cause a well-marked vasodilatation which lasts for hours, and together with polymorph lysosomal enzymes they are the present contenders for the role of mediators of the prolonged phase of acute inflammation. Prostaglandins can be synthetized in human platelets, and this action is inhibited by aspirin. Here then may be a clue to the action of this well-used but poorly understood anti-inflammatory agent.

### Other Agents

Many other agents—lactic acid, proteins, nucleic-acid derivatives, etc.—have been isolated from inflamed tissue, and may play some part in the pathogenesis of inflammation. The relative importance of all these substances is not known. Although many drugs are used which will influence the acute inflammatory response (e.g. corticosteroids, aspirin, etc.), their precise mode of action is not clearly understood. The pathogenesis of acute inflammation is thus very complex.

Although much stress has been placed upon the uniformity of the inflammatory reaction regardless of its cause, it must not be forgotten that there is, in fact, also very considerable individual diversity, both in the amount of exudate and in the type of cell involved. This was stressed by Kettle who recognized that the individuality of an inflammatory reaction was a reflection of the individuality of the causal agent.[33] It would be hard to deny the importance of many bacterial products—the leucocidins, haemolysins, kinases, permeability factors, etc. must all influence the final outcome and modify the actions of the mediators produced by tissue damage. Recent observations of the details of the vascular response to injury have revealed that it is a multiphased response with both early and delayed components affecting capillaries and venules. The precise changes vary according to the type of injury and the species of animal involved. The uniformity of the inflammatory response is more apparent than real, and it is therefore not surprising that no single common chemical mediator is involved. So far much research has been directed to the vasodilatation and increased vascular permeability of acute inflammation caused by trauma and chemical agents. The complex cellular changes and the intricacies of infection have been largely neglected.

# References

1. RATHER, L. J. (1971). *Bull. N.Y. Acad. Med.*, **47**, 303.
2. COHNHEIM, J. (1889). In "Lectures on General Pathology", p. 248. London: New Sydenham Society. (This is a translation of the 2nd edition of Cohnheim's book published in 1882.)
3. ZWEIFACH, B. W., GRANT, L. and McCLUSKEY, R. T. (1965). Edrs. "The Inflammatory Response", 931 pp. New York: Academic Press.
4. MILES, A. A. (1966). In "Wound Healing", Edr. Illingworth, C., p. 3. London: Churchill.
5. WELLS, F. R. and MILES, A. A. (1963). *Nature (Lond.)*, **200**, 1015.
6. HURLEY, J. V. and SPECTOR, W. G. (1965). *J. Path. Bact.*, **89**, 245.
7. DAVSON, H. (1970). "A Textbook of General Physiology", 4th ed., p. 526. London: Churchill.
8. PAPPENHEIMER, J. R. (1953). *Physiol. Rev.*, **33**, 387.
9. MAJNO, G. and PALADE, G. E. (1961). *J. biophys. biochem, Cytol.*, **11**, 571.
10. MAJNO, G., PALADE, G. E. and SCHOEFL, G. I. (1961). *J. biophys. biochem. Cytol.*, **11**, 607.
11. MARCHESI, V. T. (1962). *Proc. roy. Soc. B.*, **156**, 550.
12. PAPPAS, G. D. and TENNYSON, V. M. (1962). *J. cell. Biol.*, **15**, 227.
13. MOVAT, H. Z. and FERNANDO, N. V. P. (1963). *Lab. Invest.*, **12**, 895.
14. HARRIS, H. (1960). *Bact. Rev.*, **24**, 3.
15. BOYDEN, S. (1962). *J. exp. Med.*, **115**, 453.
16. WARD, P. A., REMOLD, H. G. and DAVID, J. R. (1969). *Science*, **163**, 1079.
17. DAVID, J. R. (1973). *New Engl. J. Med.*, **288**, 143.
18. HOWARD, J. G. (1963). In "Modern Trends in Immunology", Vol. 1, p. 86. Edr. Cruickshank, R. London: Butterworth.
19. WOOD, W. B. (1960). *Bact. Rev.*, **24**, 41.
20. BERLIN, R. D. and WOOD, B. W. (1964). *J. exp. Med.*, **119**, 715.
21. Editorial (1973). *New Engl. J. Med.*, **288**, 212.
22. SPECTOR, W. G. (1966). In "Wound Healing", p. 17. *loc. cit*
23. REBUCK, J. W. and CROWLEY, J. H. (1955). *Ann. N.Y. Acad. Sci.*, **59**, 757.
24. MOVAT, H. Z. (1971). "Inflammation, Immunity and Hypersensitivity", New York: Harper and Row.
25. MOVAT, H. Z. (1972). *Medical Clinics of North America*, **56**, 541.

26. LEWIS, T. (1927). "The Blood Vessels of the Human Skin and Their Responses.'
    London: Shaw & Sons Ltd.
27. KELLERMEYER, R. W. and GRAHAM, R. C. (1968). *New Engl. J. Med.*, **279**,
    754, 802 and 859.
28. KEELE, C. A. and ARMSTRONG, D. (1964). "Substances Producing Pain and
    Itch", p. 268. London: Arnold.
29. WARD, P. A. (1971). *J. exp. Med.*, **134**, 109s.
30. HENSON, P. M. (1971). *J. exp. Med.*, **134**, 114s.
31. WEISSMANN, G. *et al.* (1971). *J. exp. Med.*, **134**, 149s.
32. Leading Article (1971). *Brit. med. J.*, **3**, 61.
33. ROBB-SMITH, A. H. T. (1957). *Lancet*, **1**, 699.

*Chapter 6*

# THE BODY'S DEFENCES AGAINST INFECTION

## Introduction

Micro-organisms can cause disease in two ways. Either they gain access to the tissues of the host, multiply, and cause *infection*, or they manufacture powerful toxins which are subsequently introduced into the body and produce an *intoxication*.

Staphylococcal enterotoxic food-poisoning provides an important and typical example of an intoxication. If staphylococci from a suitable strain are allowed to grow for a few hours in a sample of food, e.g. a meat pie, the unfortunate person who eats it develops an acute attack of diarrhoea and vomiting. This occurs even if the pie is cooked, because although the heat kills the staphylococci, it does not affect the stable toxin. It is obvious that anyone with staphylococcal skin lesions should be excluded as a food handler.

By far the most important method whereby micro-organisms cause disease is by their *invasion of and multiplication in the living tissues of the host*. This is the definition of *infection*, and organisms capable of producing it are termed *pathogens*.

## Transmission of Organisms to the Body

With the exception of certain rare congenital infections, all infection is derived from the external environment. The organisms may be injected directly into the host, but more usually they are first *transmitted* to the surface of the body which thereby becomes contaminated. *Contamination* is defined as the transfer of organisms on to any object. It may be a surgical instrument, clothing, food, or a body surface.

Usually, when a body surface is involved, the organisms are destroyed, but occasionally they penetrate into the living tissues and cause infection.

The following modes of transmission are important:

### Transplacental Spread

During the early stages of pregnancy the fetus is particularly susceptible to the damaging effect of infection transmitted by the mother. Rubella (German measles) may give rise to fetal infection and deformities. The protozoan disease toxoplasmosis may result in hydrocephalus, mental defect, and blindness when transmitted across the placenta.

### Ingestion of Contaminated Food

Food may be contaminated directly by a human carrier or indirectly by flies. These insects carry many pathogenic organisms on their hairy legs.

Diseases transmitted by food include typhoid fever, bacillary dysentery, and amoebiasis. Poliomyelitis is acquired by ingestion. Milk and eggs may contain bacteria because the animal itself is diseased, e.g. bovine tuberculosis and brucellosis, and *Salmonella* infections of fowls.

### Inoculation

The agent may be an insect whose bite transmits pathogenic organisms, e.g. arboviruses, *Y. (Past.) pestis*, and rickettsiae. The iatrogenic disease* serum hepatitis is caused by the introduction of the virus by means of a contaminated needle or instrument (p. 427).

### Direct Skin Contact

Wound infection may result from contact with a staphylococcal carrier or by contamination with soil containing clostridia. The venereal diseases, e.g. syphilis and gonorrhoea, are also transmitted by direct contact.

### Spread by Droplets and Dust[1]

Droplets are produced when air, passing rapidly over a mucous membrane, causes atomization of the secretion which covers it. A few of these droplets are large, and due to the effect of gravity have a limited range. The vast majority are smaller than 100 $\mu$m in diameter, and dry up almost instantaneously to form *droplet nuclei* which stay suspended in the air for many hours.

Droplet formation occurs during talking, coughing, and particularly sneezing; the main source is from the *saliva in the front of the mouth*. Only during snorting is the nose an important source of droplets. It is possible for aerosols from high-speed dental handpieces to spread infection from the patient to the dentist; precautionary measures, such as wearing a mask and spectacles, or goggles, are recommended. The viruses of mumps, measles, smallpox, and chickenpox are found in the saliva, and these diseases may well be spread in this way.

However, bacteria residing in the nose (*Staph.pyogenes*), nasopharynx (*Strept.pyogenes*), or lung (tubercle bacilli) do not commonly reach the front of the mouth, and it is very unlikely that droplets are an important vehicle of their spread. Some may be spat out as sputum, but the most important means of dissemination is by the fingers and handkerchief. Using fluorescein or test organisms as markers, it has been found that normal human beings frequently dispense nasal secretions and saliva to their hands, face, and clothing, and to every object that is touched. After desiccation the organisms are readily disseminated in the form of dust particles, and it is these which are important in the transmission of many infections.

### Hospital Infection[2]

Whenever people are living together in confined quarters, there is always the danger that in the group there will be carriers of pathogenic organisms. Although not suffering from clinical illness themselves, they may pass on

---

* Iatrogenic from the Greek *iatros*, meaning physician, and *genein* to produce. The term is applied to a disease produced by the physician as a consequence of his treatment. Drug reactions are the commonest example.

the organisms to others who, having no resistance, develop the disease. In their turn they further transmit the disease. This is called *cross-infection*. In the past there have been many examples of epidemics of meningococcal meningitis and dysentery occurring in nurses' homes, army camps, etc. In hospitals it is not uncommon for patients to acquire severe infections from their environment; this is not surprising, because many of the patients are debilitated and their resistance to infection is lowered. Furthermore surgical incisions provide a ready avenue for the invading bacteria.

A particular feature in hospitals is that the staff acquire pathogenic organisms from their patients, become carriers, and further disseminate the bacteria. Often the strain of organism is one that is resistant to the antibiotics which are in common use in that particular hospital.[3] The infection is therefore all the more serious.

In the past *streptococcal infections* have been troublesome, particularly in labour wards. Identification of the strain of organism involved, using the Griffith method of typing (p. 179), and a subsequent search for the source of infection has usually incriminated the throats of a few members of staff. The exclusion of such carriers and general measures designed to improve aseptic techniques have usually brought such an epidemic to a halt. Penicillin therapy is very effective in streptococcal infections, since resistant organisms do not occur. It follows that outbreaks of streptococcal hospital infection are not a problem at the present time.

The staphylococcus has, on the other hand, attained a much more prominent position. Outbreaks of postoperative wound infection are not uncommon, and the methods of control which proved effective with streptococcal outbreaks are quite inadequate. Often the majority of the staff are found to be carriers, and in addition the hospital itself—the floors, air-conditioning plant, bedclothes, etc.—is also contaminated with a virulent strain of staphylococcus. Although human carriers provide the reservoir, the hardy staphylococcus often infects patients by indirect means, for instance in airborne dust particles. The problem of control is not easy; indeed there is no simple answer to an outbreak of staphylococcal wound infection.

Other organisms which sometimes cause hospital infection are the coliform group, *Proteus* species, and *Ps. pyocyanea*. As with the staphylococcus, the transfer of these organisms is usually indirect, *via* dust, contaminated articles, and fomites*. The source of organisms is often a patient with urinary tract infection who contaminates his immediate environment—bedclothing, urine bottle, etc.

### Defences of Individual Body Surfaces

It is evident that there may be contamination of the body, both externally on the skin and internally in the intestinal, respiratory, and other tracts. Many of these surfaces are habitually colonized by organisms of low-grade pathogenicity, e.g. *Staph. albus* in the skin and *Strept. viridans* in the mouth and throat. Such organisms are called *commensals*, or "resident flora", and as will be shown later, play an important role in the decontamination of

* Fomites are articles, such as bedding or clothing, capable of acting as a medium for the transmission of organisms which may give rise to infection.

these surfaces against pathogenic organisms. Contamination with virulent organisms is a common event, but infection is rare. Whether contamination is followed by infection is dependent upon:

1. *The mechanical integrity of the body surface.*
2. *Its powers of decontamination,* i.e. its ability to remove organisms.

These protective mechanisms vary greatly from one tissue to another, and each will therefore be considered separately.

## The Skin

The skin is frequently contaminated, and its exposed position renders it liable to both major and minor physical trauma. Its protective function is carried out mainly by the epithelial cells, and indeed the inability of the subepithelial tissues to resist infection was one of the limiting factors in pre-Listerian surgery. Its defences are:

### Mechanical Strength

The many layers of epithelial cells, the tough outer layer of keratin, and the distinct basement membrane all play a part in the formation of a mechanical barrier, which if impaired, may result in infection. For example, excessive sweating softens the keratin layer, and for this reason skin infections are very common in the tropics, and boils are frequently seen in moist areas like the axillae and groins.

The skin when intact appears to be completely impervious to invasion by organisms, but following trauma it becomes the portal of entry for staphylococci, streptococci, and the clostridia. In the tropics insect bites penetrate the skin barrier, and serve to introduce the causative agents of plague, typhus, yellow fever, malaria, dengue, etc.

### Decontamination[4]

The powers of decontamination of the skin may be demonstrated by deliberately contaminating the hands with haemolytic streptococci, and estimating their rate of disappearance by subsequently taking swabs at regular intervals. It is found that the organisms can no longer be recovered after 2–3 hours. The actual time taken for the skin to rid itself of organisms depends upon the organisms concerned, and in some cases is as short as 10 minutes. The mechanisms involved may be considered under three headings—mechanical, biological, and chemical:

**Mechanical.** The *desquamation* of surface squames removes some of the superficial organisms.

*Desiccation* is probably of some importance in destroying organisms on the surface of the skin.

**Biological.** It is probable that the resident flora plays an important part in the decontaminating mechanism both by producing antibiotic substances* and by competing with other organisms for essential foodstuffs. The *resident flora* includes *Staph. albus,* diphtheroids, sarcinae, and aerobic sporing

* An antibiotic is a substance produced by one organism which is inimical to the growth of another. Thus *penicillin* is produced by the mould *Penicillium notatum.*

bacilli. In addition about 25 per cent of people harbour *Staph. pyogenes* particularly on the hands, face, and perineum. It is impossible to remove all the resident organisms from the skin; they survive in the gland ducts, and though the surface may be disinfected, the organisms are soon replaced. It is for this reason that sterile rubber gloves must always be worn while performing any surgical operation.

**Chemical.** *Acidity of Sweat.* The sweat is normally acid and is unsuitable for the growth of most pathogens. The bactericidal activity is probably due to its lactic acid content. There are certain gaps in this acid coat; these are the alkaline areas where infection is quite common, e.g. axillae, groins, and interdigital clefts of the toes.

*Unsaturated fatty acids.* These are present in the sebaceous secretion and are bactericidal; it is interesting that some of the diphtheroids grow only in the presence of these fatty acids, so well are they adapted to their environment.

There is no doubt that the mechanical strength together with the decontaminating mechanisms are of great importance in maintaining the integrity of the skin. When one remembers how often it must be contaminated with all types of organisms, and, apart from staphylococci how rarely it is invaded, one appreciates its efficiency as a protective coat.

### The Alimentary Tract

#### The Mouth and Throat

As in the case of the skin the defence mechanism may be considered under two headings:

**Mechanical strength.** The toughness and integrity of the mucous membrane is important; this mechanical barrier is weakest at two points:

The *gingival margin* has only a thin epithelium, and is therefore easily traumatized. This is particularly so in the interdental region, where it is believed that a covering epithelium is present only in young healthy adults.[5]

The *tonsillar crypts.* Here the epithelium is very thin; it has been shown that carmine powder dusted on to the tonsils appears in the underlying cells and connective tissue within 20 minutes. Probably the dye is transported there by phagocytes which are normally resident on the surface. Organisms may similarly reach the subepithelial tissue. It is therefore no wonder that these two sites, the tonsils and the gingivae, are the places where infection occurs when the general body defences are impaired, e.g. in acute leukaemia and agranulocytosis. Nevertheless, it is remarkable how the tissues of the mouth, including the bone, can resist infection even with the contamination that follows injuries or dental extraction. On the other hand, skin wounds caused by bites often become infected, and they heal very badly. Some form of "tissue immunity" in the oral cavity must be postulated, but its nature is quite unknown.

#### Decontamination

A regular flow of saliva is of importance for its mechanical action in keeping the mouth clean.

**Mechanical.** The continual backward flow of saliva traps organisms, which are then swallowed. Carbon particles placed on the mucosa are removed from the mouth in 15–30 minutes.[4]

**Biological.** As in the skin the resident flora is important. These organisms are α-haemolytic streptococci (*Strept. viridans*), *Neisseria pharyngis*, diphtheroids, pneumococci, *Borrelia vincenti*, actinomyces organisms, yeasts, and various *Bacteroidaceae*. Many strains of α-haemolytic streptococci produce hydrogen peroxide, and this has been thought to play some part in the decontaminating mechanism*.[4]

**Chemical.** The saliva inhibits many pathogens: this may be due to its lysozyme or possibly its mucus content. As with other secretions, saliva contains antibodies of the IgA class; these are produced locally and passed into the secretions as a dimer linked to a distinct secretory polypeptide.[6] Saliva is therefore of importance, as will be appreciated when secretion is suppressed as in states of shock, dehydration, and fever, or as a result of infective processes, neoplasia, and irradiation.

Under these circumstances the lips, tongue, teeth, and remainder of the mouth become coated with a mixture of food particles and dead epithelial cells, which if not actively removed, become the site of bacterial infection. This may result in an ascending infection of the salivary glands terminating in suppurative sialadenitis.

In spite of the defence mechanisms of the mouth potent pathogens can adapt themselves to the mouth and throat, e.g. meningococci, diphtheria bacilli, *H. influenzae*, and *Strept. pyogenes*. These may lead to infection, but if the person has considerable immunity, they may remain as "transients" for a period of time. Such carriers are of great importance in the spread of streptococcal infections, diphtheria, and meningococcal meningitis.

### The Stomach

The stomach stands guard over the intestines and it deals not only with food, but also with the secretions of the mouth and swallowed sputum. Its defence mechanisms are:

### Mechanical Strength

The continuity of the epithelium is probably not important. Acute ulcers are common, and neither these nor the more serious chronic ulcers appear to provide points of entry for organisms.

### Decontamination

**Mechanical.** Vomiting removes chemical and bacterial irritants, but is of little value in combating infection.

**Biological.** Under normal conditions the gastric juice is sterile.

**Chemical.** Without doubt the bactericidal activity of gastric juice is due to its hydrochloric acid content, and not to its enzymes.[7] Gastric juice loses its bactericidal activity when neutralized.

* In this connexion the rare Japanese hereditary disorder of *acatalasia* is of interest. The enzyme catalase which normally breaks down $H_2O_2$ is absent from the blood, and peroxide formed in the mouth produces sufficient damage to cause ulcerating gangrenous lesions in the mouth.

Coliform organisms and tubercle bacilli can withstand the acidity of the stomach, and are able to reach, and occasionally infect, the lower intestinal tract.

Staphylococci and *Salmonella* organisms will probably pass through the stomach if ingested with food or large quantities of fluid; likewise entero-viruses can withstand moderate acidity. Milk with its potent antacid properties is a particularly favourable vehicle for organisms, e.g. *Brucella abortus*, though in fact any food is liable to have a protective action.

*Strept. pyogenes* and pneumococci are very easily killed by acid, and these organisms almost never reach the intestine nor cause infection there.

### The Intestine

The intestine undoubtedly relies upon the stomach's protective action. The minor intestinal upsets of infancy may be in part related to the low gastric acidity in this age-group. The intestine has, however, its own defence mechanism.

### Mechanical Barrier

As in the stomach this is probably not important. It is interesting that some organisms, e.g. *S. typhi* and the tubercle bacillus, can penetrate the mucosa without causing obvious damage. Probably phagocytes are normally present on the surface of the gut ready to ingest passing organisms. These are carried into the tissues, so that infection follows.

### Decontamination

**Mechanical.** Irritation of the intestine, whether it affects the small intestine (e.g. typhoid fever) or large gut (e.g. bacillary dysentery) usually causes diarrhoea. This mechanism expels organisms during an established infection, but it seems doubtful whether it plays any part in the prevention of infection.

**Biological.** The small intestine generally contains few organisms, while the colon is heavily contaminated with coliforms, *Bacteroides* organisms, faecal streptococci, and clostridia. Although the importance of the flora is well known, the exact mechanisms involved are not established. However, when the flora is altered by the broad-spectrum antibiotics, infection with *Staph. pyogenes* may be a fatal complication (p. 178).

**Chemical.** It has been shown that intestinal as well as other secretions, e.g. milk, contain specific IgA antibodies. They are secreted locally by plasma cells, and are important in providing the mucous membranes with local immunity (p. 137). It should also be noted that the lymphoid tissue of the intestine is thought to act as the central organ responsible for the development of the peripheral lymphoid tissues destined to produce all classes of immunoglobulins (p. 143).

The appendix is one of the weakest links in the alimentary tract, but the reason for this is not known. Possibly damage by hard concretions and the ease with which its lumen can be obstructed play a part, but it is humiliating to admit how little we know about the cause of such a common disease as acute appendicitis.

## The Conjunctival Sac of the Eye

Large particles are prevented from contaminating the eye by the action of blinking. This also is important as it ensures that the conjunctiva and cornea are always covered by a thin protective layer of lacrimal secretion.

In the absence of the *blink reflex* the cornea desiccates, and repeated trauma leads to its ulceration and infection. Impairment of this reflex occurs under two circumstances:

1. Motor loss—in facial nerve paralysis, e.g. Bell's palsy.
2. Sensory loss—with trigeminal nerve lesions, e.g. following zoster.

In order to prevent corneal ulceration and ocular infection, the eye should either be covered with a pad or else the lids should be sutured together.

The lacrimal secretions have other important functions, for if the cornea is irritated the volume of secretion is increased. The tears so produced mechanically wash away the irritant. The other important protective function of tears is due to their content of *lysozyme* (*muramidase*);[8,9] they contain the highest concentration of lysozyme of any body fluid. First described by Fleming, this bactericidal enzyme, a polysaccharidase, is capable of lysing some organisms and inhibiting the growth of others. It acts on the muramic acid of bacterial cell walls, but with many organisms the outer coat must first be damaged by other means, e.g. complement activation or the action of peroxide, before the organism is killed.

## The Respiratory Tract

The respiratory tract acts as a whole, the upper part functioning as an air-conditioner for the lungs. The vibrissae filter off large particles, but the main filter is the nasal mucosa itself, covering as it does the complicated ramification of the turbinates. Not only is the inspired air warmed and humidified, but the mucus-covered surface traps organisms and particles just as flies are trapped on fly-paper. The anterior nares are distinct from the remainder of the respiratory tract, because their epithelium and bacterial flora resemble that of the skin. Their great importance lies in their frequent colonization by *Staph. pyogenes*.

## The Nose and Nasopharynx

### Mechanical Barrier

The epithelium of the respiratory tract does not provide an adequate barrier against local infection. This is well demonstrated by the ease with which rhinoviruses and adenoviruses cause acute upper respiratory tract infection. Meningococci are apparently able to penetrate the mucosa of the nasopharynx without much difficulty.

### Decontamination

Irritants are expelled by the act of sneezing. If organisms are deliberately implanted in the nose, they disappear within 15 minutes. One of the main mechanisms involved is the continuous flow of mucus backwards to the nasopharynx. The nasal secretion is both bactericidal and virucidal: some antibodies have been demonstrated in it against influenza and poliomyelitis viruses. Lysozyme is also present. Nevertheless, pathogens like meningococci and diphtheria bacilli can colonize the nose, and carriers of these constitute an important reservoir of human infection. The fact that the olfactory mucosa is non-ciliated and has beneath it much lymphoid tissue has been held to explain why some organisms gain entry through this area. Experimentally dye, proteins, and viruses can be shown to penetrate the olfactory mucosa and enter the underlying lymphoid tissue.

The nasopharynx has a resident bacterial flora similar to that of the throat (especially *Strept. viridans* and *Neisseria pharyngis*), and this has a biological decontaminating function.

### The Trachea and Lower Respiratory Tract

#### Mechanical Barrier

Below the larynx the respiratory tract should normally be sterile. The mucosa itself forms a poor mechanical barrier as in the nose, and is frequently infected by the influenza virus.

#### Decontamination

The cough reflex initiated by stimulating the larynx or upper trachea expels irritants, but may also disseminate organisms within the lung. Although the diameter of the air passages decreases steadily with each division from the trachea downwards, the total cross-sectional area of all the respiratory bronchioles is over a hundred times that of the trachea.[10] It follows that the velocity of the inspired air steadily decreases as it passes down the air passages, and this allows particles to fall out of the stream and adhere to the mucus-covered walls. The film of fluid which covers the mucosa is derived partly by transudation and partly from the secretions of surface goblet cells and the underlying mucous glands. By its chemical composition it protects the epithelial cells from dangerous gases, e.g. $SO_2$, and its proper consistency allows the cilia to move it on as a continuous sheet.[11] The sheet of mucus ever moving upwards by ciliary activity is an important decontaminating mechanism, and any obstruction to it impairs the defences of the respiratory tract. This frequently leads to infection, and is well seen in the broncho-pneumonia which follows the obstruction caused by carcinoma or a foreign body, e.g. an inhaled tooth or root.

In the respiratory bronchioles and alveoli, mucociliary streams play little part in the defence of the lung, and it is here that the macrophages, or *septal cells*, are important.[12] Bacteria are phagocytosed by these RE cells and killed in their cytoplasm.

### Summary

An important aspect of the defence mechanism against infection is the manner whereby the various body surfaces are able to rid themselves of contaminating bacteria. But apart from this it appears that each surface has an intrinsic ability to resist infection which cannot easily be explained. Thus the skin is frequently colonized by *Staph. pyogenes*, and yet infection is relatively uncommon. These organisms when introduced into the subcutaneous tissues readily cause infection. The skin itself is able to resist infection, and therefore exhibits some type of local tissue immunity. The nature of this is unknown. Nowhere is this type of immunity more important than in the mouth. Subepithelial tissues, muscle, and bone may be exposed and contaminated, and yet no infection ensues. Were it not for this defence mechanism dental extraction and oral surgery would be impossible.

## References

1. HARE, R. (1964). *Proc. roy. Soc. Med.*, **57**, 221.
2. WILLIAMS, R. E. O., BLOWERS, R., GARROD, L. P. and SHOOTER, R. A. (1966). "Hospital Infection." 2nd ed., London: Lloyd-Luke.
3. BARBER, M. (1966). In "Wound Healing", ed. Illingworth, C., p. 89. London: Churchill.
4. WILSON, G. S. and MILES, A. A. (1964). In Topley & Wilson's "Principles of Bacteriology & Immunology", 5th ed., p. 1251. London: Arnold.
5. COHEN, B. (1959). *Brit. dent. J.*, **107**, 31 and *Dent. Pract.*, **9**, 167.
6. TOMASI, T. B. and DECOTEAU, E. (1970). *Adv. Int. Med.*, **16**, 401.
7. KNOTT, F. A. (1923). *Guy's Hosp. Rep.*, **73**, 429.
8. CHIPMAN, D. M. and SHARON, M. (1969). *Science*, **165**, 454.
9. GLYNN, A. A. (1968). *Sci. Basis Med. Ann. Rev.*, 31.
10. STAUB, N. C. (1963). *Anesthesiology*, **24**, 831.
11. Interdepartmental Colloquium (1964). *Ann. roy. Coll. Surg. Engl.*, **34**, 400.
12. KASS, E. H., GREEN, G. M. and GOLDSTEIN, E. (1966). *Bact. Rev.*, **30**, 488.

*Chapter 7*

# THE BODY'S RESPONSE TO INFECTION

## Patterns of Infectious Disease

When organisms gain access to the tissues of the body, their fate depends on the resultant of two factors: the *immunity* of the host and the *virulence* of the organism. Immunity and virulence are in effect two descriptive approaches to the encounter between an organism and its host. The possible end-results of such an encounter are:

(1) Rapid destruction of the organisms, e.g. non-pathogens.
(2) The organisms grow for a time, but are soon destroyed, e.g. minor or subclinical infection.
(3) The organisms enter into a symbiotic state with their host, e.g. herpes-simplex virus and adenovirus.
(4) There is a local proliferation of organisms to produce tissue damage, but there is little spread of the infection, e.g. a boil due to *Staph. pyogenes*.
(5) Organisms may proliferate locally and produce severe damage to distant tissues by means of a soluble exotoxin. The local lesion may be insignificant, as in tetanus, or severe as in diphtheria.
(6) A local lesion is produced, but rapid spread of organisms follows, so that a diffuse, ill-defined inflammation results. This is called *cellulitis*, and is most commonly caused by *Strept.pyogenes*.
(7) No local lesion forms but the organism spreads rapidly, e.g. European typhus due to *Rickettsia prowazeki*.
(8) No local lesion forms initially, but the organisms spread rapidly and later a lesion develops at the portal of entry, e.g. syphilis, typhoid fever, and typhus due to *R. rickettsi*.
(9) The organisms induce cellular proliferation, e.g. Rous's sarcoma. Proliferation may occur and be followed later by necrosis, e.g. smallpox.

This list is by no means complete. Thus, the slow viruses produce a type of infection which appears to be unique, but is not well understood (p. 227). Cholera is peculiar in that the organisms multiply in the gut, produce a toxin which damages the epithelium, but yet never penetrate beyond the basement membrane. It is obvious in this example how difficult it is to separate true infection from intoxication. Some of these possibilities must now be examined in more detail.

## Pathogenicity of Organisms—Virulence

An organism is described as *non-pathogenic* if it is unable to multiply in the tissues and produce disease. Such an organism is usually phagocytosed by the polymorphonuclear leucocytes and macrophages, and destroyed in the cytoplasm of these cells.

**Pathogens.** Some organisms, on the other hand, are capable of causing disease (i.e. are *pathogenic*) and have the ability to grow in the tissues where they produce *infection*. Disregarding for the moment the immune state of the host, the severity of this infection depends on the intrinsic nature of the organism, and the factor concerned is generally described as its *virulence*. This may be manifest in two ways:

(1) The ability of the organism to spread throughout the tissues.
(2) The ability of the organism to cause tissue damage, for instance by the production of toxins.

The ability to spread, in respect of many organisms, is inversely proportional to the tendency to produce initial local damage and a subsequent inflammatory reaction. Thus an organism like *Staph. pyogenes* produces severe tissue damage, a marked inflammatory response, and usually has little tendency to spread. On the other hand, some organisms, e.g. many viruses, *Mycobacterium leprae*, etc., excite little immediate inflammatory reaction, and are able to spread widely without leaving any trace of the site of entry. Other organisms, although behaving essentially in the same manner, produce disease in which a lesion develops later at the site of entry. Syphilis is an excellent example of this, and it should be noted that the local lesion (chancre) occurs *long after the organisms have spread throughout the body.*

Sometimes an organism may live in a symbiotic state with its host and produce no damage. Such a relationship exists between man and the virus of herpes simplex. The virus lives harmlessly in the skin around the mouth until the subject develops a "cold". Then it multiplies and produces the familiar "cold sores", or herpes febrilis. Such latent virus infections are probably quite common—probably many tumour-producing viruses behave in a similar manner. This is considered in Chapter 19.

The existence of L-forms (p. 212) raises many possibilities. They are generally considered to be non-pathogenic, but following an overt infection they might remain in the tissues in a dormant form and provide sufficient antigen to sustain an immunological response. Rheumatic carditis and chronic post-streptococcal glomerulonephritis are obvious candidates for such a pathogenesis. L-forms might also revert to type; this could explain recurrent infections, e.g. chronic pyelonephritis and infective endocarditis.

From this brief review it is evident that micro-organisms are capable of initiating a great number of disease patterns, and that no simple generalizations will suffice to describe the types of host response that occur with infection.

## Manner by which Organisms Produce Damage[1]

In the early days of bacteriology it seemed reasonable to suppose that organisms produced damage by elaborating potent chemical substances which were termed toxins. The *exotoxins* were the first bacterial products to be identified. They are freely diffusible and therefore found in the medium of a bacterial culture. They can be purified, identified, and estimated with relative ease. Their mode of action is known in many cases, and it is very specific. On a quantitative basis exotoxins are very potent; thus botulinum toxin is the most poisonous substance known. Bacteria whose main offensive weapon is an exotoxin are called *toxic organisms*. Examples of these are the causative organisms of *diphtheria, tetanus, gas-gangrene*, and *scarlet fever*. Although the infection which they produce remains localized, distant tissues of the host are damaged as a result of circulating toxins.

With most other organisms no such powerful toxins have been demonstrated. Cultures may be toxic to animals, but the responsible substances seem to be derived from the bodies of the organisms. These have been called *endotoxins*, but it is probable that in reality they are the complex constituents of the bacterial body. Many substances have been isolated—lipids, carbohydrates, and proteins. On the whole, these chemicals are of low potency and their action on the tissues is non-specific.

Further investigations of the endotoxic group of organisms have shown that some substances do indeed diffuse out of the living cell body. The coagulase of *Staph. pyogenes* and hyaluronidase of *Strept. pyogenes* are two such substances. Some microbiologists call these exotoxins, but this is probably an error of judgment. It is even debatable whether coagulase and hyaluronidase are toxins at all. Therefore whatever the theoretical argument, in practice the term exotoxin should be restricted to those substances which diffuse easily out of the organism, are highly toxic, and cause some or many of the lesions of the disease. Organisms which do not produce exotoxins as described above are called *invasive*. They are characterized by the tendency to spread widely throughout the body and enter the circulation. The pyogenic organisms, *S. typhi*, and *B. anthracis* are good examples. This term serves a useful purpose, because it emphasizes that lesions can be produced only in the actual presence of the organism.*

The manner whereby the invasive organisms produce damage is not clearly understood. Some seem to have a direct action on the tissues, and produce necrosis and acute inflammation. The pyogenic organisms fall into this group. In infection with other organisms the situation is much more complicated. *Typhoid fever* illustrates this particularly well.

## Typhoid Fever

The pathogenesis of mouse typhoid (infection with *Salmonella typhimurium*) has been studied in considerable detail, and by analogy the sequence of events in man is probably as follows[1]:

Typhoid fever is contracted by the ingestion of food contaminated with *Salmonella typhi*. The organisms reach the lumen of the small intestine, and on its mucosal surface they are taken up by phagocytes. They are carried into the mucosa itself and thence to the local lymphoid tissue (Peyer's patches). Scarcely any local damage occurs, and little or no inflammation results. The organisms multiply, and some pass on through the lymphatics to the mesenteric nodes and finally reach the blood stream *via* the thoracic duct. In this way there develops a *bacteraemia, which is defined as the transient presence of*

---

* There are certain exceptions to this, as when invasive organisms produce lesions by some hypersensitivity mechanism, e.g. acute rheumatic fever.

*organisms in the blood stream.* The phagocytic cells of the RE system are well able to deal with this, and the organisms are engulfed by them. However, the organisms are able to live and multiply in these cells. By about the tenth day the parasitized cells undergo necrosis, and the blood stream is flooded with large numbers of bacilli. This is the end of the incubation period (usually 10–14 days), and the patient becomes seriously ill with *septicaemia, which is defined as the presence of organisms in the blood stream*

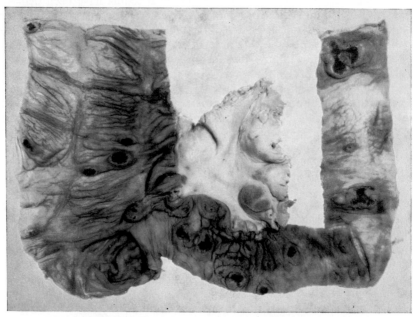

FIG. 7.1. Typhoid ulceration of the bowel. The ileum and ascending colon contain many ulcers which have retained the shape and size of the Peyer's patches and lymphoid follicles from which they have arisen. The walls are punched-out, and the bases are darkly staining due to the bile-pigmented necrotic debris in them. In the mesentery there is an enlarged lymph node.

(A 50.3, *reproduced by permission of the President and Council of the Royal College of Surgeons of England.*)

(*proven by a positive blood culture*) *which are causally associated with severe constitutional upset.* This differs from *bacteraemia* in the following ways:

(*a*) It is associated with severe clinical symptoms.
(*b*) There are more organisms in the blood.
(*c*) It indicates that the host's resistance to the organism is very inadequate.

The septicaemic phase lasts about one week and is characterized clinically by a progressive rise in temperature (step-ladder pattern) and severe constitutional symptoms. Death may occur at this stage.

The next phase of the disease is marked by the onset of diarrhoea, ulceration of the small intestine, and the appearance of organisms in the faeces. The bacilli reach the gut *via* the bile, which is heavily contaminated as a result of passage of the bacteria from the RE cells of the liver. The ulceration occurs over the inflamed Peyer's patches, and is associated with mesenteric adenitis (Fig. 7.1). In both the ulcers and the lymph nodes there is an accumulation of macrophages, while polymorphs are not present (Fig. 7.2). The most likely explanation of these events is that the local lymphoid tissue of the gut has become sensitized to the organism, and that subsequent contact with it produces damage. The local production of sensitizing anti- bodies must be postulated, because the blood level of antibodies detectable (agglutinins) does not rise till later in the course of the disease. During the second week diagnosis depends upon finding the organism in the faeces. By

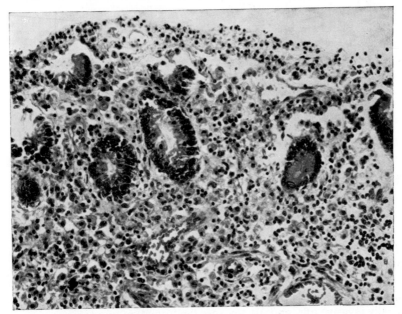

FIG. 7.2. Typhoid ulceration of the small bowel. The mucosa is ulcerated, and an inflammatory infiltration consisting of lymphocytes and swollen macro- phages is present around the remaining glands, Polymorphs are not present. × 200.

the third week the level of antibodies in the serum rises (Widal reaction), and the patient gradually recovers (Fig. 7.3).

Many viruses, e.g. smallpox, behave in a way similar to the typhoid bacillus. They produce no lesion on entry, but after dissemination and multiplication in the body cause extensive tissue damage as a result of some type of tissue hypersensitivity (see also syphilis, p. 202).

### Septicaemia

The cause of death in septicaemia is poorly understood. It has been most extensively studied in anthrax.[2] B. anthracis infection in animals leads to a fatal septicaemia, and the animals die with vast numbers of organisms in the blood. The early administration of a suitable antibiotic will save them, but it

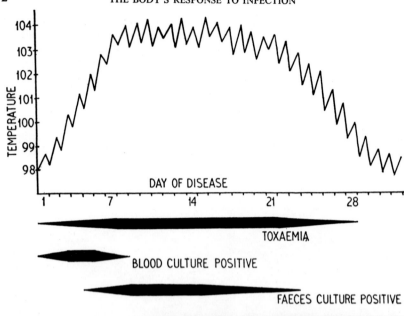

Fig. 7.3. Chart correlating the clinical course of a typical case of typhoid fever with the principal methods of bacteriological diagnosis.

(*After Harries, E. H. R. and Mitman, M.* (1947). *Clinical Practice in Infectious Disease, 3rd edition, p. 464. Edinburgh: Livingstone.*)

is found that there is a critical time after which treatment is of no avail. Although the organisms may be destroyed the animal still dies. This may be correlated with the observation that the blood of guinea-pigs dying of anthrax contains a toxin which can kill other animals. The organism, although a typically invasive one, appears to cause the formation of a toxin *in vivo*.

In septicaemia due to streptococci and staphylococci, death can reasonably be attributed to intense toxaemia consequent on the release of endotoxins. However, with other organisms, e.g. pneumococci, the symptoms are less easily explicable, because these organisms do not appear to produce toxic substances.

### The Generalized Shwartzman Phenomenon[3]

Gram-negative bacilli, e.g. *Salmonella typhi* and coliform organisms, produce an ill-defined endotoxin of lipoprotein nature. Experimentally it has been shown that this substance can produce shock if injected intravenously, especially if the dose is repeated *twenty-four hours later*. This enhancing effect of a previous dose is known as the *generalized Shwartzman phenomenon*,* and

* This should not be confused with the *localized Shwartzman phenomenon*. To demonstrate this, a quantity of Gram-negative bacterial endotoxin is injected into the skin of an animal and 24 hours later an intravenous dose is given. The site of the skin injected then undergoes necrosis. The pathogenesis is not understood, and there is little evidence that a similar reaction ever occurs in any human disease.

may be the experimental counterpart of the shock which is seen in some human cases of coliform septicaemia. The mechanism of the Shwartzman phenomenon is not well understood. It is probable that the endotoxin causes endothelial-cell damage and that this initiates intravascular clotting. The occlusion of the vessels in the kidney leads to cortical necrosis with subsequent acute renal failure. The effect of the first injection of endotoxin is probably to block the reticulo–endothelial system so that the second injection of endotoxin is less quickly removed. The generalized Shwartzman reaction is not an immunologically mediated hypersensitivity reaction.

### Types of Acute Inflammation

Although all examples of acute inflammation have many features in common, certain types have been categorized, depending upon some particular feature. The terms are useful for descriptive purposes but are of no fundamental significance.

**Suppurative Inflammation.** Certain organisms, termed the pyogenic organisms, as well as some chemicals, produce considerable tissue destruction. This is associated with a marked neutrophil infiltration, and the disintegrating phagocytes liberate proteolytic enzymes which cause liquefaction of the dead area. The fluid produced is *pus*, and the inflammation is called *suppurative*. Suppuration occurring in infection generally indicates that localization is becoming established, and therefore in the days before chemotherapy it was regarded as a favourable sign; hence the origin of the term "laudable pus". The presence of pus in a natural cavity is called an *empyema*, and this occurs most frequently in the pleural cavity.

While suppuration is usually localized, pus formation may occasionally occur in a spreading cellulitis. Such a diffuse suppurative process is generally caused by *Strept.pyogenese*, and this type of inflammation is called *phlegmonous*.

**Serous Inflammation.** In inflammation of loose tissues and in serous sacs the fluid component of the inflammatory exudate exceeds the cellular one, because the limiting factor of increased tissue tension (p. 63) is absent. There results a large accumulation of inflammatory oedema, and this is termed *serous inflammation*.

**Fibrinous Inflammation.** Fibrin formation is a feature of inflammation in serous sacs and in the lungs. It is well marked in most forms of pericarditis and peritonitis. It is also frequent in pneumococcal and staphylococcal infections. Often there is considerable serous exudate, and the inflammation is then termed *sero-fibrinous*.

**Haemorrhagic Inflammation.** A blood-stained exudate indicates that the irritant has caused severe vascular damage. It is seen in the lungs in phosgene poisoning and acute influenzal pneumonia.

**Catarrhal Inflammation.** This is seen when a mucous membrane is involved in an acute inflammatory reaction. There is some destruction of the epithelial cells, and a profuse mucus secretion from those that remain as well as from the underlying glands. The common cold provides an excellent example.

**Membranous Inflammation.** A membrane of mucus and fibrinous exudate covering an inflamed area of mucosa is seen in *membranous bronchitis*. It may be coughed up as a cast.

**Pseudomembranous Inflammation.** This differs from the above in that the membrane contains necrotic epithelium as well as fibrin and inflammatory cells. It is seen typically in diphtheria.

**Gangrenous Inflammation.** Gangrene occurs in inflammation when the dead tissue is invaded by putrefactive organisms (p. 54).

**Variability of the Cellular Exudate.** Certain inflammations do not show the usual neutrophil polymorph response. In typhoid the inflammatory reaction has virtually no polymorphs, but instead is characterized by macrophages. Why this is so is not at all clear, but it may well be that the development of a delayed-type of hypersensitivity is involved, since the mononuclear response is characteristically seen in this condition. Eosinophils are usually plentiful in inflammations produced by parasitic worms, and also in some allergic conditions (e.g. hay-fever).[4] Lymphocytic infiltration is frequent in inflammatory lesions produced by viruses, even in the early stages. It is also a feature of acute inflammation in many skin diseases. The reasons for this variation in cellular response are not known.

### Mode of Destruction of Organisms in the Inflammatory Exudate

Although a completely teleological view of the inflammatory reaction is unjustifiable, it is generally accepted that the reaction is an adaptive response having survival value for the species. It creates around the invading organisms a micro-environment unfavourable for their multiplication and survival.[5] *Local inflammation is therefore the first line of defence against the spread of infection.* An inhibition of the inflammatory reaction generally decreases the resistance to infection.

The manner in which organisms are killed in the exudate must now be considered:

**Part Played by Phagocytes.** *The polymorphonuclear leucocytes.*[6] Although many pathogenic organisms can multiply in the cytoplasm of the polymorphonuclear leucocytes and even be spread by them, the ultimate destruction of the organism often takes place within these cells. How this happens is not at all clear. Proteolytic enzymes, lysozyme, and acidic compounds like lactic acid have all been suggested as the likely bactericidal components of the polymorph cytoplasm. Other bactericidal substances isolated from polymorphs are phagocytin[7] and a group of basic proteins isolated from the lysosomal fraction of rabbit polymorphs.[8] *Peroxide* formation in polymorphs is an important step in the destruction of certain bacteria. Defects in this lead to chronic granulomatous disease (p. 152).

*The mononuclears.* Even less is known about the mechanism whereby these cells destroy bacteria. It is interesting that general conditions, like shock and haemorrhage, impair the RE system's phagocytic activity. This may well explain the lowered resistance under these circumstances.

**Part Played by the Fluid Exudate.**[5] The inflammatory oedema contains complement and other antibacterial substances present normally in the plasma. It contains lactic acid in considerable quantities. This may be a factor in the destruction of invading organisms.[9] Indeed, the conditions may be so unfavourable that some of the host cells as well as the bacteria are destroyed. To some extent this may actually be beneficial, because necrotic tissue has been shown to contain bactericidal substances.

**Part Played by Acquired Immunity.** Antibodies, e.g. opsonins, are present in the inflammatory exudate and aid phagocytosis. Activation of complement is another important mechanism whereby antibodies assist in the destruction of organisms.

It is also probable that the immune response affords protection by producing some degree of tissue hypersensitivity, such that there is acceleration of the inflammatory reaction and with it the normal mechanism of destruction.

The macrophages of an immune animal are more adept at destroying organisms, but the mechanism is poorly understood (p. 140).

## Spread of Infection

### Local Spread

The natural cohesion of tissues tends to prevent the spread of organisms. The tissue fluids are, however, in constant motion under normal conditions. Organisms are carried in any stream of fluid which may be present. The activity of muscles causes considerable movement of tissue fluids, and it is for this reason that the time-honoured treatment of inflammation is to rest the part. It should be noted that the motility of the organism itself appears to play no part in its spread. There is no correlation between the motility of the organism and the rapidity with which it spreads. Thus, *Clostridium tetani* is a motile organism but tetanus is a localized infection, whereas *Clostridium welchii* is non-motile and yet produces the rapidly spreading gas-gangrene.

Local spread may also occur in an entirely different way. Organisms ingested by phagocytes may be transported by these cells. This is an important means of spread in tuberculosis, and almost certainly occurs in many other infections.

*The Local Defence Mechanism.*[10] The acute inflammatory reaction must be regarded as a defence mechanism, although as we have seen, it is called forth only in the case of certain infections. With these infections the acute inflammatory reaction, including the laying-down of fibrin, plays an important part in the destruction of the organism. It has been thought that the fibrin forms a barrier and is important in limiting the spread of infection. However, it seems much more likely that it is the whole inflammatory response which is important rather than the fibrin itself. The presence of a fibrin barrier around the zone of infection is thus indicative of a severe inflammatory response which causes destruction of the organism, and is probably not the prime mover in the destruction itself.

**Spread by Natural Channels.** If local spread implicates a natural passage, infection may spread by this route. The following examples are important: *peritoneum*—infection may spread rapidly throughout the peritoneal space from localized lesions; it is for this reason that acute appendicitis is serious. Following perforation of the organ, the whole peritoneal cavity becomes infected, and as a large surface is involved, there is a rapid absorption of toxic substances. Infection may likewise spread through the *pleura, subarachnoid space, pericardium,* and *joint spaces.*

Infection may also spread along tubes, like the *bronchi* (in broncho-pneumonia and tuberculosis), the *ureter*, and the *gut*.

**Spread by Lymphatics.** In acute inflammation lymphatic vessels are held open by the increase in tissue tension.[11] The permeability of their walls is increased, as is also the flow of lymph. Invading organisms frequently gain access to the lymphatics, and are carried to the nearest lymph node. Phagocytes which have ingested the organisms but which are unable to destroy them, also travel by the same route. Here the RE cells lining the sinuses phagocytose the organisms and prevent their further spread. The lymph nodes may be regarded as the *second line of defence* against the spread of infection. Toxins may also be absorbed by the lymphatics. *Lymphangitis* is therefore a common event in spreading lesions, and when the vessels are superficial, as in the forearm, they appear as bright red streaks.

**Spread by the Blood Stream.** The blood stream forms the *third and last line of defence* against the spread of infection. It has two main defence mechanisms.

(1) The circulating blood itself contains a wide array of antibacterial substances. These include complement and opsonins, as well as antibodies of specific acquired immunity.

(2) The RE system, especially the sinus-lining cells of the liver (Kupffer cells), bone marrow, and spleen, forms the main defence against generalized infection. Organisms injected experimentally into the blood stream are rapidly removed. In natural infections with highly invasive organisms like the typhoid bacillus early invasion of the blood stream occurs, and the circulating organisms are rapidly taken up by the RE system.

### Mode of Entry of Organisms into the Blood Stream

The presence of organisms in the blood stream is a common event. It occurs under several conditions.

**1. Direct Invasion of Blood Vessels.** A few organisms may invade blood vessels in the course of any local infection, e.g. a boil. The infection is often quite trivial, but the adjacent blood vessels may be ruptured by trauma, thereby allowing organisms to enter. Gingival infection or abscesses related to the apices of the roots of teeth are common lesions in which this is thought to occur, e.g. following dental extraction, scaling of teeth, or even chewing hard food. When small numbers of organisms enter the blood stream in this way, they are rapidly removed by the phagocytes of the RE system and are destroyed. Bacteraemia usually causes few symptoms, but rigors may occur in the bacteraemia which follows catheterization. Its real importance, however, is that under certain conditions it may lead to serious sequelae.

*Metastatic Lesions.* Experimentally it has been shown that when an animal has a bacteraemia, histamine injected at any site will precipitate a local infection with the organism concerned. Trauma has a similar effect. Staphylococci may be localized in a bone in this way and set up osteomyelitis (p. 127). Another danger is that the organisms are filtered off by the kidneys, and if there is a coincidental obstruction to the outflow of urine, pyelonephritis may result. A further hazard of bacteraemia is that the organisms may colonize a damaged heart valve and cause endocarditis (p. 397).

*Transplacental Spread.* If the patient is pregnant, organisms may cross the placenta and reach the fetus (p. 77).

2. **Septic Thrombophlebitis.** When infection spreads to a vein, its wall becomes inflamed and thrombosis may occur, a condition called thrombophlebitis. If the thrombus is invaded by pyogenic organisms, it may soften and parts of it become detached, leading to the condition of *pyaemia*.

*Pyaemia* is the presence in the circulation of infected thrombi which are carried to various organs where they produce metastatic abscesses or septic infarcts. Which of these occurs depends on the vascular arrangements of the organ in which the emboli become lodged (p. 382). Pyaemia was a common complication of the staphylococcal osteomyelitis before the days of chemotherapy. It is now much less frequent. It sometimes follows suppuration of the gastrointestinal tract, e.g. acute appendicitis and infected piles, and the *portal pyaemia* produces multiple abscesses in the liver.

3. **Spread from the Lymphatic System.** Organisms which are not held up in the tissues at the site of entry or in the lymph nodes, reach the venous circulation *via* the lymphatic ducts. Bacteraemia produced in this way is a common event with many invasive organisms, e.g. *S. typhi*. If the cells of the RE system, having phagocytosed the organisms, are unable to destroy them, the bacteria proliferate and are subsequently liberated into the circulation which is flooded with them. The patient becomes gravely ill with septicaemia.

**Spread along Nerves.** Some viruses, e.g. rabies virus, are believed to travel up the nerves to reach the central nervous system. Whether they pass up the axoplasm or in the periaxonal space is uncertain.

### Factors Determining the Localization or Spread of Infection

It is convenient at this point to summarize the factors which determine whether a particular organism is likely to spread from the site of infection or remain localized.

#### Factors Involving the Organisms

**Virulence.** It should be appreciated that within each species of organism there are many strains, each with differing degrees of virulence. Thus certain staphylococci produce severe infection, while others produce trivial skin lesions.

**Dose.** With many organisms a large dose produces a severe spreading lesion while a small one produces a minor lesion which heals. This is seen in tuberculosis produced experimentally in animals. It is probably not true of virus infections.

**Portal of Entry.** This is a most important factor. Some organisms will cause infection only if administered by a particular route, e.g. *Vibrio cholerae* is non-pathogenic if injected, but may cause cholera if swallowed.

**Synergism.** The combined effect of two infecting organisms may be greater than either one alone. The best known example is Vincent's infection, which is a common cause of gingivitis and in which two organisms, the *Fuso-*

*bacterium fusiforme* and the *Borrelia vincenti*, are in association. (See also clostridial infections, p. 184).

**Products of the Organisms.**[10] Certain organisms produce factors which may aid their spread; streptococci produce an enzyme *hyaluronidase* which acts by depolymerizing the ground substance, and probably aids in spreading the infection. *Strept. pyogenes* also produces the enzyme *streptokinase* which aids in the lysis of the fibrin barrier by activating the plasmin system (p. 357).

### Factors Involving the Host

**General Factors.**[12,13,14] *The general state of health* of the host is important. Starvation and haemorrhagic shock have been shown experimentally to render animals more liable to infection. It is frequently observed that patients with chronic debilitating diseases, like chronic nephritis and diabetes mellitus, are less capable of resisting infection. The factors involved are complex, and probably involve both humoral factors, e.g. a low complement level, and an impaired activity of the phagocytes.

*The Immune State.* This involves both non-specific factors like complement and the specific antibodies of acquired immunity. Primary infections tend to spread much more widely than do subsequent ones due to the absence of active immunity (see tuberculosis, p. 165).

*Low White-cell Count.*[15] Infections tend to spread whenever the neutrophil polymorphonuclear leucocytes count is low, e.g. in agranulocytosis or acute leukaemia.

**Local Factors.** The local blood supply is important. Ischaemia from whatever cause, e.g. injection of adrenaline, peripheral vascular disease, etc., adversely affects the inflammatory response designed to destroy the organism. Similarly, foreign bodies and chemicals which cause necrosis are harmful. Thus silica potentiates the pathogenic action of the tubercle bacillus, and ionic calcium aids the inception of anaerobic infections in wounds (p. 184).

It is evident from this account of the various patterns of infection that the relationship between the host and his infecting organism is extremely complex. This is well illustrated in the case of man and the *Brucella* organism. The infection can vary from an acute illness to a chronic disease, or even a symptomless carrier state in which a symbiotic relationship has been established. Only in the case of the exotoxin-producing organisms is the pathogenesis of the disease which they cause at all clearly understood. It is not surprising therefore that it is in this group of infections that our understanding of immunity is also most complete.

### References

1. WILSON, G. S. and MILES, A. A. (1964). In Topley and Wilson's "Principles of Bacteriology and Immunology", 5th ed., pp. 1228 and 1836. London: Arnold.
2. SMITH, H. (1960). In "Biochemical Response to Injury", a C.I.O.M.S. Symposium, p. 341, ed. Stoner, H. B. and Threlfall, C. J. Oxford: Blackwell.
3. FINE, J. et al. (1960). p. 377 in C.I.O.M.S. Symposium, *loc. cit.*
4. ARCHER, R. K. (1963). "The]Eosinophil Leucocytes". Oxford: Blackwell.
5. DUBOS, R. J. (1955). *Lancet,* **2,** 1.

6. ROBB-SMITH, A. H. T. (1957). *Lancet*, **1**, 699.
7. COHN, Z. A. and HIRSCH, J. G. (1960). *J. exp. Med.*, **112**, 983.
8. ZEYA, H. I. and SPITZNAGEL, J. K. (1968). *J. exp. Med.*, **127**, 927.
9. HOWARD, J. G. (1963). In "Modern Trends in Immunology", Vol. 1, p. 86, ed. Cruickshank, R. London: Butterworth.
10. HADFIELD, G. and GARROD, L. P. (1947). Edrs., in "Recent Advances in Pathology", 5th ed., p. 1. London: Churchill.
11. WRIGHT, G. P. (1953). In "Recent Advances in Pathology", 6th ed., p. 1, ed. Hadfield, G. London: Churchill.
12. DUBOS, R. J. and SCHAEDLER, R. W. (1959). *J. Pediat.*, **55**, 1.
13. Annotation (1954). *Lancet*, **2**, 908.
14. SMITH, W. (1949). *Proc. roy. Soc. Med.*, **42**, 11.
15. Annotation (1959). *Lancet*, **2**, 1134.

*Chapter 8*

# WOUND HEALING

The word *healing*, used in a pathological context, refers to the body's replacement of destroyed tissue by living tissue. It is therefore useful, at the outset, to enumerate the causes of tissue loss or destruction:

## Causes of Tissue Loss:

*Traumatic excision*, whether accidental or surgical.

*Physical, chemical, and microbial agents.* These all give rise to inflammation, and in sufficient amount lead to necrosis.

*Ischaemia*, which leads to infarction.

*Hypersensitivity reactions* to foreign proteins, or to products of organisms, are instances when the body's response to external agents can itself engender necrosis (see Arthus phenomenon, p. 163, caseation in tuberculosis, p. 192).

## Mechanisms of Healing:

The healing process has two aspects:

**Contraction,** a mechanical reduction in the size of the defect occurring in the first few weeks (see below).

**Replacement of lost tissue,** which is brought about by migration of cells as well as division of adjacent cells to provide extra tissue to fill the gap. This can be accomplished in three ways:

*Repair*, the replacement of lost tissue by granulation tissue which matures to form scar tissue. This is inevitable when the surrounding specialized cells do not possess the capacity to proliferate, e.g. muscle and neurones.

*Regeneration*, the replacement of lost tissue by tissue similar in type. There is a proliferation of surrounding undamaged specialized cells. Regeneration is predominant when the cells comprising the tissue are capable of multiplication, and is well illustrated by the healing of a damaged liver.

*Reconstitution* is the co-ordinated regeneration of several types of lost tissue resulting in the reformation of whole organs or limbs. Many examples are to be found in amphibians and crustaceans. If, for instance, the limb of a newt be amputated, a new limb-bud appears. Its growth results in the production of a new limb from the stump of the old. The process is well developed in lower forms of life, and crustaceans are capable of reforming limbs, claws, and eyes. These are complicated processes resembling embryonic development or asexual reproduction, and have no exact counterpart in the higher vertebrate animals. The reformation of liver following partial hepatectomy is the nearest approach to reconstitution seen in mammals.

It should be noted that the word repair is used in a rather arbitrary way by some surgeons and pathologists. Surgeons refer to the union of fractures or the closure of defects by various inert materials as examples of repair, but the latter is not even true healing, though it has an ameliorative effect. Some pathologists equate repair with healing and recovery, and describe "repair by resolution", "repair by granulation tissue," and "repair by regeneration". There is no doubt that such variation in the nomenclature is confusing, and in this book the terms resolution, regeneration, and repair are used strictly in accordance with the definitions given previously. The processes involved in healing may best be understood if each aspect is described in as clear a form as possible. The first of these is wound contraction.

## Wound Contraction[1]

**Measurement.** This is conveniently studied by excising a small, circular, full-thickness disc of skin from the back or flank of an animal. Figures 8.1 and 8.2 show the results of such an experiment. The size of the wound is measured

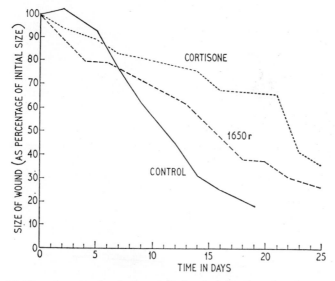

FIG. 8.1. Wound contraction in the rat. Daily administration of cortisone acetate causes considerable delay in the process. Irradiation with 1 650r immediately after inflicting the wounds has a similar delaying effect.

at regular intervals, and it can be seen that after an initial period of 2–3 days there follows a period of rapid contraction which is largely completed by the 14th day. New tissue formation is not included, since the measurements are made from the original wound edges. The wound is reduced by approximately 80 per cent of its original size in the rat, but the actual extent of the contraction varies with the species of animal, and with the shape, size, and site of the wound. Contraction results in much faster healing, as less new tissue has to be formed. If contraction is prevented, healing is slow and a large ugly scar the result.

Contraction probably plays a similar role in the healing of wounds of the oral mucosa. In the non-keratinized mucosa scarring persists as on the skin, but in wounds of the keratinized mucosa of the gingiva, edentulous

CONTROL             DAYS             1 650 r

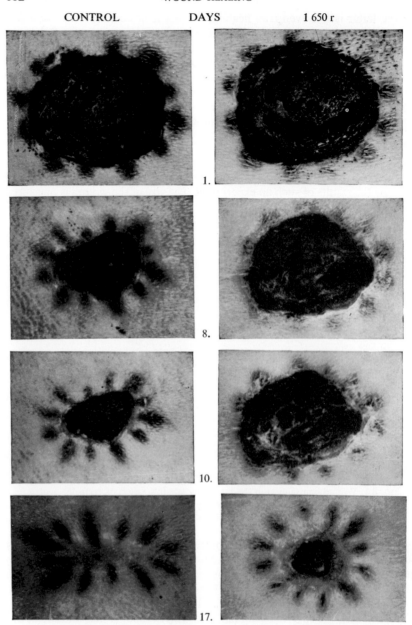

Fig. 8.2. Wound contraction in the rat and the effect of x-irradiation. The edges of the skin wounds have been tattooed with carbon so as to render them easily visible. Note how the delivery of 1 650r to the wound on the right has delayed the contraction process.

*(From Blair, G. H., Slome, D. and Walter, J. B.* (1961). *Review of Experimental Investigations on Wound Healing,* British Surgical Practice: Surgical Progress, *edited by Paterson Ross, J. London: Butterworths.)*

ridge, and the palate, only a small amount of scar tissue forms during healing and it soon becomes so inconspicuous that the actual site of the wound can no longer be found.

**Cause of Wound Contraction.**[2,3] Contraction occurs in wounds at a time when granulation tissue is being actively formed, and it is generally agreed that it is in the granulation tissue at the edge of the wound that the mechanism for contraction lies.[4] It seems that it is caused by a general remodelling of the tissues rather than by a shortening of cells or fibres comparable to contraction of muscle. It might be thought that collagen contracts, but although it does so when boiled, there is no evidence that it is capable of doing so *in vivo*.

**Inhibition.** Interference with the formation of granulation tissue, e.g. by *irradiating the wounded area* or administration of *corticosteroids* causes considerable delay in wound contraction[2] (Fig. 8.1). Interference with the formation of collagen, on the other hand, as in the Vitamin C deficient animal, has no such effect.[5] The contraction of wounds may also be impaired following burns, and also if the raw area of the wound is skin-grafted.[2]

## Organization

Organization is one of the fundamental processes in pathology, and can be defined as *the replacement of necrotic tissue, fibrin, and blood clot by living*

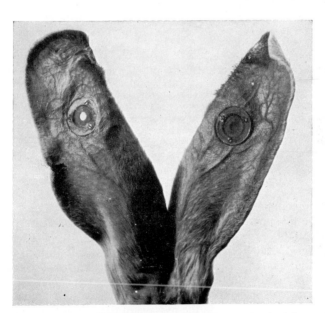

FIG. 8.3. Two rabbit ear-chambers in position. The one in the left ear shows the clear central area in which observations are made. In the chamber on the right the area of the central table is still filled with blood clot.

(*From Blair, G. H., van den Brenk, H. A. S., Walter, J. B. and Slome, D. (1961). "Wound Healing", pp. 46–53, in a symposium organized by Smith and Nephew Research Ltd. Oxford: Pergamon Press.*)

*granulation tissue.* In addition to being a feature of wound healing, organization also occurs in *inflammatory exudates, thrombi, haematomata,* and *infarcts.* It plays an important part in chronic inflammation.

The growth of granulation tissue can be studied experimentally using the rabbit ear-chamber technique[6] (Figs. 8.3, 8.4, 8.5). Four phases may be observed.

**Haematoma Formation.** Blood clot soon occupies the table area of the chamber.

**Traumatic Inflammation.** The damage caused by inserting the chamber sets in motion the phenomenon of acute inflammation in the surrounding tissue. An exudate containing fibrin and polymorphs therefore accumulates.

**Demolition.** The dead tissue cells liberate their autolytic enzymes, and other proteolytic enzymes come from disintegrating polymorphs. There is an

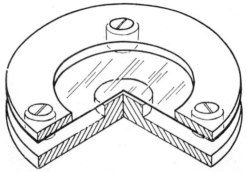

FIG. 8.4. Diagrammatic representation of one type of rabbit ear-chamber; a wedge has been cut out to show its construction. The chamber is composed of a Perspex base plate which has a raised central table and three peripherally arranged pillars. The cover-slip consists of a disc of mica supported at the edge by a ring of Perspex. The cover-slip is placed upon the three pillars, and held in position by screws which are inserted into threaded holes in the pillars. The height of the pillars is such that the gap between the top of the table and the mica is 50–100 $\mu$m.

(Drawing by Mr. S. P. Steward.)

associated mononuclear infiltration with macrophages. These are mostly derived from the blood monocytes, and their function is to ingest particulate matter, which they either digest or remove (p. 70).

**Granulation-Tissue Formation.** Granulation tissue is formed by the proliferation and migration of surrounding connective tissue elements. It is composed, in the first instance, of *capillary loops* and *fibroblasts* together with a variable number of inflammatory cells (Fig. 8.6). Initially this is a highly vascular tissue, but with the passage of time it develops into avascular scar tissue. The manner of its formation must be considered in more detail. Two stages may be recognized: there is first a stage of *vascularization,* and this is subsequently followed by *devascularization.*

Buds of endothelial cells grow out from the existing blood vessels at the wound margin, undergo canalization, and by joining with their neighbours

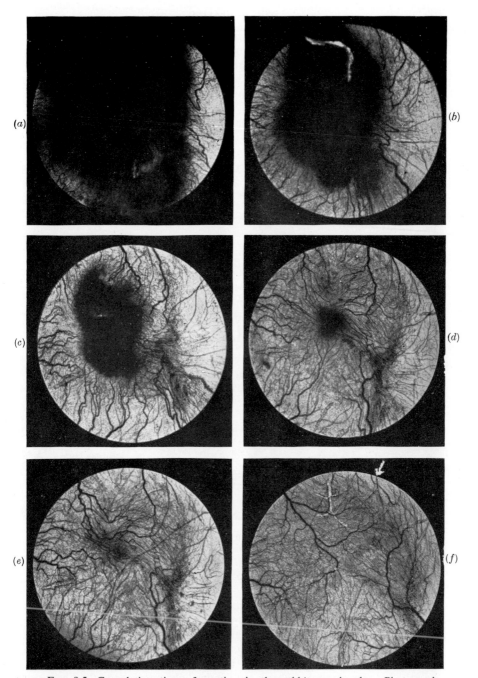

Fig. 8.5. Granulation tissue formation in the rabbit ear-chamber. Photographs taken at the following times after the insertion of the chamber: (a) 9 days, (b) 12 days, (c) 17 days, (d) 21 days, (e) 24 days, and (f) 44 days. At 9 days vessels are seen to be invading the dark clot in the centre, and by 24 days organization is complete. The large tortuous vessels are venules; the arterioles are more difficult to see at this magnification. The arrow in (f) indicates an arteriole which divides almost immediately. Note how by 44 days changes have occurred in the course of many blood vessels, although the original pattern of certain venules can still be recognized on the left-hand side of the picture. A lymphatic vessel is now visible at the top of the chamber. × 8.5.

form a series of vascular arcades. At first the newly-formed vessels all appear similar; the electron microscope shows gaps between the endothelial cells and a poorly-formed basement membrane.[7] Protein escapes from these newly-formed vessels, and it is easy to imagine that the tissue fluid around them forms a very suitable medium for cellular growth. Very soon differentiation occurs. Some vessels acquire a muscular coat and become arterioles, while others form thin-walled venules. The remainder either disappear, or persist as part of the capillary bed.

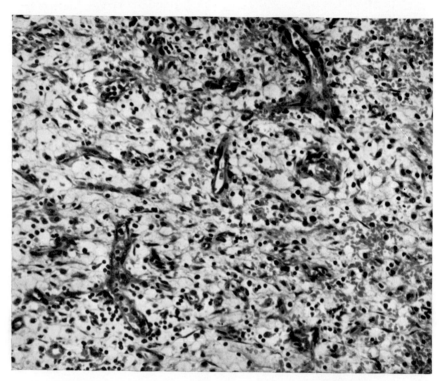

FIG. 8.6. Section of young granulation tissue composed mostly of thin-walled capillaries. Several arterioles are also present, but at this stage have only a thin muscular coat. Fibroblasts appear as elongated cells, and the small dark round cells are mostly lymphocytes. × 200.

At the same time as the vessels grow into the clot, the fibroblasts at the wound edge multiply and accompany the vascular invasion. Thus the clot is converted into a living vascular granulation tissue, and the process is known as *organization*. The fibroblasts which accompany the capillary loops are large and plump, but gradually, as collagen fibrils form around them, the cells become elongated fibrocytes. Under light microscopy the fibrils are first detected as reticulin, but this gradually changes to mature collagen fibres. During this process of fibrogenesis the pH becomes alkaline. The fibroblasts are thought also to be responsible for the formation of the ground substance. Lymphatic vessels grow into the maturing granulation tissue in much the same manner as do the blood vessels, only later. The two sets of vessels do not anastomose. At the same time there is an ingrowth of nerve fibres to supply the arterioles, which are then capable of exhibiting contraction.

As maturation proceeds some vessels undergo atrophy and disappear. Others show thickening of their intimal coats and eventual obliteration of the lumen (*endarteritis obliterans*). This process of devascularization results in the formation of a pale avascular scar. Coincident with the devascularization there is often *cicatrization* of scar tissue with much local tissue distortion. This process must be clearly distinguished from contraction. *Cicatrization* (or *contracture*, as it is sometimes called) is a diminution in the size of a *scar* and is a late event; *contraction* is a diminution in the size of a *wound* and is an early event.

Although it is generally considered that collagen once formed remains for life, experimental evidence in animals suggests that it can be removed.[8] The mechanism is not known, but that it does occur in man is suggested by the way in which scars gradually become less obvious.

### Tensile Strength[9]

Another method of examining a wound is the estimation of its tensile strength. The strength of the wound is of great practical importance because it is the main safeguard against *wound disruption*, or *dehiscence*. Three stages may be recognized.

At first the strength of a skin wound is only that of the fibrin cementing the cut surfaces together. It is for this reason that skin wounds are held together by sutures, clips, or tapes. There then follows a period of increasing tensile strength which corresponds to the amount of collagen produced by the granulation tissue uniting the cut wound edges.[10,11] Thus the increase in tensile strength parallels the increase of hydroxyproline in the wound area, since this is a reflection of the amount of collagen present (p. 26). Finally as the months go by the strength of a wound increases further, due apparently to a reorientation of collagen rather than an absolute increase in its amount.[9]

Many factors influence the rate of increase of tensile strength. These are both local and general, and in the main are related to granulation tissue and collagen formation.

## HEALING OF SKIN WOUNDS[12-14]

The histological changes which occur in healing skin wounds have recently been reinvestigated by various workers, and their findings are incorporated in the account that follows.

### Healing of a Clean Incised Wound with Edges in Apposition[15]

This process is described as *healing by primary intention*, and is the desired result in all surgical incisions.

The following changes occur:

*Initial haemorrhage* results in the formation of a fibrin-rich haematoma.

*An acute inflammatory reaction* occurs, and the fibrinous exudate helps to cement the cut margins of the wound together.

*Epithelial Changes.* Within 24 hours of injury epithelial cells from the adjacent epidermis migrate into the wound and insinuate themselves between the inert dermis and the clot (Fig 8.7 (b)). With well-approximated wounds by 24 hours a continuous layer of epidermal cells covers the surface. Overlying the area there is a crust or scab of dried clot. During the next 24–48 hours the epidermal cells invade the space where connective tissue will eventually develop; in this way a spur is formed (Fig. 8.7 (c)). The migrating cells of the

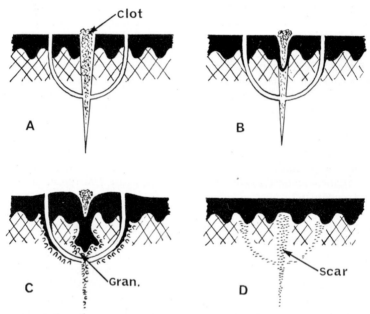

FIG. 8.7. Diagrammatic representation of the healing of an incised wound held together by a suture, the track of which alone is shown. The wound rapidly fills with clot (A) and shortly afterwards the epithelium migrates into the wound and down the suture tracks (B). Epithelial spurs are formed, and granulation-tissue (gran) formation proceeds (C). In D the suture has been removed, and scar tissue remains to mark the site of the incision and the suture tracks. The epithelial ingrowths have degenerated.

epidermis do not divide. Mitotic activity occurs in the basal cells a short distance from the edge of the wound, and in the mouse this activity is maximal at 36 hours. Epidermal cells also migrate along suture tracks, and where the suture or the incision encounters a sweat gland or other skin appendage, epithelial cells are contributed from this source (Fig. 8.7 (c)). The stimulus for this epithelial growth and migration is not known. Experimentally it has been noted that cells in tissue culture continue to divide until they establish contact with similar cells, at which point mitosis stops. This has been called *contact inhibition* by Abercrombie, but the mechanism is obscure.

*A demolition phase* follows the acute inflammatory reaction in the area of the wound.

*Organization.* By about the third day the wound area is filled with fibroblasts and capillary buds growing in from the cut surfaces. This ingrowth occurs mainly from the subcutaneous tissues, with little or no contribution from the reticular layer of the dermis, which is inert. There may be some contribution from the papillary layer of the dermis. Collagen appears a day or two later. This granulation tissue appears to prevent excessive epithelial migration into the wound, and the epithelial cells which form the spurs and the lining of suture tracks degenerate and are replaced by granulation tissue. Only the surface epithelial cells persist, and these divide and differentiate so that a multilayered covering of epidermis is reformed. It first covers a vascular granulation tissue, but as devascularization proceeds the scar shrinks in size and changes in colour from red to white.

Epithelial cells are thus the first cells to be stimulated, and their presence excites a connective tissue response which in its turn inhibits the epithelial growth. The early role that epithelium plays in the process of wound healing has been stressed by Gillman, and explains the formation of an epidermoid cyst from epithelial remnants, and also the ugly punctate scars which appear if sutures are left in position for any length of time. Punctured wounds due to injections do not form such scars, because the wound is not held open and therefore no epithelial "invasion" occurs. The use of adhesive tapes instead of sutures for closing wounds avoids these marks and produces a better cosmetic result.[16,17]

## Healing of Wounds with Separated Edges (*Healing by Secondary Intention*)

Although stress is sometimes laid on the difference between healing by primary intention and secondary intention, the pathological changes in both are very similar. When there is extensive tissue loss, either by direct trauma, inflammatory necrosis, or simply failure to approximate the wound edges, a large defect is present which must be made good. The main bulk of tissue which performs this service is granulation tissue, and this type of healing is therefore sometimes known as *healing by granulation*. The term is, however, a poor one, since it wrongly implies that granulations are not formed in the simple incised wound. The differences between healing by primary and secondary intention are quantitative not qualitative.

In healing by secondary intention the wound edges are widely separated, so that healing has to progress from the base upwards as well as from the edges inwards. From the clinical point of view healing of a well-approximated incised wound (primary intention) is fast and leaves a small, neat scar. Healing by secondary intention is slow and results in a large, distorted scar. The difference lies in the type of wound and not in the type of healing.

The following account of the healing of a large uninfected wound is illustrated in Fig. 8.8.

1. There is an initial inflammatory phase affecting the surrounding tissues. The wound is filled with coagulum, as described in simple incisions. This coagulum dries on its surface, and forms a scab in some wounds.

2. An important feature is *wound contraction*, which has already been fully

described (see p. 101). Fig. 8.2 (p. 102) shows the changes in size of full-thickness skin loss.

3. As with incised wounds, the epidermis adjacent to the wound shows hyperplasia, and epithelial cells migrate into the wound. They form a thin tongue which grows between pre-existing viable connective tissue and the surface clot with necrotic material. The epithelial cells secrete a collagenase which probably aids their penetration between living and dead connective tissue.

4. Demolition follows acute inflammation, and the clot in the centre of the wound is invaded and replaced by granulation tissue. This grows from the subcutaneous tissues at the wound edge, and is important in causing

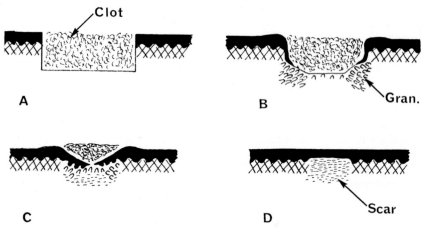

FIG. 8.8. Diagram to illustrate the healing of an excised wound. The wound is rapidly filled with clot (A). Epithelium soon migrates in from the margins to undermine the clot, which dries to form a crust. Granulation tissue (gran) grows into the wounded area, and is most profuse around the circumference where it is derived from the subcutaneous fat (B). Epithelial ingrowth continues and spurs are produced (C); these, however, do not persist, and the end-result (D) is a scar covered by epidermis which lacks rete ridges. During the healing process contraction has taken place so that the final scar is considerably smaller than the original wound.

wound contraction. Granulation tissue is also formed from the base of the wound, the amount from this source depending upon the nature and vascularity of the bed.

When the wound is viewed with a magnifying glass, the surface (under the scab) is deep red and granular, the capillary loops forming elevated mounds. It is very fragile, and the slightest trauma causes bleeding. It was this granularity which was responsible for the name "granulation tissue". The covering of the wound by granulation tissue serves an important protective role. If organisms are introduced into a recent wound, infection is likely to result, but not, however, if the wound is first allowed to granulate. Thus granulation tissue forms a temporary protective layer until the surface is covered by epithelium.

5. The migrating epidermis covers the granulation tissue, and in this way a mushroom-shaped scab is formed with a central attachment, which finally becomes nipped off (Fig. 8.8(c)).

6. The regenerated epidermis becomes thicker, and sends short processes into the underlying tissue. These are transient structures and do not persist as rete ridges, for neither these nor the skin appendages are reformed in man. The epidermal incursions appear to stimulate the formation of granulation tissue, so that the scar gains thickness and is eventually level with the surface of the skin. The scar is at first pink, but the subsequent devascularization leaves it white.

It can be seen that with full thickness skin loss, part of the clot occupying the wound is organized but much of it is cast off. With partial thickness skin loss, as may occur following burns or at the donor site of a Thiersch graft, the area of the wound is covered by epithelium both from the wound edges and from the cut remains of hair follicles and sweat glands. Epithelialization is therefore very fast, and the granulation tissue which is formed is produced beneath the new epithelium.

### Factors Influencing Repair

Although it would be desirable to analyze the factors which influence repair according to whether they affect granulation tissue formation, collagen production, contraction, etc., it must be admitted that in many instances we have insufficient information to adopt this policy. In practice, the factors which affect wound healing may be divided into two groups—those which act locally, and those whose influence is general or systemic. There are many factors which delay wound healing, but few are known which accelerate it. The following account consists therefore largely of the causes of delayed wound healing.

#### Local Factors

**Blood Supply.** Wounds in an ischaemic area, i.e. where there is a poor blood supply, heal slowly; for this reason injuries heal much more slowly in the pre-tibial region than in parts with a good blood supply, such as the face. The poor circulation in the skin of the leg in patients with varicose veins predisposes them to slow wound healing. Ischaemia secondary to pressure is an important factor in the causation and poor healing of *bedsores*. Any condition of chronic inflammation is liable to be accompanied by endarteritis obliterans and a poor blood supply to the part; perhaps the best example of this is previous x-irradiation. Finally, the slow wound healing of old age may in part be related to a poor circulation.

**Continued Tissue Breakdown and Inflammation.** Any condition causing continued tissue breakdown leads to persistent inflammation, and therefore delays completion of the healing process.

The most important examples are infection, the presence of a foreign body or irritant chemical, and excessive movement.

**Infection.** In an infected skin wound a scab does not form, and often the base is composed of dead tissue and inflammatory exudate forming a slough. Underlying this there is chronic inflammatory granulation tissue.

**Foreign Bodies and Other Irritants.** The presence of a foreign body in a wound, even in the absence of infection, may delay healing. The over-enthusiastic use of irritating disinfectants may cause considerable delay in the healing of skin ulcers, and indeed, if hypersensitivity develops, may lead to extensive necrosis.

**Movement.** This delays healing by submitting the delicate granulation tissue to repeated trauma.

**Adhesions to Bony Surfaces.** These, by anchoring the wound edges, prevent contraction. This is well seen in wounds over the tibia, and also in chronic varicose ulcers.

**Direction of the Wound.** Skin wounds made in a direction parallel to the lines of Langer heal faster than those made at right angles to them. *The lines of Langer*, first described in fact by Dupuytren in 1832, are due to the orientation of the collagen bundles in the dermis.[18] The skin is less tensile in the direction of the lines than at right angles to them. In general they correspond to the direction of the crease lines, although the latter are in fact related also to the movements of the underlying muscles and joints. Skin incisions made across the crease lines tend to gape, and their healing is delayed. Therefore, when planning a surgical incision these should be taken into consideration. Wounds parallel to or in the crease lines are more satisfactory and the scars less visible.

**Effects of Previous Wounding.** Pre-existing wounds at a distance do not influence the healing of an additional skin wound. There is therefore no evidence of a circulating wound hormone. Re-sutured wounds do, however, heal faster than do those sutured primarily, because the reparative process has already commenced.[19] Severe trauma delays wound healing, presumably because of the adrenocortical response to the stress.

**Exposure to Ionizing Radiation.** Previous x-irradiation may reduce the vascularity of the part. Apart from this, x-rays inhibit wound contraction if given at the same time as the injury. The formation of granulation tissue is also delayed.

### General Factors Affecting Wound Healing

**Age.** Wound healing is fast in the young, but is normal in old age unless there is some associated debilitating disease or ischaemia.

**Nutrition.** (*a*) *Protein deficiency.* Animals starved of protein show poor wound healing and deficient collagen formation. This abnormality may be corrected by administering proteins containing methionine or cystine, or by supplementing the diet with these amino acids only. Although cystine is not present in the collagen molecule, it accumulates in the wound area, and its increase parallels collagen formation. Cystine is therefore necessary for normal wound healing and collagen formation (see p. 29). Apart from an inadequate intake of protein the body may be deficient if there is excessive loss, as when there is a chronic discharging osteomyelitis or empyema.

(*b*) *Vitamin-C deficiency.* The observations of Lind on the effect of scurvy in sailors, and the finding that citrus fruit cured the condition is one of the classic descriptions in medicine. In spite of much research there are few who could not re-echo the words of Dr. Grainger, who, writing to Lind concerning scurvy, noted that it was "a subject of which I had read much but knew little".[20]

Experimentally in guinea-pigs (scurvy does not occur in other rodents because they can synthetize vitamin C), wound contraction and epithelial regeneration proceed normally. Granulation tissue is produced, but is abnormal:[21,22] the fibroblasts are arranged in an irregular manner and although they produce a little reticulin, normal collagen fibres are not formed. The wound is therefore very weak. Capillaries are unduly fragile and haemorrhages occur. In those who have teeth, swelling of and bleeding from the gingivae are characteristic. Vitamin C appears to be necessary for the hydroxylation of proline prior to its incorporation into the collagen molecule[23] (p. 28).

Although frank scurvy is uncommon, minor degrees of vitamin-C deficiency are not infrequent in patients who are on a marginal intake and who are in other ways stressed.[24,25]

(c) *The Role of Zinc*.[26] The addition of zinc to the diet of rats has been shown to promote the healing of thermal burns and excised wounds. The mechanism is not known, but the fact that zinc is an important component of several enzymes may be related. The oral administration of zinc sulphate has been tried in man, and a beneficial effect on wound healing claimed.

**Glucocorticosteroids.** In excessive amounts these inhibit the formation of granulation tissue and also delay wound contraction.

**Temperature.**[27] It is the general experience that wounds of the exposed parts heal much more slowly in cold weather, and experiments on animals have supported this observation.

## Complications of Wound Healing

Apart from *infection* and *delayed healing* other complications may occur.

**Wound Dehiscence.** The bursting open of a wound is described as *dehiscence*, and it occurs when stress is applied before the wound has healed sufficiently. It is particularly serious in abdominal incisions, because it results in the exposure of the abdominal contents to the atmosphere outside. Increased intra-abdominal pressure combines with poor wound healing to precipitate this catastrophic event.

**Cicatrization.** This is a frequent complication of extensive burning of the skin, and may produce great deformity. Cicatrization involving hollow viscera, e.g. the intestine or the urethra, is an important cause of narrowing (*stenosis*) of the lumen.

**Keloid Formation.** Occasionally an excessive formation of collagenous tissue results in the appearance of a raised nodule of scar tissue called a keloid. The cause of this is unknown. Repeated trauma and irritation caused by foreign bodies, hair, keratin, etc., may play a part. Keloids are more common in the young, especially girls, in Negroes, in tuberculous subjects, and during pregnancy. They are found most commonly in the region of the neck. They are especially frequent after burns.

**Weak Scars.** If scar tissue is subjected to continuous strain, stretching may result. In elderly people the abdominal viscera may bulge through a weak scar to produce a local protrusion, or *incisional hernia*.

4 WOUND HEALING

**Implantation (or Epidermoid) Cysts.** Epithelial cells which grow into the wounded area may persist, and their subsequent growth results in the formation of a small cyst. This should not be confused with a dermoid cyst.

**Painful Scars.** Pain either local or referred may be experienced if a nerve is included in the scar tissue.

**Pigmentary Changes.** Coloured particles introduced into the wound may persist and cause colouring or tattooing. Healed chronic ulcers sometimes have a russet colour due to staining with haemosiderin.

## The Mechanism of Wound Healing[28,29]

When one considers that in a healing wound there is cell and tissue production proceeding at a rate which exceeds that seen in most malignant tumours, it is humiliating to admit how little we know of the mechanisms involved. We understand neither the signal which starts the process, nor the mechanisms which maintain and control it. Many workers have claimed that local wound hormones, or *trephones*, are responsible for healing, but none has been isolated from animal tissue. In the plant world growth factors have, however, been found. Alternatively it has been postulated that removal of an inhibiting substance (*chalone*), normally present, is responsible for stimulating cell division. Physical factors may play some part; for instance epithelial cells tend to maintain contact with each other and spread over surfaces. The migration of squamous epithelium in wound healing can be easily understood. However, the subsequent division of cells, and the formation of a multicellular epidermis cannot be so explained. Although some general factors, such as food supply and hormones, affect wound healing, local factors far outweigh them in potency and probably in importance. In the control of cell division and maturation it is therefore local factors which are most likely to play the dominant role.

## General Reading

BLAIR, G. H., SLOME, D. and WALTER, J. B. (1961). Review of experimental investigations on wound healing. In "British Surgical Practice: Surgical Progress", p. 462–505, ed. by Rock Carling, E. and Paterson Ross, J. London: Butterworths.
DeVITO, R. V. (1965). "Healing of Wounds". The Surgical Clinics of North America, ed. by Moyer, C. A., **45**, 441. Philadelphia and London: Saunders.
DOUGLAS, D. M. (1963). "Wound Healing and Management: A Monograph for Surgeons". Edinburgh: Livingstone.
NEWCOMBE, J. F. (1965). In "The Scientific Basis of Surgery", ed. by Irvine, W. T., p. 371. London: Churchill.
PATTERSON, W. B. (1959). Edr. "Wound Healing and Tissue Repair". Chicago: University of Chicago Press.
PEACOCK, E. E. and VAN WINKLE, W. (1970). "Surgery and Biology of Wound Repair", 630pp., Philadelphia, London and Toronto: Saunders.
RUSSELL, P. S. and BILLINGHAM, R. E. (1962). "Some Aspects of the Repair Process in Mammals". *Progr. Surg. (Basel)*, **2**, 1–72.
SLOME, D. (1961). Edr. "Wound Healing". Oxford: Pergamon.
WILLIAMSON, M. B. (1957). Edr. "The Healing of Wounds". New York: McGraw-Hill.

## References

1. VAN DEN BRENK, H. A. S. (1956). *Brit. J. Surg.*, **43**, 525.
2. BILLINGHAM, R. E. and RUSSELL, P. S. (1956). *Ann. Surg.*, **144**, 961.
3. ABERCROMBIE, M., JAMES, D. W. and NEWCOMBE, J. F. (1960). *J. Anat.*, **94**, 170.
4. WATTS, G. T., GRILLO, H. C. and GROSS, J. (1958). *Ann. Surg.*, **148**, 153.
5. GRILLO, H. C. and GROSS, J. (1959). *Proc. Soc. exp. Biol. (N.Y.)*, **101**, 268.
6. CLIFF, W. J. (1963). *Phil. Trans. B.*, **246**, 305.
7. SCHOEFL, G. I. (1963). *Virchow Arch. path. Anat.*, **337**, 97.
8. PÉREZ-TAMAYO, R. (1970). *Lab. Invest.*, **22**, 137 and 142.
9. DOUGLAS, D. M. (1966). In "Wound Healing", ed. Illingworth, C., p. 233. London: Churchill.
10. DUNPHY, J. E. and UDUPA, K. N. (1955). *New Engl. J. Med.*, **253**, 847.
11. VILJANTO, J. (1964). *Acta Chir. Scand. Suppl.*, 333.
12. GILLMAN, T. and PENN, J. (1956). *Med. Proc., Suppl.*, **2**, 121.
13. ORDMAN, L. J. and GILLMAN, T. (1966). *Arch. Surg.*, **93**, 857, 883 and 911.
14. GILLMAN, T. (1968). *Glaxo Volume*, **31**, 5.
15. LINDSAY, W. K. and BIRCH, J. R. (1964). *Canad. J. Surg.*, **7**, 297.
16. ROTHNIE, N. G. and TAYLOR, G. W. (1963). *Brit. med. J.*, **2**, 1027.
17. MURRAY, P. J. B. (1963). *Brit. med. J.*, **2**, 1030.
18. KAZANJIAN, V. H. and CONVERSE, J. M. (1959). In "Surgical Treatment of Facial Injuries", 2nd ed., p. 28. London: Baillière, Tindall and Cox.
19. OGILVIE, R. R. and DOUGLAS, D. M. (1964). *Brit. J. Surg.*, **51**, 149.
20. HUNT, A. H. (1940). *Brit. J. Surg.*, **28**, 436.
21. STEIN, O. and WOLMAN, M. (1958). *Brit. J. exp. Path.*, **39**, 418.
22. DUNPHY, J. E., UDUPA, K. N. and EDWARDS, L. C. (1956). *Ann. Surg.*, **144**, 304.
23. UDENFRIEND, S. (1966). *Science*, **152**, 1335.
24. GOLDSMITH, G. A. (1961). *Ann. N.Y. Acad. Sci.*, **92**, 230.
25. CRANDON, J. H. *et al.* (1961). *Ann. N.Y. Acad. Sci.*, **92**, 246.
26. PORIES, W. J., *et al.* (1967). *Lancet*, **1**, 121.
27. BILLINGHAM, R. E. and SILVERS, W. K. (1960). *Ann. Surg.*, **152**, 975.
28. BULLOUGH, W. S. (1966). In "Wound Healing", p. 43, ed. by Illingworth, C. London: Churchill.
29. BULLOUGH, W. S. (1968). In "The Biological Basis of Medicine", vol. 1, p. 311, ed. by Bittar, E. E. and Bittar, N. London and New York: Academic Press.

*Chapter 9*

# HEALING IN SPECIALIZED TISSUES

It is generally stated that the greater the degree of specialization of a tissue, the less well developed are its powers of regeneration. Certainly nerve cells are highly specialized and incapable of division, but degrees of specialization in cells are as difficult to define as they are amongst human beings. Is a liver cell more or less specialized than a simple unstriped muscle fibre? Liver cells show remarkable powers of proliferation, yet perform functions of which they alone are capable. Similarly, it is impossible to compare the degrees of specialization of the different types of epithelium, each of which has its own peculiar characteristics. It seems more likely that the power of regeneration is best developed in those organs and tissues which are most liable to injury, and the replacement of which has survival value for the individual and species.

## EPITHELIAL TISSUES

All covering epithelia show good regenerative power. This is hardly surprising since they are being continuously subjected to trauma, and their integrity depends upon their ability to replace the lost cells. Glandular epithelia, on the other hand, show erratic regenerative capacity.

### Covering Epithelia[1,2]
#### Squamous Epithelium of Skin

This shows good regeneration, although specialized structures like the rete ridges, hair follicles, sweat glands, and sebaceous glands are not replaced in man. The details of the epithelial changes in skin wounds, involving both movement and division of cells, have already been described (Chapter 8).

#### Oral Epithelium

Complete regeneration occurs. The lamina propria and submucosa heal by repair, and scar tissue may remain in the lining mucosa but not in the masticatory mucosa.

#### Intestinal Epithelium

Complete regeneration results in perfect replacement of lost epithelium, including, in the case of the small intestine, the crypts and villi. It is noteworthy that because there is normally a very high rate of mitotic activity in the epithelium of the small intestine, no further increase occurs at the wound margins. In passing, it should be noted that the remainder of the gut wall, including the muscularis mucosae, heals by scar tissue.

#### Stomach

Here epithelial regeneration is good. Acute ulceration of the mucosa of the stomach is a common event, but healing occurs rapidly and without any scarring, because the underlying specialized connective tissue and muscle are not destroyed. In chronic peptic ulcers epithelial regeneration is inhibited, the reason for which is not known. When healing does occur, the newly-formed epithelium may be of intestinal type, even showing well-marked villi.

## Respiratory Tract

Loss of epithelium, such as occurs in acute influenzal tracheobronchitis, is quickly followed by the division of basal cells leading to a reformation of ciliated pseudostratified columnar epithelium. Sometimes after repeated damage the new epithelium may change to simple columnar or squamous type (see metaplasia, p. 237).

## Glandular Epithelium

### Liver[3,4]

The liver has remarkable powers of regeneration. In the rat resection of three-quarters of the organ results in such active division of the remaining cells that within two weeks the organ is restored to its original weight. The process could be regarded as a simple type of reconstitution, because it involves the co-ordinated growth of liver cells, blood vessels, bile ducts, etc.

In man regeneration of liver cells is seen following any type of necrosis, provided the patient survives. The end-results of this regeneration vary so widely, depending upon the type of hepatic necrosis, that this important subject will be considered in Chapter 31.

### Kidney

The renal tubular epithelium has considerable powers of regeneration; thus in acute tubular necrosis, in spite of extensive damage, complete return to normal may occur. This type of lesion is therefore most eligible for treatment with the artificial kidney, since recovery is quite possible. When damage to the kidney results in destruction of a complete nephron, regeneration does not occur. Glomeruli once destroyed cannot be replaced.

## CONNECTIVE TISSUES

When conditions are favourable many of the specialized connective tissues show excellent regeneration. However, not infrequently adverse factors operate and these result in healing by repair.

### Mesothelial Lining of Peritoneum and Other Serous Cavities[5,3]

Lost mesothelial cells are replaced from underlying connective tissue cells, which take on the appearance of flattened mesothelium. It has also been suggested that desquamated mesothelial cells can alight on the raw surface.

### Synovium[6]

Synovial lining cells are also replaced from underlying connective tissue. The adjacent uninjured synovial cells are inert, and play no part in the process of healing.

### Vascular Endothelium[7,8,9]

In large arteries, e.g. the aorta, new endothelial cells arise by mitotic division of pre-existing ones, and slowly spread over the denuded area. It has been suggested that endothelial cells can also develop from deposited circulating mononuclear cells, but the evidence for this is not good.[10]

## Fat

Although fat cells may appear in fully mature granulation tissue, defects in fatty tissue are usually made good by fibrous tissue. The process of repair shows a remarkable feature during the demolition phase; the macrophages ingest large quantities of fat, becoming greatly swollen in the process. These *foam cells* form a prominent feature of traumatic fat necrosis (p. 54).

## Cartilage[11]

Regeneration in cartilage is generally poor. In the case of the hyaline cartilage of joint surfaces small defects are made good by regeneration. With larger injuries which involve damage to the underlying vascular bone, there is formed a haematoma which becomes vascularized and converted either into fibrous tissue or bone.

## Tendon[12]

Regeneration in tendon is good, but the process is slow. It is said that the tendon ends should be accurately opposed and under some tension, otherwise union is by scar tissue.

## Muscle[13,14]

It is generally taught that damaged muscle is not replaced, and that union is by scar tissue. In large destructive lesions of unstriped muscle a permanent scar remains to mark the site of the original injury, and this is well illustrated by the appearance of a healed chronic gastric ulcer. Although unstriped muscle cells appear incapable of division in postuterine life, the arterioles of granulation tissue acquire a muscular coat; the origin of these fibres is not known. There is also experimental evidence that smooth-muscle regeneration occurs when the taenia of the guinea-pig caecum is crushed.[15] Thus it would appear that smooth (unstriped) muscle has limited powers of regeneration.

In respect of striated muscle, when part of an individual muscle fibre is damaged, there may be limited regeneration with the production of new myocytes which later fuse to form a syncytial mass.[16] In a clean surgical wound of voluntary muscle, the sarcolemmal masses on either side of the incision may unite, so that the continuity of the muscle is restored, and in time no indication of the site of injury can be found. However, with extensive damage to muscle the architecture is destroyed, and healing is by scar tissue; this is seen following infarction.

Cardiac muscle shows no regenerative capacity, and once necrosis has occurred, as in infarction, a permanent scar remains. Under special circumstances cardiac muscle cells may form giant cells similar to those seen in voluntary muscle. It has been suggested that the Aschoff giant cell of rheumatic fever is of this nature (p. 395).

## Bone Marrow

Bone marrow provides an excellent example of tissue in which regeneration is complete.

## Bone

The regeneration of bone as seen in the healing of a fracture is described in Chapter 33.

### Nervous Tissue

Adult nerve cells are unable to divide and therefore when ·a part of the brain or spinal cord is destroyed, new neurones are not produced.

## Peripheral Nervous System[17-19]

Following section of the axis cylinder the nerve cell shows changes described as *chromatolysis*. The cell swells and its Nissl granules disappear. These bodies are zones of endoplasmic reticulum studded plentifully with ribosomes, and their disappearance reflects dysfunction in the protein-synthetizing system of the nerve cell. The axis cylinder becomes irregular and varicose, and by 48 hours has broken up. The surrounding myelin shows splitting of the laminae, and later fragmentation. The Schwann cells enlarge, proliferate, and become filled with lipid droplets from the degenerated myelin. These changes were originally described as *Wallerian degeneration*. They affect the nerve fibre distal to the point of section and also, in myelinated fibres, a short area proximally up to the first node of Ranvier. The next stage is described as regeneration, but it should be remembered that it entails rather more than mere replacement of the lost part of an individual cell. From the proximal portion of the cut axon numerous neurofibrils sprout out, and are seen to lie invaginated into the cytoplasm of the Schwann cells. They push their way distally through the Schwann cells at the rate of about 1 mm. per day. Many of the fibrils lose their way and degenerate, but some reach an appropriate end-organ, and persist to form the definitive replacement axon. It is evident that accurate apposition of the cut ends of the nerve is of great importance in facilitating this process. The final process involves the reformation of the myelin sheath as the regenerating axon matures and increases in diameter.

The functional end-result of nerve damage depends on various factors: if the axons are damaged but the nerve trunk itself is not severed, an excellent result may be expected. When the nerve is severed, careful suturing and absence of infection are important. Functional recovery is more complete when a pure motor or sensory nerve is cut. Recovery from a lesion of a mixed nerve, like the median nerve of the forearm, is often poor.

## Central Nervous System[20-22]

Here oligodendroglia take the place of the Schwann cells in relation to nerve fibres. It is often stated that regeneration of central nerve fibres does not occur. The affected nerve cells show chromatolysis often followed by necrosis, and the destroyed tissue is replaced by proliferating neuroglia to form a dense glial scar. Nevertheless, there is considerable evidence that some regeneration is possible. In the clinical field it is noticeable that in patients with partial spinal-cord lesions, voluntary muscle strength seems to increase steadily for 9–12 months. This is generally attributed to improved utilization of residual undamaged pathways. In the lower animals regeneration of the long-tract axons in the spinal cord is a usual feature, and it is possible that some regeneration may occur in the higher animals, including man.

## References

1. McMinn, R. M. H. (1960). *Ann. roy. Coll. Surg. Engl.*, **26**, 245.
2. Johnson, F. R. and McMinn, R. M. H. (1960). *Biol. Rev.*, **35**, 364.
3. Harkness, R. D. (1961). In "The Scientific Basis of Medicine Annual Reviews", p. 236. London: Athlone Press.
4. Weinbren, K. (1966). In "Wound Healing", ed. Illingworth, C., p. 69. London: Churchill.
5. Russell, P. S. and Billingham, R. E. (1962). *Progr. Surg. (Basel)*, **2**, 1.
6. Levene, A. (1957). *J. Path. Bact.*, **73**, 87.
7. Poole, J. C. F., Sanders, A. G. and Florey, H. W. (1958). *J. Path. Bact.*, **75**, 133.
8. Poole, J. C. F., Sanders, A. G. and Florey, H. W. (1959). *J. Path. Bact.*, **77**, 637.
9. Ghani, A. R. and Tibbs, D. J. (1962). *Brit. med. J.*, **1**, 1244.
10. Leading Article (1967). *Lancet*, **2**, 1239.
11. Bennett, G. A., Bauer, W. and Maddock, S. J. (1932). *Amer. J. Path.*, **8**, 499.
12. Buck, R. C. (1953). *J. Path. Bact.*, **66**, 1.
13. Adams, R. D., Denny-Brown, D. and Pearson, C. M. (1962). "Diseases of Muscle", 2nd ed. New York: Hoeber.
14. Gay, A. J. and Hunt, T. E. (1954). *Anat. Rec.*, **120**, 853.
15. McGeachie, J. K. (1971). *Experientia*, **27**, 436.
16. Editorial (1971). *New Engl. J. Med.*, **284**, 1033.
17. Seddon, H. J. (1954). Edr. "Peripheral Nerve Injuries". Medical Research Council Report, London H.M.S.O.
18. Guth, L. (1956). *Physiol. Rev.*, **36**, 441.
19. Nathaniel, E. J. H. and Pease, D. C. (1963). *J. Ultrastruct. Res.*, **9**, 511.
20. Windle, W. F. (1955). Edr. "Regeneration in the Central Nervous System". Springfield, Ill: Thomas.
21. McMasters, R. E. (1962). *J. comp. Neurol.*, **119**, 113.
22. Clemente, C. D. (1964). *Int. Rev. Neurobiol.*, **6**, 257.

*Chapter 10*

# CHRONIC INFLAMMATION

Although the concept of chronic inflammation is in part a clinical one implying that the inflammatory process persists for a long period, pathologically it is best defined as *a process in which destruction and inflammation are proceeding at the same time as attempts at healing.*

The tissue response to injury has been divided into three phases: the initial vascular and exudative phenomena of *acute inflammation* are followed by a second phase of *demolition* which is accomplished by macrophage activity. The third and final phase is one of *healing*, by which lost tissue is replaced by the processes of *repair* and *regeneration*.

It is evident that complete healing can occur only when the acute inflammation and demolition phases are themselves completed. Since these are the consequences of the initial damage, it follows that healing results only when the cause of the inflammation is itself removed. If tissue damage continues, a disease process develops in which there is present a mixture of the phenomena of acute inflammation, demolition, repair, and regeneration. To such a lesion the term chronic inflammation is applied.

## Causes of Chronic Inflammation

Since all agents which cause cell damage initiate an acute inflammatory response, they may, if they persist, also lead to chronic inflammation. In this way insoluble particles such as silica and asbestos may readily cause chronic inflammation. Organisms, like the tubercle bacillus, against which the body has only a limited resistance, are other important causes. Moreover, if local or general conditions impair the body's defences, an organism which usually produces a transient acute inflammation may persist to cause a chronic one. Any of the causes of delayed healing (p. 111) may so load the scales against the host that there develops the frustrated healing which chronic inflammation has so aptly been called. Finally a state of hypersensitivity, if persistent, may lead to exuberant chronic inflammatory reactions. This is seen in many chronic infective diseases of which tuberculosis is a prototype, and is also important in non-infective conditions, such as allergic contact dermatitis (p. 133) and rheumatoid arthritis.

## Classification of Chronic Inflammation

Chronic inflammation may be classified in several ways, none of which is ideal.

(1) Clinical.
(2) Specific and non-specific.
(3) Histological.
(4) Granulomatous and non-granulomatous.

**Clinical.** Although chronic inflammation may follow in the wake of obvious acute inflammation, some irritants (e.g. tubercle bacillus) cause a mild or fleeting acute reaction which clinically may be completely missed. Nevertheless, they persist and lead to the development of a chronic disease. Clinically therefore two types of chronic inflammation may be described:

(a)  Secondary to acute inflammation.
(b)  Starting *de novo*.

**Specific and Non-specific.** It is customary to subdivide chronic inflammation in another way. Certain irritants cause a tissue reaction which is histologically characteristic. By examining such a lesion one can deduce its cause without either seeing or isolating the causative agent. Such a lesion is said to be *specific*. Tuberculosis, leprosy, and syphilis are included under this heading, and may be contrasted with the lesions of pyogenic organisms which are *non-specific*. Unfortunately, many lesions encountered in the specific diseases are not histologically characteristic, and therefore, strictly speaking, the term specific should not be used. Thus while the histological appearance of a gumma is fairly typical, the lesions of secondary syphilis are by no means diagnostic. The reaction is non-specific. Nevertheless, syphilis is still called a specific infection even though this is not justified in terms of the original conception. The distinction between "specific" and "non-specific" is now quite artificial.

**Histological.** The histological features of a chronic inflammatory lesion may be used in descriptive classification. Where polymorphs abound and abscess formation is present, the lesion may justly be called a *chronic suppurative inflammation*. Likewise when epithelioid cells are found grouped together in follicles resembling those found in tuberculosis, the term *tuberculoid* is frequently applied. Three variants occur:

*Non-caseating tuberculoid reaction*, as seen in sarcoidosis (Fig. 15.6).
*Caseating tuberculoid reaction*, as commonly seen in tuberculosis (Fig. 15.2).
*Suppurative tuberculoid reaction*, in which small abscesses filled with polymorphs are formed and are surrounded by a mantle of epithelioid cells. This is an uncommon reaction and is seen in coccidioidomycosis and lymphogranuloma venereum.

**Granulomatous and Non-granulomatous.** Some chronic inflammations are characterized by the formation of tumour-like masses composed of granulation tissue which is heavily infiltrated with inflammatory cells. These inflammations are sometimes called *granulomatous*, and such a reaction is frequently to be found in tuberculosis. By convention this disease and certain other chronic infections are often called the *specific infective granulomata*. It must be stressed that in fact not all lesions in these diseases are granulomatous, and that tumour-like masses can occur in other chronic inflammations not generally called granulomata, e.g. silicosis.

*Granulomatous inflammation* is a term frequently used but rarely defined with precision. To some, including Virchow, it implies the presence of granulation tissue, but most writers use the term to describe a chronic inflammatory reaction in which there is a *preponderance of macrophages*. A diffuse accumulation of parasitized macrophages as occurs in lepromatous leprosy and histoplasmosis may therefore be called a granulomatous reaction. However, other writers imply that a tuberculoid reaction with epithelioid cells and giant cells is a prerequisite of granulomatous inflammation. Nevertheless, they usually include actinomycosis in this group even though the lesions are typically suppurative. It is evident that granulomatous inflammation as a term has no generally accepted precise meaning, and it is wise not to use it, unless its application is first defined. Indeed, it is obvious that many of the terms used in the classification of chronic inflammation are both ambiguous and imprecise.

## Features of Chronic Inflammation

These are best considered under the headings of the three component reactions which together constitute chronic inflammation.

### Acute Inflammation

This is particularly well marked in chronic suppurative disease, for example osteomyelitis, empyema, and chronic brain abscess, to mention only a few examples. It is also typical of actinomycosis. Pus, rich in polymorphonuclear leucocytes, is very evident, and fibrin may not only be seen microscopically, but on occasions forms large masses easily visible to the naked eye. Fluid exudation is also a feature of chronic suppurative disease, and if drained the continued protein loss may lead to hypoalbuminaemia (p. 329). Accumulations of protein-rich fluid are frequent in chronic inflammation of the serous sacs, e.g. tuberculous peritonitis.

Eosinophils are sometimes present in large numbers in the exudate in chronic inflammation. Whether this is a manifestation of hypersensitivity is not known.

### Demolition

This is accomplished by *macrophages*. The source of these cells is disputed. They could be formed by division of local histiocytes, and on this assumption chronic inflammatory lesions which have a marked macrophage reaction are called *proliferative*. The small lymphocyte has also been regarded as a parent cell of the macrophage (see p. 69), but the current view is against this, and under special circumstances other tissue cells may well become phagocytic, e.g. Schwann cells.

On the other hand, it is now accepted that the macrophages are altered monocytes which have migrated from the blood as an exudative phenomenon; recent evidence has shown that these cells also divide. Whatever may be the truth, an *exudative lesion* is by common consent defined as one showing acute inflammation with an exudate of plasma, fibrin, and polymorphonuclears. The term "proliferative" is still retained for mononuclear reactions regardless of the origin of these cells.

In some chronic inflammatory lesions the macrophages enlarge, develop abundant eosinophilic cytoplasm, and lose their phagocytic power. They are then called *epithelioid cells* because of the superficial resemblance they bear to the cells of squamous epithelium. Such cells tend to be grouped into follicles or tubercles.

When macrophages encounter insoluble material they frequently fuse together to form *giant cells*. This occurs around exogenous foreign bodies like silk and talc, as well as around endogenous debris such as pieces of dead bone (sequestra), cholesterol crystals, and uric acid crystals. They are also formed in response to certain organisms such as the tubercle bacillus and many fungi. Two forms of these giant cells have been described.

*Langhans Giant Cell*. The nuclei are disposed around the periphery of the cell in the form of a horseshoe or a ring. These cells are particularly frequent in tuberculous lesions (see Fig. 15.1).

*Foreign-body Giant Cell*. In this type the nuclei are scattered haphazardly throughout the cytoplasm. In many lesions giant cells of both Langhans and foreign-body type are present, and the two should not be regarded as distinct types (Fig. 10.4).

## Features of Healing

**Repair.** Granulation tissue is prominent in many chronic inflammatory lesions. It contains:

(1) Endothelial cells forming blood and lymphatic vessels.
(2) Fibroblasts forming collagen.
(3) Small round cells—lymphocytes and plasma cells.

The vascularity of the granulation tissue may give rise to haemorrhage. Thus bleeding occurs from the base of chronic peptic ulcers, the inflamed dilated bronchi in bronchiectasis, and in chronic gingivitis.

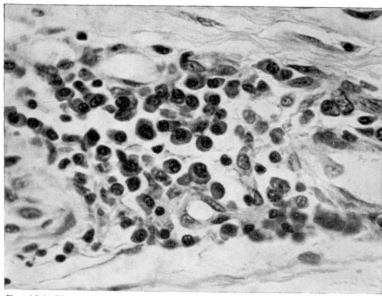

Fig. 10.1. Plasma cells. Note the round or pear-shaped contour of the cells and their eccentric nuclei with the cart-wheel disposition of clumped chromatin. The rather darkly-staining nature of the cytoplasm is due to its high content of RNA. The section was taken from an area of chronic inflammation. × 400.

In chronic suppuration, the pus-filled cavity is lined by acutely inflamed granulation tissue which forms a pyogenic membrane.

Fibroblasts are prominent in most chronic inflammations. They lay down collagen, and the resulting scar formation is characteristic of many chronic inflammatory lesions. It is seen in fibroid tuberculosis, chronic ulcerative colitis, deep in the base of a chronic peptic ulcer, and in the wall of an abscess. If fibrin is the hallmark of acute inflammation, fibrosis can be considered the salient feature of chronic inflammation. As scarring proceeds the lumina of small arteries and arterioles are gradually obliterated by thickening of the tunica intima. This process is called *endarteritis obliterans*. Ultimately a mass of dense avascular scar tissue is formed. Cicatrization may ensue and produce serious effects. For instance a chronic ulcer of the pylorus may lead to narrowing and obstruction of the lumen (pyloric stenosis).

A feature of chronic inflammation which is worthy of special note is the accumulation of lymphocytes and plasma cells (Fig. 10.1). Together these are called the cells of chronic inflammation, or *small round cells*. Their significance is poorly understood. Although they are present in small numbers in the granulation tissue of a healing wound, they are more abundant in chronic inflammatory granulation tissue. Frequently they assume a perivascular distribution, e.g. in syphilitic aortitis, and are presumably derived from the blood rather than from local lymphoid tissue or stem cells. There is little doubt that the plasma cells are concerned with the local production of immunoglobulins. They are particularly prominent in inflammatory lesions involving the skin adjacent to mucocutaneous junctions and the mucous membranes themselves. Chronic gingivitis is characterized by a massive plasma-cell infiltration. Occasionally a plasma cell is seen to contain one or more spherical, eosinophilic, PAS-positive, hyaline structures called *Russell bodies*. When the cell dies these are released into the stroma. They are of no great significance, but should not be mistaken for fungi.

The function of the lymphocytes is less well understood. They may form a mobile reserve for other cells, and some authorities regard them as precursors of plasma cells, macrophages, and fibroblasts. They also play a part in the immune response (p. 144), and as noted elsewhere cells which have the morphology of small lymphocytes may have different origins and functions. For this reason the term "small round cells" is convenient, for it distinguishes them from polymorphs and obvious macrophages.

**Regeneration.** When the tissue destroyed in chronic inflammation is of a type capable of division, regeneration rather than repair takes place. This is particularly obvious in surface epithelia. Indeed, regeneration may become so exuberant that the line of demarcation between it, hyperplasia, and neoplasia may be difficult to define. For this reason, cancer has frequently been ascribed to "chronic irritation" (pp. 233 and 275).

The epithelial overgrowth at the edge of a chronic ulcer is sometimes quite remarkable, and may be misinterpreted by the unwary as cancer. The greatly divergent views expressed in the past on the frequency of malignant change in chronic peptic ulcer are largely due to the difficulties in interpreting the microscopic appearances at the edge of the ulcer.

The position is complicated by the fact that malignancy may indeed supervene on the exuberant regeneration of chronic inflammation. This is sometimes seen in chronic ulcerative colitis.

## General Effects of Chronic Inflammation

The general effects of chronic inflammation depend upon the nature of the responsible agent and the extent of the lesion. In a localized foreign-body reaction there is no noteworthy response at all. On the other hand, in chronic infective disease like tuberculosis or actinomycosis there may be widespread changes in the RE system and in the blood stream. Remarkably little is known about the exact mechanisms involved.

### Changes in the Reticulo-Endothelial System

Apart from the local accumulation of RE macrophages already described, the lymph nodes draining a chronic inflammatory lesion show hyperplasia. This may sometimes affect the sinus-lining cells ("sinus catarrh"), while at other times there is a marked increase in the number of germinal centres or small lymphocytes. These changes are related to the development of an immune response.

If organisms or their toxins gain access to the blood stream there may be a more generalized hyperplasia of the RE cells, producing enlargement of the spleen (splenomegaly) and lymph nodes (lymphadenopathy). Sometimes this is related to formation of antigen-antibody complexes in the blood stream, which are subsequently removed by the RE system. In other instances, e.g. leishmaniasis, there is a widespread parasitization of the RE cells.

### The Immune Response

Antibody production is a prominent feature of most chronic inflammatory diseases. The antibodies may be immunoglobulins or of the cell-bound variety. The importance of hypersensitivity in chronic inflammation is described in Chapter 13.

The immune response may be reflected in definite morphological changes, and is an additional factor in the production of splenomegaly and generalized lymphadenopathy. Hypergammaglobulinaemia may occur, and finally the long-continued stress on the antibody-producing mechanism can lead to amyloid disease (p. 332).

### Changes in the Blood

The white cells frequently show changes which are related to the causative agent and to the extent of infection. These are considered later (p. 349). *Anaemia* is frequent, and is usually of the normochromic normocytic type. Repeated haemorrhages may lead to a hypochromic microcytic anaemia.

A rise in the erythrocyte sedimentation rate (ESR) occurs in many chronic inflammatory diseases, and is commonly used as an aid both to diagnosis and in assessing progress, e.g. in tuberculosis and rheumatoid arthritis (p. 331).

### Other Changes

Although "toxaemia" is put forward as the explanation of many of the general symptoms, it cannot be regarded as anything more than a cloak for our ignorance. The following signs and symptoms are frequent and attributed to this state: tiredness, malaise, headaches, loss of appetite (anorexia), loss of weight, anaemia, loss of libido, and pyrexia.

Toxaemia is often assumed to be due to the liberation of endotoxins, but although such substances have been isolated from some organisms, e.g. *Esch. coli*, there are others, like the *Tr. pallidum*, in which no such endotoxins are known. Possibly toxic substances are formed when tissue is damaged either as a result of bacterial action or hypersensitivity. However, there is no direct evidence as to the nature of the endotoxins or the products of tissue damage which are responsible for the "toxaemia" of infection.

## Examples of Chronic Inflammation

The types of chronic inflammation can be graded as follows; those due to:

(*a*) Non-specific, pyogenic bacterial agents like *Staph. pyogenes* and *E. coli*.
(*b*) Inanimate foreign bodies.
(*c*) "Specific" organisms, e.g. tubercle bacillus. This third group is so important that it is dealt with separately in Chapter 15.
(*d*) Ionizing radiation. This is described in Chapter 21.
(*e*) Hypersensitivity. This is discussed in Chapter 13. The collagen diseases can be conveniently included in this group, though their aetiology is obscure.

The first group embraces a wide collection of conditions which are very commonly encountered in clinical practice. For the purpose of this discussion two important examples have been selected.

### Osteomyelitis

Acute osteomyelitis occurs most often in children at the metaphysis of one of the long bones of the lower limbs. This is the area which is most easily traumatized, and should this occur during the course of a *Staph. pyogenes* bacteraemia, the organisms become lodged and produce a metastatic lesion. A typical acute inflammatory reaction occurs, and owing to the rigidity of the bone the increased tension produced by the exudation causes compression of the blood vessels and subsequent ischaemia. Necrosis of marrow and bone therefore follows: pus is formed, and it tracks under the periosteum, thereby further imperilling the blood supply to the cortex. In this way quite extensive necrosis may occur, sometimes involving the whole shaft. This sequestrum acts as a foreign body; it cannot be easily removed, and it not only provides a focus for growth of organisms but also prevents adequate drainage of pus. Conditions are ideal for the development of chronic infection.

Pus ruptures through the periosteum into the muscular and subcutaneous compartments. Usually it is discharged on to the skin surface through sinuses.* The vascular periosteum attempts to reform the shaft of the bone by producing bone. This encases the sequestrated shaft, and is called the *involucrum* (Fig. 10.2). The shaft is bathed in pus which escapes through holes, or *cloacae*, in the involucrum, and is then discharged to the surface. Osteoclasts

---

* A *sinus* is an abnormal channel, often lined by epithelium, which leads from the interior of the body to a free surface.

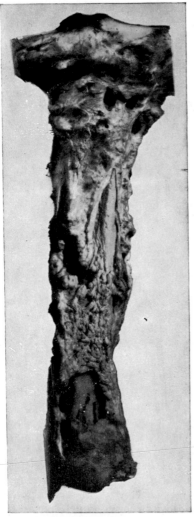

FIG. 10.2. Osteomyelitis of tibia. The extensive central sequestrum is largely encased in an exuberant involucrum formed from the detached periosteum. There is a cloaca at the base of the shaft, and through it the pitted sequestrum is clearly visible.

(HS44.1. *Reproduced by permission of the President and Council of the Royal College of Surgeons of England.*)

slowly erode the sequestrum, detaching it at each end from living bone and slowly destroying it. This must be completed before healing can be accomplished. In practice this is seldom possible without elaborate surgical intervention. If nothing is done, the condition may lead to death as the result of pyaemia, "toxaemia", or amyloid disease.

Chronic osteomyelitis is fortunately uncommon nowadays since the advent of antibiotic therapy, which is used in combination with early surgical drainage in the acute stage.

From a pathological point of view the disease illustrates many points. It shows how an acute infection can become chronic due to inadequate drainage of pus, as well as to the presence of a foreign body, in this case the sequestrum. Moreover, all the features of chronic inflammation are present. Acute inflammation is evident by the polymorphonuclear and fluid exudate, demolition by macrophages and osteoclastic activity, regeneration by bone formation, and repair by the surrounding scarring.

### Chronic Ulcerative Colitis[1]

Chronic inflammatory lesions of the colon may follow specific infections by the *Shigella* species (bacillary dysentery) or *Entamoeba histolytica*, but the commonest lesion of this type in temperate climates is idiopathic ulcerative colitis. This disease may commence as an acute fulminating condition which may either lead to rapid death, or else follow a more chronic course. Often the lesion is insidious and chronic from the beginning.

The first changes involve the mucosa, which is acutely inflamed. Small abscesses in the crypts are characteristic.

As the disease progresses, the mucosa becomes ulcerated, and the inflammation spreads into the submucosa, which is gradually destroyed and replaced by granulation tissue containing lymphocytes and plasma cells. The colon becomes rigid and shortened due mainly to hypertrophy of the muscle coat. Fibrosis is not marked. An increase of subserous fat may also occur—this is quite common in chronically-inflamed, shrunken organs. The cause is unknown.

The mucosal disease causes chronic diarrhoea in which blood, pus, and mucus are present in the faeces. This is an example of catarrhal inflammation. The surviving islets of epithelium regenerate profusely, and may produce the appearance of pedunculated nodules (Fig. 10.3). In about 4 per cent of cases cancer of the colon supervenes.[2,3]

### Tissue Response to Insoluble Inanimate Foreign Materials

The tissue response to these substances is very complex, but with the increasing use of metals and plastics in reconstructive surgery, it is a matter of considerable importance. In the root treatment of non-vital teeth a variety of compounds have been used. As they are in contact with vital tissues in the apical region, it is important that they should be non-irritant. Research on some of these compounds shows that, although most of them cause an inflammatory response when first inserted, this usually subsides within a few weeks.[4] It is probably true to state that all foreign materials are capable of producing an inflammatory response under certain circumstances. Nothing is truly inert. The factors which determine the severity of the inflammatory response are not completely understood, but the following are important:[5]

**The Chemical Nature of the Material.** The chemical stability and solubility are of great importance; thus stainless steel is more inert than ordinary steel.

**Physical State of Substance.** Smooth, highly-polished surfaces provoke much less reaction than do rough, irregular surfaces. It is important to bear this in mind when inserting metal prostheses or pins. Finely divided or colloidal substances are particularly irritating. Nylon has been used in joint reconstruction, but the scratching and powdering which occur during use lead to a brisk foreign-body reaction.[6]

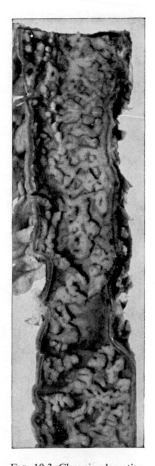

FIG. 10.3. Chronic ulcerative colitis with pseudopolyposis. Note that the intervening mucosa is roughened and inflamed, and that the bowel wall is considerably shortened. The regenerative pseudopolyps are to be distinguished from true neoplastic polyposis coli by the accompanying inflammatory change.

(EA70.1. *Reproduced by permission of the President and Council of the Royal College of Surgeons of England.*)

**Electro-Chemical Potentials.** These are set up by the close proximity of dissimilar metals, and cause tissue damage. This is particularly important in orthopaedic and traumatic surgery. Plates and screws must all be of exactly the same composition, otherwise there is sufficient reaction to cause loosening of the screws. Even the metal scraped off the screwdriver may be enough to produce this effect.

The relatively insoluble foreign materials cannot be removed by the inflammatory reaction which they excite, and it follows that the lesions induced are typically chronic in character. Giant cells abound, and while most of these are of the foreign-body type, Langhans giant cells are also seen.

The extent of the reaction to foreign material depends on the nature of the material itself. A few important examples will be cited.

**Carbon.** Tattooing consists of introducing carbon or cinnabar into the dermis. It excites a mild inflammatory response and is soon taken up by macrophages, in which it remains in the tissues indefinitely. The small amount of carbon which is deposited in the lungs of city-dwellers likewise causes little damage.

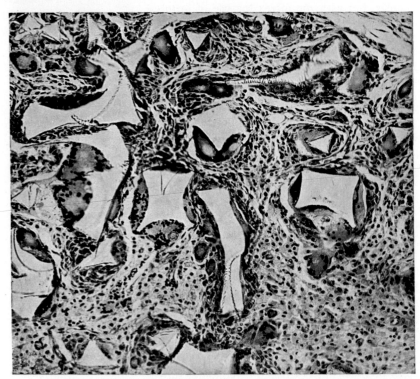

Fig. 10.4. Foreign-body reaction to an Etheron sponge implanted for 40 days subcutaneously in a rat. The clear areas were occupied by fragments of sponge which have been dislodged during processing. They are surrounded by giant cells, mostly of the Langhans type with peripherally disposed nuclei. Only a few resemble typical foreign-body giant cells. × 150.

**Metals.**[7] Vitallium and stainless steel cause little reaction when used in the form of polished plates, pins, arthroplasty cups, dental implants, etc. Tantalum, titanium, and zirconium are also used for their inertness. Other metals, e.g. iron, produce much more reaction, and in certain situations, e.g. the eye, can lead to serious damage.

**Dental Implants.** There are four main types of dental implants: the subperiosteal implant, the needle (or pin), the screw, and the blade. These implants are inserted beneath the oral mucosa with a break in continuity, where a post projects through to support a crown, bridge, or denture. The material usually used is chrome cobalt.

Histological examination shows fibrous tissue around the subperiosteal implant. Probably it is the contracture of this tissue which causes physical retention of the implant.

**Suture Material.**[8,9] Catgut excites a brisk acute inflammatory reaction which is soon followed by an infiltration of macrophages and giant cells. The strength of the plain catgut is reduced to half within two days, while for chromic catgut the time is 10 days. Plain catgut is therefore unreliable, and should be discarded from general use. Fine chromic catgut should be used whenever absorbable material is indicated. The tissue reaction to nylon, linen, etc. does not readily remove the material, which therefore persists for a long period (Fig. 10.4).

**Silica.**[10] Small particles of silica are inhaled during the course of certain occupations like mining. An inflammatory response ensues in the interstitial tissues of the lungs, and this is later followed by dense nodular fibrosis. The precise manner by which silica causes such extensive destruction of lung is not known. It is thought that an immunological reaction is involved. The silica may react with tissue proteins to form an antigen which stimulates antibody formation. The subsequent antigen-antibody reaction causes tissue damage.

Many other dusts when inhaled into the lungs induce an inflammatory response which terminates in fibrosis. Such diseases are called the *pneumoconioses*. Silicosis and asbestosis are the most important.

### References

1. LUMB, G. and PROTHEROE, R. H. B. (1955). *Lancet*, **2**, 1208.
2. HINTON, J. M. (1966). *Gut*, **7**, 427.
3. Leading Article (1967). *Brit. med. J.*, **1**, 322.
4. FRIEND, L. A. and BROWNE, R. M. (1968). *Brit. Dent. J.*, **125**, 291.
5. WATSON-JONES, R. (1955). In "Fractures and Joint Injuries", 4th ed., p. 205. Edinburgh: Livingstone.
6. SCALES, J. T. (1953). *J. Bone Jt. Surg.*, **35B**, 6.
7. Various Authors (1957). *Lancet*, **1**, 1174.
8. LAWRIE, P., ANGUS, G. E. and REESE, A. J. M. (1959). *Brit. J. Surg.*, **46**, 638.
9. LAWRIE, P., ANGUS, G. E. and REESE, A. J. M. (1960). *Brit. J. Surg.*, **47**, 551.
10. GOUGH, J. (1959). In "Modern Trends in Pathology", p. 273, ed. by Collins, D. H. London: Butterworths.

*Chapter 11*

# THE IMMUNE RESPONSE

## Introduction

One of the characteristic features of the adult animal is its ability to distinguish between its own constituents ("self") and those of external, or foreign, origin ("non-self"). Foreign material excites a reaction which results in the elimination of the alien matter. Since many of the foreign substances encountered are living organisms or their toxins, it follows that the reaction results in immunity to infection or limitation of its spread. For this reason the reaction is called the *immune response*. Presumably it has been evolved by animals during evolution as a means of self-preservation in a world teeming with micro-organisms.

The immune response is a reaction to foreign material which results in the formation of antibodies. These may be either *immunoglobulins* or *cell-bound*. It is believed that at least two separate systems are involved. The lymphoid tissue with *T lymphocytes* is associated developmentally with the *thymus* and is responsible for the production of cell-bound antibodies. Immuno-globulins are formed in lymphoid tissue, containing *B lymphocytes*, which is developmentally dependent on the *bursa of Fabricius* in birds, or possibly the gut-associated lymphoid tissue in animals.

Under certain circumstances the elimination of foreign material is accom-panied by a severe reaction—sometimes more severe than that caused by the material itself. The term *hypersensitivity* is therefore applied to such a reaction. It is evident that the "immune response" is not concerned solely with immunity to infection, and for this reason it will be considered first in a general way rather than being linked with either immunity or hypersensitivity.

## Properties of Antigens[1]

Any agent which is regarded as non-self is called an *antigen*, and is capable of causing an immune response. This is often manifested by the development of specific globulins in the plasma called *antibodies*. These will be considered in detail later in this chapter, but it should be noted here that *antibodies are highly specific*, i.e. they react with the antigen which gave rise to them but to no other.

Antigens are high-molecular-weight substances, nearly always proteins, and are recognized as foreign by special features of their chemical structure—probably by particular configurations of their external shape. The areas of the molecular surface which are concerned are called *determinant sites*, or *epitopes*.[2] It is possible to add new epitopes to a protein by the addition of quite simple chemical substances called *haptens*. The antigenic properties of the protein are altered by this procedure such that if it is introduced into a

132

suitable animal, the antibodies which are produced are specific for the hapten. Thus haptens are substances which are not antigenic in themselves, but which behave as antigens when combined with a suitable carrier protein. They are of great importance in human pathology as a simple example will illustrate: iodine is not an antigen, but if applied to the skin of some individuals it acts as a hapten, and will combine with body proteins so that a new antigenic complex is formed. This stimulates the production of antibodies which are specific for iodine. The next occasion on which iodine is applied to the skin a damaging antigen-antibody reaction occurs and this produces a severe inflammatory response (*allergic contact dermatitis*).*

Between the two extremes of simple chemical hapten and true protein antigen there are many intermediate compounds, often polysaccharides and lipids, which are weakly antigenic when acting alone but powerfully so when combined with protein.

## The Antibody Response[3,4]

The antibodies formed as a result of an antigenic stimulus are of two types:

1. *Cell-bound Antibodies.* These are related to changes in lymphocytes. They are difficult to detect.

2. *Plasma Antibodies.* These are the classical antibodies of immunology, and will be described in some detail.

When antigen is introduced into the body it is taken up by large phagocytic cells of the RE system.[5,6] Following subcutaneous injection this occurs both locally and in the regional lymph nodes. With intravenous injection it is the sinus-lining cells of the bone marrow, spleen, and liver which are principally involved. This taking up by the RE cells appears to be the first step in the immune response.[5] The next step is the *recognition* of the antigen as non-self, and there is considerable evidence that this is performed by cells which do not themselves manufacture antibodies. The final step is the production of antibodies.

## The Immunoglobulin Response to Antigenic Stimulation

### Factors Influencing the Antibody Response

1. **Previous Contact with Antigen.** *Primary Response.* When an antigen is introduced into an animal for the first time, there is an interval of about 10 days before antibody can be detected in the plasma (Fig. 11.1). There then follows a slow rise in titre which climbs to a maximum and then diminishes. This is the typical *primary response*, and it should be noted that the antibody titre reached is comparatively low.

*Secondary Response.* When the same animal is injected with the same antigen on a second occasion, there is an immediate drop in circulating antibody due to its neutralization by the injected antigen. After 2–3 days there is a rapid rise in antibody titre which reaches a peak and again falls off, rapidly at first

* If it is proposed to use iodine as a preoperative skin disinfectant, a patch test should *always* be performed beforehand to eliminate the possibility of this reaction. This is done by applying iodine to a small patch of skin and reading the result 24 hours later.

and later more slowly (Fig. 11.1). The final level of antibody is usually above the previous one. The secondary response is thus *quicker, of greater magnitude,* and *of longer duration.*

It is evident that the first encounter with an antigen produces a change (termed *potential immunity*), such that future contact with the same antigen produces a big immune response.

2. **Type of Antigen.** Antigens vary considerably in their ability to elicit antibody production. As a general rule those in particulate or insoluble form produce a better response than does soluble material. For this reason antigen precipitated with alum is used for diphtheria immunization (APT or alum precipitated toxoid). Freund's adjuvant is considered on p. 168.

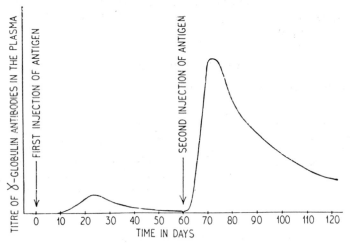

FIG. 11.1. Diagram to show the differences between the primary and the secondary response to an antigenic stimulus.

3. **Age of Animal.** This is a most important factor. The description of the immune response so far given applies only to the mature animal.

During early fetal life animals will accept foreign proteins without antibody production. In addition, they may be rendered incapable of reacting to the same antigen throughout adult life. This is called *specific immunological tolerance* and will be described in more detail later in this chapter.

4. **Treatment Designed to Reduce Antibody Response.** Several methods are available for suppressing the immune response. Some have been used in man in attempts to prolong the life of homografts and treat diseases, such as systemic lupus erythematosus, in which tissue damage is thought to be caused by an immunological mechanism.[7] All methods tend to be more effective in suppressing a primary response than a secondary one, and affect both cell-bound and immunoglobulin antibody production.

*Glucocorticosteroid Administration.* Continuous administration is commonly used, and it reduces the immune response particularly to primary antigenic stimulation.

*Administration of Antimetabolite Drugs,*[8] such as are used in the treatment of cancer, e.g. 6-mercaptopurine, cyclophosphamide, and azathioprine (Imuran).

*Administration of Antilymphocytic Serum.*[9] Antilymphocytic serum, prepared by the injection of lymphocytes from an animal of one species into one of another species, has been found to inhibit the production of antibodies, especially the cell-bound type. Its use in man for inhibiting the graft reaction is under active study, but in a number of patients malignancy has followed its use.

*Total Body Exposure to Ionizing Radiation.*[10] This suppresses a primary response more than a secondary one. The dose necessary to suppress the immune response is dangerously close to the lethal dose and the method is not now commonly used in man.

*Depletion of Small Lymphocytes.* Chronic drainage of these cells from the thoracic duct by establishing a fistula in the experimental animal causes depletion of lymphocytes and impairment of the immune response.[11]

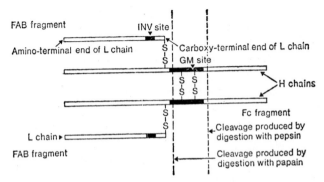

FIG. 11.2. Diagrammatic representation of the structure of IgG antibody. The molecule is composed of two light polypeptide chains and two heavy chains joined together by disulphide bonds. Digestion with the enzyme papain splits the molecule into three fragments, as indicated by the dotted lines. Two fragments are similar and have one antibody-combining site each (Fab fragments). The third fragment (Fc) can be crystallized, and has no antibody activity. The splitting action of pepsin is also shown. The sites for the antigenic determinants governed by the *Inv* and *Gm* genes are shown.

## Properties of the Immunoglobulins[12,13]

Antibody activity in the plasma is due to a group of globulins which, on electrophoretic separation, form a broad band in the $\gamma$ fraction together with some activity in the $\alpha$ and $\beta$ regions. They are highly specific and react with their corresponding antigens in various ways, although this action may not always be demonstrable *in vitro*. The specificity of each antibody is thought to be determined by the precise amino-acid sequence of its polypeptide chains.

The in-vitro reactions between antigens and antibodies are considered later in this chapter, but it may be noted at this stage that in general the antibodies tend to neutralize their antigens and lead to their elimination. The antibody produced in an animal after the injection of an antigen is not a single distinct protein, for one antigenic compound may have several epitopes, and therefore antibodies of different specificities are produced. Furthermore, even the antibody possessing a single specificity is heterogeneous and consists of a group of proteins differing somewhat in molecular composition and size, and in electrophoretic mobility.

**Nomenclature and Chemical Structure**[12, 13] The plasma antibodies are now called *immunoglobulins*, with the designation Ig regardless of their electrophoretic mobility. Each molecule consists of four polypeptide chains—two light and two heavy chains held together by disulphide bonds. As explained in Fig. 11.2, the antibody properties of the molecule are associated with the Fab fragments, a fact which harmonizes well with the bivalent properties of most antibodies.

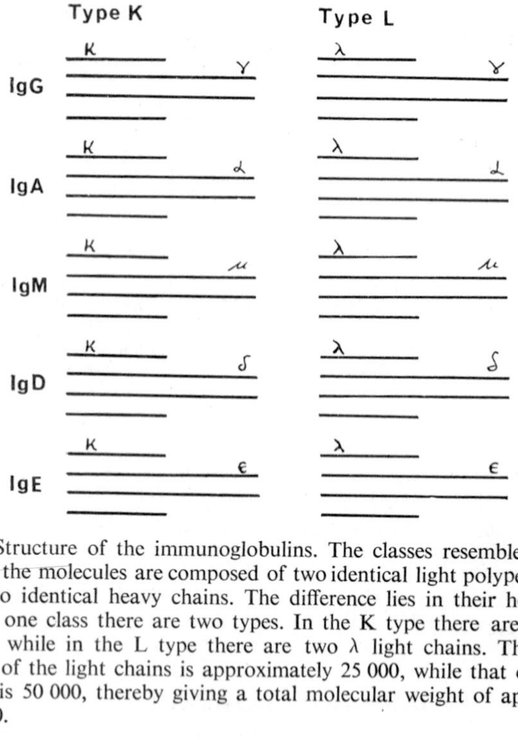

FIG. 11.3. Structure of the immunoglobulins. The classes resemble each other in that the molecules are composed of two identical light polypeptide chains and two identical heavy chains. The difference lies in their heavy chains. In any one class there are two types. In the K type there are two κ light chains, while in the L type there are two λ light chains. The molecular weight of the light chains is approximately 25 000, while that of the heavy chains is 50 000, thereby giving a total molecular weight of approximately 150 000.

The immunoglobulins are themselves antigenic when injected into other species, and immunoelectrophoretic studies have revealed that the light and heavy chains are not homogeneous. Human antibodies can be divided into classes depending upon specific antigenic determinants on the light and heavy chains. There are five types of heavy chains, which are named: γ, α, δ, ε, and μ. Each antibody molecule has a pair of identical heavy chains, and therefore five *classes* are recognized: IgG, IgA, IgD, IgE, and IgM respectively. Each class has been further subdivided into two groups: K for Korngold and L for Lipari, after the two workers who first recognized them. The difference lies in the light chains which are termed κ (kappa) and λ (lambda). Each molecule, whether IgG, IgA, IgM, IgD, or IgE, has either two $\kappa$ or two $\gamma$ chains, *but never one of each*. (See Fig. 11.3).

Variants of the heavy chains have been found. Thus there are four of the $\gamma$ chains, so that there are four subtypes of IgG—IgG1, IgG2, IgG3, and IgG4. Similarly, there are two subclasses each of IgA and IgM to add to the remarkable heterogeneity of the immunoglobulins.

*IgG* is the most abundant immunoglobulin present in the plasma. It is a 7S protein*, with a molecular weight of about 150 000 and a structure as depicted in Figs. 11.2 and 11.3. It is the only immunoglobulin to cross the placenta.

*IgA* is present in the plasma, but its highest concentration is found in secretions (mucus, colostrum, etc.) and it is an important factor in preventing infection of mucous membranes. It is made locally in plasma cells and secreted as a dimer with a third polypeptide chain called the *secretory* or *transport piece* which may serve to stabilize the IgA against proteolysis. IgA does not fix complement, and its main function may be to react with antigens absorbed from the gut and other mucous membranes, and neutralize them without the damaging effects of complement activation.[14]

*IgD* is of unknown function.

*IgE* is a 7S fraction which is responsible for human anaphylaxis (p. 160) as well as for hypersensitivity states such as asthma and hay-fever.

*IgM* is a 19S globulin with a molecular weight of 900 000—hence it is also called a *macroglobulin*. It can be dissociated into five 7S subunits each of which has a similar structure to that of IgG except that the heavy $\mu$ chains are present instead of $\gamma$. Because of its size, IgM is largely restricted to the intravascular compartment. In an immune response it is often the first immunoglobulin to be produced; this is later augmented by IgG.

## Antigen-Antibody Union[15]

There is only one way in which antibodies may be recognized and measured, and that is by their specific union with antigen.

When antibody is mixed with antigen a *primary union* occurs.[16] Frequently there is no visible change but if the physicochemical conditions, e.g. pH, temperature, electrolyte concentration, etc., are appropriate, the primary union is followed by a variety of *secondary phenomena*, which can be seen or detected. They are therefore of great practical importance and are used to identify and measure antibodies. *Agglutination, precipitation,* and *complement fixation* are the most important.

**Agglutination.** When a particulate antigen, e.g. a bacterial suspension, is added to its antibody, the particles may adhere to each other to produce large visible clumps. This clumping is called *agglutination,* and the antibody is called an *agglutinin.* The detection of agglutinins in the serum of patients is frequently of value in the diagnosis of infectious disease. The highest

* The sedimentation constant is measured in Svedberg units, and is a measure of the rapidity with which macromolecules move when subjected to centrifugal force in an ultracentrifuge. The higher the constant the larger and heavier is the molecule. The 7S fraction of plasma contains the $\gamma$-globulins of MW 150 000, while the 19S fraction contains those of MW $10^6$.

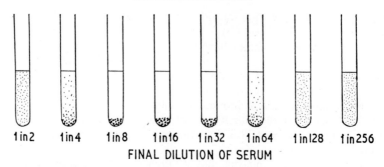

1 in 2    1 in 4    1 in 8    1 in 16    1 in 32    1 in 64    1 in 128    1 in 256
FINAL DILUTION OF SERUM

FIG. 11.4. Agglutination test. The titre of the antibody is 1 in 64. The failure of the first tube (1 in 2 dilution) to show agglutination is known as the prozone phenomenon, and is not uncommonly seen in *Brucella* agglutination tests.

dilution of serum which produces agglutination is called its *titre*, and a rising value is particularly significant (Fig. 11.4).

When the organism used is of the *Salmonella* group, the test is known as the *Widal reaction*.

It should be noted that agglutination tests may be used to *identify unknown organisms*, provided a supply of known antisera is available.

Agglutinins to red cells (*haemagglutinins*) are of great importance in haematology, and both the "complete" and "incomplete" types are described on p. 346.

**Precipitation.** Precipitation is the formation of an insoluble product when two soluble substances are mixed together. If a soluble antigen (e.g. a protein, a toxin, or an extract of an organism) is added to its specific antibody, a precipitate may form. The antibody is called a *precipitin*, and probably acts by virtue of the divalent antibody molecules joining up the antigen molecules to form a lattice.[17] Precipitins may be demonstrated simply by mixing the reagents in a test-tube, but the most sensitive method is to perform the reaction in an agar gel (Ouchterlony). Two cups are cut in an agar plate; into one is placed the antigen and into the other the antibody. Each now diffuses towards the other, and where they meet in optimal proportions a white line of precipitation appears (Fig. 11.5). Precipitin reactions are used in streptococcal grouping (Lancefield), in the identification of human blood and semen, and in the diagnosis of syphilis (Kahn test).

**Complement Fixation.** This type of antibody, also called an *amboceptor*, produces an effect on its antigen only in the presence of a component of the blood called complement. *Complement* has been defined as the heat-labile activity in plasma which, in the presence of haemolysin, is cytotoxic to red cells. It is described in detail on page 153.

Amboceptors may unite with their corresponding antigens in the presence of complement to produce some visible effect—for instance *lysis*. Antibodies which lyse red cells (*haemolysins*) or bacteria (*bacteriolysins*) are both of the complement-fixing variety. With some amboceptors the union is invisible but can nevertheless be detected indirectly. The *Wassermann reaction*, employed to detect syphilitic antibodies, is a good example of this. The test is

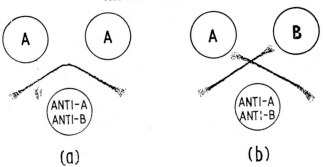

FIG. 11.5. Ouchterlony plates showing precipitin reactions. In (a) the precipitin lines join together, as they are both due to the same A-anti-A reaction. In (b) the lines cross, as they are formed by different antigen-antibody reactions.

explained diagrammatically in Table 11.1, in which it is seen that serum, heated to 56°C for 30 mins., is mixed with a standard quantity of complement and syphilitic antigen.* The object of heating ("inactivating") the serum is to inactivate the unknown quantity of complement which is normally present, so that a known, measured amount can be added to the reaction. The serum-complement-antigen mixture is allowed to incubate for a standard length of time. If the syphilitic antibody is present in the patient's serum, the antigen combines with it, and at the same time fixes the added complement. The detector system is then added. It is also of antigen-amboceptor type, and utilizes red cells with their corresponding haemolysin. If complement has not been used up in the first reaction it is available for the second system. Therefore haemolysis of the red cells denotes an absence of syphilitic antibody, and the Wassermann reaction is negative. On the other hand, the absence of haemolysis indicates a positive reaction. Similar complement fixation tests are employed in the diagnosis of many other infections—being particularly useful in virology.

**Neutralizing Antibodies.** If the antigen has a particular biological property, for instance if it is a toxin, the corresponding antibody neutralizes this activity. Thus antibodies to toxins are called *antitoxins*.

### TABLE 11.1. WASSERMANN REACTION

| First Reaction | Second or Detector Reaction (Haemolytic System) |
|---|---|
| Patient's serum with ? antibody heated to 56°C for 30 mins. (to destroy any complement which is present).<br>+<br>Antigen (standard quantity).<br>+<br>Complement (carefully measured amount). | Red cells (sheep).<br>+<br>Haemolysin (serum of rabbit immunized against sheep red cells). This is inactivated commercially to remove its complement.<br>? Complement unused. |

* The antigen is in fact a cholesterolized extract of heart muscle. This has been found to work in practice, but the precise reason for this is not clear. Treponemal protein can be used to make the test more specific.

It must be stressed that the immunoglobulins have been named according to the nature of the test used to detect them. In many cases a single antibody can perform several functions depending upon the conditions under which it is tested. For instance, an antibody may be capable of neutralizing toxin, e.g. diphtheria toxin, in an *in-vivo* experiment. It is therefore rightly called an *antitoxin*. However, *in vitro* it will produce a precipitate with its antigen and therefore be labelled a *precipitin*. Similarly a single antibody may perform the functions of precipitin, agglutinin, and lysin.

### Cell-bound Antibodies[18]

Following the introduction of antigen, particularly if combined with Freund's adjuvant (p. 168) or in the form of a living organism, an animal produces cell-bound antibodies. These are in the form of *sensitized lymphocytes* which morphologically are small lymphocytes. They react specifically with antigen, undergo blast transformation, and release a number of agents called *lymphokines*[55] which have a variety of actions. These are ill-defined chemically, and it is not known whether there are a few agents having many actions or separate substances each with a specific effect. They may be listed:

1. *Migration Inhibition Factor* (*MIF*). This acts on macrophages and prevents them migrating in a tissue-culture system (see Fig. 13.2). It is probably the same as the *macrophage activating factor*, which makes the cells more phagocytic and better able to kill organisms. It may be supposed that MIF is important as a mediator of the demolition phase of acute inflammation and in chronic inflammation. This has yet to be proved.

2. *Transfer Factor*. This substance specifically transfers sensitization to previously uncommited lymphocytes. It therefore recruits new cells to the site involved, e.g. a site of infection.

3. *Lymphotoxin*. This agent has a cytopathic effect on cells, such as a monolayer of fibroblasts in culture.

4. *Skin Reactive Factor*

5. *Chemotactic Factors*. Probably several types are produced, and these affect either neutrophils, monocytes, or eosinophils.

6. *Mitogenic Factor*. This causes blast transformation and stimulates mitosis.

7. *Interferon*.

8. *Immunoglobulin*.

An important feature of sensitized lymphocytes is that, while they are sensitized to a specific antigen, the subsequent events (such as cell damage due to lymphotoxin and macrophage activation) are quite non-specific.

### Effect of Antibodies in the Living Animal

Antibodies can produce important effects in the living animal. They may provide *immunity* to infection, or cause *hypersensitivity*, immediate-type in the case of immunoglobulins and delayed-type with cell-bound antibodies. These effects are considered in the chapters which follow.

## The Antibody Forming Tissues

Before describing the cellular features of the immune response it is essential to understand the structure and development of the lymphoid tissues of the body.

### The Lymphoid Tissues[19-21]

**The Thymus.** The first lymphoid tissue to develop in mammals is the thymus. It contains an epithelial element in the form of reticular cells and Hassall's corpuscles. In addition there are many thymocytes which morphologically resemble lymphocytes.

**The Bursa of Fabricius.** In birds the next lymphoid organ to develop is the *bursa of Fabricius*. This is situated near the cloaca, and, like the thymus, has an epithelial as well as a lymphoid element. It is suspected that mammals have an equivalent tissue, perhaps more widely distributed, and forming the lymphoid tissue of the appendix and colon, and the Peyer's patches of the small intestine.

**Lymph Nodes.** Lymph comes into the lymph node through the peripheral sinus, traverses the cortex, enters the sinusoids of the medulla, and finally leaves through the efferent duct. The sinuses are lined by plump, *littoral*, or *sinus-lining cells*, which have eosinophilic cytoplasm and are phagocytic. Reticulum cells are present and appear to be concerned with the formation of reticulin, which constitutes the connective tissue framework of the node. In the outer part, or *cortex*, of the node there are densely packed lymphocytes which are focally aggregated into *follicles*. In the centre of each follicle there is often a well-defined *germinal centre of Flemming*.[22] This contains large cells which are generally called lymphoblasts. They show a high turn-over rate and therefore mitoses are abundant. In addition, the centres contain large macrophages which usually contain nuclear debris in their clear, abundant cytoplasm. On microscopy the macrophages produce clear spaces which have been likened to the stars in a starry sky.

The *medulla* of the node shows prominent sinuses and medullary cords of cells between them. These cells are mainly small lymphocytes together with a variable number of plasma cells and granulocytes.

Between the cortex with its germinal centres and the medulla there is a third zone which is packed with lymphocytes but less densely so than the cortex. There are no follicles in this *paracortical zone*.

Small lymphocytes from the blood normally enter the lymph node *via* the post-capillary sinusoids in the paracortical zone and subsequently leave the node in the efferent lymph.[23] The lymphocytes therefore re-enter the blood stream through the thoracic duct. It follows that if this duct is exteriorized and drained, the body is steadily depleted of lymphocytes.

**Blood Lymphocytes.**[24] The lymphocytes in the blood range from the large to the small variety. The latter have a dense spherical nucleus and little cytoplasm. Originally thought to be a differentiated cell, the lymphocyte is now known to be a resting cell capable of being stimulated to remarkable activity. In the circulating blood many of the lymphocytes are long-lived cells and continuously re-circulated through the lymph nodes. At present the relationship between the various types of lymphocytes found in the blood, lymph nodes, marrow, and thymus is speculative, and there is no way of distinguishing between them on morphological grounds. The differences can be detected only by their varying behaviour. It is now thought that there are two populations of cells in the blood. The long-lived, thymic dependent *T lymphocytes* form the majority, and continually recirculate through the paracortical zone of the lymph nodes. These cells are mobile and participate in cell-mediated immune responses. The second group are short-lived cells derived from the bone marrow and are bursal dependent. These *B lymphocytes* tend to be sessile, and are found in the primary follicles of the lymph nodes. They can be induced to secrete immunoglobulin.

**Spleen.** In the spleen the blood passes through the central (malpighian) arterioles to enter the sinusoids which are, as in the lymph nodes, lined by phagocytic cells. In the red pulp there are reticulum cells, lymphocytes, and plasma cells as well as occasional granulocytes and megakaryocytes. The lymphoid cuffs are situated around the malpighian arterioles, and the lymphocytes are thought to be derived from the blood as part of the re-circulation of cells as in the paracortical zones of the lymph nodes.[25] Germinal centres may be prominent.

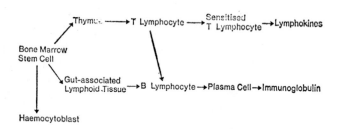

Fig. 11.6. Diagram showing the postulated development of the peripheral lymphoid tissue of the lymph nodes.

**Development of the Peripheral Lymphoid Tissues.** The thymus, and in birds the bursa, is well developed and large before the peripheral lymphoid tissue matures. There is considerable evidence that both these organs are necessary for the development of the peripheral lymphoid tissues. The thymus is the central organ responsible for the formation of the paracortical zone of the lymph nodes and for the sheath of lymphocytes around the central arterioles in the spleen. These are the *thymus-dependent areas*. The bursa is necessary for the formation of the germinal centres in the spleen and in the cortex of nodes, and also for the cells, presumably B lymphocytes, which differentiate into plasma cells in the splenic red pulp and the medullary cords of the nodes. It has been supposed that the earliest immunological cell is to be found in the bone marrow (*reticular anlage*). This cell may differentiate to a haemocytoblast or develop into a lymphoid cell (Fig. 11.6). It is not known whether the marrow cells migrate to the peripheral tissues and there develop under the influence of a thymic or bursal hormone, or whether the cells migrate first to the thymus or bursa, develop for a while, and then are released to populate the peripheral lymphoid tissue.

## The Thymus in Relation to the Immune Response[25–27]

Thymectomy performed shortly after birth can produce dramatic effects in some species. Mice, for example, appear normal for 3–4 weeks, and then a wasting syndrome usually develops which closely resembles runt disease (p. 170). This is probably a result of microbial infection, for it does not occur in germ-free animals. Significantly there is a deficiency of small lymphocytes in the splenic white pulp, the paracortical zones of lymph nodes, and in the circulating blood. The animals exhibit impaired ability to develop delayed-type hypersensitivity, and are tolerant of allografts and sometimes even of xenografts. The production of immunoglobulins to some antigens is normal, but to others, e.g. sheep red cells, it is impaired.

## The Bursa of Fabricius in Relation to the Immune Response

Removal of the bursa, especially if combined with non-lethal total body irradiation, results in an immunologically deficient state characterized by a failure to produce immunoglobulins when suitably challenged by an antigen.[28] It is possible that in mammals the intestinal lymphoid tissue corresponds to the bursa, for its removal in rabbits produces a similar failure in immuno-globulin production. This may be regarded as the *gut-associated central lymphoid tissue*. It is presumed to be responsible for the development of that part of the peripheral lymphoid tissue which is responsible for the production of immunoglobulins, namely germinal centres and plasma cells (*bursal*, or *bursal-equivalent, dependent cells*).

## Lymphocyte Transformation

One of the most remarkable observations of recent times is that the small lymphocytes of the blood and lymph can be stimulated *in vitro* to become large cells with basophilic, pyroninophilic cytoplasm containing many free ribosomes, while their nuclei have nucleoli. These cells have been called *immunoblasts*, pyroninophilic cells, and blast cells. They exhibit DNA synthesis and mitotic activity, a feature which has led to them being intensively used in studies of human chromosomes.

Agents which lead to lymphocyte transformation are:

*Phytohaemagglutinin.* This is contained in an extract of broad bean, but the active agent has not been identified. Phytohaemagglutinin was used originally to produce agglutination of red cells in experiments designed to facilitate the isolation of white cells from the blood.

*Antilymphocytic serum.*

*Antigen-antibody complexes.*

*Other allogeneic lymphocytes.* If small lymphocytes from another individual are mixed with test lymphocytes, both groups of cells undergo blast transformation.

*Antigen,* if added to the lymphocytes from a sensitized individual. This occurs regardless of whether the sensitization is of the immediate or delayed type.[29] Although many agents can cause transformation, it does not follow that the process is the same in each instance. Phytohaemagglutinin causes a high percentage of lymphocytes to transform rapidly. Other agents affect fewer cells, and the transformation is slower.

The blast cells are cytotoxic to cells grown in tissue culture, an effect which is non-specific since it occurs regardless of the agent used to produce the transformation. The precise role of the blast transformation phenomenon in the intact animal is not known, but various suggestions have been made:

1. The proliferating cells form the germinal centres. The function of these is not known.

2. The cells can develop endoplasmic reticulum, manufacture immuno-globulin, and thereby differentiate into plasma cells.

3. They can revert to a type of lymphocyte. Such a cell could have various functions. It could act as a memory cell, so that when next stimulated by antigen it could transform and produce antibody. It could also contain cell-bound antibody and act as an effector cell in cell-mediated immune reactions.

### Functional Steps in the Immune Response

The following steps may be postulated as occurring after the introduction of an antigen:

**The Recognition System.** A mechanism must exist for recognizing an antigen as foreign. Furthermore, the system must have a *memory* so that the same antigen can be recognized again.

**The Processing System.** Once having been recognized as an antigen, its determinants must be processed in such a way that specific antibody can be produced.

**The Production System.** The final outcome of the immune response is the manufacture of antibody. This involves the synthesis of a range of specific proteins as well as the formation of immune lymphocytes. The production system must be *regulated* in some way, so that the immune response can be turned off when the antigenic stimulus is withdrawn.

### Anatomical Site of Antibody Production[30,31]

Antibodies are not produced in any one organ or site. With intravenously administered antigens they are produced in the spleen, liver, and lymph nodes, while locally introduced antigen stimulates antibody production at the local site and in the regional lymph nodes.

Since all antibodies are either cellular or else proteins produced by cells, a complete understanding of the immune response entails an understanding of the cellular events involved. It is generally agreed that the lymphoreticular tissues are of prime importance and that two morphological cell types are concerned. There are the large mononuclear, potentially phagocytic cells grouped together as the RE system, and the lymphocytes. Detailed knowledge about the origin, morphology, and function of these cells is unfortunately lacking, and much confusion has been caused in the past by making wholly unwarranted assumptions. Cells which look alike, e.g. small lymphocytes, do not necessarily have the same origin or function.

## The Recognition System

A cell which is capable of recognizing antigen and of initiating an immune response, although not necessarily producing antibody itself, is termed an *immunologically competent cell*.[32] There is considerable evidence that such a cell is morphologically a small lymphocyte. The evidence may be summarized as follows: Procedures which deplete the population of small lymphocytes also inhibit the development of a primary response to antigenic stimulation. The following may be mentioned: total body irradiation, administration of cytotoxic drugs (p. 134), thoracic-duct drainage (p. 135), and thymectomy in the neonate (p. 143). Animals rendered tolerant to an antigen (p. 147) can have their immunological responsiveness restored by the injection of lymphocytes from a non-tolerant adult syngeneic animal.

There is evidence that both B and T lymphocytes have immunoglobulin on their surfaces.[33,34] It may be in this way that they recognize antigen, especially in a secondary response.

## Cells Involved in Immunoglobulin Synthesis

There is abundant evidence that immunoglobulins are present in plasma cells. If sections from various organs of an immunized animal are treated with labelled antigen, it is found that the antigen becomes firmly localized to the cytoplasm of the plasma cells. The labelling may be done with fluorescent dye, radioactive iodine or, for electron microscopy, with ferritin.[35, 36] The well-developed endoplasmic reticulum with its ribosomes and the high concentration of cytoplasmic RNA all suggest that the plasma cell is actively engaged in protein synthesis. The evidence all points to its being the major source of immunoglobulin. Nevertheless, some antibody may also be demonstrated in the germinal centres and in cells which appear to be lymphocytes.

In the lymph nodes immunoglobulin production is related to the formation of germinal centres, and the greatest amount of antibody is formed in the cells of the medulla which finally appear as plasma cells. These are the bursal, or bursal-equivalent, dependent areas. Whether lymphocytes transform directly into plasma cells perhaps through an intermediate pyroninophilic cell stage, as suggested by Gowans, is not settled. Nor is it clear whether cells from the germinal centres migrate into the medulla and differentiate into antibody-producing cells.

**Number of Cell-Types Involved in Immunoglobulin Production.** There is considerable evidence that immunoglobulin formation does not occur as the result of the activity of one cell type acting alone. T cells are thought to act as helper cells needed for the manufacture of immunoglobulin,[37] but whether they do this by acting as recognition cells for a specific antigen[38,39] or in some other way is not known. The T cells being mobile are certainly well adapted to acting as recognition cells. Macrophages from a normal mouse, when primed by incubating them with a *Shigella* antigen, will cause specific antibody to be formed when injected into a second, sub-lethally irradiated (550 r) animal. The antibody is formed by host lymphoid tissue. Injection of antigen alone, or irradiated primed macrophages, cause no antibody response in such an animal.[40] Furthermore, primed macrophages injected into a *heavily* irradiated mouse (900 r) fail to lead to antibody production since the host's lymphoid tissue is damaged. If the cells are injected together with lymphocytes, an immune response follows. It is thought that macrophages play a vital role by ingesting antigen and manufacturing a specific RNA which evokes antibody formation in lymph-node cells.[41]

If following a primary response to an antigen in an animal, the small lymphocytes are drained from the thoracic duct, it is found that these cells will transfer immunological memory if injected into another animal: administration of antigen will produce a secondary response. Furthermore, the small lymphocytes from the thoracic duct, if incubated with antigen *in vitro*, will themselves evoke a secondary response when injected in another animal. This type of evidence suggests that, *so far as the secondary response is concerned*, an intermediate cell like a macrophage is not required for antibody production.

**Cell-Bound Antibody Production.** The site of cellular antibody is the small lymphocyte. The evidence for this is that this is the only cell which has the ability to transfer delayed-type hypersensitivity from one animal to another (p. 166).

### Theories of Antibody Production

**The Instructive Theory.**[42] It has been postulated that antigens play an instructive role, and that the extraordinary specificity of antibodies is related to the fact that antigens act as moulds, or templates, during antibody formation. The theory, although superficially satisfying, has many drawbacks. It assumes that the antigen persists in the body throughout the period of antibody production—a period which is often measured in months or even years. There is little direct evidence that antigens can remain in the body for such long periods; indeed, the immune reaction is responsible for their rapid elimination.[43, 44] It is possible that antigenic determinants, rather than the whole molecule, are retained to provide the jolt for immunological memory, but this is unproven. It is possible to envisage that by becoming attached to RNA, they might modify protein synthesis, i.e. lead to specific antibody production.[45] An alternative explanation is that contact with antigen produces a permanent modification of the antibody producing cells. The postulated change must be of a self-reduplicating nature, for it seems to be handed down to the progeny of the cells for many generations. The nature of this hypothetical change is quite unknown.

**The Selective Theory.**[46] This supposes that in the adult there are cells capable of mounting an immune response against any non-self antigen which the individual is likely to meet. The antigen *selects* these cells and stimulates them to grow and produce antibody. The antigen thus determines the *quantity* of antibody produced but not directly its *specificity*.

This theory, formulated by Jerne and elaborated by Burnet, provides one explanation of the phenomenon of specific immunological tolerance. It may be supposed that during the early stages of embryonic development there occur many somatic mutations in the immunologically competent cells. This results in the formation of a whole range of cells which between them are capable of mounting an immune response specific for any antigen which the body may subsequently meet. In the adult contact with antigen stimulates growth of these cells, and in this way a body of cells, or *clone*,* develops, and as it multiplies in size, so does antibody production increase.

It is obvious that if somatic mutation occurs so frequently that cells are produced which can form antibodies against all possible antigens, then inevitably some mutations will produce cells capable of forming antibodies against the host's own developing tissues. It must therefore be postulated that there exists some mechanism *during embryonic life* for the destruction of these harmful, or *forbidden clones*. Any antigen present in the developing embryo is recognized as self, and at birth there are no cells present which could make antibodies against it. It is apparent that if normally foreign antigens are introduced into an embryo, they will be accepted as "self" and the animal will exhibit *specific immunological tolerance*.

In fact, this statement is an over-simplification, for the fetus can produce antibodies if stimulated, especially towards the end of intrauterine life. Infants infected *in utero* with rubella and other virus and bacterial diseases show a considerable titre of IgM, an antibody which is not normally present since it does not cross the placenta.[47]

### Specific Immunological Tolerance[48,49]

The administration of an antigen to an embryo results not in the formation of antibodies but in the acceptance of the foreign substance as "self". The phenomenon was first noticed when embryos were grafted with allogeneic cells, i.e. from an animal of the same species but of a different genetic constitution. So long as the grafted cells survived in the host the animals were tolerant of further grafts from the same donor, but not from those of any other donor. The tolerance was therefore *specific* and not due to a generalized depression of the immune response.

Specific immunological tolerance to non-living antigens can also be induced, but it persists only for so long as the antigen remains.[50] Repeated injections are therefore usually required.

The theory of Burnet explains how early contact with antigen could destroy the appropriate clone, but in order to explain why tolerance is lost when the antigen is dissipated, it must be assumed that the capacity to relearn "self" from "non-self" is also present during adult life. It could be that new immunologically competent cells are being formed throughout life, and that at an early stage in their development they learn to recognize as "self" those antigens which are present at that time[48]. Thus, during embryonic life when antibody-forming cells are few and many immunologically competent cells are being formed, tolerance is easy to establish with relatively small doses of antigen. In the adult, on the other hand, there are many antibody-forming cells and few developing immunologically competent cells; therefore tolerance is difficult to establish.

**Induction of Tolerance.** There are various ways in which tolerance may be induced.

(1) Administration of antigen to a fetus or immature animal.

* A clone is a group of cells of like hereditary constitution which has been produced asexually from a single cell. The word is derived from the Greek *klon* meaning a cutting used for propagation.

(2) Administration of massive doses of antigen to a mature animal.
(3) Administration of very small, often repeated, doses of antigen to young animals[48].
(4) Administration of antigen following extensive damage to the lympho-reticular system by ionizing radiations or cytotoxic drugs. Antibody formation is temporarily in abeyance, and regeneration of the immuno-logically competent cells occurs in the presence of antigen.
(5) Administration of antigen in an immunologically defective animal such as one subjected to a neonatal thymectomy.
(6) Administration of certain antigens, e.g. picryl chloride by mouth.[51, 52]

**Maintenance of Tolerance.** To maintain the state of tolerance the antigen must usually persist in the body, and this can be ensured either by injecting living cells as antigen or by the repeated injection of non-living antigens.

**Explanation of Tolerance.** Two major theories have been put forward.

*Production of Tolerant Cells.* Under some circumstances antigen can act on immunologically competent cells to render them unresponsive. It has been suggested that if antigen acts directly on the cells they are rendered tolerant. If antigen is taken up by macrophages first, the immunologically competent cells are stimulated to initiate an immune response. This concept explains how *very large doses* of antigen can produce tolerance, for antigen can act directly on cells. Likewise *very small doses* of antigen may fail to initiate antibody production and yet can act on the immunologically competent cells to render them tolerant.[48] Another possibility is that antigen-antibody complexes stimulate the immunologically competent cells to divide and lead to further antibody production. Tolerance is easier to produce if specific antibodies are absent and if the animal's capability of producing them is impaired, e.g. in fetal life and following x-irradiation and the administration of cytotoxic drugs.

*Elimination of Potentially Reactive Cells.* It is possible that there is no such thing as a tolerant cell, but rather that the appropriate cell has been eliminated as suggested by Burnet's theory.

An essential clue towards deciding between these two theories would be a knowledge of whether a single cell could produce one or many antibodies. By the use of specific fluorescent antibodies to immunoglobulin, it has been shown that a particular cell always produces one class of antibody, i.e. one type of heavy chain and one type of light chain. As to whether a single cell can produce antibodies specific to more than one antigen is not clear. When an animal is immunized with several antigens, most plasma cells produce an antibody against only one of the antigens.[53] However, some early experiments have shown that some cells produce antibodies against two antigens but not more.[54] Nevertheless, these observations tend to support the theory that tolerance is due to the elimination of the appropriate clone. Although it is usually assumed that the essential recognition unit of immunological competence is a cell, it is quite possible that it is in fact a subcellular component or a chemical mechanism.

It must be concluded that we are very ignorant about the manner in which antigens bring about a lifelong change in immunoglobulin synthesis. Probably the processing of antigen by macrophages or some other helper cell is important in producing a primary response, but the stimulation for a secondary response is a direct action of the antigen on sensitized cells, possibly with the formation of an antigen-antibody complex. Tolerance is a state in which a particular antibody mechanism is in abeyance, but whether this is due to chemical repression or to physical elimination of the appropriate mechanism is undecided.

## Conclusion

When antigen gains access to the tissues of the body a complex series of events occur. It is taken up by the phagocytic cells of the RE system, and this is followed by some permanent change in the immunologically competent cells. In this way the macrophages, lymphocytes, and plasma cells are altered, and under some circumstances specific immunoglobulins pass into the blood stream.

The appearance of these circulating antibodies is therefore the final event in a sequence of changes, the whole of which constitutes the "immune response".

### General Reading

BELLANTI, J. A. (1971). "Immunology", 584 pp. Philadelphia: Saunders.
HUMPHREY, J. H. and WHITE, R. G. (1970). "Immunology for Students of Medicine", 3rd ed., 757pp., Oxford: Blackwell.
MIESCHER, P. A. and MÜELLER-EBERHARD, H. J. (1968 and 1969). edrs. "Textbook of Immunopathology", in two volumes, 805 pp. New York and London: Grune and Stratton.
WEIR, D. M. (1970). "Immunology for Undergraduates", 140 pp. Edinburgh and London: Livingstone.

### References

1. DAVIES, D. A. L. (1963). In "Modern Trends in Immunology", I, ed. by Cruickshank, R. London: Butterworth.
2. KABAT, E. A. (1966). *J. Immunol.*, **97**, 1.
3. Various Authors (1966). *Ann. int. Med.*, **64**, 687.
4. UHR, J. W., FINKELSTEIN, M. S. and BAUMANN, J. B. (1962). *J. exp. Med.*, **115**, 655.
5. FISHMAN, M. and ADLER, F. L. (1963). *J. exp. Med.*, **117**, 595.
6. FRIEDMAN, H. P., STAVITSKY, A. B. and SOLOMON, J. M. (1965). *Science*, **149**, 1106.
7. SKINNER, M. D. and SCHWARTZ, R. S. (1972). *New Engl. J. Med.*, **287**, 221 and 281.
8. TURK, J. L. and STONE, S. H. (1963). In "Cell Bound Antibodies", p. 51, ed. by Amos, B. and Koprowski, H. Philadelphia: Wistar Inst. Press.
9. WOLSTENHOLME, G. E. W. and O'CONNOR, M. (1967). Edrs. "Antilymphocytic Serum", Ciba Foundation Study Group No. 29. London: Churchill.
10. TALIAFERRO, W. H., TALIAFERRO, O. L. G. and JAROSLOW, B. N. (1964). "Radiation and Immune Mechanisms". New York: Academic Press.
11. McGREGOR, D. D. and GOWANS, J. L. (1963). *J. exp. Med.*, **117**, 303.
12. Various Authors (1967). Cold Spring Harbor Symposium on Quantitative Biology, vol. 32, "Antibodies". New York: Cold Spring Harbor Laboratory of Quanitative Biology.
13. MARTIN, N. H. (1969). *J. clin. Path.*, **22**, 117.

14. Editorial (1971). *New Engl. J. Med.*, **284,** 552.
15. Ackroyd, J. F. (1964). Ed. "Immunological Methods", a C.I.O.M.S. Symposium. Oxford: Blackwell. Various authors describe most of the techniques used in detecting antibodies.
16. Weir, D. M. (1963). In "Modern Trends in Immunology", p. 53, *loc. cit.*
17. Pauling, L. (1964). *J. Amer. chem. Soc.*, **62,** 2643.
18. David, J. R. (1973). *New Engl. J. Med.*, **288,** 143.
19. Yoffey, J. M. (1967). Edr. "The Lymphocyte in Immunology and Haemopoiesis", 376 pp. London: Arnold.
20. Elves, M. W. (1972). "The Lymphocytes", 2nd ed., 604 pp. London: Lloyd-Luke.
21. Smith, R. T. and Miescher, P. A. (1966). "Phylogeny of Immunity", 276 pp. University of Florida Press.
22. Cottier, H. *et al.* (1967). Edrs. "Germinal Centers in Immune Responses", 449 pp. New York: Springer-Verlag.
23. Gowans, J. L. and Knight, E. J. (1964). *Proc. roy. Soc.* B, **159,** 257.
24. Craddock, C. G., Longmire, R. and McMillan, R. (1971). *New Engl. J. Med.*, **285,** 324 and 378.
25. Miller, J. F. A. P. (1967). *Lancet*, **2,** 1299.
26. Miller, J. F. A. P. and Osoba, D. (1967). *Physiol. Rev.*, **47,** 437.
27. Wolstenholme, G. E. W. and Porter R. (1966). Edrs. "The Thymus: Experimental and Clinical Studies", Ciba Foundation Symposium. London: Churchill.
28. Cooper, M. D. *et al.* (1966). *J. exp. Med.*, **123,** 75.
29. Loewi, G., Temple, A. and Vischer, T. L. (1968). *Immunology*, **14,** 257.
30. Stavitsky, A. B. (1961). *Advanc. Immunol.*, **1,** 211.
31. White, R. G. (1961). In "The Scientific Basis of Medicine Annual Reviews", pp. 31–46. London: Athlone Press.
32. Wolstenholme, G. E. W. and Knight, J. (1963). Edrs. "The Immunologically Competent Cell" (Ciba Foundation Study Group No. 16). London: Churchill.
33. Bankhurst, A. D., Warner, N. L. and Sprent, J. (1971). *J. exper. med.*, **134,** 1005.
34. Unanue, E. R. *et al.* (1971). *J. exper. med.*, **133,** 1188.
35. Singer, S. J. (1959). *Nature*, **183,** 1523.
36. de Petris, S., Karlsbad, G. and Pernis, B. (1963). *J. exp. Med.*, **117,** 849.
37. Lesley, J. F., Kettman, J. R. and Dutton, R. W. (1971). *J. exper. med.*, **134,** 618.
38. Lischner, H. W. and DiGeorge, A. M. (1969). *Lancet*, **2,** 1044.
39. Miller, J. F. A. P. *et al.* (1971). *J. exper. med.*, **134,** 1266.
40. Feldman, M. and Gallily, R. (1967). In Cold Spring Harbor Symposium on Quanitative Biology, p. 415, *loc. cit.*
41. Fishman, M. and Adler, F. L. (1967). In Cold Spring Harbor Symposium on Quantitative Biology, p. 343, *loc. cit.*
42. Haurowitz, F. (1965). *Nature (Lond.)*, **205,** 847.
43. Benacerraf, B., Sebestyen, M. and Cooper, N. S. (1959). *J. Immunol.*, **82,** 131.
44. Weigle, W. O. (1961). *Advanc. Immunol.*, **1,** 283.
45. Campbell, D. H. and Garvey, J. S. (1963). *Advanc. Immunol.*, **3,** 261.
46. Burnet, F. M. (1959). "The Clonal Selection Theory of Acquired Immunity". London: Cambridge University Press.
47. Annotation (1966). *Lancet*, **2,** 1403.
48. Medawar, P. B. (1960). In "Cellular Aspects of Immunity", Ciba Foundation Symposium, ed. by Wolstenholme, G. E. W. and O'Connor, M. p. 134. London: Churchill.
49. Hašek, M., Lengerová, A. and Hraba, T. (1961). *Advanc. Immunol.*, **1,** 1.
50. Smith, R. T. (1961). *Advanc. Immunol.*, **1,** 67.

51. CHASE, M. W. (1959). In "Cellular and Humoral Aspects of the Hypersensitive States", p. 251, ed. by Lawrence, H. S. New York: Hoeber-Harper.
52. CHASE, M. W. and BATTISTO, J. R. (1959). In "Mechanisms of Hypersensitivity", p. 507, ed. by Shaffer, J. H., LoGrippo, G. A. and Chase, M. W. London: Churchill.
53. MÄKELÄ, O. (1967). In Cold Spring Harbor Symposium on Quantitative Biology, p. 423, *loc. cit.*
54. MÄKELÄ, O. and NOSSAL, G. J. V. (1961). *J. Immunol.*, **87**, 457.
55. Leading Article (1973), *Lancet*, **1**, 1490.

*Chapter 12*

# IMMUNITY TO INFECTION

Immunity, or the ability to resist infection, is a property of all living creatures, and is highly complex. It has two components:
(1) Immunity not dependent upon previous contact with the organism or its antigens.
(2) Immunity which is dependent upon previous contact with the organism or its products. This is acquired as a result of an immune response, and is mediated by antibodies.

## Immunity not Dependent upon Previous Contact with the Organism

All individuals possess an inherent ability to destroy invading micro-organisms, which is not dependent on the presence of antibodies or on the individual's previous contact with the organism or its antigens. The main characteristic of this basal immunity is its non-specificity. Its nature is poorly understood but it may be considered under three headings.

     1. *Cellular factors.*
     2. *Humoral factors.*
     3. *Genetic factors*—innate immunity.

**Cellular Factors.** Organisms are phagocytosed by, and ultimately destroyed in, the polymorphs and macrophages. If there is a decrease in the number of circulating polymorphs, liability to bacterial infection is increased. For this reason gingivitis and ulcerative pharyngitis are often a prominent feature of agranulocytosis or acute leukaemia. Inhibition of the acute inflammatory response reduces the numbers of phagocytes available locally. Glucocortico-steroid therapy has this effect, and predisposes to infection.

There is a rare but interesting group of diseases in which polymorphs are able to phagocytose bacteria but have an impaired ability to kill them. As noted previously (p. 94), intracellular bactericidal activity in polymorphs is related to oxidation of glucose *via* the hexosemonophosphate shunt and the formation of hydrogen peroxide.[1] In *chronic granulomatous disease* there is an inherited defect in one of the required enzymes, and the afflicted child has repeated, chronic infections of the skin, lymph nodes, lung, and other organs.[2,3]

**Humoral Factors.** It has been known for a long time that blood and serum possess bactericidal power. For this reason blood is always well diluted with broth when it is cultured bacteriologically. The substances involved are not well understood, and in fact only three have been identified with any degree of certainty. *Natural oposonins* aid the phagocytosis of organisms of low-grade virulence (p. 68); *complement* and *properdin* have more complex actions.

*Complement.*[4] Complement was originally conceived as a plasma component which aided, or complemented, the union of antigen to antibody. It is now known to consist of at least nine components,* designated C1, C2, etc., which can be sequentially activated in a cascade manner similar to that described in the clotting of blood. There are two sequences described:

*The Classical Sequence for the Activation of Complement.* The most intensively studied complement reaction is that of immune haemolysis initiated by the interaction of a site on the membrane of an erythrocyte E with a specific antibody A. The complex EA binds the first component of complement C1 and sets in action the stages illustrated in Fig. 12.1. The final result is damage to the red-cell membrane which leads to haemolysis. It should be noted that bacteriolysis also involves the activation of complement, and it is

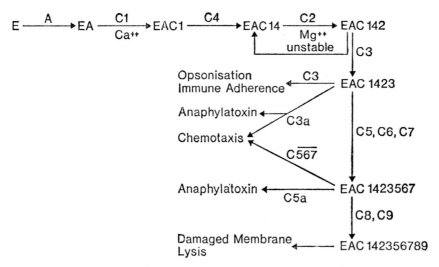

FIG. 12.1. Diagram to illustrate the stages in the activation of complement, the components of which are designated C1, C2 etc. E represents a receptor site on a red cell, while A is a specific antibody. The complete reaction results in lysis of the red cell, but intermediate products are formed which result in the formation of anaphylatoxin, and in opsonization, chemotaxis, and immune adherence. The last is a process whereby organisms are induced to adhere to red cells.

in this way that antibodies can lyse and kill organisms. The complement system therefore is an important factor in host defence, and a number of cases are on record of individuals susceptible to infection lacking a particular complement component, e.g. C5. Nevertheless, defects of C2 produce no ill-effects, and the alternate pathway is presumed to compensate for this (see below).

It should be noted that during the activation of complement a number of soluble active components are formed and these are designed with a bar over the component number, e.g. C576. Active fragments of a component are

*C1 itself consists of three components, C1q, C1r, and C1S.

indicated by a lower case letter, e.g. C3a. These products are important because they are thought to play a vital role in the pathogenesis of acute inflammation, the Arthus phenomenon, anaphylaxis, and immune-complex disease. Thus C3a and C5a are histamine-releasing agents (anaphylatoxins), while C567 is a chemotactic agent (p. 74).

*The Alternate Pathway for the Activation of Complement.*[5] In the classical pathway C3 is activated by C24, also known as C3 convertase. In the alternate pathway this service is performed by a C3 activator which is produced in a manner outlined in Fig. 12.2. The activating agents are lipoprotein, bacterial endotoxin, and aggregates of IgA, IgM, and IgG, including IgG4. This pathway is probably important, because IgA and IgE can activate complement only by this route.

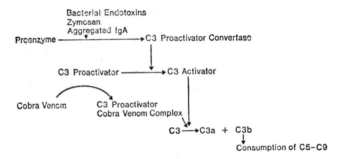

FIG. 12.2. The alternate pathway for the activation of complement.

*Properdin.*[6,7] This substance was described by Pillemer in 1954 as an important bactericidal agent in plasma. Its very existence has been questioned in the past, but it is now thought to play a role in the activation of C3 and the terminal complement sequence. Properdin and three other factors react sequentially, and finally activate C3 in much the same way as the alternate pathway described above. Indeed, the two systems are very similar and it is probable that when the separate components are categorized they will be found to be identical.

**Genetic Factors.** The immunity which is related to inherited constitution is known as *innate*, or *inborn*, *immunity*. It is manifest as *species*, *racial*, and *individual*.

*Species Immunity.* This is the most absolute type of immunity known. Thus the spirochaete of syphilis infects man with prodigious ease, and yet nearly all other animals are immune. Likewise animals suffer from diseases to which man exhibits immunity (e.g. distemper). It should be noted that saying an animal has innate immunity to an organism is an alternative way of saying the organism is avirulent to that animal.

*Racial Immunity.* It is well established that different strains of an animal species may vary in their susceptibility to particular infections, e.g. tuberculosis in rabbits.[8] Similar differences between human races probably exist, but are difficult to substantiate—Negroes and the Irish are said to have a poor innate immunity to tuberculosis. Dark-skinned races are more immune to malaria than are Northern Europeans. This is related to their possession of an abnormal type of haemoglobin[9,10] (p. 37).

*Individual Immunity.* Individuals differ considerably in the degree of immunity which they exhibit, but it is difficult to prove that this is innate and not acquired. Nevertheless, innate differences almost certainly exist.[11]

## Immunity Dependent upon Previous Contact with the Organism or its Antigens —Acquired Immunity

This type of immunity is always associated with the presence of antibodies, which may be of a humoral or cellular nature. When the animal produces its own antibodies, the immunity is said to be *active*. When the antibodies are donated from another animal the immunity is described as *passive*.

**Active Immunity.** This is produced as a result of the individual's own immune response.

*Natural active immunity* follows a natural infection with the organism. The subject may have been aware of the disease, or it may have been subclinical and have passed unnoticed. Subclinical attacks are very common with some infections, e.g. poliomyelitis and tuberculosis.

*Artificial active immunity* follows the injection of toxoids or vaccines.

**Passive Immunity.** Preformed immunoglobulins may be passively transferred either naturally or artificially.

*Natural passive immunity* is seen in the newborn.[12-14] The human fetus does not manufacture immunoglobulins unless infected *in utero* (see p. 147), and those which are normally present at birth are derived from the mother, having crossed the placenta. They are of the IgG variety, and confer some degree of immunity to infection on the baby for 3–6 months. Thus common virus diseases like measles and mumps are rare during this period.

*Artificial passive immunity* is deliberately induced by injecting immunoglobulin antibodies for prophylactic or therapeutic purposes. The antibodies may be obtained from the serum of an animal, usually the horse, or from another human. The protection afforded is short lived.

*Adoptive Immunity*[15,16] This is the passive immunity acquired by transference of cells from an immunized individual. It has been demonstrated in the experimental animal, but not in man because of the danger of producing a graft versus host (GVH) reaction (p. 170). The immunoglobulins are manufactured by the progeny of the transferred cells. This differs from the manner by which cells can transfer delayed hypersensitivity, in which it is the host cells that are changed (p. 166).

## Mechanism of Acquired Immunity

The manner whereby acquired immunity protects the body against infection depends upon the type of organism concerned. With the toxic organisms (p. 89) the immunity is due to *antitoxins*, while with the invasive group it is due to *antibacterial antibodies*.

**Antitoxic Immunity.**[17] Toxic organisms produce their effects by means of powerful, diffusible exotoxins which are highly antigenic. The antibodies (antitoxins) are capable of neutralizing the toxin, and act in the body by intercepting the toxin before it reaches susceptible tissues. Diphtheria provides a good example.

*Immunity in Diphtheria.* Diphtheria bacilli alighting on a mucous membrane produce their effect, and indeed the disease, by elaborating an exotoxin. This acts on the local tissues, causing necrosis of epithelium and pseudo-membrane formation, and is also absorbed by the blood stream and produces damage at such sites as the heart, adrenals, and peripheral nerves. If the host has a high antitoxin level in the circulation, and therefore in the tissues and mucus, the toxin is rapidly neutralized, thereby depriving the organism of its main offensive weapon. It then becomes in effect avirulent, and is removed by the normal decontaminating mechanism of the part. A virulent organism attacking a host with a high antitoxin level is in the same position as an avirulent organism attacking a normal host.

*Passive immunization* consists of giving diphtheria antitoxin (prepared from the serum of an immunized horse), so that no further damage is produced by the toxin. The organism itself is not directly affected, but is soon destroyed by the host's defence mechanism. This treatment is effective only if given early in the course of the disease.

*Active Immunization.* Since immunity to diphtheria is conferred by circulating antitoxin, active immunization is performed by inducing the subject to manufacture antitoxin. This is done by a series of *toxoid* injections. Toxoid consists of toxin treated with formaldehyde so that its toxicity is lost while its antigenicity is retained.

The other important toxic organisms, those causing tetanus and gas-gangrene, are described in Chapter 14. Immunity to them is also conferred by antitoxin, and closely resembles that seen in diphtheria.

**Antibacterial Humoral Immunity.**[17] Invasive organisms contain a great number of antigens, and during the course of an infection many types of antibody appear in the plasma. Thus towards the end of the second week in typhoid fever antibodies appear which are specific for the surface and flagellar antigens of *Salmonella typhi.* They are easily detected as agglutinins (see Widal reaction, p. 138). Similarly, in syphilis precipitins and complement-fixing antibodies appear, and are detected by the Kahn and Wassermann tests respectively. The appearance of these antibodies is often of *diagnostic value,* especially if their titre continues to rise.

In infection with invasive organisms the antibodies which appear are *antibacterial,* in the sense that they are directed against bacterial components. They are detected as agglutinins, precipitins, complement fixers (amboceptors), antibacterial haemolysins, antihyaluronidase, etc. Which test is employed to detect them in clinical practice is arbitrary—it is often the one which is most convenient, or merely the one which was first discovered! The antibodies detected are not necessarily the ones which destroy the organism *in vitro* or *in vivo.* Therefore they do not necessarily provide immunity. A syphilitic patient with a strongly positive Wassermann test is not immune—he is quite likely to be highly infectious!

Invasive organisms are destroyed in the body by two mechanisms: either they are digested by polymorphs or the phagocytic cells of the RE system, or they are lysed by the activation of complement. Antibacterial antibodies can provide immunity, and they do it by aiding one of these two mechanisms.

(*a*) They can act as *opsonins*. These neutralize the noxious surface antigens of certain virulent organisms, e.g. the capsular polysaccharide of pneumococci and the M protein of *Strept. pyogenes* (pp. 181 and 179), which repel or kill phagocytes at close quarters. An opsonized bacterium is easily phagocytosed.

(*b*) They can act as *amboceptors* (*bacteriolysins*) and activate complement. This bacteriolysis is seen in infections with *S. typhi*, *Vibrio cholerae*, and probably many other organisms. In many bacterial infections we have no satisfactory methods of detecting or estimating the titre of these protective antibodies. Hence *passive immunization*, produced by the administration of horse or human immunoglobulin, is not uniformly successful. The advent of chemotherapy as an alternative treatment has rendered serum therapy obsolete.

*Active immunization* can be induced by injecting a suspension of whole organisms called a *vaccine*. With some organisms a dead vaccine is used (e.g. TAB, which is a suspension of *S. typhi* and *S. paratyphi A and B*), but with others dead material is ineffective, and use is made of an attenuated (rendered avirulent) living vaccine (e.g. BCG in tuberculosis). Unfortunately, the factors which determine the virulence of invasive organisms are not clearly understood. Vaccines are prepared by a process of trial and error. Some are useful and others are not. Whooping-cough vaccine provides some protection, while staphylococcal vaccines do not. Moreover bacteria show considerable variation in their antigenic make-up, and a vaccine made with one strain will not protect against infection by another. Typhoid epidemics have occurred in troops "immunized" with TAB.

The local immunity produced by the presence of IgA in secretions is described on pages 83, 137, and 222.

**Cellular Antibacterial Immunity.**[18,19] Infection with some invasive organisms leads to the formation of cell-bound antibodies, so that the macrophages of the body are better able to ingest and destroy the organisms. This change is closely related to the development of *delayed-type hypersensitivity* (p. 165).

**Antiviral Immunity.** Circulating immunoglobulins play an important part in the destruction of viruses. By coating the virus, they prevent its attachment to the receptor site of the susceptible cell. Such a virus is soon destroyed by the humoral and cellular defences of the host. Other aspects of

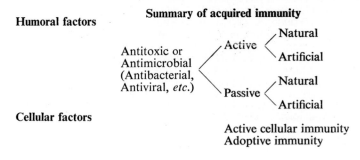

**Summary of acquired immunity**

Humoral factors

Antitoxic or Antimicrobial (Antibacterial, Antiviral, *etc.*)

Active — Natural / Artificial

Passive — Natural / Artificial

Cellular factors

Active cellular immunity
Adoptive immunity

antiviral immunity, i.e. cellular immunity and interferon, are considered in Chapter 16.

## Immunological-Deficiency Diseases[20,21]

The primary group of immunological-deficiency diseases is uncommon, but its study has strengthened the view that the immune response has two separate components. In one group, typified by *congenital sex-linked agammaglo-bulinaemia*, there is a failure in development of the B lymphocytes and the subject is susceptible to repeated bacterial infections often resulting in early death. In another group there is thymic aplasia and a complete failure in T lymphocyte development. These individuals suffer from virus, fungous, and acid-fast bacterial infections. In the most severe type there is a complete failure of both T lymphocytes and B lymphocyte development, and life is limited to a year or two.

*Acquired immunological deficiency* is of much greater practical importance, and occurs in generalized lymphoma (particularly Hodgkin's disease), leukaemia, multiple myeloma, and occasionally in other types of malignant disease. It is also a feature of therapy with cytotoxic drugs and glucocortico-steroids.

An interesting feature of the immunological-deficiency diseases, particularly the primary group, is the tendency for the subjects to develop malignant disease, particularly lymphoma. This lends support to the concept that the immune reaction plays a role in eliminating malignant cells from the body.

## References

1. McRipley, R. J. and Sbarra, A. J. (1967). *J. Bact.*, **94**, 1417.
2. Editorial (1969). *New Engl. J. Med.*, **280**, 1355.
3. Pincus, S. H. and Klebanoff, S. J. (1971). *New Engl. J. Med.*, **284**, 744.
4. Ruddy, S., Gigli, I. and Austen, K. F. (1972). *New Engl. J. Med.*, **287**, 489, 545, 592 and 642.
5. Götze, O. and Müller-Eberhard, H. J. (1971). *J. exp. Med.*, **134**, 90s.
6. Editorial (1972). *New Engl. J. Med.*, **227**, 716.
7. Lepow, I. H. and Rosen, F. S. (1972). *New Engl. J. Med.*, **286**, 942.
8. Lurie, M. B. (1950). *Amer. J. Med.*, **9**, 591.
9. Allison, A. C. (1954). *Brit. med. J.* **1**, 290.
10. Roberts, J. A. F. (1970). In "An Introduction to Medical Genetics", 5th ed. p. 67. London: Oxford University Press.
11. Kallmann, F. J. and Reisner, D. (1943). *Amer. Rev. Tuber.*, **47**, 549.
12. Cruickshank, R. (1963). In "Modern Trends in Immunology", I, p. 107. London: Butterworths.
13. Brambell, R. W. R. (1961). *Proc. roy. Soc. Med.*, **54**, 992.
14. Bangham, D. R. (1961). *Proc. roy. Soc. Med.*, **54**, 993.
15. Harris, T. N. and Harris, S. (1960). In "Cellular Aspects of Immunity" (Ciba Foundation Symposium), p. 172, ed. by Wolstenholme, G. E. W. and O'Connor, M. London: Churchill.
16. Cochrane, C. G. and Dixon, F. J. (1962). *Advanc. Immunol.*, **2**. 205.
17. Wilson, G. S. and Miles, A. A. (1964). In "Topley and Wilson's Principles of Bacteriology and Immunity", 5th ed., p. 1261. London: Arnold.
18. Howard, J. G. (1963). In "Modern Trends in Immunology", p. 86, *loc. cit.*
19. Rowley, D. (1962). *Advanc. Immunol.*, **2**, 241.
20. Editorial (1970). *New Engl. J. Med.*, **283**, 656.
21. Gatti, R. A. and Good, R. A. (1970). *Medical Clinics of North America*, **54**, 281.

*Chapter 13*

# HYPERSENSITIVITY, TISSUE GRAFTS, AND AUTOIMMUNITY

## Hypersensitivity

Hypersensitivity is a state in which, having experienced a primary response to an antigen, an animal reacts in an excessive way to a subsequent exposure to the same antigen. *Allergy* is sometimes used to denote a second response which is altered in quality rather than being simply excessive. It is very doubtful whether such a distinction is valid. Furthermore, both terms are used quite indiscriminately in the literature; in this book they will be used synonymously.

Two distinct types of hypersensitivity can be recognized. In one, the reaction to administration of antigen is immediate (within minutes), while in the other it is delayed for 24 to 48 hours. The distinction between these two types is of fundamental importance. The *immediate-type* hypersensitivities are related to the formation of sensitizing immunoglobulins. In *delayed-type* hypersensitivity the reaction is cell mediated.

It is now realized that immunoglobulins can cause hypersensitivity in various ways, and that in only one of these is the reaction immediate in the sense that this term is usually used. Indeed, injury due to immunoglobulins can be caused in three distinct ways, and these have been classified thus:

*Type I, or immediate-type hypersensitivity.* This is commonly mediated by IgE, and is typified by acute anaphylaxis in man.

*Type II, or cytotoxic reaction.* Antibodies, IgG or IgM, are directed against cellular or tissue antigens, e.g. as in haemolytic anaemia due to haemolysins.

*Type III, due to antigen-antibody complexes.* IgG is mainly involved.

In the *delayed-type hypersensitivities*, no such sensitizing antibodies can be demonstrated, and the hypersensitivity is cell-mediated. This type of hyper-sensitivity is classified as *type IV*.

## TYPE I—IMMEDIATE HYPERSENSITIVITY

The features of this type of hypersensitivity have been the subject of intensive experimental study in animals. Anaphylaxis, which represents the most severe manifestation, will be described first as it illustrates the main features of this group.

### Anaphylaxis[1-3]

#### Generalized Anaphylaxis in the Guinea-Pig

If a guinea-pig is given an injection of a simple protein, e.g. egg albumin, it shows no obvious discomfort. After about two weeks specific immuno-globulins appear in plasma. If a second injection of egg albumin is then given intravenously, antigen reacts with sensitizing antibody on the cells and the animal dies of generalized anaphylaxis (*anaphylactic shock*) within a few minutes. The following features should be noted:

1. Generalized anaphylaxis can be elicited by giving a single large *shocking dose* of antigen at a suitable interval after one or more sensitizing doses.

2. The reaction is highly *specific* for the antigen.

3. The shocking dose must be administered quickly, and the intravenous route is generally employed.

4. The serum, or purified specific immunoglobulin, of a sensitized animal will passively sensitize a previously normal animal. The passive sensitization is not immediate but is made manifest after a time interval of several hours. Thus the presence of specific immunoglobulin in the plasma alone does not confer sensitivity—present evidence suggests that the antibody must become fixed to cells.

5. The cells which are sensitized (*target cells*) are mast cells; it is uncertain whether other cell types are also involved.

6. An important mediator of generalized anaphylaxis is *histamine*.[4] It can be detected in the blood during anaphylactic shock and is released when antigen is applied to sensitized tissue *in vitro*. Antihistamine drugs will inhibit the acute manifestations of anaphylaxis, but the animal may still die some hours later of *protracted anaphylaxis*. The pathogenesis of this is not known for certain, but *kinin* formation has been suggested. Histamine is not the only agent released from sensitized tissue when acted upon by antigen. Another vasoactive substance can be detected: this, when applied to isolated uterine muscle, produces a slow, sustained contraction quite unlike the rapid kick produced by histamine. The agent is a lipoprotein and is called *slow reacting substance of anaphylaxis* (*SRS–A*)[4]. It is probably an important mediator in human anaphylaxis.

**Cytotropic Anaphylaxis.** Anaphylaxis as described in the actively sensitized guinea-pig is called *cytotropic*, because it is the result of antigen reacting with antibody fixed to cells. The sensitizing antibody concerned migrates in the $\gamma_1$ band, and is of the 7S IgG type and has in the past been called a reagin. Other animals produce a similar type of sensitizing antibody, and in man the most important belongs to the IgE class. A person sensitized by this type of antibody will exhibit erythema and a weal if a small quantity of antigen is injected into the skin (*cutaneous, or local, anaphylaxis*).

**Aggregate Anaphylaxis.** This type of anaphylaxis occurs in the actively sensitized rabbit, and is due to the formation of antigen-antibody aggregates in the circulation. The antigen-antibody complexes *fix complement*, and the chemotactic $C\overline{567}$ is released. Polymorphs join the aggregates and release their damaging lysosomal enzymes. The sensitizing 7S IgG antibody migrates in the $\gamma_2$ band on electrophoresis. In aggregate anaphylaxis there is *no cell fixation, histamine is not released*, and *antihistamine drugs do not protect*. Both *complement* and *polymorphs* are essential and the phenomenon falls into the type III, or immune-complex, group.

Cytotropic and aggregate anaphylaxis are best studied in pure form in animals passively sensitized with purified antibody of the appropriate type.

Actively sensitized animals usually produce antibodies of both types, and anaphylactic shock in them is often a mixture of the two types. This accounts for the confusing past literature on this subject.

Although the manifestations of anaphylactic shock vary in different species, and even in the same species under separate conditions, two main effects are seen. These are:

1. *Spasm of smooth muscle*—either blood vessel or bronchial.
2. *Damage to small blood vessels.*

When the reaction occurs in man the manifestations are:

(1) *Bronchospasm*, with great difficulty in expiration. This sudden onset of wheezing dyspnoea is characteristic.
(2) *Oedema*, due to a generalized increase in vascular permeability. Sometimes *oedema of the larynx* adds to the respiratory difficulty.
(3) *Pallor and low blood pressure. Death often follows.*

The sensitizing IgE has a great affinity for cells to which it becomes firmly attached. Very little need be present in the blood. Hence, unlike the situation in the guinea-pig, very small doses of antigen can cause acute anaphylactic shock. Although rare in man, it is seen under two circumstances:

(*a*) When horse γ-globulin is given to patients who are sensitized to horse protein, e.g. in passive immunization against diphtheria and tetanus, whether prophylactic or therapeutic.
(*b*) When a drug which is capable of acting as a hapten is injected into a patient who is sensitive to it. *Penicillin* is such a drug, and each year a number of people die of anaphylaxis from this therapy.

The danger of anaphylaxis should always be kept in mind by anyone administering animal serum or drugs by injection. At the first sign of anaphylaxis, 1·0 ml. of a 1 in 1 000 solution of adrenaline should be given by *intramuscular* injection and 0·5 ml. repeated as necessary. Oedema of the larynx may necessitate an emergency tracheotomy.

### Dust and Food Hypersensitivity[5]

This group of hypersensitivity reactions occurs after the *ingestion* of certain foods and the *inhalation* of antigens like pollen and dust. The symptoms differ according to the route of absorption. The offending chemical may be a complete antigen or a hapten; the latter presumably combines with tissue or plasma protein to produce a complete antigen.

#### Types

*Inhalation* of antigens like pollen, horse dander, and dust usually produces watering of the eyes (*hay-fever*), symptoms referable to the respiratory tract, e.g. congestion of the nasal mucosa (*allergic rhinitis*), and *asthma* (p. 410).

*Ingestion* of certain foods produces either *gastrointestinal symptoms* or *skin eruptions*. Shellfish, mushrooms, strawberries, and milk are among the numerous foods to which some people are allergic. Hypersensitivity to drugs is considered later.

## Nature of the Lesions

The lesions are *exudative* in type and sometimes contain *eosinophils*. Histamine is almost certainly a mediator, and antihistamine drugs have an ameliorative effect.

## Genetic Influence: Atopy

Patients with this type of hypersensitivity frequently give a family history of similar complaints. One may have hay-fever, another asthma, etc. It is the capacity to react to antigens in this peculiar way which is inherited, and the condition is called atopy. The subjects manufacture IgE which has a marked capacity of adhering to cells and sensitizing them to the subsequent contact with antigen. These antibodies, although present in the plasma, cannot easily be detected by the conventional methods of precipitation, complement fixation, etc. They can, however, be demonstrated by *passive transfer*. Serum from a hypersensitive patient injected into the skin of a normal person renders that portion of skin sensitive to the antigen. This test is called the *Prausnitz-Küstner reaction*, after the two workers who demonstrated it in experiments on themselves. Küstner was sensitive to cooked fish and transferred his sensitivity to Prausnitz.

Sensitive people can be detected by injecting a minute dose of the offending antigen into the skin. Erythema and a weal appear *within a few minutes*. It should be noted that if a large dose of antigen is given, especially if it is injected intravenously, the subject may exhibit anaphylactic shock. Unfortunately, the results of skin tests are not a reliable indication of a possible sensitization to anaphylaxis. The safest procedure, when administering foreign sera, is to give a small test dose subcutaneously and watch for any mild general reaction.

Atopic subjects are particularly liable to develop sensitization to anaphylactic shock. It therefore follows that before any injection is given to a patient, enquiry should be made into any personal or familial liability to hypersensitivity (infantile eczema, hay-fever, asthma, etc.).

## Desensitization to Immediate-Type Hypersensitivity

If it is desired to give an antigen (e.g. serum) to which an individual is sensitive, this may be done by giving small doses at frequent intervals. Although this procedure may avoid immediate serious complications, e.g. anaphylactic shock, and is loosely referred to as "desensitization", it is doubtful whether it is ever justified. The injected antigen is rapidly eliminated, and is therefore of little therapeutic value. Furthermore, an accelerated type of serum sickness (p. 163) may result and symptoms appear after a few days.

Another type of desensitization is sometimes attempted in patients with asthma, hay-fever, etc. Minute doses of antigen (e.g. pollen extracts) to which the subject is sensitive are injected at weekly intervals. The aim is to induce the formation of "blocking antibodies" in excess. When the individual is next exposed to antigen, it combines with the circulating blocking antibody, which therefore protects the sensitized cells from the damaging effect of antigen. Unfortunately this procedure is not uniformly successful.

## HYPERSENSITIVITY MEDIATED BY ANTIGEN-ANTIBODY COMPLEXES[9]

### Arthus Phenomenon[1]

Repeated weekly subcutaneous injections of an antigen, even into different areas, lead to progressively more severe local reactions; later injections produce haemorrhagic necrosis and ulceration. The reaction is due to the interaction of injected antigen with circulating sensitizing immunoglobulins.

Damaging antigen-antibody complexes are formed in the vessel wall, the complement system is activated, and this induces polymorphs to accumulate and release damaging lysosomal enzymes. The vessels become blocked, the wall is damaged, and haemorrhage and ischaemic necrosis follow. The pathogenesis of the Arthus phenomenon bears some resemblance to that of aggregate anaphylaxis. However, in the Arthus reaction the antibody concerned is probably different, it must be present in much larger quantities, and finally the damaging antigen-antibody interaction is believed to take place in the vessel wall itself. The Arthu phenomenon is an example of a type III reaction, and is of interest to the experimental pathologist, but the reaction is difficult to implicate in any common human disease.

### Serum Sickness[1]

Serum sickness is a condition characterized by *fever*, *joint pains*, and *urticarial eruptions* that occurs 10–14 days after the administration of a *large dose* of foreign serum, e.g. horse $\gamma$-globulin. The pathogenesis is explained in Fig. 13.1. The injected antigen persists in the blood until the 10th day. At this time the immune response becomes evident by the disappearance of antigen from the blood (immune catabolism) and the appearance of immunoglobulins in the plasma. At first they form complexes with antigen, but as these are eliminated, free antibody appears in the plasma. The lesions of serum sickness are due to the damaging effect of immune complexes deposited at certain sites—skin, etc. Complement is activated, and polymorphs accumulate and release damaging lysosomal enzymes.

Microscopically the lesions of serum sickness are similar to those of the Arthus reaction, but are less severe. There is an acute vasculitis with polymorphs infiltrating the vessel walls. In addition, a glomerulonephritis is characteristic.

*Chronic Immune-Complex Disease.* If daily injections of antigen are given to an animal in doses such that antigen-antibody complexes with antigen excess are formed in the blood, a chronic glomerulonephritis develops. It is believed that some types of human glomerulonephritis have a similar pathogenesis, for example the renal lesions of systemic lupus erythematosus.

### Drug Hypersensitivity[35-37]

Hypersensitivity to drugs is a common clinical event, and is due to the drug, or one of its degradation products, acting as a hapten and stimulating the formation of sensitizing antibodies. Virtually any drug can produce a reaction, but common offenders are penicillin, sulphonamides, aspirin, barbiturates, and quinine. Relatively few people given a drug manifest hypersensitivity, and the tendency to develop IgE-mediated effects is particularly marked in atopic individuals.

**Types of Drug Reaction.** The reaction may be *immediate* (type I reaction), and range from urticaria to severe, fatal anaphylactic shock. Sensitizing IgE antibodies are responsible. *Later drug reactions* begin several days after the

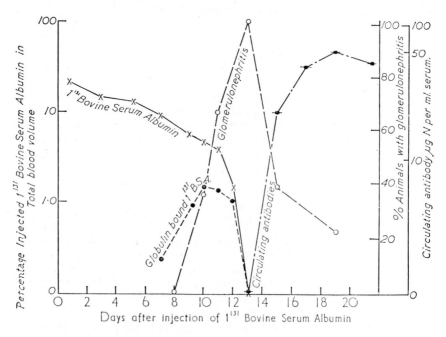

FIG. 13.1. Time relations between fall of circulating antigen, formation of antigen-antibody complexes, lesions of serum sickness (glomerulonephritis), and rise of circulating antibody in rabbits injected with large doses of [131]I-labelled bovine serum albumin.
(*From Gladstone, G. P.* (1961). *In Florey, H. W.* "General Pathology" 3rd ed.; *after Dixon, J. F. et al.* (1959). *In Lawrence, H. S.* "Cellular and Humoral Aspects of the Hypersensitivity States", p. 345. *New York: Harper and Row.*)

administration of the drug, and have the features of immune–complex disease (type III reaction). Urticarial, papular, and petechial skin eruptions are common in addition to arthralgia and fever. The antibodies concerned are IgG or IgM. *Late drug effects* are thrombocytopenia, haemolytic anaemia, erythema multiforme, jaundice, and a syndrome resembling systemic lupus erythematosus. The pathogenesis of many reactions is unclear. In some instances, e.g. haemolytic anaemia, cytotoxic antibodies are present (type II reaction); they may be directed against the drug, as in penicillin-induced haemolytic anaemia, or against the red-cell surface antigens, an effect induced by α-methyldopa.

## DELAYED-TYPE HYPERSENSITIVITY[6-8]

The simplest example of this type is bacterial hypersensitivity (bacterial allergy) as exemplified by the *Koch phenomenon*. It should be noted that the term bacterial allergy is somewhat inappropriate, because immediate-type hypersensitivity can also occur during bacterial infections. *Delayed-type hypersensitivity* is a more acceptable term, and it can occur in response to antigens of non-bacterial origin. *Cell-mediated hypersensitivity* is the most common currently used term, since it not only indicates that the antibodies concerned are cellular, but it also distinguishes the reactions from certain immune-complex phenomena which take several hours to develop and are therefore difficult to distinguish, if the classification is based strictly on the time taken for the reaction to appear.

### The Koch Phenomenon

If tubercle bacilli are injected into a normal guinea-pig, there is an incubation period of 10–14 days followed by the appearance of a nodule at the site of injection. Ulceration follows and persists till the death of the animal. The bacilli spread to the local lymph nodes, finally reach the blood stream, and produce generalized miliary tuberculosis and death. The injection of more tubercle bacilli into an animal infected 4–6 weeks previously evokes a different type of response. A nodule appears in 1–2 days, ulcerates, and then heals. There is little tendency to spread to the local lymph nodes. This second type of response was described by Koch, and it should be noted that the reaction of a tuberculous animal to tubercle bacilli differs from that of a normal one in three important respects:

(1) The incubation period is greatly shortened—this may be described as *hypersensitivity*.
(2) The lesion heals quickly.
(3) There is no spread. These are the features of *immunity*.

The heightened tissue response of the tuberculous animal can be demonstrated not only to the living tubercle bacillus, but also to dead organisms and extracts of organism. Koch originally used "old tuberculin", a crude extract of the bacilli, but more recently a Purified Protein Derivative (PPD) has been introduced.

The injection of a small quantity of PPD into a normal animal results in a negligible inflammatory response. In the tuberculous animal, however, there develops an indurated erythematous lesion which appears within 12–24 hours and reaches a peak by 48–72 hours. This is the *tuberculin*, or *Mantoux test*, and a positive result indicates the existence of hypersensitivity to tuberculoprotein. The injection of a larger quantity of PPD into a tuberculous animal leads to a generalized reaction with *fever* and in severe cases *shock* and *death*. This occurs with a dose of tuberculoprotein which would have no serious effects on a normal, unsensitized animal.

This type of hypersensitivity differs in many important respects from the type I reactions previously described:

1. The reaction is delayed—it takes at least 12 *hours* to develop as compared with a few *minutes*.

2. Although there is some vasodilatation and oedema, the reaction is characterized by the accumulation of lymphocytes and macrophages rather than polymorphs.

3. The reaction is not mediated by histamine, serotonin, kinins, or products of complement activation. The reaction is not blocked by antihistamine drugs, but is inhibited by cortisone.

4. It is not causally related to any known types of immunoglobulins, and cannot be transferred to another animal by serum transfusion. It has been suggested that a plasma antibody with high affinity for antigen is involved, and that it is present in such low concentrations that it cannot be detected by present-day methods.[10] This explanation is possible but improbable.[11]

5. Delayed-type hypersensitivity can be transferred to a normal animal by the transfer of lymphocytes. These T cells carry cell-bound antibodies,[12] and the delayed nature of the reaction is probably due to the time taken for these cells to accumulate at the site of antigen injection. The lymphokines (p. 140) are the mediators for this reaction.

The state of passive hypersensitivity persists for as long as the injected cells live in the new host. In some way *the transplanted cells alter the host's own lymphocytes* so that these also take part in a delayed-type skin reaction which is subsequently elicited.[13,14] *In man*, delayed-type hypersensitivity can be transferred, not only by living cells, but also by extracts of white cells. Although described by Lawrence in 1955,[15] the action of the *transfer factor*, which is one of the lymphokines, is not known but it is evidently very potent, for a single injection can render the recipient hypersensitive for many months.[16,17]

**In-Vitro Detection of Cellular Antibody.**[38] In spite of the potent effects exhibited by sensitized lymphocytes *in vivo*, the manner by which they produce tissue damage is poorly understood. As described on p. 140, when T lymphocytes come into contact with specific antigen, a number of potent low-molecular-weight factors called lymphokines are liberated. Insofar as cell-mediated hypersensitivity is concerned, lymphotoxin is probably the most important, but other factors may recruit cells (migration-inhibition factor) and augment the inflammatory reaction (skin-reactive factor). The lymphokines can be demonstrated *in vitro*, and in practice two methods are commonly used to detect sensitized lymphocytes:

*Migration Inhibition Effect.*[18] Lymphocytes and macrophages from the peritoneal cavity of a sensitized guinea-pig are placed in a capillary tube, and incubated in a suitable chamber containing culture fluid. Normally the cells migrate from the free ends of the tube to form tufts. These tufts do not appear if the cells from a guinea-pig showing delayed-type sensitivity are incubated in the presence of antigen (Fig. 13.2). If cells from a normal animal, mixed with about 10 per cent of cells from a sensitized one, are placed in a tube and cultured in the presence of antigen, *none* of the cells migrate. Hence a few sensitized cells can transfer information to cells *in vitro* just as they can *in vivo*. This is due to the action of transfer factor. It should be noted that lymphocytes from an animal sensitized towards immunoglobulin

production and not delayed-type hypersensitivity do not show this phenomenon.

The effect of antigen on sensitized human cells can be assessed by using
white blood cells from the buffy coat. If these are packed into capillary
tubes, as described above, their migration is inhibited by the antigen to
which the patient is sensitive.

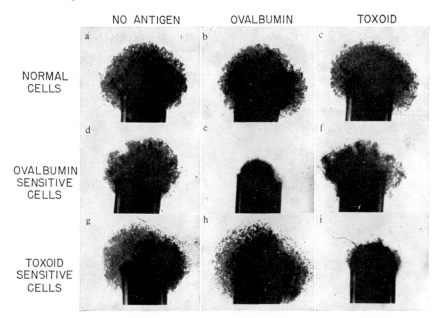

FIG. 13.2. Specific inhibition by antigen of the migration of cells from sensitized
animals. The cells, mostly macrophages and lymphocytes from a peritoneal
exudate, are placed in capillary tubes and incubated in a microchamber.
Normally the macrophages migrate from the open end and produce a
tufted appearance. The cells derived from animals with delayed-type hypersensitivity show no migration in the presence of the specific antigen.

(*From David, J. R., Al-Askarí, S., Lawrence, H. S. and Thomas, L. (1964),
J. Immunol., 93, 264*).

*Lymphocyte Transformation.* Lymphocytes from a sensitized animal, when
incubated with the appropriate antigen, show transformation (p. 143). The
number of cells transforming is not as great as with phytohaemagglutinin nor
is it as rapid.

## Examples of Cell-Mediated Hypersensitivity

1. *Following infection.* A positive Mantoux reaction means past or present
infection with the tubercle bacillus. Similar tests are available for other
infections, e.g. leprosy, histoplasmosis, and coccidioidomycosis. Quite apart
from their diagnostic value, delayed hypersensitivity reactions are probably
responsible for many of the features of chronic infection. Much of the damage
produced by the organisms is due to the host's own reaction.

2. *Allergic contact dermatitis.*[19] This follows the application of a sensitizing chemical to the skin. The pathogenesis has been described previously (p. 133). The reaction is typically that of an acute dermatitis, and should not be confused with the erythematous, itchy, wealing type of skin reaction seen in immediate-type hypersensitivity.

3. *The Graft Reaction.* See below.

4. *Experimental.*[20] It has also been described after certain experimental procedures in which antigen is injected with *Freund's adjuvant.* The latter consists of an oil-in-water emulsion mixed with tubercle bacilli. It is not known how this curious mixture can potentiate the sensitizing effect of an antigen.

**Retest Reaction.**[21] If a positive tuberculin skin test is performed on a sensitive person, and the *same site* is retested with tuberculin at a later date, an accelerated reaction is observed. It appears at 2 hours and is maximal at 8 hours. The lesion is characterized by exudation of *fluid* and massive accumulation of *eosinophils.* Immediate-type hypersensitivity is not involved, but the mechanism concerned in the retest reaction is not known. Nevertheless, this phenomenon deserves further study, for many human diseases of an "allergic" nature are also characterized by exudation and eosinophil infiltration, and some are curiously unresponsive to antihistamine drugs (e.g. asthma, allergic rhinitis, nasal polyps, etc.).

## TISSUE GRAFTS[22]

In addition to its practical value in surgery, the transplantation of tissue has done much to extend our knowledge of the body's response to foreign tissues. To a considerable extent the fate of a graft depends upon its origin— the three types, autografts, homografts, and heterografts, will therefore be described separately.

### Autografts

An *autograft* is a graft of tissue made from one site to another site in the same individual. Provided the graft attains an adequate blood supply it usually lives and functions normally.

Autografts have found extensive use in plastic surgery. Whole-thickness flaps of skin may be used as pedicle grafts from one part of the body to another, or alternatively free grafts may be applied to raw surfaces, e.g. following burns.

In dentistry, teeth have been transplanted successfully from one part of the mouth to another.[23,24]

### Homografts

A *homograft* is a transplant made from one individual to another of the same species. If the two individuals are *syngeneic (isogeneic)*, i.e. of identical or nearly identical genetic structure, then the term *syngeneic*, or *isogeneic homograft* is used. Such a graft is accepted as "self", does not provoke any immune response, and provided it attains an adequate blood supply persists indefinitely. In man this situation occurs only with grafts exchanged between identical twins.

An *allogeneic homograft*, or *allograft*, (often simply called a homograft), is a graft made between individuals of the same species but of different genetic constitutions.

As a general rule such a graft is always rejected due to the destruction of its cellular component by antibodies manufactured by the host. Three patterns of rejection are seen:

*Hyperacute*, due to the presence of preformed immunoglobulin, as in the white graft reaction.[25]

*Acute*, the most common reaction, and cell mediated.

*Chronic*, occurring after a year.

If, following the rejection of a allograft, another graft is applied to the same animal from the same donor, this second graft is rejected even more rapidly. This is known as the *second set phenomenon*.

The application of a second skin graft within a short time (about 12 days) of the rejection of the first results in the *white graft reaction:* the graft is not vascularized, but becomes pale, undergoes necrosis, and is cast off. The rejection is mediated by immunoglubulins, and a human counterpart is seen when a kidney graft undergoes hyperacute rejection due to a major ABO incompatibility or the pre-existence of antibodies to the graft.

If the second graft is applied after a longer interval, it shows early vascularization, but suddenly by the fourth or fifth day it becomes cyanosed and the surrounding skin shows marked erythema and oedema. The vessels thrombose and the graft undergoes necrosis. This is termed the *accelerated graft rejection phenomenon*, and is mediated by cell-bound antibodies in the form of small lymphocytes. These cells are also responsible for the rejection of a first graft, and is presumably mediated by lymphokines. This accelerated graft rejection reaction can be transferred from one animal to another by the transfer of small lymphocytes. Graft immunity therefore resembles very closely the tuberculin-type of cell-mediated hypersensitivity.

*Chronic rejection* has been seen in human heart and kidney transplants. A year or more after apparent acceptance, the vessels of the graft become obstructed by intimal thickening and the organ suffers from progressive ischaemia. Humoral as well as cellular antibodies are involved in this type of rejection.

The vigour with which a graft is rejected is related to the type and amount of *transplantation antigens*[26] present in the graft but not represented in the host. Some tissues contain much antigen and these are rejected rapidly—thus in man skin and heart transplants have met with little success. Renal grafts, on the other hand, are of great value. A start has been made on identifying the transplantation antigens in man, and it is now possible to match the host and graft more closely. The antigens are determined by genes which are part of a single complex called the HL-A system.

Various attempts have been made to prolong the life of allografts[27,28] (p. 134). In general these involve suppression of the immune response by ionizing radiation and the administration of cytotoxic drugs, but although the graft, e.g. a kidney, may live for several years, indefinite survival is very difficult to attain using present methods. Thus grafts whose function is dependent upon the continued survival of their cells (*homovital grafts*) are of limited value. This contrasts with a *static* graft, in which the cells die, but the matrix persists and performs an important function. The best example of this is a bone graft.[29] The cells die, but the matrix remains and is gradually replaced by living host bone. Bone homografts are in fact as useful as auto-grafts, because the osteocytes of the latter usually die through their failure to acquire an adequate blood supply in time. *Cornea* and *heart valves* are also used as homostatic grafts.

Homotransplantation of tissues in animals has provided much useful basic knowledge. The observation by Medawar that foreign cells injected into fetal or newborn mice were accepted as self and persisted indefinitely, led to the concept of *specific immunological tolerance*, since grafts from the same donor were accepted throughout the life of the treated animal. Furthermore, it was noted that if the injected foreign cells were immunologically competent (i.e. were small lymphocytes taken from adult animals), although they were recognized as "self" and accepted, they themselves reacted against the host. The injected animals failed to thrive, and often died of a wasting disease called runt disease. This is an example of a *graft versus host (GVH) reaction*.[30] It is occasionally seen when children suffering from an immunological deficiency disease are transfused with fresh blood containing living white cells, incompatible so far as the HL-A antigens are concerned.[31]

### Heterografts

A *heterograft*, or *xenograft*, is a transplant from one animal to another of a different species. Vital grafts are invariably rejected.

## AUTOIMMUNITY

Although it is evident that under normal conditions the body does not make antibodies against its own tissues, the mechanisms which prevent their formation may on occasion break down.

In theory antibodies could be made against the individual's own tissues (*autoantibodies*) under three circumstances:

1. **Alteration in Antigenicity of Tissue Protein.** This may be due to:

*Degenerative lesions.* Following necrosis of tissue, e.g. the skin in burns, antibodies may be produced. It is evident that these antibodies are an effect of the disease and not its cause.

*Attachment of hapten*, e.g. allergic contact dermatitis (p. 133). A similar mechanism has been held to explain the aetiology of acute rheumatic fever. Streptococcal antigen might become attached to body proteins (e.g. of heart), and the antibodies produced against the altered proteins could cause damage. An alternative explanation is that the streptococci share a common antigen with the heart, so that antibodies to the organisms also react with the heart.[32] Nevertheless, the most likely explanation of acute rheumatic fever is that it is an immune-complex disease involving streptococcal antigen in excess.

2. **Release of an Antigen Which has Always been Isolated.** It may be that some tissue products are anatomically isolated from the immunologically competent cells, and are therefore not recognized as "self" when released into the blood stream following injury or disease. It has been postulated that

thyroglobulin in the thyroid acini is one such substance, and that antibodies to it could damage the thyroid cells to produce Hashimoto's disease (p. 475). The evidence is not convincing.

3. **Altered Reactivity of the Immune Mechanism.** In this case "self" proteins would no longer be recognized. There is little doubt that this does sometimes occur. In chronic lymphatic leukaemia haemolysins are sometimes produced, and these may cause haemolytic anaemia. This is a good example of a condition caused by autoantibodies, and it indicates that the lymphoid tissue plays an important role in the immune response.

**Experimental Autoimmune Disease.** The injection into an animal of normal syngeneic or allogeneic tissue mixed with Freund's adjuvant may result in a disease of the respective organ, which is presumed to be due to autoantibody production. If thyroid is used, a condition resembling Hashimoto's disease is produced.[33] If brain tissue is used, allergic encephalomyelitis results.

**Types of Antibody.** It may be postulated that the autoantibodies will either be immunoglobulins or cell-bound. The immunoglobulins might be of any class and of one or two types:

1. *Organ-specific* immunoglobulins, whose specificity is directed against a determinant present in one organ, e.g. haemolysins and antithyroid antibodies.

2. *Non-organ-specific.* Antibodies directed against DNA, mitochondria, smooth muscle, and immunoglobulin determinants (rheumatoid factor) fall into this group.

### Role of Autoantibodies in Disease Processes

Antibodies may directly attack a tissue and cause damage. The immunoglobulins acquire destructive properties by activating complement, e.g. acute haemolytic anaemia due to a haemolysin. Cell-bound antibodies can also destroy cells, e.g. experimental allergic encephalomyelitis. Autoantibodies can also combine with antigen and form damaging antigen–antibody complexes; sometimes complement is activated. The lesions of this immune-complex disease resemble serum sickness if acute, but if the process is chronic, the kidney is the organ most often affected[9] (see p. 163). Diseases in which the major lesions are caused by an immune mechanism may with justification be called autoimmune diseases. However, it must be stressed that the autoimmunity merely provides a mechanism in the pathogenesis of a disease. It does not provide the cause, which as noted below may be inherited or acquired.

### Aetiology of Immunologically Mediated Diseases

1. *Genetic factors.* There is a definite tendency for some autoimmune diseases, e.g. systemic lupus erythematosus and rheumatoid arthritis, to be familial. This is probably due to the fact that the ability to produce sensitizing antibodies, or antibodies in such quantity or of such a type that immune-complex disease can occur, is genetically determined.

2. *Acquired factors.* Any extrinsic cause of disease can precipitate an autoimmune process. Certain drugs and sunlight can precipitate the onset of lupus erythematosus, and viral infections will on occasions produce autoimmune haemolytic anaemia (e.g. in mycoplasmal pneumonia). When the aetiology of a disease is clearly established, as in smallpox, the immunologi-

cally mediated manifestations of the disease, such as the skin eruption, are readily accepted as part of the whole condition. It is when the cause of a disease is not known, e.g. rheumatoid arthritis, that stress is laid on the autoimmune component of the illness. The label "autoimmune disease" should not, however, delude one into thinking that one knows the cause of the disease—one has only described part of its pathogenesis.

## The Collagen Diseases

This term has been a convenient respository for a number of conditions of obscure aetiology in which there is a chronic inflammatory reaction and widespread parenchymatous destruction. Fibrinoid necrosis of collagen is a feature of most of them, and the presence of autoantibodies in these diseases has led to them being regarded as autoimmune. These antibodies play some part in the pathogenesis of the lesions of the diseases, but the precise aetiology of each of them is unknown.

*Lupus erythematosus* is described in Chapter 36. It is the disease in which the greatest array of autoantibodies is found, and immune complexes are an important feature in the pathogenesis of some of the lesions, e.g. the glomerular lesions. In *polyarteritis nodosa*, medium-sized arteries are involved and their damaged walls show acute inflammation, necrosis, and aneurysm formation.

*Acute rheumatic fever* and *rheumatoid arthritis* may also be included among the collagen diseases; in them the connective tissue of the joints is particularly affected. *Scleroderma* is the most indolent of these collagen diseases, and is described in Chapter 36.

## Summary

From this brief account of the immune response and its relationship to hypersensitivity and immunity to infection, it is evident that the body's response to foreign material is very complex.

In response to antigenetic stimulation, two types of antibodies can be produced: the immunoglobulins and the cell-bound type. Which variety is formed depends upon the nature of the initiating antigen and the method whereby it is presented to the body.

With *simple protein antigens*, or haptens which combine the body proteins, it is the immunoglobulin type of antibody which is produced. If the antigen is a bacterial toxin or component of a bacteria, the antibody can afford immunity to infection. Sometimes, the immunoglobulin antibodies are of such a type (IgE in man) that they can sensitize the cells of the body to the action of antigen—this mediates hypersensitivity of the anaphylactic type. Sometimes antibodies form damaging complexes with antigen, and this leads to non-specific injury in various parts of the body; commonly the kidney and blood vessels are involved. This is immune-complex disease, or type III reaction. Occasionally antibodies are specific for a particular tissue, as when haemolysins are formed. This is the type II reaction.

When the body is invaded by *foreign living cells*, cell-bound antibodies are formed and these reside in the lymphocytes. Such sensitized lymphocytes when confronted with the appropriate antigen release a variety of lymphokines. These may attack the target cells directly or recruit macrophages and enhance the inflammatory response. The cell-mediated immune response can lead to the rejection of grafts and cause damage to the skin in acute allergic contact dermatitis. It can also mediate immunity to microbial infection, not only by directly affecting the organisms but also by exciting an inflammatory response and recruiting macrophages.

The role of the immune response appears clear enough when considering the action of immunoglobulins. Bacteria and their toxins are killed or neutralized. Hypersensitivity appears to be an unfortunate side-effect, but even this may have some beneficial effect in that it excites an acute inflammatory response.

The role of the cell-mediated immune response is less clear. Sensitized cells are thought to be important in the destruction of intracellular organisms and are therefore of survival value. The advantage of type IV hypersensitivity is, however, difficult to understand, since it seems to be a factor in prolonging the effect of some infections which thereby become chronic. Also the value of a response which eliminates foreign, grafts is of no obvious evolutionary advantage. It has been suggested that the immune response, particularly the cell-mediated type, has evolved as a mechanism for eliminating invading organisms and also for the destruction of abnormal cells which have been produced in the body as a result of damage or genetic change. This scrutinizing action of the lymphocytes may therefore be an important homeostatic mechanism whereby neoplastic cells are destroyed and eliminated. Although there has been no dramatic increase in the incidence of malignancy in patients on immunosuppressive therapy, some increase in the incidence of lymphoma has been reported.[34] Another suggested role of cellular immunity is that it has been evolved in mammals to prevent the invasion of the mother by fetal cells during gestation.

## General Reading

SAMTER, M. and ALEXANDER, H. L. (1965). Edrs. "Immunological Disease", 966 pp. Boston: Little, Brown & Co. In addition to describing the diseases associated with hypersensitivity this book also contains sections on basic immunology.

## References

1. DAVIS, B. D., DULBECCO, R., EISEN, H. N., GINSBERG, H. S. and WOOD, W. B. (1967). "Microbiology". New York: Harper and Row-Hoeber.
2. MIESCHER, P. A. and MÜLLER-EBERHARD, H. J. (1968 and 1969). "Textbook of Immunopathology", vols. 1 and 2. New York and London: Grune and Stratton.
3. AUSTEN, K. F. and HUMPHREY, J. H. (1963). Advanc. Immunol., 3, 1.
4. BROCKLEHURST, W. E. (1968). In "Clinical Aspects of Immunology", 2nd ed. p. 611, ed. by Gell, P. G. H. and Coombs, R. R. A. Oxford: Blackwell.
5. Various Authors (1968). In "Clinical Aspects of Immunology", pp. 633–659 and 693–755. loc. cit.
6. TURK, J. L. (1967). "Delayed Hypersensitivity". Amsterdam: North-Holland.
7. UHR, J. W. (1966). Physiol. Reviews, 46, 359.
8. CHASE, M. W. (1965). Med. Clin. N. Amer., 49, 1613.
9. Various Authors (1971). Journal of Experimental Medicine, 134, 1S.

10. KARUSH, F. and EISEN, H. N. (1962). *Science*, **136**, 1032.
11. SILVERSTEIN, A. M. and BOREK, F. (1966). *J. Immunol.*, **96**, 953.
12. AMOS, B. and KOPROWSKI, H. (1963). Edrs. "Cell Bound Antibodies". Philadelphia: Wistar Inst. Press.
13. MCCLUSKY, R. T., BENACERRAF, B. and MCCLUSKEY, J. W. (1963). *J. Immunol.*, **90**, 466.
14. TURK, J. L. and OORT, J. (1963). *J. Immunol.*, **6**, 140.
15. LAWRENCE, H. S. (1955). *J. clin. Invest.*, **34**, 219.
16. LAWRENCE, H. S. (1960). In "Cellular Aspects of Immunity" (Ciba Foundation Symposium), p. 243, ed. by Wolstenholme, G. E. W. and O'Connor, M. London: Churchill.
17. LAWRENCE, H. S. *et al.* (1963). *Trans. Assoc. Amer. Physicians*, **76**, 84.
18. DAVID, J. R. (1968). *Proceedings of the National Academy of the Sciences of the United States of America*, **56**, 72.
19. CALNAN, C. D. (1968). In "Clinical Aspects of Immunopathology", p. 756, *loc. cit.*
20. UHR, J. W. (1966). *Phys. Rev.*, **46**, 359.
21. ARNASON, B. G. and WAKSMAN, B. H. (1963). *Lab. Invest.*, **12**, 737.
22. RUSSELL, P. S. and WINN, H. J. (1970). *New Engl. J. Med.*, **282**, 786, 848 and 896.
23. JONCK, L. M. (1966). *Brit. J. oral Surg.*, **4**, 137.
24. SHULMAN, L. B. (1964). *Oral Surg., Oral Med. and Oral Path.*, **17**, 389.
25. Editorial (1968). *New Engl. J. Med.*, **279**, 657.
26. DICK, H. M. and CRICHTON, W. B. (1972). "Tissue Typing Techniques", 152 pp. Edinburgh and London: Churchill Livingstone.
27. Leading Article (1966). *Lancet*, **2**, 951.
28. MICKLEM, H. S. and LOUTIT, J. F. (1966). "Tissue Grafting and Radiation". New York and London: Academic Press.
29. BURWELL, R. G. (1969). In "Recent Advances in Orthopaedics", p. 115, ed. by Apley, A. G. London: Churchill.
30. NISBET, N. W. and HESLOP, B. F. (1962). *Brit. med. J.*, **1**, 129 and 206.
31. GRAW, R. G. *et al.* (1970). *Lancet*, **2**, 1053.
32. KAPLAN, M. H. (1963). *J. Immunol.*, **90**, 595.
33. KOSUNEN, T. U. and FLAX, M. H. (1966). *Lab. Invest.*, **15**, 606.
34. Leading article (1972). *Brit. med. J.*, **3**, 713.
35. LEVINE, B. B. (1968). *Ann. N.Y. Acad. Sci.*, **151**, 988.
36. DASH, C. H. and JONES, H. E. H. (1972). "Mechanisms in Drug Allergy," 208 pp. Edinburgh: Churchill Livingstone.
37. LEVINE, B. B. (1972). *New Engl. J. Med.*, **286**, 42.
38. DAVID, J. R. (1973). *New Engl. J. Med.*, **288**, 143.

# Chapter 14

# SOME IMPORTANT BACTERIAL INFECTIONS

## ACUTE PYOGENIC INFECTIONS

The organisms responsible for acute inflammation and the formation of pus account for some of the most important lesions seen in surgical practice.[1] Although it is these bacteria which have responded most encouragingly to antibiotic therapy, it is still common for the surgeon to be called upon to drain abscesses formed as a result of their pathogenic action. The most important members of this group are:

**The pyogenic cocci**, e.g. *Staphylococcus pyogenes*, *Streptococcus pyogenes*, pneumococcus, meningococcus, and gonococcus.

**The Gram-negative intestinal bacilli**, viz. *Escherichia coli*, *Proteus* species, and *Pseudomonas pyocyanea*.

Of these it is the staphylococcus, streptococcus, and Gram-negative bacilli which are of greatest surgical moment because of their capacity to produce infections in many different sites. Furthermore, they are of cardinal importance because they not only infect wounds and burns, but also act as secondary invaders in chronic ulcerative lesions from other causes, e.g. cancerous and tuberculous lesions of the skin and mucous membranes. By contrast the pneumococcus, meningococcus, and gonococcus tend to affect the lungs, meninges, and genital tract respectively.

The pathological effects of these bacteria are all essentially similar. There is an acute inflammatory response culminating in the accumulation of an exudate crowded with neutrophil polymorphs, which attempts to destroy the organisms. If it is successful, the inflammation abates, but if the organisms gain the upper hand, the condition proceeds to tissue destruction and suppuration. The abscess so formed may burst spontaneously on to a free surface or else be drained surgically. The destroyed tissue is then replaced either by the regeneration of specialized tissue or by the formation of fibrous scar tissue. Sometimes if the body's resistance is very poor or if the organism is extremely virulent, there may be rapid local spread and generalized dissemination of organisms. In this case a fatal septicaemia or pyaemia may ensue.

Not infrequently an impasse is reached when the body's defences are incapable of completely overcoming the organism. At the same time the organism is not virulent enough to spread rapidly throughout the tissues. In this case destruction of tissue and the subsequent inflammation coincide with attempts at healing. This is the condition of *chronic inflammation*. Indeed, these organisms are responsible for the chronic non-specific bacterial inflammation that plays such an important role in everyday clinical practice.

Except in very localized infections there is a general body response reflected in a polymorphonuclear leucocytosis with an increased proportion of immature neutrophils in the blood. If the infection is spreading to any extent there is a variable constitutional reaction with pyrexia and an elevation of the ESR (p. 331).

## General Bacteriology of Pyogenic Organisms

It is important to note the salient bacteriological features of these organisms because only by investigating their properties can a logical attempt be made to understand the diseases which they cause.

### STAPHYLOCOCCI[2]

**Morphology.** They are Gram-positive, spherical organisms about 1$\mu$m in diameter, which tend to be arranged in grape-like clusters. They are non-motile, non-sporing, and non-capsulate.

**Cultural Characteristics.** They grow easily on most media. They are aerobic organisms, but can tolerate an anaerobic atmosphere quite well, i.e. they are facultative anaerobes. They grow best at 37°C. On blood agar, conspicuous, shiny, convex colonies appear within 24 hours, and these are pigmented, some golden yellow and others white. The former, called *Staphylococcus aureus*, is always pathogenic, whereas the latter, *Staphylococcus albus*, is often found as a harmless commensal, especially on the skin. However, pathogenicity is not infallibly related to pigment production, because some white strains are virulent. Nowadays little importance is attached to the colour of a colony.

**Coagulase Production.** The important laboratory criterion of pathogenicity is the production of coagulase, an enzyme which coagulates plasma even in the absence of calcium. All pathogenic staphylococci produce coagulase, and are called *Staph. pyogenes*. Some bacteriologists have retained the name *Staph. aureus* for coagulase-positive staphylococci irrespective of their pigment production. In this book the name *Staph. pyogenes* will be used for all pathogenic strains.

Not all coagulase producers are equally virulent. Some produce mild skin lesions only, whereas others are responsible for epidemics of hospital infection of the most severe intensity. It is extremely important to type the organisms in such an epidemic, so as to ascertain whether they are all of one strain or of many different strains (p. 79).

**Typing.** The basis of staphylococcal typing lies in the use of staphylococcal bacteriophage*, a virus which specifically lyses colonies of staphylococci. Any one bacteriophage can lyse only a few susceptible strains, thus each staphylococcus exhibits a distinct pattern of lysis: for example, a well-known epidemic strain of staphylococcus is lysed by phages 47, 53, 75, and 77, and is therefore typed 47/53/75/77. One of the most notorious epidemic strains is the phage type-80 staphylococcus. This was first recognized in Australia in 1953,[3] and has since then wreaked havoc in many hospitals throughout the world.

**Toxin Production.** The staphylococcus is an invasive organism, but the essential factors responsible for its virulence are not clearly defined. Nevertheless, some toxins are known, and these mainly have the characters of endo-

* Bacteriophage is often abbreviated to "phage."

toxins. The most important of these is the α-*toxin*, which produces local tissue necrosis, and is lethal when injected intravenously. It is also haemolytic to red cells, and destroys white cells, i.e. it is a *haemolysin* and a *leucocidin*.

There is another staphylococcal toxin, the action of which is confined to white cells. It is called the *Panton-Valentine leucocidin*. Three other endotoxins are also described, and these have haemolytic and necrotizing actions.

In this list the three enzymes produced by staphylococci can be included:

*Coagulase*, which has already been described.

*Staphylokinase*, which lyses fibrin by activating the plasmin system.

*Hyaluronidase*. Both staphylokinase and hyaluronidase are produced only by some strains and seldom in large amounts.

In addition some strains produce an exotoxin, called *enterotoxin*, which produces symptoms of food-poisoning when ingested. It is the only exotoxin produced by the staphylococcus, and unlike most exotoxins it is thermostable.

**Lesions Produced by Staphylococci**[1,4] The typical staphylococcal lesion is a *circumscribed area of inflammation with suppuration*. Coagulase production has been suggested as an important factor in the localization of the infection by virtue of the copious fibrin formation that it induces. On the other hand, other authorities regard coagulase as a factor aiding spread of infection, because the deposition of fibrin acts as a protective covering for the organism and prevents its phagocytosis. It is evident that our ideas on the importance of coagulase in staphylococcal infection are still purely speculative. It seems likely that the local damage inflicted by the α-toxin leads to a considerable inflammatory reaction which in its turn successfully localizes and overcomes the infection.

Staphylococcal skin lesions are very frequent and include boils, carbuncles, paronychia (inflammation of the nail-fold), impetigo, and pemphigus neonatorum.

In *impetigo contagiosa* the organisms invade the superficial layers of the skin and produce characteristic subcorneal bullae and pustules. This is common on the face and in children. The blisters soon rupture and become covered by a honey-coloured crust.

*Folliculitis*. Infection of the hair follicles is common, and the type of lesion produced depends on how deeply the organisms penetrate. Since pus is produced, the term *pyoderma* is sometimes employed to include impetigo and folliculitis. In *superficial folliculitis* (*Bockhart's impetigo*) numerous small pustules are seen at the openings of adjacent hair follicles; the face and scalp are common sites. A somewhat deeper infection is seen in the beard area (*sycosis barbae*), and in addition to involvement of the hair follicle itself, there is much perifollicular inflammation. The lesions are very liable to become chronic.

A deeper more destructive infection of the hair follicle is the *boil*, or *furuncle*. Suppuration is the usual result, and pus is discharged from a single opening. A well-known regional type of boil is the *stye*, in which an eyelash is implicated. Boils are particularly common in the axillae and on the back of the neck, and they are often multiple in these sites due to the regional concentration of hair follicles and sebaceous glands. Nevertheless, each boil has its own "head" through which it discharges its pus.

In a *carbuncle* the infection extends to the underlying fatty subcutaneous tissue and spreads laterally in this plane. The subcutaneous tissue is divided into compartments by fibrous septa which extend from the deep fascia to the dermis. It therefore follows that when infection spreads a loculated abscess forms. The pus reaches the surface through hair follicles or sweat glands, and each abscess has its own "head". Thus a single carbuncle has multiple heads, each with one loculus. Extensive areas of skin become undermined, and they eventually slough off; a large granulating surface is produced as healing occurs.

Staphylococci are the commonest causal organisms in *infected wounds*, usually the result of cross infection in hospital.

*Bullous impetigo of the newborn*, also called pemphigus neonatorum, is the result of similar cross infection in maternity wards. Infected infants may transmit the staphylococci to their mothers during breast feeding. A *breast abscess* may be the result.

Two other important examples of cross infection are *bronchopneumonia* (p. 407) and *enterocolitis*.

*Staphylococcal enterocolitis*[5,6] is an occasional complication in patients who have been given a broad-spectrum antibiotic. There is an acute inflammation of the bowel mucosa which is sloughed off in long strips. Clinically there is severe diarrhoea and intense shock. In the worst cases death may occur with dramatic speed.

Staphylococci are the most important causal agents in *acute osteomyelitis* (p. 127).

If the blood stream is massively invaded during the course of a staphylococcal infection, fatal *septicaemia* will ensue.[7] *Pyaemia* is not uncommon, and follows suppurative thrombophlebitis which may complicate any staphylococcal infection.

*Staphylococcal food-poisoning* is the only condition due entirely to the enterotoxin.

**Occurrence.** The reservoir of pathogenic staphylococci is the anterior nares. About 40 per cent of healthy adults are nasal carriers and in a hospital population the figure may rise to over 70 per cent. From the nose they are transferred to the skin, particularly of the hands and perineum, where they multiply and spread. Staphylococci are also present in the faeces, though this is probably not an important source of infection except in patients with enterocolitis.

**Staph. albus** (coagulase negative) is a universal commensal of the skin and nose, and rarely produces infection. It occasionally leads to urinary-tract infections, and has recently gained prominence as a cause of opportunistic infection especially following surgery when foreign material is inserted. Thus it may cause endocarditis after open-heart surgery.

### STREPTOCOCCI[8]

**Morphology.** These too are Gram-positive, spherical organisms, slightly smaller than staphylococci. They tend to be arranged in chains which vary in length. They are non-motile and non-sporing. Some strains possess very thin capsules called microcapsules.

**Cultural Characteristics.** They grow less easily than staphylococci, but are also aerobes and facultative anaerobes. A few strains are obligatory anaerobes.

They can be cultured on blood agar at 37°C, and within 24 hours, tiny, transparent, dewdrop colonies develop. Around these there may be a zone of haemolysis, and according to this the organisms are classified into three main groups:

α-*haemolytic streptococci*, which produce an ill-defined zone of partial haemolysis, which may be yellow or green in colour. These organisms are often reported as *Strept. viridans* or *Strept. salivarius*.

β-*haemolytic streptococci*, which produce a sharply demarcated zone of complete haemolysis. These organisms are loosely called "*Strept. haemolyticus*", a confusing name.

*Non-haemolytic streptococci*. These are also called γ-type streptococci.

β-haemolytic streptococci are particularly important in producing serious pyogenic infections. Not all, however, are pathogenic to man; some produce disease only in cattle and other animals. It is therefore important to distinguish between the different groups of β-haemolytic streptococci. This is done by Lancefield's method.

**Lancefield Grouping.** Lancefield found that β-haemolytic streptococci could be divided into 15 groups according to the presence of a specific carbohydrate hapten (called the C antigen) present in the wall of the organism. The vast majority of human pathogens fall into Lancefield's group A, and are called *Strept. pyogenes.*

**Griffith Typing.** As described with staphylococci, *Strept. pyogenes* may also give rise to epidemics of hospital infection, particularly in labour wards. The necessity for typing the organisms may then arise. The technique used was first described by Griffith, who discovered that group-A streptococci could be subdivided into over 50 different types depending on the presence of protein antigens on the surface of the organisms. These are called M and T antigens, and the M antigen[9] is particularly important. It is type-specific, and is responsible for the virulence of the organism. Typing is carried out by means of agglutination tests using specific rabbit antisera. Nowadays a more complex agglutination-precipitation procedure is used, because some of the antigens are revealed better by precipitation than by agglutination.

**Toxin Production.** Like the staphylococcus, *Strept. pyogenes* is an invasive organism that produces powerful endotoxins and a single exotoxin. There are two haemolysins designated *streptolysin O* and *streptolysin S*. Streptolysin O is also cardiotoxic and leucocidic, whereas streptolysin S is a pure haemolysin. As the chemical nature of endotoxins is generally so poorly understood, it is reasonable to include the *M protein* among them. This is powerfully antigenic. It acts by interfering with phagocytosis, and the antibody formed against it is an opsonin (p. 157).

The organisms produce three enzymes:

*Hyaluronidase.*

*Streptokinase*, which induces fibrinolysis by activating the plasmin system.

*Streptodornase*, which lyses DNA. The peculiar name streptodornase is derived from the first letters of the syllables **deoxyribonuclease.**

The exotoxin referred to is the *erythrogenic toxin* responsible for the generalized punctate erythema characteristic of scarlet fever. It is produced by some strains only.

**Lesions Produced by Strept. pyogenes.**[10] The typical streptococcal lesion is a *spreading infection of the connective tissue called a cellulitis.* The poor localizing tendency has been associated with the hyaluronidase and streptokinase produced by most strains, often in large amounts. Abscesses occur much later than in staphylococcal infections, and the pus is watery and often blood-stained. It is probable that the streptodornase and streptokinase are responsible for this, because the viscosity of the pus is due to DNA and fibrin.

In recent years the virulence of *Strept. pyogenes* has declined so markedly that many of the classical streptococcal lesions which produced so much damage in years gone by are now rarely seen. By contrast staphylococcal lesions are commoner and more severe than ever.

Streptococci are occasional causes of *wound* and *burn infections,* and are also responsible for some cases of *impetigo contagiosa. Erysipelas,* a spreading infection of the dermis, is a classical streptococcal lesion.

Streptococci are still important causes of *tonsillitis* and *pharyngitis* (streptococcal sore throat) and these may be complicated by infection of the middle ear (*otitis media*). Streptococci have a great tendency to invade the blood stream, with the development of *septicaemia.* This is quite a common complication of streptococcal infection of the uterus following labour (*puerperal sepsis*), which killed thousands of women as recently as 30 years ago, but now is very uncommon.

If an infecting streptococcus produces the erythrogenic exotoxin, and the patient has no circulating antitoxin, the local lesion will be complicated by the effects of this toxin. A generalized punctate erythema appears, and the condition is called *scarlet fever.*

There is an indirect relationship between streptococcal infections on the one hand and *acute rheumatic fever* and *acute glomerulonephritis* on the other. Acute nephritis occurs about 10 days after an attack of streptococcal pharyngitis; after impetigo the period is often three weeks or longer. Acute rheumatic fever follows only on streptococcal pharyngitis, almost never on skin infections;[11] the current view is that both are manifestations of immune-complex reactions.

**Occurrence of Strept. pyogenes.** *Streptococcus pyogenes* is found in the throats of about 10 per cent of people, and in from 2 to 5 per cent it is also present in the anterior nares.

**Lesions Produced by α-Haemolytic Streptococci.** The α-haemolytic streptococcus (*Strept. viridans*) is an invariable commensal of the mouth and throat, and has been incriminated in apical tooth infections. The relationship to infective endocarditis is considered on page 397.

**Lesions Produced by Non-Haemolytic Streptococci.** The non-haemolytic streptococcus is always present in the colon, hence its alternative names *Strept. faecalis* and *enterococcus.* If it leaves its normal habitat this organism can cause suppurative lesions of a type and distribution similar to *E. coli.* It is a common cause of urinary-tract infection.

**Anaerobic Streptoccal Infections.** Anaerobic streptococci are normal inhabitants of the bowel, vagina, and mouth (particularly the gingival sulci). These were important causes of puerperal sepsis in the past,[12] and occasionally are associated with *wound infection*. They may also be found in gangrenous lesions (p. 55).[13]

## THE PNEUMOCOCCUS[14]

*Diplococcus pneumoniae* is closely related to the streptococci, and is sometimes called *Strept. pneumoniae*, but in fact it is better to regard it as a separate genus.

**Morphology.** It is an oval or lance-shaped coccus. The organisms are arranged in pairs with the long axes in line with each other. It is the same size as the streptococcus, and like it is Gram-positive, non-motile, and non-sporing. An important feature is the presence of a prominent capsule.

**Cultural Characteristics.** It resembles the α-haemolytic streptococcus very closely, and both produce a diffuse greenish haemolysis of the surrounding blood agar.

**Typing.** Type-specificity depends on the polysaccharide hapten (the specific soluble substance, or SSS) present in the capsule of the organism, and it is this that causes its virulence. Over 70 different types of pneumococci have been recognized, but in practice pneumococcal typing is seldom carried out nowadays. Types 1, 2, and 3 are the most virulent, and are responsible for most cases of lobar pneumonia (p. 403). Types 5, 7, and 14 are also quite virulent, but the remainder appear to be commensals of the nose and throat, and cause little harm in healthy people.

**Lesions Produced.** The most important pneumococcal lesion is *lobar pneumonia*, which is caused by one of the virulent strains, either type 1, 2, or 3. Other types of pneumococci are sometimes implicated in bronchopneumonia (p. 405). Other primary pneumococcal conditions are *otitis media* and *suppurative sinusitis*, both of which may lead to *meningitis*.

## THE GRAM-NEGATIVE INTESTINAL BACILLI[15]

The members of this group, which are important producers of pyogenic infections, are *Escherichia coli*, *Proteus* species, and *Pseudomonas pyocyanea* (also called *Ps. aeruginosa*). Most of these organisms belong to the family *Enterobacteriaceae*[16] which includes the numerous genera conveniently grouped together as the "coliform organisms". Of these the most important is the genus *Escherichia*. *Proteus* is included, but *Pseudomonas* is excluded from it, because *Ps. pyocyanea* is only occasionally found as a commensal of the bowel, whereas the true *Enterobacteriaceae* are all native to the intestinal tract.

**Morphology.** They are all Gram-negative rods 1–4 μm long. Most of the "coliforms" are vigorously motile, but some of them, e.g. *Klebsiella* species, are non-motile.

**Cultural Characteristics.** They grow easily at 37°C, being aerobic and facultatively anaerobic. On blood agar, large greyish-white, irregular, shiny colonies are produced within 24 hours.

Colonies of some *Proteus* species tend to spread over the surface of the agar as a thin film submerging other bacterial colonies, a feature called "swarming".

*Ps. pyocyanea* produces a bluish-green pigmentation due to the formation of fluorescin and pyocyanin.

**Biochemistry.** The most important biochemical property of these organisms is their ability to ferment various sugars. This is used in their laboratory identification.

**Occurrence.** Unlike the pyogenic streptococci and staphylococci, these organisms may be regarded as normal inhabitants of the body, causing disease only when they leave their normal environment.

*Escherichia coli* is always present in the bowel, and about a third of all human faeces harbour *Proteus*. *Ps. pyocyanea* is a more foreign type of organism, being found in only 3–16 per cent of faeces.

**Pathogenicity.** The pathogenic action of these organisms is believed to be due to an endotoxin, which as yet has been poorly defined. When they escape from the lumen of the bowel and invade the tissues, suppurative lesions ensue. Endotoxin is probably responsible for shock when large numbers of Gram-negative organisms enter the circulation (p. 312).

**Lesions Produced by the Coliform Organisms.** *E. coli* and the other coliform organisms are always predominant in infective lesions derived from the bowel contents, e.g. *appendix abscess* and *generalized peritonitis following perforation of a hollow viscus*. It frequently infects *penetrating wounds of the abdomen*. It is furthermore the commonest agent in *urinary-tract infections*, reaching the kidney as part of a normal bacteraemia from the colon, or else being introduced into the bladder following maladroit catheterization.

*E. coli* is not infrequently present in sputum, and it may be an agent in producing *pneumonia*.

It should be noted that although *E. coli* is an inevitable and harmless inhabitant of the bowel, in recent years certain enteropathogenic strains have been isolated.[17] These are of no special importance as causes of suppuration but they may produce epidemics of *infantile gastroenteritis*. The condition is most common in artificially-fed babies, and is probably spread by fomites and contaminated food.

*Proteus* organisms and *Ps. pyocyanea* have a similar range of pathogenicity, but as they are less frequently commensals of the bowel, they are much more frequently transmitted by cross-infection.

Both are important causes of urinary-tract, respiratory, ear, and wound infections.

## THE ANAEROBIC WOUND INFECTIONS

These infections are of great importance in clinical practice, not because they are common but because when they do occur they are serious. With the exception of infections with the anaerobic streptococci, bacteroides, and actinomyces, all are due to the clostridial group of anaerobic spore-bearers. The clostridial organisms are responsible for two extremely serious conditions, *gas-gangrene* and *tetanus*. Gas-gangrene is produced by the combined action of a number of clostridia, the most important of which are *Cl. welchii*, *Cl. oedematiens*, and *Cl. septicum*, whereas tetanus is caused by a single orga-

nism, *Cl. tetani*. The rare, lethal form of food-poisoning, botulism, is produced by another clostridium, *Cl. botulinum*. This is not a wound infection but an intoxication which follows the ingestion of a heat-stable, potent exotoxin produced by the organism in poorly prepared food during its period of storage.

## Bacteriology of the Clostridial Organisms[18]

**Morphology.** They are large, Gram-positive bacilli approximately 5 $\mu$m long. The most characteristic feature is the spore, which is produced whenever the organism finds itself in adverse conditions. It is usually central or subterminal, but in the case of *Cl. tetani* it is situated terminally, so that *Cl. tetani* is sometimes called the "drum-stick bacillus". These organisms are all motile and non-capsulate, with the exception of *Cl. welchii* which is nonmotile and possesses a capsule.

**Cultural Characteristics.** They all grow quite easily but most of them demand anaerobiosis, i.e. they are obligatory anaerobes. They are most conveniently cultured at 37°C on blood agar in the anaerobic atmosphere afforded by a McIntosh and Fildes jar. Robertson's meat broth is an alternative medium.

**Biochemical Reactions.** These are of considerable importance. Clostridia are divided into two categories, saccharolytic and proteolytic.

*Saccharolytic clostridia.* These ferment many sugars, e.g. lactose and glucose. They do not break down proteins, and they merely turn the meat in Robertson's medium a pink colour, due to the production of acid. The true pathogens of gas-gangrene, viz. *Cl. welchii*, *Cl. septicum*, and *Cl. oedematiens*, come into this category.

*Proteolytic clostridia.* These break down protein, and produce foulsmelling gases like hydrogen sulphide and ammonia. The meat in Robertson's medium becomes black due to the formation of iron sulphide. These organisms are also able to ferment sugars, but they are less active than the first group. The secondary putrefactive saprophytes of gas-gangrene, e.g. *Cl. sporogenes* and *Cl. histolyticum*, come into this category.

**Toxin Production.** The clostridia are excellent examples of toxic organisms, the lesions they produce being due entirely to exotoxins. The infection is localized, but the systemic effects are far-reaching.

In the gas-gangrene group most work has been done on *Cl. welchii*, and a number of toxins have been identified. Of these the $\alpha$-*toxin*, a lecithinase, is by far the most important. In animals a local injection causes tissue necrosis, and larger doses are lethal. By virtue of its lecithinase activity it destroys the phospholipid components of red-cell envelopes, and is thus a powerful haemolysin.

The other toxins of *Cl. welchii* include a *hyaluronidase*, a *deoxyribonuclease*, and a *collagenase*. These enzymes play an important part in breaking down the intercellular ground substance and collagen fibres of tissues which are infected with *Cl. welchii*, and so aid the local spread of the organism.*

* The description of proteolytic enzymes in saccharolytic organisms seems to be a contradiction in terms. But "proteolytic" refers to the putrefaction of complex protein, and this is not done by the saccharolytic group.

*Cl. septicum* and *Cl. oedematiens* produce powerful haemolytic and necrotizing exotoxins. *Cl. oedematiens* also yields small amounts of a lecithinase.

By contrast, *Cl. tetani* produces only two exotoxins. The important one is a neurotoxin called *tetanospasmin*, which is, of course, responsible for the convulsions of tetanus. Tetanospasmin has been separated in a pure crystalline form. It is an immensely potent poison, being second only to the exotoxin of *Cl. botulinum* in this respect. The other exotoxin is haemolytic, and is known as *tetanolysin*.

**Occurrence.** The spores of these organisms are widely dispersed in nature, and are especially plentiful in soil. They are commensals of the human and animal intestine, and are excreted in the faeces and returned to the soil in the form of manure. *Cl. welchii* is almost invariably present in the human bowel, but tetanus spores occur somewhat more sporadically. These organisms must be expected in all environments, including the air and furniture of wards and even operating theatres.[19]

By virtue of their ability to form spores in adverse circumstances, these organisms are resistant to heat and desiccation. Only well-devised sterilizing methods can destroy them.

Apart from the role played by *Cl. welchii* in gas-gangrene, certain specific strains are an important cause of *food-poisoning* when they contaminate meat in heavy culture.[20,21]

### GAS-GANGRENE[22]

Gas-gangrene may follow the contamination of a wound with the spores of the pathogenic clostridia. Considering the ubiquitous presence of these spores and the rarity of gas-gangrene in civilian practice, it is evident that healthy incised wounds so contaminated do not develop infection. The essential factor necessary for spore germination is a reduced oxygen tension. This is present in irregularly contused or lacerated wounds containing much dead tissue, which has been devitalized as a result of compression or impaired blood supply. Foreign bodies like shrapnel or pieces of clothing will exert local pressure, and also favour pyogenic infection. Soil is particularly dangerous, in that the ionizable calcium salts in it lead to considerable tissue necrosis. Finally, any coincidental infection by aerobic pyogenic organisms serves to augment the anaerobiosis. The local injection of adrenaline has a similar effect by causing vasoconstriction.

It therefore follows that most gas-gangrene is exogenous in origin, and is due to the gross contamination of severely lacerated wounds. It is usually seen in battle casualties or in agricultural accidents. Occasionally gas-gangrene is endogenous, and occurs when a wound is contaminated with the patient's faeces.

Spores of clostridia have been known to remain dormant in healed wounds, and to have germinated following surgical intervention. This is particularly important with regard to tetanus, and immunization is always advisable before surgery is performed on old war and agricultural wounds.

**Pathogenesis and Lesions.** Gas-gangrene is never due to infection by a single type of clostridial organism; it is the result of a combined assault by numerous saccharolytic and proteolytic organisms working together. The true pathogens, *Cl. welchii, Cl. septicum,* and *Cl. oedematiens,* germinate, and the powerful exotoxins which they liberate produce local tissue necrosis. At this stage the proteolytic saprophytes, such as *Cl. sporogenes* and *Cl. histolyticum,* flourish on the dead material, and break it down into putrid products.

If the wound is merely superficial, it will discharge foul-smelling fluid in which there are bubbles of gas, but if it is extensive enough to implicate the underlying muscles, the florid anaerobic myositis typical of gas-gangrene develops.[23,24]

(*a*) There is a rapidly progressive necrosis of muscle fibres due to the necrotizing exotoxins of the saccharolytic clostridia.

(*b*) The muscle carbohydrate is fermented by these organisms. Lactic acid and gas (mostly hydrogen and carbon dioxide) are formed. This is the origin of the "gas" in gas-gangrene. At this stage it is odourless.

(*c*) There is rapid spread of infection due to the destruction of local tissue barriers (e.g. endomysium and perimysium) by the hyaluronidase and collagenase present as components of the exotoxins. A whole muscle bundle may be affected with great rapidity. Indeed, gas-gangrene resembles an invasive infection in the extent of its local spread, but the organisms remain localized to one area. They show no tendency towards blood-stream invasion, except occasionally just at the time of death.

(*d*) As the infection spreads, so the necrosis increases, due not only to the liberated exotoxins, but also to the effect of ischaemia engendered by the pressure of the gas and exudate on the surrounding blood vessels. The area is tense, oedematous, and crepitant, and the muscle is odourless and brick-red in colour.

(*e*) Following in the wake of the extensive necrosis there is progressive putrefaction, which is brought about by the proteolytic clostridia. These thrive on and decompose the dead muscle, which becomes greenish-black in colour. Necrosis with superadded putrefaction is called gangrene (p. 54), and in this way these saprophytes complete the evolution of "gas-gangrene". It is at this stage that the characteristically foul odour appears.

(*f*) During this local process there is a profound general toxaemia due to the presence of circulating exotoxins. It is manifested by shock and a rapidly-developing haemolytic anaemia, which is secondary to the effect of the lecithinase on the red-cell envelopes. It is this toxaemia which brings about the death of the patient.

The local pathological effects of gas-gangrene are those of acute inflammation with much muscle necrosis and spreading oedema.[25,26] Polymorph infiltration is not conspicuous, at least not while the process is advancing. In the oedema fluid there are large numbers of organisms. The absence of polymorphs is strange; perhaps the powerful exotoxins exert a negative chemotactic influence.

**Treatment.**[27] In the treatment of gas-gangrene it is usual to give a poly-valent antiserum against the exotoxin of the three main pathogens, as well as penicillin or tetracycline. For prophylaxis in cases of grossly contaminated wounds penicillin has replaced antiserum therapy. There is no doubt, however, that a complete wound toilet is the most important aspect of prevention.

## TETANUS[28]

The spores of *Cl. tetani* not infrequently contaminate wounds, but as with the gas-gangrene organisms a reduced oxygen tension is essential for germination. The conditions conducive to tetanus infection are therefore similar to those already described. Quite often the degree of trauma appears to be very mild, because an insignificant punctured wound, like the prick of a contaminated thorn, has quite commonly been the site of origin of a fatal tetanus infection.

Exogenous infection has also resulted in *surgical tetanus*,[29,30] i.e. the introduction of spores into a wound during the course of a surgical operation. For such spores to germinate they must be presented with a nidus where conditions are relatively anaerobic. Foreign materials embedded in the tissues, e.g. contaminated catgut, talc, or cotton-wool, provide the necessary nidus, and these are the causes of surgical tetanus, which nowadays is fortunately very rare indeed owing to modern methods of sterilization.

**Clinical Features.** The incubation period varies from a few days to several weeks, and the shorter it is, the worse is the prognosis. Tetanus developing from wounds of the upper extremities, neck, and face is said to be more frequently lethal than that arising after injuries to the lower parts of the body.

Tetanus is clinically a disease of the central nervous system. The local lesion may be so mild that only very careful search will reveal it, yet the exotoxin produced may be sufficient to cause death.

After peripheral absorption, the toxin reaches the central nervous system probably by passing along the motor trunks; it acts by interfering with the inhibitory impulses reaching the motor neurones. This accounts for the generalized increase in tone, and also explains *local tetanus*. This is the early tendency to spasms of those muscles controlled by the same spinal segment as that supplying the area infected. At first there is stiffness, but this is soon followed by increase in muscular tone and spasms. Spasm of the masseter muscles results in trismus (inability to open the mouth, or "lockjaw").

Spasm of the facial muscles produces the characteristic *risus sardonicus*. Finally generalized tetanic convulsions occur. Death is due to asphyxia following involvement of the respiratory muscles.

**Prophylaxis.**[31] Since tetanus may occur following quite trivial wounds, by far the best method of prophylaxis is active immunization. This is carried out by a course of three injections of tetanus toxoid, a formolized preparation of the exotoxin adsorbed on to aluminium hydroxide or phosphate. The second injection is given about 8 weeks after the first, and the third from 6 to 12 months after the second. This regime should be carried out on all infants, and is mandatory for people whose occupation carries a hazard of injury.

In cases of deep wounds, particularly those with much ragged laceration of tissue or of a punctured type, prophylaxis is essential, and the procedure to be adopted depends on whether there has been previous active immunization or not. If there has been previous active immunization, all that needs to be given is a further dose of the toxoid. If, on the other hand, there has been no previous immunization, the advisability of passive immunization with antitoxin must be considered. In the past the administration of horse anti-tetanic serum (ATS) has been advised, but the danger of inducing anaphylactic shock or serum sickness is considerable. Furthermore the duration of passive immunity is short, especially if the subject has had previous injections of horse serum. The use of human antitetanic serum obviates these difficulties, and it should, wherever possible, be given when passive immunization is indicated.[32]

Following successful passive immunization the patient should be instructed to return 2 months later for a course of active immunization with toxoid. The first dose can, in fact, be given at once now that the adsorbed type of toxoid is used. Its antibody response is not interfered with by the high titre of circulating immunoglobulin introduced passively.[33]

## Gram-Negative Anaerobic Intestinal Bacilli

The Gram-negative intestinal organisms of the genus *Bacteroides* form the bulk of organisms in the faeces, and are present also as part of the normal flora of the mouth and vagina. They are non-spore-bearing, strict anaerobes. They cause wound infection, pelvic abscesses, otitis media, puerperal sepsis, and oral infections (p. 55), but in these instances their role is probably secondary to infection with more pathogenic organisms. Their presence should be suspected in any infection associated with a foul odour. The organisms may invade the blood stream and cause septicaemia and Gram-negative shock.

## References

1. WILSON, G. S. and MILES, A. A. (1964). In Topley and Wilson's "Principles of Bacteriology and Immunity", 5th ed., p. 1788. London: Arnold.
2. GOULD, J. C. (1965). In "Medical Microbiology", 11th ed., p. 134, ed. by Cruickshank, R. Edinburgh: Livingstone.
3. ROUNTREE, P. M. and FREEMAN, B. M. (1955). *Med. J. Aust.*, **2**, 157.
4. ROGERS, D. E. (1956). *Ann. intern. Med.*, **45**, 748.
5. ALTEMEIER, W. A., HUMMEL, R. P. and HILL, E. O. (1963). *Ann. Surg.*, **157**, 847.
6. GARDNER, R. J., HENEGAR, G. C. and PRESTON, F. W. (1963). *Arch. Surg.* **87**, 58.
7. SKINNER, D. and KEEFER, C. S. (1941). *Arch. intern. Med.*, **68**, 851.
8. GILLIES, R. R. (1965). In "Medical Microbiology", 11th ed., p. 149, ed. by Cruickshank, R. Edinburgh: Livingstone.
9. LANCEFIELD, R. C. (1962). *J. Immunol.*, **89**, 307.
10. WILSON, G. S. and MILES, A. A. (1964). p. 1763, *loc. cit.*
11. WANNAMAKER, L. W. (1970). *New Engl. J. Med.*, **282**, 23 and 78.
12. COLEBROOK, L. and HARE, R. (1933). *J. Obstet. Gynaec.*, **40**, 609.
13. MELENEY, F. L., FRIEDMAN, S. T. and HARVEY, H. D. (1945). *Surgery*, **18**, 423.
14. GILLIES, R. R. (1965). p. 165, *loc. cit.*
15. GILLIES, R. R. (1965). p. 249, *loc. cit.*
16. WILSON, G. S. and MILES, A. A. (1964). p. 806, *loc. cit.*
17. HUTCHINSON, R. I. (1957). *J. Hyg. (Lond.)*, **55**, 27.
18. COLLEE, J. G. (1965). In "Medical Microbiology", 11th ed., p. 308, ed. by Cruickshank, R. Edinburgh: Livingstone.
19. LOWBURY, E. J. L. and LILLY, H. A. (1958). *J. Hyg. (Lond.)*, **56**, 169.
20. HOBBS, B. C. *et al.* (1953), *J. Hyg. (Lond.)*, **51**, 75.

21. Annotation (1963). *Lancet*, **2**, 991.
22. WILSON, G. S. and Miles, A. A. (1964). In Topley and Wilson's "Principles of Bacteriology and Immunity", 5th ed., p. 2124. London: Arnold.
23. MacLENNAN, J. D. (1943). *Lancet*, **2**, 63, 94 and 123.
24. WILSON, T. S. (1960). *Canad. J. Surg.*, **4**, 35.
25. ROBB-SMITH, A. H. T. (1945). *Lancet*, **2**, 362.
26. GOVAN, A. D. T. (1946). *J. Path. Bact.*, **58**, 423.
27. ALTEMEIER, W. A. *et al.* (1957). *Arch. Surg.*, **74**, 839.
28. WILSON, G. S. and MILES, A. A. (1964). In Topley and Wilson's "Principles of Bacteriology and Immunity", 5th ed., p. 2095. London: Arnold.
29. WILLIAMS, R. E. O., BLOWERS, R., GARROD, L. P. and SHOOTER, R. A. (1966). "Hospital Infection", 2nd ed. London: Lloyd-Luke.
30. Report of the Public Health Laboratory Service (Medical Research Council, London). (1959). *Brit. med. J.*, **1**, 1150.
31. Annotation (1966). *Lancet*, **2**, 482.
32. RUBBO, S. D. and SURI, J. C. (1962). *Brit. med. J.*, **2**, 79.
33. EDSALL, G. (1963). In "Modern Trends in Immunology", I, p. 161, ed. by Cruickshank, R. London: Butterworths.

*Chapter 15*

# TUBERCULOSIS, SYPHILIS, ACTINOMYCOSIS, AND SOME FUNGOUS DISEASES

## Introduction

Whereas the pyogenic infections which have just been discussed manifest themselves by an overt acute inflammatory reaction which may or may not terminate in resolution, there are a great number of other organisms which tend to set up the condition of chronic inflammation. In these there is usually great tissue destruction so that resolution is impossible and a chronic course invariable. During the progress of these infections acute exacerbations of an exudative type are not infrequent, and these are usually due to allergy. The most important infections of this type are tuberculosis, syphilis, and actinomycosis, but the whole range of fungous, protozoan, and helminthic infections of the tissues come into the same category.

There are no histological features common to all these lesions; in tuberculosis and histoplasmosis the macrophage is the prominent cell type, in actinomycosis there is a polymorph infiltration, while in syphilis there is a peculiarly non-specific infiltration of lymphocytes and plasma cells.

In the acute bacterial infections the causal organisms appear to produce damage by some direct action often by producing powerful toxins. From the many organisms responsible for chronic infection no satisfactory toxin has been isolated. The generally held view is that their destructive effect is the result of the development of cell-mediated hypersensitivity.

In the acute bacterial infections a long-lasting immunity is often produced, and this is usually due to the presence of immunoglobulins in the circulation. In chronic infections these may also be present, but though they may be valuable in the diagnosis of the disease, e.g. in the serological diagnosis of syphilis, they do not produce immunity against the disease. They will not passively transfer immunity when transfused into another person. There is evidence in some of these infections, notably tuberculosis, that a degree of immunity is acquired after an infection, and this appears to be cell mediated rather than due to the development of specific immunoglobulins.

The body's general reaction to these infections depends on whether they are localized or generalized. In the latter case, there is pyrexia, and severe constitutional disturbances are common. The ESR is considerably elevated and there is a tendency for a rise in the immunoglobulin fraction of the serum proteins.

## TUBERCULOSIS

There are at least five different strains of *Mycobacterium tuberculosis:* the human, bovine, murine, avian, and piscine.[1] The human and bovine strains are potential human pathogens, and the murine strain ("vole bacillus"), which is endemic in wild voles, has been used as an alternative to BCG (Bacille-Calmette-Guérin vaccine introduced in France in 1908) in active immunization against tuberculosis. The other two strains are pathogenic to birds and fish respectively, and have little human importance. The bovine organism is excreted in the milk of infected cows, and it used to be the cause of much intestinal and tonsillar infection in childhood. Nowadays bovine tuberculosis, acquired by *ingestion*, has almost completely disappeared from the list of human diseases in civilized countries owing to the eradication of tuberculous herds and the pasteurization of milk. It therefore follows that to all intents and purposes nearly all tuberculosis is caused by the human

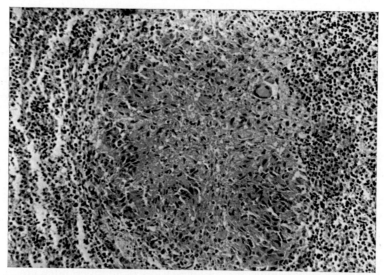

FIG. 15.1. A tubercle follicle. Note the central area of caseation surrounded by an ill-defined zone of epithelioid cells among which a Langhans giant cell is present. In the periphery there is a small round cell infiltration. × 120.

strain. The mode of infection is by the *inhalation* of organisms present in fresh droplets or the dust of dried sputum expectorated from an open case of pulmonary tuberculosis. Pulmonary tuberculosis is by far the most common type of disease encountered. *Inoculation* of the skin from *post-mortem* material is so uncommon as to be little more than a curiosity, and a primary tuberculous lesion of the oral mucosa is nowadays exceedingly rare.

**Bacteriology.**[2] *Myco. tuberculosis* is a slender bacillus about 3 μm long, non-motile and non-sporing. Its most conspicuous feature is its waxy content which makes it impermeable to the usual stains. It slowly takes up heated stains, e.g. carbol fuchsin in the Ziehl-Neelsen method, and then resists decolorization even by strong acids and alcohols, i.e. it is *acid-fast* and *alcohol-fast*. It is Gram-positive, but Gram-staining is not performed because the methyl violet penetrates only with great difficulty. It grows very slowly and then only on complex artificial media. The Löwenstein-Jensen medium is one that is commonly used, and it takes several weeks at 37°C in an aerobic atmosphere for any growth to appear.

In recent years the presence of "atypical" or "anonymous" mycobacteria have been noted in human lesions.[3] While some produce pulmonary infections, other types have been isolated from skin ulcers.[4,5]

*Myco. tuberculosis* is very resistant to drying, and it can survive in dust for several months. It is, however, very sensitive to the effect of ultraviolet radiation, and is rapidly killed in sunlight.

**Pathogenesis of the Tuberculous Lesion.**[6] The following sequence of events occurs when tubercle bacilli are introduced into the tissues.

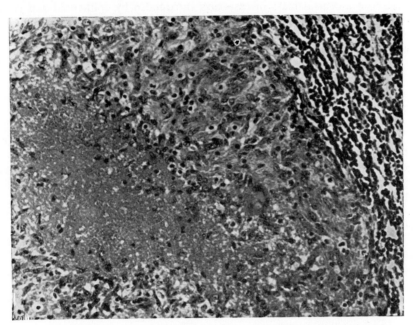

Fig. 15.2. A tubercle follicle. This is more advanced than the follicle in Fig. 15.1. There is a large area of caseation on the left-hand side, and it is surrounded by a dense zone of epithelioid cells in which a Langhans giant cell is present. At the right there is a small round cell infiltration. × 230.

1. A transient acute inflammatory reaction with an infiltration of polymorphs. These cells are rapidly destroyed by the organisms.

2. A progressive infiltration of macrophages.

3. The macrophages phagocytose the bacilli. In a short time they change their character and become converted into epithelioid cells (p. 123).

4. Some macrophages, instead of becoming epithelioid cells, form giant cells which are usually of the Langhans type.

5. Surrounding this mass of macrophages there is a diffuse zone of lymphocytes and fibroblasts.

6. Within 10–14 days necrosis begins in the centre of this mass, which consists of altered macrophages and cells peculiar to the tissue of the part.

The *caseation* of tuberculosis is a very firm, cheesy type of coagulative necrosis, and it differs from other types of necrosis in that it has a very high content of lipid material, and shows little tendency towards autolysis. Histologically, caseation is associated with such great tissue disintegration that scarcely any structure is recognizable. Everything is merged into a brightly eosinophilic mass of amorphous debris.

Caseation is probably caused by the development of hypersensitivity to products of the bacilli, notably tuberculoprotein. It is not produced directly by toxins.

There is now produced the *tubercle follicle* (Figs. 15.1 and 15.2), which consists of a central mass of caseation surrounded by epithelioid and giant cells, which in turn are surrounded by a wide zone of small round cells. The appearance is characteristic of tuberculosis, though a similar picture is sometimes seen in the deep-seated fungous infections. For definite proof of a tuberculous origin organisms must be sought in the lesion.

**Variations in the Reaction to the Tubercle Bacillus.** The common type of lesion described above is called *productive*, or *proliferative*, because its main components are cells rather than a fluid exudate.

Another well-known type of lesion is the *exudative* form of tuberculosis. It is characterized by the outpouring of an inflammatory exudate rich in fibrin. There is a considerable infiltration of lymphocytes, and often many polymorphs are present, but epithelioid and giant cells are scanty. Exudative lesions are typical of tuberculosis of serous cavities. They are not necessarily more serious than productive ones.

**The Fate of the Tuberculous Lesion.** The caseous focus may either cease to progress and heal by fibrosis, or it may soften and spread.

*The hallmark of healing* is fibrous tissue, and this is produced by the proliferating fibroblasts at the periphery of the lesion. In due course the area of caseation may be replaced by a solid fibrous nodule. Sometimes only a ring of fibrous tissue forms around the periphery, while the central mass of caseation undergoes slow *dystrophic calcification*. In this calcareous nodule organisms may still survive, and years later, when the resistance of the host breaks down, they may become active again.

*The hallmark of activity* is caseation and softening. If the lesion is spreading, bacilli are carried by macrophages into the surrounding lymphatics and tissue spaces. There they settle and set up satellite follicles, which by fusing with the primary enlarging lesion, produce a *conglomerate tubercle follicle*. Caseous material does not soften rapidly, due possibly to phosphatides that inhibit autolytic enzymes. Sometimes, however, *liquefaction* does occur, and this is attended by serious consequences.

There is no really satisfactory explanation for this softening. There is no doubt that it is associated with spread, and that the liquefied debris contains many bacilli, but it is not known whether this multiplication of organisms is the cause or the result of the softening. It has been suggested that the liquefaction is due to secondary infection, but this is untrue. Pyogenic infection may certainly complicate a tuberculous lesion, but liquefaction often occurs in the absence of such infection. The element of hypersensitivity is probably of considerable importance.

Once liquefaction has occurred, the debris contains large numbers of tubercle bacilli, and the whole is often called a *cold abscess*. Unlike a pyogenic abscess there are comparatively few cells present, and most of these are disintegrating. The term "pus" is therefore inapplicable, as there are no pus cells. The term "cold abscess" is equally inapplicable. In practice it is reserved exclusively for tuberculous lesions, even though in fact the suppurative lesions of actinomycosis may also be "cold", as neither the heat, pain, nor redness seen in acute pyogenic infection is a marked feature of them. The liquefied debris ("pus") tracks towards a free surface and discharges there. In a lesion of the lung rupture soon occurs into a bronchus, and the disease spreads to other parts of the lung; much infectious material is also coughed up. A tuberculous abscess is lined by tuberculous granulation tissue. This consists of systems of tubercle follicles irregularly disposed in a mass of newly-formed fibrous tissue which is heavily infiltrated with lymphocytes and macrophages.

Whenever a tuberculous abscess opens to the exterior, the disease becomes more serious, firstly because of its *open*, infectious character, and secondly because the tubercle bacillus is an aerobic organism and proliferates much more profusely in an atmosphere of air. These features are well illustrated in the open, cavitating type of pulmonary tuberculosis.

### Spread of Tuberculosis in the Body

The principles differ in no significant way from those of other infections.

**Local Spread.** The spread of macrophages has already been described.

**Spread in serous cavities** is seen in the diffuse pleurisy that may complicate lung lesions, the localized peritonitis found in cases of tuberculous salpingitis, and in tuberculous meningitis.

**Spread along epithelial-lined surfaces** is typified by the intrabronchial spread of tuberculosis that occurs when sputum is inhaled into adjacent lung segments. If the sputum is coughed up, it can produce *tuberculous laryngitis.* Tuberculous infection occasionally occurs on the tongue, lips, or gingivae. The ulcer so formed has an irregular outline with undermined edges. The most frequent lesion is an ulceration of the tongue, and the necrotizing tuberculous infection can spread to involve the pharynx, lips, and adjacent skin (*tuberculosis cutis orificialis*). The laryngeal and oral lesions are extremely painful, and fortunately are now rare.

If sputum is swallowed, the bacilli may infect the ileo-caecal area of the bowel and lead to tuberculous enteritis (Fig. 15.4).

**Lymphatic Spread.** This is a continuation of local spread. The result is a regional tuberculous lymphadenitis.

**Blood Spread.** Organisms may reach the blood stream in one of two ways:

1. *As an extension of lymphatic involvement.* In an overwhelming infection the organisms enter the blood stream to produce *miliary tuberculosis.* The lungs, spleen, liver, kidney, and to a lesser extent other organs, are seeded with tubercle bacilli which produce numerous follicles about 1 mm. in diameter. Clinically the patient is seriously ill and has a high fever. Sometimes only a few organisms enter the blood stream, and become lodged in various organs to produce metastatic lesions (see below).

2. *Direct involvement of a vein.* Blood spread also occurs when caseous hilar nodes directly implicate the adjacent pulmonary vein. If there is a discharge of large numbers of organisms into the blood stream, miliary tuberculosis occurs, but the lungs are often spared.

*Tuberculous meningitis* is almost invariably present in miliary tuberculosis, and is due either to involvement of the choroid plexus, or else to a small subcortical lesion (*Rich's focus*) rupturing into the subarachnoid space.[7] Miliary tuberculosis is much more common in young children than in adults.

*Metastatic lesions.* In older children and adults it sometimes happens that only a few bacilli invade the systemic circulation. These may be destroyed by the RE system, or else become lodged in various sites to give rise to metastatic disease. Such a lesion may progress immediately to produce clinical effects, or else remain quiescent, only to undergo reactivation years later. This type of lesion is called *local metastatic tuberculosis*, and it accounts for most of the disease seen in surgical practice. Organs sometimes involved in this way are the *kidneys, adrenals, fallopian tubes, epididymes,* and the *bones, joints,* and *tendon sheaths.*

### Morphology of Tuberculous Infections

It has been recognized for a long time that the behaviour of tuberculous infection is quite different in children as compared to adults. At all ages the lung is the organ principally affected.

**Childhood.** In childhood the primary focus (*Ghon focus*) is a small wedge-shaped area situated at the periphery of the lung field. This subpleural focus may heal and produce no clinical illness, or else the infection spreads to the hilar lymph nodes, which become greatly enlarged and caseous. A conspicuous *primary complex* is the result. It either heals and calcifies, or else it spreads and the child dies of *miliary tuberculosis with meningitis.*

In days gone by the primary lesion was frequently in the pharynx, tonsil, gingiva, or palate. It appeared as a painless ulcer and was acquired by the ingestion of contaminated milk. Sometimes the primary lesion was in the oesophagus or small intestine and usually escaped clinical attention. In most cases the primary lesion was small and the major feature was the enormous enlargement of the regional lymph nodes—*mesenteric* or *cervical.* In all childhood lesions the feature in common is the small size of the primary focus and the tendency to extensive lymph-node involvement with the danger of spread to the blood stream and a fatal termination.

**Adult Life.** In adult life the pulmonary focus is almost always apical or subapical (*Assmann focus*). The lesion either heals, or else it progresses, softens, and produces a cavity. Haemoptysis (the coughing up of blood), chronic cough, low-grade fever, and a raised ESR are the main clinical features. Depending on the resistance of the patient there is a tendency for either fibrosis or extensive cavitation to occur. In severe cases great destruction of lung tissue eventually results (Fig. 15.3). A large cavity may be produced, and a vessel in its wall may be eroded, leading to severe haemoptysis. At any time caseous debris may be inhaled into other bronchi to produce tuberculous bronchopneumonia. This may occur on a small scale and result in extension of the disease, but if widespread it causes rapid caseation of a great area of lung tissue. The latter is associated with intense hypersensitivity, and the disease remains localized to the lungs. Lymph-node involvement is inconspicuous, and blood-spread dissemination is unusual. Death is the result of the local lung lesion which is called *acute caseous*

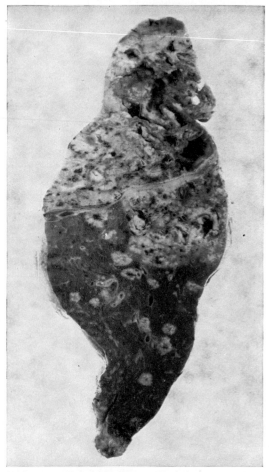

FIG. 15.3. Caseous tuberculosis of lung. The entire upper lobe and part of the apex of the lower lobe have been destroyed by caseous tuberculosis with extensive cavitation. Discrete areas of infection are present in the remainder of the lower lobe.

(R37.1, *Reproduced by permission of the President and Council of the Royal College of Surgeons of England.*)

*bronchopneumonia* ("galloping consumption"). There are severe constitutional symptoms due probably to the effects of hypersensitivity—these are described clinically as toxaemia, but no definite toxins have been isolated.

*Chronic tuberculosis.* Here the immunity of the host is adequate to cause some destruction of the bacilli, and healing by repair (fibrosis) occurs side

by side with caseous destruction. Three types of chronic pulmonary tuberculosis are recognized: caseous, fibro-caseous, and fibroid, depending on the
relative degrees of caseation and fibrosis. In long-standing fibroid tuberculosis
the lung may be converted into a contracted mass of dense fibrous tissue, in
which there may be little recognizable evidence of active tuberculous infec-

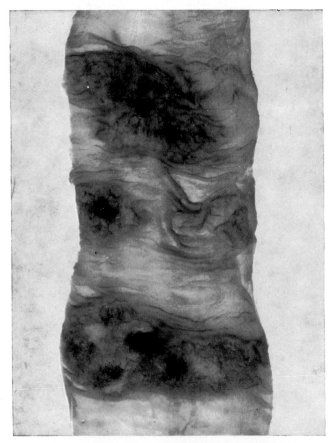

FIG. 15.4. Tuberculous ulceration of small bowel. There are three ulcers, two of
which have spread laterally to encircle the lumen. Their edges are undermined, and in their floor there is caseous debris.

(A51.1, *Reproduced by permission of the President and Council of the Royal
College of Surgeons of England.*)

tion. Bronchiectasis is a frequent complication of this type of disease, which
is characterized clinically by dyspnoea, respiratory failure, and right-sided
heart failure.

A similar type of pathogenesis occurs in other organs in the adult. Tuberculous enteritis due to the swallowing of infected sputum in open pulmonary
tuberculosis is characterized by a spreading ulceration of the wall of the
ileum (Fig. 15.4).

Another type of cutaneous tuberculosis, apart from tuberculosis cutis orificialis (p. 193), is *lupus vulgaris*. It nearly always involves the face with the ears and nose being commonly affected. The dermis shows a typical non-caseating tuberculoid reaction and the disease spreads by continuity. The course of lupus vulgaris is prolonged, and ultimately great tissue destruction and scarring result. Nevertheless, few organisms can be found in the lesions

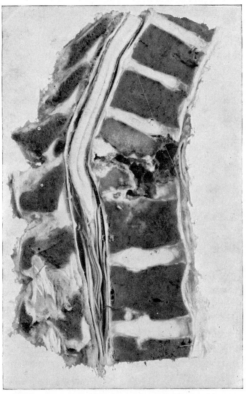

FIG. 15.5. Tuberculosis of spinal column (Pott's disease of the spine). There has been destruction of two adjacent vertebral bodies and the intervening inter-vertebral disc. The result has been collapse of the vertebrae, acute angulation of the spine, compression of the cord, and paraplegia.

(S.49a.48, *Reproduced by permission of the President and Council of the Royal College of Surgeons of England.*)

and the disease appears to be an infection in a person with considerable immunity. The source of the infection may be from a previous pulmonary lesion, but often no other active tuberculosis can be detected.

Skeletal tuberculosis usually starts in the metaphyseal area of a bone, and it causes great local destruction. Unlike pyogenic osteomyelitis it destroys the epiphyseal cartilage with ease, and soon the neighbouring joint is affected. When softening occurs a "cold abscess" is produced. Tuberculosis of the spine used to be quite common (Pott's disease), and was responsible for collapse of the affected vertebrae and great deformity (Fig. 15.5). Tuberculous "pus" sometimes entered the psoas muscle sheath and tracked down, discharging on to the skin of the groin below the inguinal ligament.

The feature that all these adult lesions have in common is the tendency to extensive local destruction without much lymphatic involvement.

It is traditionally believed that the adult lesion is always secondary to a "primary" lesion acquired during childhood, and that the difference in course of the two infections can be explained on the basis of allergy and immunity acquired during the "primary" infection. Just as in the Koch phenomenon (p. 165), where the second dose of organisms remained localized and did not spread to the regional nodes, so it is that the "secondary" adult lesion remains localized to the lungs and does not spread further afield.

It is becoming increasingly apparent that more and more young adults are Mantoux negative, a proof that they have not had tuberculosis in childhood, yet the incidence of the "primary" Ghon type of lesion with massive hilar lymphadenopathy is not increasing in the adult population. It seems that even primary infections in adults start at the apex of the lung and do not produce much lymphatic involvement. Furthermore, there are very definite differences between the adult lesion and the Koch phenomenon. There is lymph-node involvement in the adult, though it is of microscopic extent only, and the lesion shows no particular tendency to heal as in the second infection of the tuberculous guinea-pig. The essential difference in behaviour between childhood and adult lesions appears to be due to tissue maturation;[6] the older the patient the less is the tendency towards gross lymph-node involvement. The effect of a previous infection as an additional modifying factor cannot be excluded, but it is unjustifiable to label all adult lesions as secondary. The terms childhood and adult tuberculosis are much more accurate than "primary" and "secondary" tuberculosis.

The source of the organisms causing adult-type tuberculosis has been the centre of much discussion in the past. The pulmonary lesions were regarded as due either to *reactivation* of a quiescent primary lesion or to the development of a new lesion produced by a *reinfection* from some external source. In the past reinfection was probably of great importance, but nowadays it seems that adult-type lesions are themselves primary infections. In the case of other organs, e.g. kidney and bone, it is almost certain that tuberculosis is due to the reactivation of small lesions which were produced during a bacteraemic phase of a previous primary infection.

### Factors Determining the Response of Tissues to Tuberculous Infection[1]

It is apparent that sometimes there is healing by fibrosis of a small tuberculous focus, and on other occasions there is caseation, liquefaction, and even a rapidly spreading fatal disease. The factors that determine the tissue response are:

(a) the dose and virulence of the organism;

(b) the innate and acquired resistance of the body. It is this latter consideration which must be examined; the former is self-evident.

Innate immunity is of great importance in tuberculosis but is poorly understood (p. 154).

**Age and Sex.** During the first five years of life the body's resistance is poor and the mortality rate is high. From 5–15 years resistance is at its peak, but it breaks down during the early adult period of 15–30 years, particularly in women. After the age of 30 years resistance is quite high, but it breaks down again in old age, particularly in men.

**General Health of the Individual.** Malnourished people in concentration camps or slums have a poor resistance, and, of course, the overcrowding germane to such conditions predisposes to the rapid spread of disease throughout the community. Psychological stress and chronic debilitating diseases also lower the resistance. In this respect diabetes mellitus is particularly notorious in predisposing to a rapidly spreading type of infection. So also is administration of glucocorticosteroids.[8]

**Occupational Factors.** Those whose work carries the hazard of atmospheric pollution by particulate *silica*, e.g. tunnellers, miners, and quarrymen, are liable to a spreading type of disease. The same applies, to a lesser extent, to those who manufacture *asbestos* products.

**Acquired Immunity and Hypersensitivity.** The effect of previous infection with tuberculosis was first described by Koch using guinea-pigs.[1] Undoubtedly a primary infection with tubercle bacilli induces a state of immunity which is accompanied by delayed-type hypersensitivity to tuberculoprotein.

The really inscrutable feature of the Koch phenomenon is the immunity to the second infection. It is a very important consideration, because on it depends the advocacy of protective active immunization with BCG vaccine. It is clear that the immunity produced is in no way as effective as that seen in diphtheria or smallpox following an attack of the disease. It is certain that whatever type of immunity is produced, it is not due to specific immuno-globulins. The serum of a cured patient will not passively immunize another patient, as in diphtheria or measles. In fact, the serum of a tuberculous patient contains agglutinating, precipitating, and complement-fixing antibodies, but these have no protective action against the organism.

The acquired immunity in tuberculosis appears to be cellular in type: the macrophages not only accumulate more rapidly but also destroy the organisms more efficiently than they do in the course of a primary infection. The actual change which takes place in the cells is unknown.

The relationship between hypersensitivity and immunity has been much debated. Some authorities regard them as distinct and separable components, with hypersensitivity, by causing caseation and necrosis, being a harmful factor. On the other hand, it has been argued that the acute inflammation which hypersensitivity induces, does serve to bring many macrophages into contact with the bacilli very rapidly, and these are the essential agents in destroying the bacilli. Whatever may be the truth, it is generally acknowledged that so far as BCG vaccination is concerned, the benefits of immunity more than outweigh any possible harmful effects of hypersensitivity.

It should finally be noted that not only is the acquired immunity of partial degree, but also that it seems to have no effect in overcoming the primary infection. Even in Koch's phenomenon, though the second dose is overcome successfully, the animal still dies of its first infection. This may indicate that an important mechanism of the immunity is the localization of the organism at a very early stage of the infection.

## Treatment

Treatment with the chemotherapeutic agents streptomycin, para-amino-salicylic acid (PAS), and isonicotinic acid hydrazide has greatly improved the prognosis of tuberculosis. Nevertheless, the great improvements in social and economic conditions combined with facilities for early diagnosis have played the major role in the abolition of tuberculosis as an important cause of death in civilized countries.

## Sarcoidosis[9]

Although of unknown aetiology it is convenient to consider sarcoidosis at this point. The unit of sarcoidosis is a discrete follicle composed of plump epithelioid cells, in the midst of which a few giant cells may be found. The follicle is surrounded by a rim of lymphocytes and is therefore very like a tubercle follicle, but differs in that there is rarely any central caseation (Fig. 15.6).

Sarcoidosis is a generalized disease and affects the lungs, producing miliary lesions, the bones, especially those of the hands, the skin, eye, spleen, liver, lymph nodes, salivary glands, heart, and nervous system.

The lesions tend to heal with fibrosis, and in certain situations, e.g. the eye, brain, and lung, they can produce serious effects. The disease is not

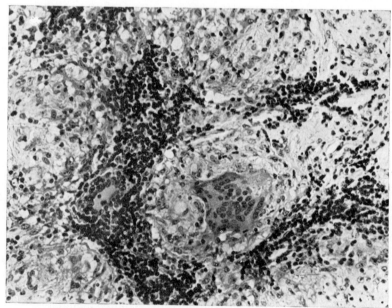

Fig. 15.6. Sarcoidosis. In this lymph node there are semi-confluent follicles of epithelioid cells without central caseation. A large giant cell is present, and is unusual in resembling that found in foreign-body reactions rather than a typical Langhans cell. × 230.

uncommon in Northern European countries. It has been regarded as an atypical form of tuberculosis, but proof of this is lacking.

## SYPHILIS

**Bacteriology and Serology.** The causative organism *Treponema pallidum*[10] is a delicate spiral filament, or spirochaete, about 10 μm long. It cannot be stained by the usual techniques, and is demonstrable in exudates by means of dark-ground illumination. In histological sections it is stained by special silver impregnation methods.

The organism has never been cultured artificially even in fertile eggs or tissue-culture systems, nor does animal inoculation play any part in the diagnosis of the disease. In fact, rabbits develop acute orchitis after the intratesticular inoculation of the organisms. This method is used to obtain a supply of spirochaetes for such procedures as the *Treponema pallidum immobilization* (TPI) *test*. An allied organism, the Reiter strain of spirochaete, can be cultured *in vitro*, and is used as a source of antigen in the Reiter Protein Complement Fixation (RPCF) test.

During the course of infection the patient develops immunoglobulins which are of great diagnostic importance. The best known is the *Wassermann antibody*, which fixes complement in the presence of a phosphatide extract of heart muscle (*Wassermann reaction*), or produces a flocculent type of precipitate in the presence of a similar type of antigen (*Kahn reaction*, the *Venereal Disease Research Laboratory* (*VDRL*) *test*, and other variants). As this "antigen" can hardly be considered specific for the organism of syphilis, it is not surprising that a positive reaction is sometimes found in other diseases, viz. yaws, trypanosomiasis, leprosy, malaria, infectious mononucleosis, mycoplasmal pneumonia, and systemic lupus erythematosus. Pregnancy too is occasionally associated with a false positive reaction.

In recent years it has been found that syphilitics develop a more specific *treponemal antibody* in their sera. It reacts specifically with the treponema or its products. When mixed with a concentrated suspension of *Tr. pallidum* in the presence of complement, it leads to the immobilization of the spirochaetes viewed under dark-ground illumination (TPI test).[11] It is also capable of fixing complement in the presence of a specific antigen made from *Tr. pallidum*.[12] Protein from the Reiter strain may be used (see RPCF test above). Specific treponemal antibody adheres to *Tr. pallidum*, and this can be detected by applying fluorescein-labelled anti-human γ-globulin. This *fluorescent treponemal antibody* (*FTA*) *test* can be made even more specific if the serum is first absorbed by Reiter treponemes, the *FTA-ABS test*, and is as sensitive and specific as the TPI test. These tests are not performed routinely, but they are of great value in verifying ambiguous results and eliminating false positive reactions.*

* They cannot distinguish between syphilis and *yaws*, a disease which has much in common with syphilis and is caused by *Tr. pertenue*. It is frequent in some tropical countries, and is not venereal in origin. The primary lesion is extra-genital, and this is followed by a secondary and tertiary stage. In the latter there are destructive skin and bone lesions, and these may affect the face and nose. Significant cardiovascular and central-nervous-system involvement is rare compared with syphilis. It is possible that *Tr. pallidum* developed as a variant of *Tr. pertenue* which became adapted to venereal transmission.

## The Disease[13,14]

Apart from congenital syphilis, the infection is almost always acquired venereally. But on rare occasions it is transmitted by a blood transfusion, and a primary lesion can occur on the finger of an unfortunate dentist or physician who examines an infected patient. Nevertheless, considering how frequent it must be for the hands to come in contact with the treponema, the rarity of cutaneous chancres is curious. Evidentally the organism cannot easily infect the skin. Unlike the tubercle bacillus, *Tr. pallidum* is very rapidly destroyed both in water and by drying. Intimate direct contact is therefore necessary for infection to occur. The spirochaete is one of the most invasive organisms known. Once it penetrates the surface integument, it spreads along the lymphatics to the regional lymph nodes, and finally reaches the blood stream within a matter of hours. There is therefore systemic dissemination long before any local manifestation appears.

The disease is divisible into three stages with a latent period between each of them.

**Primary Syphilis.** The typical lesion of primary syphilis is the *chancre*, which usually appears on the genital region 2–4 weeks after infection. It is an indurated nodule which breaks down to form an ulcer. It is characteristically painless, and is accompanied by a considerable *regional lymphadenitis* which is also painless. Extragenital chancres are not uncommon, e.g. around the anus in homosexuals, and on the lips, tip of tongue, tonsils, gingiva, or other part of the oral cavity.

The histological appearance is quite non-specific, consisting merely of a dense infiltration of lymphocytes, plasma cells, and a few macrophages in the dermis.

Even without treatment the chancre gradually heals, usually with little scarring.

The fact that the spirochaetes become disseminated in the blood stream long before there is any local lesion suggests that hypersensitivity plays an important part in the process. The chancre is not comparable with a boil, for it is not a local inflammatory reaction tending to limit the infection. A possible explanation is that sensitizing antibodies are first formed in the cells at the site of entry and in the regional lymph nodes. During the incubation period the spirochaetes multiply in the RE system, and when liberated react with the sensitized tissue. This would explain the chancre and the lymphadenopathy quite well.

At a later stage the other tissues of the body become sensitized, and then the generalized lesions of secondary syphilis become manifest. Nevertheless, our knowledge about allergy and immunity in syphilis is woefully inadequate.

*Diagnosis.* The laboratory diagnosis depends on demonstrating spirochaetes in the exudate from the chancre by dark-ground illumination.

About two weeks after the appearance of the chancre, antibodies first appear in the blood. Blood serology should never be neglected in practice.

**Secondary Syphilis.** Within 2–3 months after exposure the disease becomes clinically generalized. When syphilis was first introduced into Europe, this stage was severe enough to warrant the name, "the great pox". Nowadays it is much milder, and is characterized by a low-grade pyrexia, "rheumatic" pains, moderate anaemia, and a generalized painless lymphadenopathy. Mucocutaneous involvement is conspicuous, and it takes the form of symmetrical eruptions of various types. In moist areas, e.g. the vulva, anal region, and axillae, plateau-like excrescences are formed (*condylomata*). In the buccal mucosa the flat lesions are called *mucous patches,* and shallow serpiginous ulceration also occurs (*snail-track ulcers*). The histology of these is essentially

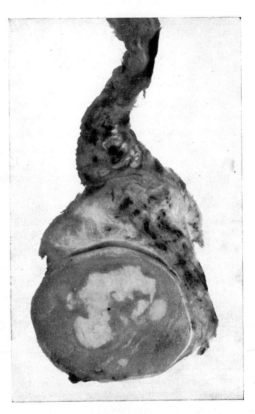

FIG. 15.7. Gumma of testis. The testis is replaced by an ill-defined area of gummatous necrosis, but the epididymis and spermatic cord are not affected.

(EM6.1, *Reproduced by permission of the President and Council of the Royal College of Surgeons of England.*)

similar to that of the chancre, and once again there is a tendency towards spontaneous healing.

Secondary lesions do not form scars. This is the phase of maximal infectivity; spirochaetes ooze out of condylomata and mucous patches.

*Diagnosis.* The serological tests are always positive in overt secondary syphilis, and organisms can be demonstrated in the exudates from mucous and cutaneous lesions.

**Tertiary Syphilis.** Local destructive lesions of a truly chronic inflammatory nature may appear 2–3 years after infection and continue to erupt sporadically for at least 20 years. The lesions are presumably due to marked hypersensitivity, since spirochaetes are few and the reaction is excessive. Two forms

of lesions occur: *localized gummata* and *diffuse inflammatory lesions* characterized by parenchymatous destruction.

*Localized gummata.* The *gumma* is the classical lesion of tertiary syphilis.
It is usually solitary, and consists of a large area of coagulative necrosis very
similar in appearance to caseation, except that the tissue destruction is usually
not quite so complete. Details of architecture can therefore still be faintly
distinguished amid the debris. It is surrounded by an extensive zone of
lymphocytes, plasma cells, and macrophages. Proliferating fibroblasts are
plentiful, and much reparative fibrous tissue is laid down. Giant cells are
much less numerous than in tuberculosis. The arteries in the vicinity show
marked endarteritis obliterans.

Gummata are particularly liable to occur in the liver, testes (Fig. 15.7),
subcutaneous tissues, and in bones, notably the tibia, ulna, clavicle, calvaria
of skull, and the nasal and palatal bones. The destruction produced by
gummata is exemplified by the perforated palate and the saddle-shaped
nasal deformity so characteristic of tertiary syphilis.

*Diffuse lesions.* The really baneful effects of tertiary syphilis fall on the
cardiovascular and nervous systems. In the former it is the thoracic aorta
which usually suffers first. An infiltration of lymphocytes and plasma cells
accumulates around the vasa vasorum of the tunica adventitia, and soon
spreads inwards into the tunica media, where it destroys much of the elastic
tissue which is essential for the integrity of the aorta.

The *syphilitic aortitis* that results weakens the wall so much that aneurysmal
dilatation eventually ensues. Sometimes the disease spreads down to the
aortic ring, which dilates and leads to aortic regurgitation. If the ostia of the
coronary arteries are occluded at the same time, there is severe myocardial
ischaemia as well.

Cerebral syphilis may be *meningo-vascular* or *parenchymatous*. In the former
type there is focal meningitis and vascular occlusion due to endarteritis
obliterans of the small vessels. Isolated cranial nerve palsies are quite common.

Parenchymatous neurosyphilis includes the two well-known conditions,
general paralysis of the insane and tabes dorsalis. *General paralysis of the
insane* is a chronic syphilitic meningoencephalitis in which the frontal lobes
are particularly severely affected. This results in progressive dementia and
often paralysis. *Tabes dorsalis* is a degenerative condition of the posterior
columns of the spinal cord and the posterior roots of the spinal nerves. There
is severe demyelination of the sensory tracts. This results in loss of sensation
leading to trophic disturbances, and loss of postural sense, which produces
the typical staggering gait.

The bones are sometimes affected by a diffuse type of syphilitic inflammation.[15] There may be widespread periostitis, involving especially the tibia
and the bones of the calvaria of the skull. The irregular thickening that is
very apparent clinically is due to the laying down of new bone. This gives
rise to the classical *sabre tibia*, and in the skull a rather typical worm-eaten
appearance.

*Diagnosis.* The diagnosis of tertiary syphilis is primarily clinical, but it may
often be substantiated by serological examination of the blood and cerebro-
spinal fluid. In most cases of overt syphilis this examination is strongly

positive, and in neuro-syphilis the cerebrospinal fluid is generally more helpful than the blood.

### Congenital Syphilis

During the first two years of infection an untreated syphilitic mother is very liable to transmit the disease to her fetus, particularly after the fourth month of pregnancy, when the Langhans layer of the placenta becomes attenuated. Abortion may result, or else a severely affected infant may die soon after birth.

More frequently the child survives, and it may then exhibit early stigmata of infection like skin eruptions, snuffles, epiphysitis of the elbows, and wasting. Sometimes stigmata appear only in later childhood. The notched, peg-shaped Hutchinson's incisor teeth and mulberry molars (Moon's molars) due to syphilitic infection of the tooth germs during fetal life are well-known examples of this type of lesion, as are also interstitial keratitis (inflammation of the cornea), tibial periostitis (sabre tibia), and nerve deafness.

The histological appearances of these various lesions are all very similar, being combinations of the heavy cellular infiltration of secondary syphilis together with the gummatous destruction typical of the tertiary phase. In fact, congenital syphilis may be regarded as a combined secondary and tertiary syphilis occurring in a child whose primary lesion was placental.

The incidence of syphilis showed a decline during most of the twentieth century, but since 1957 there has been an upward trend in many parts of the world. Its prognosis has greatly improved since the advent of penicillin,[16] and *tertiary lesions are now very infrequent.*

## ACTINOMYCOSIS[17]

Actinomycosis is characterized by chronic, loculated foci of suppuration occurring particularly in the region of the lower jaw. The human disease is caused by *Actinomyces israeli*,[18,19] while a similar condition in cattle ("lumpy jaw") is caused by another organism, *Actinomyces bovis*.

**Bacteriology.**[20] These organisms are Gram-positive filaments which have a tendency to branch. They grow in a colonial, bunched form particularly in animal tissues, where a densely felted mass of branching filaments matted together in an amorphous matrix is characteristic. It is called a *mycelium*. A mycelium of this type appears in the pus of actinomycotic lesions in the form of a small granule which is greyish-white in colour. This is called a *sulphur granule*. It is in fact a single colony of the actinomyces organism, comprising many individual filaments matted together. In the diagnosis of actinomycosis it is important to search for and culture these sulphur granules. "Blind" culture of the pus is unlikely to grow the organism.

A mycelium formed in the tissues tends to be surrounded by club-shaped excrescences (*clubs*) which radiate outwards in the form of a ring. These "clubs" are produced as the result of deposition on to the mycelium of lipid material derived from the host's tissues. This radiating appearance of "clubs" around the mycelium explains the alternative name *ray fungus* which is loosely applied to *Actinomyces bovis* or *Actinomyces israeli*.

**Pathogenesis.** *Actinomyces israeli* is a normal commensal of the mouth, and it is found especially in the tonsils and in carious teeth. Actinomycosis is an endogenous infection,[21] and is not transmitted by contaminated pieces of straw and grass that have been sucked by cattle. It can follow a dental extraction,[22] though considering the widespread distribution of the organism, the disease is surprisingly infrequent. It is not understood what local conditions must be fulfilled before the organism can invade the tissues and set up a progressive inflammatory reaction. It has been known to produce infection in a hand wound caused by hitting an assailant in the teeth ("punch actinomycosis").[23]

**The Lesions.** Actinomycosis commonly occurs in the *cervico-facial* region. Primary *ileo-caecal* infection is uncommon, and *pulmonary* lesions are rare.

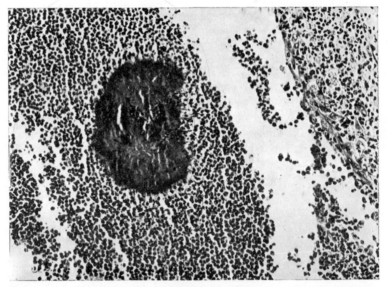

FIG. 15.8. Actinomycotic pus. This section shows a colony of actinomyces ("sulphur granule") in a dense mass of pus cells. × 150.

The actinomycotic lesion starts as an acute suppurative inflammation, which then persists and progresses to intractable chronicity. As the organisms spread by direct continuity, large numbers of abscesses are produced. Some of these fuse together, but there is a tendency for individual foci of suppuration to remain discrete owing to the persistence of fibrous septa. This produces a characteristically loculated appearance, which is seen most typically in actinomycotic lesions of the liver (*honeycomb liver*).

Histologically the abscess cavities are crowded with pus cells which surround actinomycotic colonies (Fig. 15.8). The narrow septa between the abscesses are composed of fibrous tissue which is heavily infiltrated by polymorphs, lymphocytes, macrophages, and plasma cells. These fibrous septa are not merely the remains of destroyed parenchyma; they are produced by attempts at healing by repair, and the entire lesion is surrounded by a similar dense zone of fibrous tissue.

**Spread of Infection.** The main mode of spread of the disease is by direct contact. Whereas other organisms move in the tissue spaces along preformed planes, the actinomyces extends slowly and inexorably onwards through the tissues. In cervico-facial actinomycosis there is direct spread to the adjacent muscles and bones. The mandible is the bone usually involved, but sometimes there is extension to the maxilla, and eventually the meninges and brain become infected.[24] There is also progressive cutaneous involvement, and the abscesses discharge with the production of many sinuses. The appearance of a diffuse, indurated, painless area of suppuration in the area of the mandible discharging to the exterior through multiple sinuses is very characteristic of actinomycosis.

Similarly ileo-caecal actinomycosis spreads through the anterior abdominal wall with the development of discharging sinuses, and pulmonary actinomycosis erupts through the wall of the chest.

Lymphatic spread does not occur in actinomycosis; perhaps the filaments are too large to be accommodated in the lymphatic channels. Any regional lymphadenitis that may occur is attributable to secondary bacterial infection by staphylococci and coliform organisms.

Blood-borne spread, on the other hand, is important, and is typified by the spread of ileo-caecal disease by the portal vein to the liver, where the loculated actinomycotic abscesses of honeycomb liver are produced.

**Treatment.**[25, 26] Actinomyces organisms are very sensitive to the commonly-used antibiotics, and in practice penicillin is the most useful.

## FUNGOUS INFECTIONS

A fungus is a member of the vegetable kingdom, devoid of roots, stems, and leaves and incapable of photosynthesis. Some are unicellular (e.g. yeasts) while others consist of branching filaments (*hyphae*) aggregated into a mass (*mycelium*). Multiplication is by budding in the case of yeasts, and spore formation in the case of the higher fungi. Some organisms are dimorphic, growing as a yeast under some conditions but producing hyphae at other times—often in artificial culture. The line of distinction between some higher bacteria (e.g. actinomyces and streptomyces) and "true" fungi is by no means clear-cut.

### Superficial Infections by Fungi

A number of fungi are able to grow in the hair and the superficial layers of the epidermis, where they produce skin diseases typified by *ringworm*. These will not be considered.

**Candidiasis.**[27] Infection with Candida species is one of the most frequent fungus infections in man. The organism most commonly involved is the dimorphic fungus *Candida albicans*. The common yeast form is seen in thrush, and is $1 \cdot 5–5 \cdot 0$ μm in diameter and intensively Gram positive. It reproduces by budding, but sometimes the bud elongates to form a mycelium. This form can occur in cultures and is also characteristic of invasive candida infections, especially the lesions of systemic candidiasis. The organism is a common commensal in the oral cavity, alimentary tract, and vagina. Infections occur when local or general conditions become suitable, but it must be accepted that the factors which govern the delicate balance between host and organism are poorly understood. The superficial infections of the mucous membranes appear as white patches called *thrush*. In the mouth this is very common in infants, especially premature ones, and may be accompanied by perianal lesions. Oral candidiasis can occur at any age during the course of any debilitating disease. It may also occur under dentures and orthodontic appliances, and can complicate other erosive disease, e.g. pemphigus vulgaris. Vaginal thrush is common during pregnancy, in those on the contraceptive pill, and in diabetes mellitus. Cutaneous candidiasis occurs around the corners of the mouth (*angular cheilosis*, or *perlèche*), in other moist intertriginous areas, and in the nail folds (*chronic paronychia*).

The important feature of candidiasis is that it is sometimes a serious opportunistic infection. With glucocorticosteroid therapy, in lymphomata, following the administration of cytotoxic drugs, and indeed in any disease in which cell-mediated immunity is impaired, oral lesions can extend down the alimentary or respiratory tracts to produce fatal results. The organism may invade the blood stream and lead to generalized systemic candidiasis in which lesions occur in many organs. Renal abscesses are usually prominent, but almost any organ may be affected and endocarditis is sometimes seen. Severe candidiasis is often a feature of the immunological deficiency diseases which affect the T lymphocytes.

Less extensive candida infections are seen in particular circumstances. Endocarditis can occur as a primary event, particularly in addicts who inject themselves intravenously with narcotics. Oral lesions can spread to produce extensive gastro-intestinal infection following the prolonged administration of oral broad-spectrum antibiotics. Finally there are some types of primary immunological deficiency disease affecting the T lymphocytes in which there is *chronic widespread mucocutaneous candidiasis*.[28] These may be familial, and endocrine abnormalities, particularly hypoparathyroidism, may coexist. These conditions persist for many years and do not tend to terminate in generalized spread, nor is there usually a tendency for other infections to occur.

The tissue reaction to candida varies. In minor and superficial infections there is some tissue necrosis accompanied by a pyogenic response. Intra-epidermal pustules are seen in the cutaneous lesions. When the infection is overwhelming, as in generalized candidiasis, there is much necrosis and very little inflammatory reaction. Indeed, the lesions show massive accumulations of fungus and few host cells.

## Deep-Seated Fungous Infections

In certain parts of the world fungus infections are of considerable importance. In general the organisms are found in the soil, and infection is acquired by inhalation. A primary lesion occurs in the lung and in the majority of people healing follows. Occasionally, however, the organisms produce more severe damage and spread to involve other organs. These diseases therefore resemble tuberculosis in their pathogenesis. Their histological appearances sometimes resemble tuberculosis quite closely.

**Cryptococcosis.**[28] The causative organism *Cryptococcus neoformans* (previously called *Torula histolytica*) is a true yeast, and of world-wide distribution. The primary lung lesion is usually small and heals by fibrosis. Occasionally the organism becomes widely disseminated and in particular causes *meningitis*. The infection is sometimes seen in patients weakened by such conditions as Hodgkin's disease and leukaemia.

**Histoplasmosis.**[30] The causative organism *Histoplasma capsulatum* has a

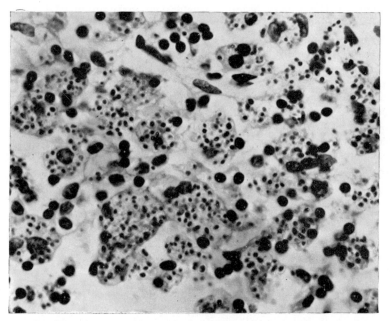

FIG. 15.9. Histoplasmosis. This section of spleen contains many macrophages crowded with *Histoplasma capsulatum* organisms. × 400.

world-wide distribution, but infection is particularly common in the Mississippi Valley of the USA. The histoplasmin test, analagous to the tuberculin test, is positive in affected individuals.

The primary lung lesion resembles tuberculosis and usually heals with calcification. Occasionally cavitation occurs, and rarely there is blood-borne dissemination. This occurs most commonly in infants, and many of the internal organs are involved. Large numbers of organisms are then found parasitizing the RE cells (Fig. 15.9). Disseminated histoplasmosis may also occur in elderly debilitated subjects, usually men, and the infection is less widespread than in the infantile type. In some cases infection of the lips, mouth, nose, or larynx is the initial manifestation. In Africa, *Histoplasma duboisii* generally infects the skin.

**Coccidioidomycosis.**[31] This disease, caused by *Coccidioides immitis*, is common in the desert regions of California and Arizona and also in the Chaco district of Argentina. Many of the inhabitants acquire a pulmonary infection, but this is either asymptomatic or accompanied by a self-limiting influenza-like illness called locally "desert fever". Occasionally the disease is progressive, and the destructive lung lesions closely resemble tuberculosis. Systemic spread to many organs may occur. Histologically the lesions show a suppurative tuberculoid reaction, the centre of each follicle being occupied by necrotic material containing many polymorphs.

**North American Blastomycosis.** This is caused by infection with *Blastomyces dermatitidis*, a yeast with a thick double-contoured capsule, which reproduces by budding. The primary lesion is usually pulmonary but may be cutaneous. It generally subsides spontaneously, but occasionally it progresses and widespread dissemination can then follow. Suppurative lesions occur in many sites, particularly the skin and bones.

**South American Blastomycosis.** The causative organism, *Blastomyces braziliensis*, multiplies by producing multiple peripheral buds so that the organism becomes surrounded by a "row of beads". The common primary site of infection is the nasopharynx, and ulcerative destructive lesions are produced. The lymph nodes are soon involved, and sometimes cervical lymphadenopathy is the presenting symptom. The disease tends to become disseminated and affect the lungs, skin, and other organs. It is commonly fatal unless treated.

## References

1. WILSON, G. S. and MILES, A. A. (1964). In Topley and Wilson's "Principles of Bacteriology and Immunity", 5th ed., p. 1588. London: Arnold.
2. CRUICKSHANK, R. (1965). In "Medical Microbiology", 11th ed., p. 194, ed. by Cruickshank, R. Edinburgh: Livingstone.
3. MARKS, J. (1964). *Proc. roy. Soc. Med.*, **57**, 479.
4. CONNOR, D. H. and LUNN, H. F. (1966). *Arch. Path.*, **81**, 183.
5. PHILPOTT, J. A. *et al.* (1963). *Arch. Derm.*, **88**, 158.
6. POOLE, J. C. F. and FLOREY, H. W. (1970). In "General Pathology", 4th ed., p. 1190, ed. by Florey, H. W. London: Lloyd-Luke.
7. RICH, A. R. and McCORDOCK, H. A. (1933). *Bull. Johns Hopk. Hosp.*, **52**, 5.
8. MOLOMUT, N. and SPAIN, D. M. (1953). *Amer. Rev. Tuberc.*, **67**, 101.
9. SCADDING, J. G. (1967). *Sarcoidosis.* London: Eyre and Spottiswoode.
10. SWAIN, R. H. A. (1965). In "Medical Microbiology", 11th ed., p. 342, ed. by Cruickshank, R. Edinburgh: Livingstone.
11. WILKINSON, A. E. and SEQUEIRA, P. J. L. (1955). *Brit. J. vener. Dis.*, **31**, 143.
12. WILKINSON, A. E. (1957). *Brit. J. vener. Dis.*, **33**, 25.
13. WILSON, G. S. and MILES, A. A. (1964). p. 2170, *loc. cit.*
14. BEERMAN, H. *et al.* (1960). *Arch. intern. Med.*, **105**, 145 and 324.
15. KING, A. J. and CATTERALL, R. D. (1959). *Brit. J. vener. Dis.*, **35**, 116.
16. Leading Article (1963). *Lancet*, **2**, 1317.
17. COPE, V. Z. (1938). "Actinomycosis." Oxford University Press.
18. WILSON, G. S. and MILES, A. A. (1964). p. 1563, *loc. cit.*
19. PEABODY, J. W. and SEABURY, J. H. (1957). *J. chron. Dis.*, **5**, 374.
20. GILLIES, R. R. (1965). In "Medical Microbiology", 11th ed., p. 303, ed. by Cruickshank, R. Edinburgh: Livingstone.
21. UTZ, J. P. (1962). *Lab. Invest.*, **11**, 1018.
22. LESNEY, T. A. and TRAEGER, K. A. (1959). *J. oral Surg.*, **17**, No. 1, 51.
23. WINNER, H. I. (1960). Quoted in *Lancet*, **2**, 907.

24. INTILE, J. A. and RICHERT, J. H. (1962). *J. Amer. med. Ass.*, **181,** 724.
25. PEABODY, J. W. and SEABURY, J. H. (1960). *Amer. J. Med.*, **28,** 99.
26. SPILSBURY, B. W. and JOHNSTONE, F. R. C. (1962). *Canad. J. Surg.*, **5,** 33.
27. WINNER, H. I. and HURLEY, R. (1964). "Candida Albicans", 306 pp. London: Churchill.
28. Leading Article (1972). *Brit. Med. J.*, **4,** 505.
29. COX, L. B. and TOLHURST, J. C. (1946). "Human Torulosis". Melbourne: Melbourne University Press.
30. SCHWARZ, J. and BAUM, G. L. (1963). *Arch. intern. Med.*, **111,** 710 and *Arch. Path.*, **75,** 475.
31. FIESE, M. J. (1958). "Coccidioidomycosis." Springfield, Ill.: Thomas.

# Chapter 16

# VIRUS DISEASES

## Introduction

The peculiar characteristics of viruses are best understood when compared with those of other organisms.

**Bacteria** are generally unicellular, but even the smallest is within the range of the light microscope (which resolves up to about $0 \cdot 2\mu m$ in diameter). They grow with variable ease on artificial cell-free media, though in this respect *Myco. leprae* and *Tr. pallidum* are exceptions, for as yet they have not been cultured artificially. The bacterial cell is complete, and contains both DNA and RNA.

**Rickettsiae**[1] are unicellular organisms about $0 \cdot 4\mu m$ (400 nm) in size, and are visible under the light microscope. They resemble bacteria in reproducing by asexual binary fission, possessing both DNA and RNA, and having a *cell wall* containing muramic acid. They differ from bacteria in that they require living cells for growth, i.e. they are *obligatory intracellular parasites*. The rickettsiae produce the *typhus group of fevers* which have a world-wide distribution, and are transmitted by arthropods like lice, fleas, ticks, and mites, e.g. Rocky mountain tick-borne typhus is caused by *R. rickettsi*. Another condition caused by a rickettsia is Q (query) fever, a febrile disease with chest symptoms. The causal organism *Coxiella burneti* is somewhat smaller than those of typhus. The organisms of trachoma, inclusion conjunctivitis, psittacosis, and lymphogranuloma venereum are now also classified among the rickettsial organisms. They are smaller even than *Cox.burneti* (about 350 nm in diameter), but like all the others are sensitive to tetracyclines.

**Mycoplasmas**[2,3] (pleuropneumonia group of organisms) comprise a group of minute organisms of doubtful systematic position. They are 100–150 nm in size, and possess no cell wall but only a limiting membrane. The result is *extreme fragility* and *pleomorphism*; granules, rings, coccoid forms, and fine filaments are all described. Because of their small size they pass through very fine filters, yet they resemble bacteria in being able to grow on artificial cell-free media.

The important human pathogen is *Mycoplasma pneumoniae*.[4] At one time it was classified as a virus, and the disease it causes was erroneously called *virus pneumonia*. It responds well to tetracyclines. Mycoplasmas are also found in the mouth and genito-urinary tract,[46] and have also been isolated from leukaemic tissue and rheumatoid joints.

**L-forms.** These were first described by Klieneberger-Nobel working at the Lister Institute, London (L stands for Lister). When certain bacteria are faced with adverse circumstances, they swell up (and possibly fuse) into a large mass which then disintegrates into irregularly spherical granules which are plastic, refractile, and very fragile. They are minute, measuring

0·1–0·5 μm in diameter. They are penicillin-resistant irrespective of the general sensitivity of the strain from which they are derived. L-forms have been described in *Strept. viridans, Esch. coli,* and many other species. They pass easily through ordinary bacterial filters, and it is possible that they are present in bacteriologically "sterile" filtrates. They bear a close resemblance to *Mycoplasma* organisms, and in fact have not been adequately separated from this group. An L-form returns to type when conditions are normal.

**Viruses.**[5, 6] Size is not a criterion in the definition of a virus because some of them are larger than the mycoplasmal organisms.

All viruses are obligatory intracellular parasites, but this is also a feature of the rickettsiae and a few bacteria.

The only feature which distinguishes viruses from all other organisms is that during the process of multiplication they enter a non-infective, or "eclipse", phase (p. 215).

Viruses possess no enzyme systems capable of synthetizing viral material; they are therefore dependent on the parasitized cell for survival and multiplication. Indeed, the essential difference between viruses and other organisms is that the synthetic processes that attend multiplication take place within the protoplasm of the infected cells in the case of viruses, but in the body of the organism itself in other infective agents.

## PROPERTIES OF TRUE VIRUSES

### Size

Among the largest of the true viruses is the pox group responsible for smallpox, vaccinia, and similar diseases in other species of animals. These are about 250 nm in size, and a single virus particle when suitably stained is just visible under the light microscope. Those smaller than this cannot be seen by light microscopy, and therefore other methods of measurement are used.

*Filterability.* Their size can be assessed by their capacity to pass through specially graded filters. This is too inaccurate for precise measurements.

*Sedimentation rate.* A more modern method is ultracentrifugation using high-speed centrifuges. The larger the particle, the faster it falls.

*Electron microscopy.* The most accurate method at present available is electron microscopy, which has also imparted fundamental information about virus size, shape, and chemical configuration. Most viruses are less than 200 nm in size—varicella virus is 150–120 nm, and one of the smallest, that of foot-and-mouth disease, is only 20 nm.

Many viruses are spherical in shape, e.g. poliovirus, herpes-simplex virus, and adenovirus, some are filamentous, e.g. tobacco-mosaic virus and influenza virus, while *E.coli* bacteriophage has a characteristic tadpole shape (Fig. 16.1).

### Chemical Constituents

The basic composition of a virus particle, or *virion* (also called an *elementary body*), is a nucleic-acid core surrounded by a protein envelope called a *capsid.* In some viruses, e.g. herpesviruses and adenoviruses, the nucleic acid is DNA, whereas in others, e.g. the enteroviruses and myxoviruses, it is RNA. The heart of a virus is its nucleic-acid portion, for this controls the synthesis of new viral material when it infects a host cell.

The protein envelope is composed of sub-units built in a compact, regular manner around the nucleic-acid core.[7,8,9] These protein sub-units are called *capsomeres*, and their arrangement is related to the shape of the virus.

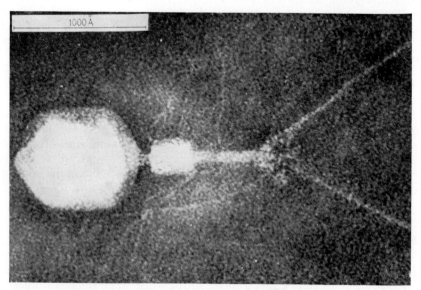

FIG. 16.1. The bacteriophage particle viewed under the electron microscope after negative staining. Note the following structures:

(*a*) The head, a bipyramidal prism. It contains the viral DNA.

(*b*) A central rigid core.

(*c*) A tail sheath which surrounds this central core. In the picture the sheath is contracted to the upper part of the core. It is attached to a hexagonal plate structure at the extreme end of the tail—it is unrecognizable in this picture.

(*d*) Tail fibres (six altogether) associated with the plate structure.

It is suggested that the plate and fibres are a means of attachment to the host. The components of bacteriophage have been compared to a micro-syringe system serving to inject the viral DNA into the host bacterium. × 300 000.

(*From Brenner, S., et al.* (1959). J. molec. Biol., **1**, 281.)

In spherical viruses they show a cubical or icosahedral symmetry, i.e. they are disposed around the core in the form of a regular icosahedron (a solid bounded by 20 plane surfaces each of which is an equilateral triangle). This is demonstrated in Figs. 16.2 and 16.3. Filamentous (or rod-shaped) viruses are surrounded by a helix of protein sub-units, i.e. they are arranged in a spiral around the central rod.

Some viruses, e.g. the herpesviruses and myxoviruses, have an additional outer envelope consisting largely of lipid material, while the most complex poxviruses also contain carbohydrates, vitamins, and even some simple enzymes.

## Life-cycle and Reproduction

The knowledge about the life-cycle of a virus in a cell is still far from complete. Much of our information has been gained from research into a few individual viruses, notably bacteriophage, and it might be fallacious to assume that all viruses behave identically.

**Attachment and Penetration.**[10] The first stage is the attachment of the virus to a specific *cell receptor*, or *receptor site*, on the cell membrane. This

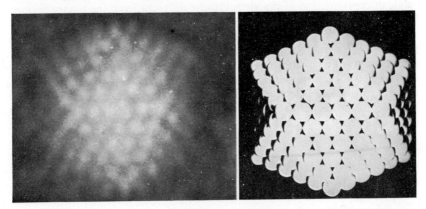

FIG. 16.2.                                         FIG. 16.3.

FIG. 16.2. A single particle, or elementary body, of adenovirus embedded in electron-opaque phosphotungstate and viewed under the electron microscope. The particle is composed of morphological units (capsomeres) of spherical shape packed in a symmetrical arrangement. × 480 000.
(*From Horne, R. W., Brenner, S., Waterson, A. P., and Wildy, P.* (1959). J. molec. Biol., **1**, 84.)

FIG. 16.3. A model of the geometrical figure formed by the capsomeres of an adenovirus. It has been calculated that the total number of capsomeres around the central core of an adenovirus is 252. They are arranged in the form of a regular twenty-sided figure all of whose faces are equilateral triangles—it is called an icosahedron.
(From the same reference as Fig. 16.2.)

*attachment phase* is followed by *penetration* of the virus into the cell. The bacteriophage attaches by its tail fibres to specific receptor sites on the bacterial wall, which is then weakened by a hydrolytic enzyme present in the phage tail. There then follows the injection of its content of DNA into the interior of the bacterium, while the protein coat of the phage, which acts as a microsyringe, remains attached externally to the bacterial wall.

This mode of entry is not seen in animal viruses, of which the myxoviruses, e.g. influenza and mumps, have been most studied. Some viruses enter the cell intact, but regardless of the mode of entry it is established that the nucleic acid is the essential infective agent.

**Eclipse Phase.**[11] Following the entry of the virus the next phase ensues;

it is called the *eclipse phase*, and is characteristic of all viruses. During this phase the virus is unidentifiable by infectivity tests, and cannot be demonstrated by electron microscopy. It appears that the free nucleic acid is engaged in redirecting the cell's metabolism so that more viral nucleic acid and protein are produced. It probably does this by producing a new mRNA, if it is a DNA-containing virus, or by acting as a new mRNA, if it is a RNA-containing virus. The eclipse phrase takes from one to thirty hours. It is indeed remarkable that a minute quantity of foreign nucleic acid can so dominate the cellular metabolism that, instead of forming normal cell substance, the cell is perverted into forming large amounts of the virus. This mode of reproduction of the virus is quite different from the binary fission of higher organisms.

**Maturation.**[11] The stages leading up to the formation of mature virus particles are complex, and vary in different viruses. The nucleic acid core and protein capsid may sometimes be formed in different parts of the cell, e.g. the nucleus and the cytoplasm, and these will then have to be assembled together into mature virus. Infective material soon becomes recognizable, and it is released from the cell as mature virus particles. These then effect entry into other cells, either by direct contact or after carriage by the tissue fluids.

In herpesvirus and myxovirus infections, as the particles are released from the cell surface, they become ensheathed by the plasma membrane of the host cell, which thus becomes an integral component of their bodies. The release of virus particles is continuous and persists for some hours. Other viruses, e.g. poliovirus, are formed completely within the cell, and are released rapidly by a burst-like process.

The escape of virus may be associated with a disintegration of the host cell, e.g. in bacteriophage and poliovirus infections. Myxovirus, on the other hand, showers off the cell surface without causing immediate damage.

Sometimes during the phase of virus development there are found large intracellular masses, or *inclusion bodies*. These are particles seen in virus-infected cells, and composed of aggregations of developing virus material bound together in a gelatinous matrix. Unlike *elementary bodies*, which are single mature virus particles, inclusion bodies are large (up to $20\mu$m in size) and easily visible under the light microscope. Some are acidophilic and others basophilic; some are intracytoplasmic and others intranuclear. At one time these structures were of great moment in the diagnosis of virus disease; nowadays they are mostly of historical interest. The *Negri body*, an acidophilic body, found in the cytoplasm of neurones in cases of rabies, is one of the best known examples. Some inclusion bodies are merely altered protein in virus-infected cells, but do not contain any virus.

## Reaction to Environment

Unlike bacteria, most viruses are easily inactivated even at room temperature, and care must be taken to keep specimens frozen, if possible at $-70°C$. A few viruses are much more stable than this, however, and the viruses of poliomyelitis and vaccinia can survive at ordinary atmospheric temperatures for some weeks. The agent of infective hepatitis appears to be particularly resistant, but the most durable agent is that of scrapie, which withstands boiling for three hours.

## Reaction to Chemicals

Viruses are destroyed without difficulty by the chemical disinfectants used against bacteria. One important difference lies in the great resistance of many viruses to a 50 per cent solution of glycerol, which kills non-sporing bacteria quite rapidly. Vaccinia virus is actually preserved in glycerol. No virus is susceptible to any antibiotic therapy in current use, but a few specific chemotherapeutic agents are now known.[44,45]

## Cultivation of Viruses[12]

Viruses multiply only in living cells, and at first the only systems that could be used were experimental animals and chick embryos. The discovery by Enders and his colleagues in 1949[13] that the virus of poliomyelitis could proliferate in tissue cultures of non-neuronal origin, e.g. human prepuce, ushered in the modern era of virus research. Nowadays the vast majority of viruses are cultivated in tissue culture, a method which is cheap, simple, and efficacious.

1. *Animal inoculation* is reserved for those viruses which do not grow satisfactorily in tissue culture, e.g. some Coxsackie viruses.

2. *Chick embryo inoculation* is still used to culture some viruses. Characteristic lesions may be produced on the chorio-allantoic membrane by the poxviruses, and the amniotic sac is used for culturing influenza virus.

3. *Tissue culture* is the method of choice. The basis of this technique is that living cells are grown on the sides of test-tubes. Many viruses are able to multiply in these cells, in which they produce destructive changes. This is called a *cytopathic effect*, and is illustrated in Figs. 16.4 to 16.6. The changes are sometimes characteristic of a specified virus, but in any case the virus can be identified by *neutralization tests* and *complement fixation* using specific rabbit antisera. If, for instance, a specific antiserum prevents a cytopathic effect in a cell system (or for that matter, if it prevents a lesion in an egg or a test animal), the virus is typed accordingly. The fluid in the tissue culture system provides the virus material. It also provides the source of antigen for performing complement fixation tests. The cell systems commonly employed in this way are monkey kidney cells, human amnion cells, and strains of cancer cells, e.g. the "HeLa cell" derived from a carcinoma of the cervix of a woman named Helen Lane.[14]

## Infectivity

Viruses produce disease even in minute quantities, and their degree of infectivity is so high that *epidemics are very common*, e.g. smallpox, influenza, and the common virus diseases of childhood.

Virus disease is by no means confined to vertebrates; there are insect infections like silkworm jaundice and sacbrood of bees, plant diseases like tobacco-mosaic disease, and also the very important group of bacterial infections due to bacteriophage.

Of the viruses pathogenic to man many seem to attack one organ speci-

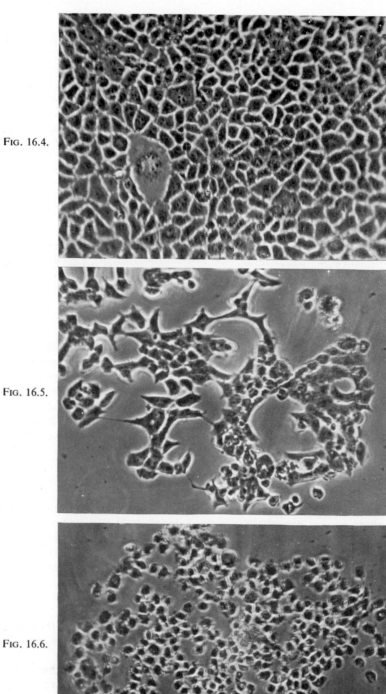

Fig. 16.4.

Fig. 16.5.

Fig. 16.6.

fically, but the once fashionable concept of *tropism* is no longer valid. A "neurotropic" virus like poliovirus multiplies in the cells of the small intestine, while the "dermatotropic" virus of herpes simplex can produce encephalitis. There is as yet no entirely satisfactory classification of viruses, and therefore it is probably still most helpful to consider virus infections in terms of the organs or tissues that they usually attack:

**Viruses attacking the skin:** vaccinia, herpes simplex, and verruca vulgaris (the common wart).

**Viruses attacking the central nervous system:** enteroviruses, zoster, rabies, arthropod-borne viruses (arboviruses), mumps, and occasionally herpes simplex, measles, and vaccinia.

**Viruses attacking the liver:** hepatitis and yellow fever.

**Viruses attacking the respiratory tract:** influenza, adenoviruses, and the common cold viruses (rhinoviruses).

**Viruses attacking the conjunctiva:** herpes simplex and adenoviruses.

**Viruses attacking the salivary glands and other secreting organs:** mumps.

**Generalized virus diseases often producing characteristic rashes:** smallpox, measles, rubella, chickenpox, dengue, and some enterovirus infections.

## Tissue Reactions to Viruses

All considerations of the effects of viruses on the tissues of the body must start at a cellular level; viruses are intracellular parasites, and the damage they produce is directed primarily at the cell. This is followed secondarily by a local inflammatory reaction.

**Cellular Reaction.** A cell infected with a virus may degenerate at once, or it may undergo proliferation which may or may not be followed by later necrosis, or it may show no change whatsoever.

This last effect is typical of what is called "latent virus" infection.[15] It is well known, for example, that the skin of the face frequently harbours herpes simplex virus without showing any lesion. Similarly, many children are infected with certain types of adenoviruses early in life, and these remain in their tonsils and adenoids without producing conspicuous damage.[16]

Whether a cell degenerates or proliferates depends on the type of cell involved and on the nature of the infecting virus. Labile cells, like those of surface epithelia, undergo continuous division throughout life, and so it is not surprising that some virus conditions of the skin have a proliferative tendency, e.g. verruca vulgaris.

---

FIG. 16.4. Normal HeLa cells. Note the confluent sheet of plump polygonal cells with a conspicuous giant form. They are derived from a malignant epithelial cell line. (McCarthy phase contrast × 200.)

FIG. 16.5. HeLa cells infected with adenovirus. The sheet has been broken up, and the swollen, refractile cells form irregular masses. (McCarthy phase contrast × 200.)

FIG. 16.6. HeLa cells infected with poliovirus. Note the severe disintegration of cells. Poliovirus has a more dest͏͏ ͏   ͏    ͏    ͏ cultures than does ovirus. (McCarthy phas͏

Other cells described as permanent, e.g. neurones, cannot divide after birth, and virus infection of these is necessarily always destructive in tendency.

The skin is usually taken as a tissue in which the gamut of changes from immediate necrosis to indefinite proliferation is possible, as the following five infections demonstrate:[17]

*Foot-and-mouth disease* causes a rapid swelling and necrosis of epidermal cells.

*Vaccinia* causes an early proliferation of the cells with necrosis following about 3 days later.

*Fowl-pox* causes a much more prolonged proliferation with necrosis supervening some weeks later.

*Verruca vulgaris* produces a massive proliferation which may last many months before involution occurs.

The *Shope papilloma of rabbits* is manifested by a neoplastic proliferation of cells, and malignancy may occur.

This is an instructive list, but many of the diseases mentioned are not relevant to man. Only in a few skin conditions, e.g. verruca vulgaris, is proliferation of cells a marked feature. There is no known example of human neoplasia directly attributable to viruses, a very important difference between human and animal virus disease. Nevertheless, some human tumours may be associated with viruses (see p. 277).

In most human virus diseases cellular destruction is the predominant lesion. The respiratory viruses destroy the surface epithelium, a tendency well marked in influenza, the viruses of serum hepatitis and yellow fever produce a characteristic necrosis of the liver, mumps produces destructive lesions of the acinar cells of the salivary glands and sometimes the pancreas, while the central nervous system may sustain permanent neuronal loss as a result of poliomyelitis and virus encephalitis.

Once the infection is overcome, there is rapid healing due to proliferation of neighbouring cells. The focal necrosis of infective hepatitis heals so rapidly that needle biopsy of the liver performed after a few months may reveal no abnormality whatsoever. Neuronal destruction can be healed only by repair, i.e. gliosis, and hence permanent damage must sometimes be expected. It should be noted, however, that not every neurone infected with poliovirus is necessarily doomed. Many recover completely.

**Inflammatory Reaction.** Secondary to the cellular damage there is a non-descript acute inflammatory reaction in the vicinity. This takes the form of vascular dilatation and an exudate containing lymphocytes and macrophages. Polymorphs are usually few in number. Most virus diseases are acute and of short duration, terminating in either rapid death or recovery. Exceptions to this are the tumour-producing viruses and perhaps certain neurotropic viruses.

Virus infections of epithelial surfaces are often complicated by secondary bacterial invasion: influenza is commonly followed by bacterial pneumonia.

## The General Body Reaction to Virus Infection

**Localization.**[18] Like other organisms, viruses first contaminate a surface integument, either by inhalation (e.g. influenza), ing poliomyelitis), or by the bite of an arthropod vector (e.g. yellow fever). Some viruses remain localized to their tissues of entry, e.g. verruca vulgaris virus and the rhinoviruses, while others become disseminated throughout the blood stream, and produce lesions in an organ remote from the sites of primary infection, e.g. poliomyelitis and yellow fever, or else lead to a generalized virus infection involving many organs, e.g. smallpox and measles. The systemic type of infection is associated with much more pronounced constitutional symptoms than the localized one, and a characteristic feature is the presence of high fever during the early viraemic phase. This is often followed by a remission, which is in turn succeeded by another spurt of pyrexia when the virus becomes clinically localized at its organ of destination. Localized diseases like the common cold and verruca vulgaris are accompanied by little, if any, constitutional upset.

**Dissemination.** The mode of dissemination of a virus in the body has been investigated with respect to mouse-pox.[19] The virus enters the mouse's body through an abrasion in its skin, and multiplies there. Within 8 hours the virus reaches the local lymph nodes, and after further multiplication it invades the blood stream and is taken up by the RE cells of the liver and spleen. There it multiplies once more, and after 6 days it invades the blood stream in large amounts, and settles selectively in the epidermal cells of the skin. This phase of viraemia is accompanied by severe constitutional effects; still another 4 days elapse before a rash appears.

The initial 6 days of infection constitute the *incubation period*; the 4 days of severe illness, which may prove fatal in overwhelming infections, are the *prodromal period*. During this time virus material may still be cultured from the blood, but once the rash appears (10th day) there is a rapidly rising level of neutralizing antibody in the circulation. Human diseases like smallpox and measles have a somewhat similar pattern of dissemination, but the route of entry is through the respiratory tract.

*Transplacental infection*[18,20] of the fetus is important in rubella infections and may lead to congenital abnormalities (p. 285). Other virus diseases transmitted across the placenta are herpes-simplex infection and Coxsackievirus myocarditis.

**Antibody Response.** Virus infections are accompanied by a high titre of circulating antibodies during the period of convalescence. The highest antibody response is encountered in those viruses which are widely disseminated in the circulation, and a life-long *immunity* may be expected after diseases like smallpox, measles, and mumps. Localized infections, like the common cold, also induce antibodies, but the degree of immunity is small, and recurrence is common. It must also be remembered that many viruses are of more than one type, e.g. there are 3 types of poliovirus and 31 types of human adenovirus. This is an additional reason for recurrent attacks of certain infections.

The element of *hypersensitivity* is also noteworthy in virus infections. The accelerated reaction following a second vaccination is a good example of allergy to vaccinia virus. The lesion appears within a day or two and resolves after about one week, whereas a primary vaccination reaction appears on the fourth or fifth day and reaches its zenith on about the tenth day.

It takes about 3 weeks to heal and is occasionally complicated by systemic lesions. The close resemblance of this to the Koch phenomenon is obvious, except that here the element of immunity is much greater than in tuberculosis.

There is a strong allergic element in the skin eruption that occurs in the course of generalized infections like smallpox and measles. In such conditions there is an incubation period of about two weeks, and the skin is sensitized to viral products before the virus reaches it in full force. The analogy to the later intestinal ulceration of typhoid fever is very close.

## Mechanism of the Pathogenic Effects of Viruses[21]

Viruses produce their harmful effects by virtue of the cell destruction they cause; no factors comparable with bacterial toxins have been demonstrated. It is believed that the cytotoxic effect of viruses is due to complex biochemical disturbances that accompany virus replication. In addition, there is also a delayed type of hypersensitivity.

The cause of death in virus disease is obvious when a vital organ is damaged directly, e.g. the liver in hepatitis. In the pox diseases the mode of death is less easily explained. Clinically there is a state of "shock" reminiscent of the toxaemia of invasive bacterial infections, and it is suggested that this is due to virus invasion and damage of vascular endothelial cells.

## Immunity to Virus Infections[22]

The mechanism of immunity to virus infection is complex and has several components.

(a) **Immunoglobulin Antibodies.** Plasma antibodies play an important part, especially in the disseminated infections. Most viruses possess several antigens, some associated with the protein envelope and others with the nucleoprotein. It is the antibodies that react with the protein coat that are important in immunity; they prevent the virus attaching itself to the cell receptor. The virus is invulnerable to antibody when it is intracellular.[23] These plasma, virus-neutralizing immunoglobulins belong to the IgG class.

It is also to be noted that after recovery from an attack of poliomyelitis or following immunization with living attenuated virus administered orally, a subsequent dose of poliovirus does not flourish in the cells of the small bowel. This is due to the action of IgA antibodies produced locally in the intestine and present in the secretions. People who have been immunized with a killed suspension of poliovirus administered parenterally usually exhibit unhindered virus multiplication in the small bowel despite a considerable antibody response.

(b) **Cellular Immunity.** There is also a cell-mediated, lymphocytic immunity. independent of circulating antibodies. Children with congenital immunoglobulin deficiency can resist virus infections, [22,24,25] but when there is a lymphocytic defect, death is often due to widespread virus disease[22]. The lymphokines liberated by sensitized lymphocytes (see p. 140) include interferon. Lymphocytic immunity is particularly important in herpesvirus and poxvirus infections.

(c) **Interference.** It has been recognized for a long time that the presence of

one virus often protects a cell from infection by a second virus. This phenomenon of *virus interference* was described in 1937 in monkeys infected with
Rift Valley fever virus who were then found to be protected against a lethal
dose of yellow fever virus.[26] The phenomenon has been intensively investigated, and in 1957 the substance responsible was isolated. It is a protein
called *interferon*, [27,28,29] which is not antigenic or toxic; it is produced by the
infected cell, and in some way alters the cellular metabolism so that further
virus production is prevented. It acts against a wide range of viruses infecting
living cells, but is inactive *in vitro*. There can be little doubt that it is an
important mechanism in checking the course of many virus infections.[30]
Whether it is also important in the acquired cellular immunity of virus
disease is not known. Its use as a therapeutic agent is still being assessed.
The administration of cortisone inhibits the production and action of
interferon[31]; pyrexia, on the other hand, stimulates it.[40] As noted above, it is
also liberated by sensitized lymphocytes in contact with virus-infected cells.

### The Diagnosis of Virus Disease[12]

In a few instances diagnostic *inclusion bodies* may be found (e.g. Negri
bodies in rabies), or characteristic *elementary bodies* may be seen by light
microscopy (e.g. Paschen bodies in the vesicles of vaccinia).

An important diagnostic procedure is the isolation of the virus from the
patient's secretions using the living cell systems already described. The
virus may then be typed by means of complement fixation and neutralization
tests using specific rabbit antisera. Some viruses with a characteristic shape
can be identified by electron microscopy, a method of diagnosis likely to be
used more extensively in the future.

In convalescent patients there is invariably a great rise in titre of antibodies
against the agent, and these too may be demonstrated by complement
fixation and neutralization tests against the specific viruses.

In practice retrospective diagnosis made on serological grounds is the most
important method of diagnosing virus disease.

## Some Common Virus Infections

### Enteroviruses[32]

The enteroviruses are a group of small, spherical, RNA-containing viruses
found particularly in the cells of the intestine. There are three subgroups:

**The Coxsackie viruses,** of which there are 30 types. They were first isolated
in the town of Coxsackie in New York State in 1948, and are found quite
frequently in the faeces of healthy children. They are responsible for a variety
of clinical pictures including an upper respiratory, cold-like condition, and
an illness which resembles paralytic poliomyelitis. They also cause *herpangina*,
a febrile disease of children in which there are shallow greyish ulcers in the
mouth and fauces, and *Bornholm disease*, in which there is agonizing chest
pain.

**The ECHO (Enteric, Cytopathic, Human, Orphan) viruses,** of which
there are 24 types. They are found quite commonly in children's faeces, and
for a long time could not be associated with any disease—hence the name

"orphan". It is now known that they produce a variety of febrile illnesses including some which mimic poliomyelitis and the common cold.

**The Polioviruses.** Poliomyelitis is caused by the three types of poliovirus, of which type 1 produces the most severe disease. The disease is contracted by the ingestion of material which has been contaminated by virus-containing faeces. Faecal pollution of drinking water or swimming baths is a possible danger, as is also fly-borne contamination of food. Indirect contact with excretors, whose dirty hands contaminate fomites, is another source of infection.

*Spread of virus in the body.* It is believed that the virus proliferates first in the cells of the pharynx and the lower part of the small bowel. If it is not arrested at this stage, it enters the general circulation *via* the lymphatics, and it then multiples in various extraneural sites like the spleen and kidneys. This marks the end of the incubation period, which usually lasts 7–14 days, but may extend up to 30 days. The next viraemic phase is ushered in by a febrile reaction, but even then the infection may be overcome. If the condition proceeds, the virus settles finally in the central nervous system which it reaches by the blood stream. It localizes itself specifically in the anterior horn cells and their medullary counterparts, and paralysis ensues.

A second mode of spread is directly up the peripheral nerve endings of the bowel and especially the pharynx. Opinions vary about the importance of this method of spread; it probably accounts for the bulbar type of disease that sometimes follows tonsillectomy and other operative procedures in the mouth.

It is evident that much has still to be learned about the pathogenesis of the disease. One thing is clear; many people are infected with poliovirus, and either show no illness at all or else have a mild febrile reaction. Only a small unlucky minority develop paralysis. Poliomyelitis is an excellent example of an infection that tends to be subclinical.

*Factors aggravating the disease.* The incubation period is shortened, and the liability to nervous-system involvement increased by the following factors: heavy exercise and fatigue, pregnancy, operative procedures, and active immunization with any antigen. When the disease follows immunization, it is called *provocation poliomyelitis*; it is believed that alum and other adjuvants in the vaccines and toxoids are the important factors. The mode of action is unknown, but it has been suggested that the focus of inflammation acts as a nidus for proliferation of the virus during the period of viraemia. It might then travel up the local nerve to the spinal cord. Active immunization procedures should be postponed during a poliomyelitis epidemic. So also should minor surgery, e.g. dental extraction.

*Immunization.* A consideration of poliomyelitis immunization is valuable as a general exercise in comparing the relative merits of dead suspensions to those of live attenuated viruses.

*Active immunization.*[33,34] The first effective vaccine was devised by Salk, who used polioviruses grown in monkey kidney cells and subsequently inactivated by formolization. At first some cases of severe poliomyelitis occurred following the use of inadequately inactivated virus suspensions, but since then the process has been so perfected that safety is assured and a potent vaccine produced. It is issued in trivalent form, containing types 1, 2, and 3, and requires at least three intramuscular inoculations, the second a month after the first, and the third about six months after the second. A high titre of circulating antibody should be produced, though often there is a disappointing response to type-1 virus, the most dangerous of the three. Immunity depends on the presence of circulating antibody. The resistance of the cells of the small bowel to subsequent infection by poliovirus is not altered.

Later Sabin produced a vaccine consisting of living attenuated strains of poliovirus which had undergone mutation after passage through mice. These attenuated viruses are given orally, and they closely simulate the natural disease except that spread does not occur to the nervous system. The immunity they produce depends not only on circulating antibody, but also on a changed resistance of the cells of the small bowel, as has already been discussed. If a triple vaccine is given, a possible snag is that one virus might infect the cells first and interfere with the entry of the other two. In practice it is found that any interfering tendency is obviated by giving three doses of trivalent vaccine at monthly intervals. It must be stressed that the Sabin type vaccine leads to an infection of the intestine and a subsequent passage of virus in the faeces. It is almost inevitable therefore that the individual will infect other people, who in turn will become immunized. The possibility that the virus might mutate back to a virulent form has caused some concern, but there appears to be little danger of this.

## The Poxviruses[35]

The poxviruses are a group of large DNA-containing viruses which produce vesicular and pustular skin lesions. Many animals have their own variety of pox disease, e.g. cow-pox, mouse-pox, etc. The human disease is smallpox.

**Smallpox.** The disease is acquired by the inhalation of infected particles from a patient directly or from fomites indirectly. The bedding is particularly dangerous, and numerous instances are on record where laundry workers have contracted the disease from contaminated bedclothes.

*Spread in the body.* It is believed that the primary lesions occur in the nasal mucosa and that this is followed by systemic spread to the RE system. After an incubation period of 10–14 days there occurs a phase of secondary viraemia during which the patient becomes ill. Some four days later the virus settles in the mucous membrane and skin giving rise to the characteristic rashes, the *enanthem* and the *exanthem*.

*Active immunization.* The first really effective attempt at smallpox immunization was performed by Edward Jenner, who discovered that the natural pox infection of bovine animals, *cow-pox*, could produce a similar lesion in human beings, and protect them against smallpox infection.

Since then a third virus has emerged, *vaccinia virus*.[36] Its origin is obscure, and although it may have arisen as a mutant of either cow-pox virus or smallpox virus, it now appears to be quite distinct from both.

In man vaccinia virus applied to the skin with firm pressure by a needle (*vaccination*) produces a localized infection, and the subsequent immune response gives good, though temporary, protection against smallpox infection.

Unfortunately vaccination is occasionally complicated by spread of the virus. either locally (*progressive vaccinia*), or to the rest of the skin (*generalized vaccinia*). A form of encephalitis with a 50 per cent mortality rate is another rare complication. For these reasons the routine vaccination of infants is no longer advocated.

### Viruses Affecting the Respiratory Tract[37]

The number of viruses incriminated in respiratory infections is legion.

**Myxoviruses.**[38] The myxoviruses are a group of medium-sized RNA-containing viruses. They are so named because they have a strong affinity for mucins. Thus, *in vitro* they can attach themselves to the mucroprotein receptors of red cells, and by forming bridges, cause the cells to agglutinate. The important human myxoviruses are the *influenza viruses* of which there are three types. The *parainfluenza viruses* and the virus of *mumps* belong to a closely related group, the *paramyxoviruses*, which are slightly larger than the myxoviruses.

**Adenoviruses.**[39] The adenoviruses are small DNA-containing viruses which have a proclivity for the mucosa of the upper respiratory tract and the conjunctiva.

**The Common Cold.** The viruses that cause the common cold are called rhinoviruses and are related to the enteroviruses. The composite name *picornaviruses* (pico = small, + RNA) is used to embrace both these groups

### The Arthropod-borne Viruses (Arboviruses)[40]

Arboviruses cause yellow fever, dengue, sandfly fever, and a number of types of encephalitis of regional geographical distribution.

### The Herpesviruses[41]

**Varicella and Zoster.** Though the well-known clinical features of varicella (chickenpox) and zoster are poles apart, there is good evidence that they are both caused by the same virus.

*Chickenpox* has a pathogenesis similar to that of smallpox, and exhibits an enanthem involving the oral mucosa and an exanthem consisting of vesicles on the skin, which subsequently become pustular.

*Zoster.* Following an attack of chickenpox it seems that the virus may lie latent in the tissues, and in later life be reactivated by some physical or mental shock. It produces lesions specifically in the posterior root ganglia of the spinal, trigeminal, or facial nerves, and from there infection spreads down the nerve fibres to the skin. Pain followed by the development of a vesicular rash restricted to an area supplied by the nerve are characteristic. Children exposed to a patient with zoster often develop chickenpox.

**Herpes Simplex.** The virus of herpes simplex is one of the most widely distributed viruses in human beings. It is estimated that about 60 per cent of the population are affected. Of these only 10 per cent exhibit primary childhood lesions, such as *gingivostomatitis*, *keratoconjunctivitis*, and *vulvovaginitis*. Rarely the infection is more widespread.

Abrasions of the skin predispose to primary herpetic infection (*traumatic*, or *inoculation*, *herpes simplex*). A good example of this is the painful *herpetic whitlow*, which is seen in nursing attendants working in neurosurgical wards. These people acquire their infection while inserting endotracheal tubes into the mouths of unconscious patients.

Usually, however, the primary infection remains subclinical, and the virus remains latent in the cells of the host. This symbiosis tends to be disturbed by intercurrent infections, e.g. the common cold, pneumonia, and malaria, and even, in very susceptible victims, by menstruation, emotional strain, and exposure to sunlight. There then develop typical *herpetic blisters*, especially around the mucocutaneous junction of the lips. The skin of the genitalia is sometimes affected, and also occasionally are the conjunctiva and cornea. It should be noted that the common aphthous ulcers are not due to this virus.

**Epstein-Barr (EB) Virus.** This herpesvirus causes classical *infectious mononucleosis* (glandular fever) with a positive Paul-Bunnell test. It is also associated with Burkitt's tumour and nasopharyngeal carcinoma (see p. 277).

## Slow Viruses[42,43]

*Scrapie* is a lethal neurological disease of sheep which appears to be caused by an agent which is very resistant to heat and chemical disinfectants. The incubation period is several *years*. The nature of the agent is not clear, but there is interesting speculation as to whether any human counterpart exists to account for certain chronic diseases of the central nervous system.

**Virus hepatitis** is considered on p. 427.

## Conclusion

The range of diseases caused by viruses is very large, and in many of them there are oral lesions; although these are often of little significance, some are useful in diagnosis. The enanthem often appears before the typical exanthem —Koplik's spots in measles are a good example of this. These resemble white grains of salt on a red background, and may be present on the buccal mucosa a day or two before the typical skin rash appears.

The increasing complexity of virus structure and reproduction which recent research has revealed is necessitating a reappraisal of the aetiology of many diseases.[47] The phenomena of virus latency and the eclipse phase indicate that a failure to isolate a virus does not necessarily signify its absence. Similarly slow viruses, mycoplasmas, and the delicate and elusive L-forms of bacteria have not yet been sufficiently investigated for their role in disease to be assessed.

### General Reading

SWAIN, R. H. A. (1965). In "Medical Microbiology", 11th Ed., pp. 54–87 and 367–502, ed. by Cruickshank, R. Edinburgh: Livingstone.

### References

1. WILSON, G. S. and MILES A. A. (1964). In Topley and Wilson's "Principles of Bacteriology and Immunity", 5th ed., p. 1134. London: Arnold.
2. WILSON, G. S. and MILES, A. A. (1964). p. 1148, *loc. cit.*
3. Various Authors (1966). *Proc. roy. Soc. Med.*, **59**, 1109.
4. CHANOCK, R. M., HAYFLICK, L. and BARILE, M. F. (1962). *Proc. nat. Acad. Sci. (Wash.)*, **48**, 41.

 5. WILSON, G. S. and MILES, A. A. (1964). p. 1161, *loc. cit.*
 6. ISRAEL, M. S. (1966). *Brit. med. J.*, **2**, 687.
 7. CRICK, F. H. C. and WATSON, J. D. (1956). *Nature (Lond.)*, **177**, 473.
 8. HORNE, R. W. *et al.* (1959). *J. molec. Biol.*, **1**, 84.
 9. HORNE, R. W. and NAGINGTON, J. (1959). *J. molec. Biol.*, **1**, 333.
10. COHEN, A. (1963). In "Mechanisms of Virus Infection", p. 153, ed. by Wilson Smith. London and New York: Academic Press.
11. ISAACS, A. (1963). p. 191, *Ibid.*
12. DUDGEON, J. A. (1961). *Brit. med. J.*, **1**, 1269.
13. ENDERS, J. F., WELLER, T. H. and ROBBINS, F. C. (1949). *Science*, **109**, 85.
14. GEY, G. O., COFFMAN, W. D. and KUBICEK, M. T. (1952). *Cancer Res.*, **12**, 264.
15. STOKER, M. G. P. (1957). *Brit. med. J.*, **1**, 963.
16. ISRAEL, M. S. (1962). *J. Path. Bact.*, **84**, 169.
17. WRIGHT, G. P. (1958). In "An Introduction to Pathology", 3rd ed., p. 184. London: Longmans.
18. DOWNIE, A. W. (1963). In "Mechanisms of Virus Infection", p. 101, *loc. cit.*
19. FENNER, F. (1948). *Lancet*, **2**, 915.
20. DUDGEON, J. A. (1966). *Proc. roy. Soc. Med.*, **59**, 1084.
21. WESTWOOD, J. C. N. (1963). In "Mechanisms of Virus Infection", p. 255, *loc. cit.*
22. GORDON SMITH, C. E. (1969). *Proc. roy. Soc. Med.*, **62**, 292.
23. ANDREWES, C. H. (1929). *Brit. J. exp. Path.*, **10**, 273.
24. JANEWAY, C. A. and GITLIN, D. (1957). *Advanc. Pediat.*, **9**, 65.
25. GOOD, R. A., BRIDGES, R. A. and CONDIE, R. M. (1960). *Bact. Rev.*, **24**, 115.
26. FINDLAY, G. M. and MACCALLUM, F. O. (1937). *J. Path. Bact.*, **44**, 405.
27. ISAACS, A. and LINDENMANN, J. (1957). *Proc. roy. Soc.*, B, **147**, 258.
28. Leading Article (1961). *Brit. med. J.*, **1**, 1745.
29. "Interferon", A Ciba Foundation Symposium (1968). Edited by Wolstenholme, G. E. W. and O'Connor, M., 271 pp. London: Churchill.
30. ISAACS, A. (1962). *Brit. med. J.*, **2**, 353.
31. KILBOURNE, E. D., SMART, K. M. and POKORNY, B. A. (1961). *Nature (Lond.)*, **190**, 650.
32. STUART-HARRIS, C. H. (1962). *Brit. med. J.*, **1**, 1779.
33. STUART-HARRIS, C. H. (1964). *Proc. roy. Soc. Med.*, **57**, 459.
34. DANE, D. S. (1964). *Ibid.*, 462.
35. WILSON, G. S. and MILES, A. A. (1964). p. 2268, *loc. cit.*
36. FENNER, F. and BURNET, F. M. (1957). *Virology*, **4**, 305.
37. STUART-HARRIS, C. H. (1962). *Brit. med. J.*, **2**, 869.
38. *Ibid.* (1959). *Brit. med. Bull.*, **15**, 216.
39. PEREIRA, H. G. (1959). *Brit. med. Bull.*, **15**, 225.
40. GORDON-SMITH, C. E. (1959). *Brit. med. Bull.*, **15**, 235.
41. DOWNIE, A. W. (1959). *Brit. med. Bull.*, **15**, 197.
42. GIBBONS, R. A. and HUNTER, G. D. (1967). *Nature (Lond.)*, **215**, 1041.
43. Leading Article (1967). *Lancet*, **2**, 705.
44. HIRSCHMAN, S. Z. (1971). *Amer. J. Med.*, **51**, 699.
45. JUEL-JENSEN, B. E. (1970). *Brit. med. J.*, **2**, 154.
46. MCCORMACK, W. M. *et al.* (1973). *New Engl. J. Med.*, **288**, 78.
47. Leading Article (1973). *Brit. med. J.*, **1**, 129.

*Chapter 17*

# DISORDERS OF GROWTH

Most organs of the body possess a considerable reserve of tissue, which can be brought into play whenever additional work is demanded of them. At rest the inactive cells are maintained by an intermittent blood flow through their supplying capillaries. This mechanism results in an economical use of the circulation and explains why noxious substances spread by the blood stream may nevertheless produce patchy effects. When more work has to be performed, the shut-down vessels dilate and the organ shows active hyper-aemia. This is well illustrated by the tremendous increase in blood flow through the salivary glands which occurs during periods of active secretion.

## Growth Potentiality of Cells

In addition to this reserve mechanism, organs or tissues subjected to pro-longed excessive strain respond by increasing their bulk. This may be done by either increasing the size of each constituent cell, or increasing the total cell number; which of these occurs depends upon the growth potentiality of the cells involved. Three classes of cells are described.

*Labile cells.* These undergo division throughout life to replace those lost through differentiation and subsequent desquamation.

The cells of lymph nodes, bone marrow, and most of the covering or pro-tective epithelia (skin, endometrium, alimentary, respiratory, and urinary mucosa) come into this category.

*Stable cells.* These cells rarely divide in adult life, but never lose their ability to proliferate if suitably stimulated. This group includes most of the secretory epithelial structures (liver, kidney, pancreas, and endocrine glands).

*Permanent cells.* These cells, typified by neurones, are incapable of multi-plication. For practical purposes muscle cells fall into this group.

Although this classification is extremely useful, it is only relative. In fact most "stable" cells, e.g. of the liver, pituitary, etc., do have specific cycles of growth, degeneration, death, and replacement, but these are gradual and inconspicuous. The term *necrobiosis* is sometimes applied to this quiet death of cells which is a part of the normal tissue turnover.

The factors which control the growth and differentiation of cells are largely unknown. Nevertheless, abnormalities in these two functions are frequent, and form an important aspect of many disease processes. They may be considered under three headings:

1. *Quantitative abnormalities of cellular growth.*
2. *Abnormalities of cellular differentiation.*
3. *Neoplasia,* a topic so important that it is considered separately in the succeeding chapters.

## QUANTITATIVE ABNORMALITIES OF CELLULAR GROWTH

**Excessive Growth**

Tissues composed of labile or stable cells respond to an increased demand
for work primarily by multiplication. Permanent cells either show no morphological change (neurones), or else only an increase in size (muscle). Even
stable and labile cells usually show some increase in size. An increase in the
cell number is called *hyperplasia*, and an increase in individual cell size is
*hypertrophy*. Both are usually related to a tangible stimulus, which is often
a basically physiological one acting to excess. The most important stimulus
is an *increased demand for function*. As will be seen, this may take the form
of increased muscular work in response to an abnormal load, an increased
production of the blood cells in response to hypoxia or infection, a thickening of protective epithelium in response to external trauma, or an increased
secretion of a gland in response to some external need.

## HYPERPLASIA

**Definition.** Hyperplasia is the increase in size of an organ or tissue due to
an increase in the number of its specialized constituent cells. Enlargements
due to congestion, oedema, inflammation, amyloid infiltration, or tumour
formation are excluded from the definition. The suffix —megaly is used to
denote a large organ or tissue regardless of its cause, e.g. cardiomegaly is
enlargement of the heart, splenomegaly is enlargement of the spleen, etc.

It is important to realize that those hyperplasias due to a specific stimulus
exist only for so long as that stimulus is applied. When it is removed, the
hyperplasia ceases and the tissue may return to normal.

Although the concept of hyperplasia is traditionally a morphological one,
it must never be forgotten that the increase in size of the organ is accompanied
by a corresponding increase in function. Nowhere is this more apparent than
in hyperplasia of the endocrine glands.

### Hyperplasia in the Endocrine Glands[1]

In endocrine hyperplasias there is enlargement of the gland (or glands, as
the case may be). Sometimes this enlargement is diffuse, but in many instances
it is circumscribed and discrete. The nodules so formed are often labelled
adenomata. In secreting epithelia generally the line of demarcation between
hyperplasia and benign neoplasia is so tenuous that a distinction is often
purely arbitrary.

*Parathyroids.* The parathyroid glands show hyperplasia in response to a
persistent hypocalcaemia (see secondary hyperparathyroidism, p. 446). In
primary hyperparathyroidism the stimulus for the hyperplasia is unknown.

*Thyroid.* Thyroid hyperplasia is sometimes the result of prolonged stimulation by pituitary thyrotrophic hormone (Figs. 17.1 and 17.2). As a primary
idiopathic condition it occurs in Graves's disease (p. 473).

Hyperplasia of the endocrine glands is described in greater detail in
Chapter 35.

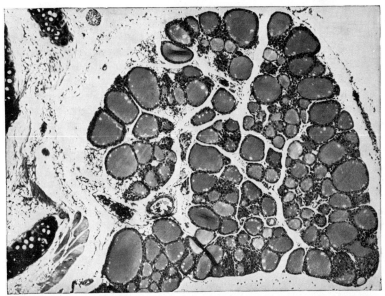

FIG. 17.1. Normal mouse thyroid. The acini are evenly disposed, and are lined by a cuboidal epithelium. They contain dense colloid. The pattern is similar to human thyroid. × 90.

(*From Israel, M. S. and Ellis, I. R.* (1960). Brit. J. Cancer, **14,** 206.)

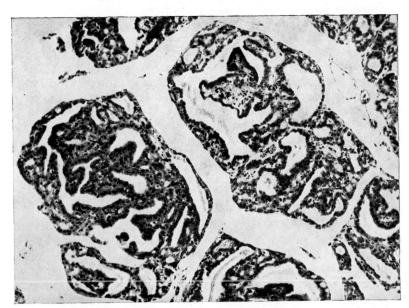

FIG. 17.2. Effect on mouse thyroid of thiouracil. There is nodular hyperplasia, and the component acini are irregular and elongated. They are distorted by papillary invaginations of exuberant columnar epithelium, and the acini are empty. × 120.

(From the same reference as Fig. 17.1.)

### Hyperplasia in the Target Organs of the Endocrine Glands

*Breasts*. Hyperplasia of the epithelial tissue and surrounding specialized connective tissue is a normal feature of the female breast at puberty, during pregnancy and lactation, and to a lesser extent towards the end of each menstrual cycle.

In *mammary dysplasia*, also called cystic hyperplasia of the breast and "chronic mastitis", there is considerable epithelial hyperplasia, and cysts often develop. It is quite a common condition, and causes discomfort as well as nodularity of the breast substance. Hormonal imbalance is presumed to be the cause, but its nature is obscure.

*Prostate*. Senile enlargement of the prostate is due to epithelial hyperplasia as well as an increase in the fibromuscular element. The condition is common over the age of 60 years, and is erroneously called "benign prostatic hypertrophy" or "adenomatosis of the prostate". It is an important cause of urinary obstruction, and surgical treatment is often necessary to relieve back-pressure effects on the bladder and kidneys. The cause is unknown, but is probably hormonal in nature.

### Hyperplasia of Skin.

Hyperplasia of the epidermis is a feature of many skin diseases. It may be caused by a wide range of physical "irritants" acting for a long time, e.g. trauma, heat, etc. The corn on the toe caused by the friction of an ill-fitting shoe is a good example of hyperplasia of a covering epithelium in response to damaging trauma. Hyperplasia may also be induced by virus infection, e.g. the common wart (verruca vulgaris).

### Hyperplasia of Bone Marrow.

Pronounced hyperplasia is seen in the haematopoietic tissue when there is a stimulus for blood cell production. The erythroid series is affected in hypoxia and in many types of anaemia, e.g. pernicious anaemia. In infection it is the white-cell precursors which are affected. The cellular marrow extends into the long bones of the adult (normally filled with fatty marrow), while in childhood extramedullary foci of haematopoiesis may occur in the liver, spleen, and other organs.

### RE System and Lymphoid Tissue.

Both undergo hyperplasia in chronic infection. This accounts for the enlargement of the spleen (*splenomegaly*) and lymph nodes (*lymphadenopathy*).

### Hyperplasia in Relationship to Chronic Inflammation

As noted previously hyperplasia is sometimes a feature of long-standing chronic inflammation (p. 125).

*In the skin* the hyperplasia may affect the epithelium or the connective tissue. Epithelial hyperplasia may be seen at the edge of chronic ulcers. Another example is *keratoacanthoma* (molluscum sebaceum), in which there is an exuberant down-growth of hyperplastic epithelium which extends as far as the level of the sebaceous glands.[2,3] The surrounding dermis shows an inflammatory reaction. It may be almost impossible to differentiate this condition from an early invasive squamous-cell carcinoma; the natural history, however, is quite different, for the keratoacanthoma grows rapidly and then involutes spontaneously after a few months, finally healing with scarring. The nature of this lesion is quite obscure, and it has in the past often been misdiagnosed as cancer.

The *granuloma pyogenicum* is another curious skin lesion in which there is such a profuse proliferation of blood vessels and fibroblasts that the elevated nodule which is produced closely resembles a haemangioma. In spite of its name, the lesion does not appear to be inflammatory, nor is it granulomatous.

*In the oral mucosa* chronic inflammation may likewise cause epithelial or connective tissue hyperplasia. Multiple warty epithelial overgrowths may occur, apparently as a result of the irritation from an ill-fitting denture (*papillomatosis*).[4,5] Chronic inflammation may produce hyperplasia of the connective tissue so that fibrous nodules are formed. These are sometimes called "fibromata", or if pedunculated, *fibro-epithelial polyps.* An *epulis* is a nodule on the gingiva, and most examples are due to connective-tissue hyperplasia induced by inflammation. Sometimes the fibrovascular proliferation and giant-cell formation is so marked that the lesion resembles a giant-cell tumour of bone. It is called the *peripheral giant-cell reparative granuloma* (*giant-cell epulis*).[6]

## Pseudoneoplastic Hyperplasia

Reference has been made to the difficulties in distinguishing nodular hyperplasia from benign neoplasia, particularly in the endocrine glands, the prostate, and the breast. From a practical point of view the distinction is unimportant since both processes are benign. There are, however, many examples of hyperplasia in which the mass of cells produced closely resembles a malignant tumour. Experience has taught that they are benign, since they either resolve spontaneously or respond to simple treatment. Their importance lies in their recognition, for a mistaken diagnosis can result in grave therapeutic errors. Almost any tissue can show such lesions, and only a few examples will be described.

## Pseudomalignant Connective Tissue Hyperplasia

*Pseudolymphoma.* Pseudolymphoma of the skin[7] appears as nodules of lymphoid tissue which histologically closely resemble the nodular type of lymphocytic lymphoma (p. 262). Unlike the latter, however, the cutaneous lesion never becomes systematized nor develops into an overtly malignant process. Similar pseudolymphomata are described at other sites, e.g. orbit,[8] rectum, and mediastinum.[9]

*Pseudosarcomatous nodular fasciitis*[10] affects the subcutaneous tissues, commonly of the arm. There is rapid growth of a highly vascular mass which diffusely infiltrates the surrounding tissues. Many mitoses are present in its spindle-cell component, but in spite of the malignant microscopic appearance the lesion is benign in its behaviour.

**Pseudomalignant epithelial hyperplasia** of the epidermis which gives an appearance of dermal invasion by squamous cells is seen from time to time in a great variety of chronic skin lesions ranging from fungal granulomata and insect bites to basal-cell carcinoma. The lesion is commonly called *pseudoepitheliomatous hyperplasia* and at times differentiation from squamous-cell carcinoma is not possible, especially when small biopsy specimens alone are available for study.

Pseudoepitheliomatous hyperplasia is well shown in the keratoacanthoma described on page 232. It is also seen over a *myoblastoma*, a somewhat controversial lesion found most often on the tongue and occasionally in the skin. It is composed of very large polygonal and strap-shaped cells, the cytoplasm of which contains coarse eosinophilic granules. The tumour is now thought to be derived from Schwann cells rather than muscle, and the cause of the overlying epithelial hyperplasia is unknown.

## HYPERTROPHY

**Definition.** Hypertrophy is the increase in size of an organ or tissue due to increase in size of its constituent specialized cells. Pure hypertrophy without accompanying hyperplasia occurs only in muscle, and the stimulus is almost always a mechanical one.

### Hypertrophy of Smooth Muscle

Any obstruction to the outflow of the contents of a hollow muscular viscus results in hypertrophy of its muscle coat. It is seen in the *bladder* when there is prostatic hyperplasia, and in any part of the *gut* above an obstruction, e.g. a stricture or a carcinoma. The *myometrium* of the uterus shows tremendous hypertrophy during pregnancy, and the stimulus, although partly mechanical, is also a hormonal action of oestrogen.

### Hypertrophy of Cardiac Muscle

Although the heart of the newborn child weighs only 30 g., it is believed that no further muscle cells are produced. The fibres increase in size tenfold by the time adult life is reached. Any demand for an increased work-load leads to hypertrophy of the fibres of the chamber affected. The stimulus is probably the stretching which results from the additional strain, and the ability of the heart to respond in this way constitutes a part of the cardiac reserve (p. 388). Hypertrophy is best seen in the left ventricle (Fig. 17.3). Systemic hypertension, aortic valvular disease, and mitral regurgitation are the common causes.

### Hypertrophy of Skeletal Muscle

The village blacksmith's brawny arms provide a simple illustration of hypertrophy due to mechanical stimulus.

### Diminished Growth

**Nomenclature.** *Agenesis* is a failure of development of an organ or tissue (p. 286). *Hypoplasia* is a state of imperfect development resulting in a small under-developed organ. *Aplasia* has been used in the context of extreme hypoplasia (short of agenesis), but in practice it is better to restrict the use of this term to the condition seen in the bone marrow (see aplastic anaemia, p. 352). *Atrophy* is the acquired diminution in size of an organ due to a decrease in size or number of its constituent elements. Only in muscle is a decrease in size the major factor. In all other instances the number of cells is also reduced. This is brought about by the periodic destruction (necrosis) of some of the

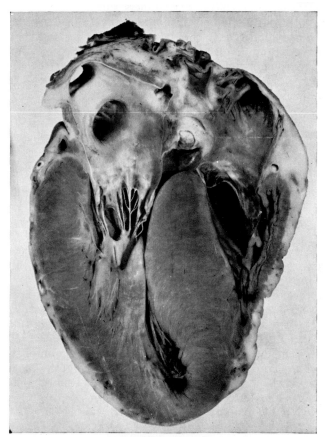

FIG. 17.3. Hypertrophy of the heart. The muscle of the left ventricle is greatly thickened. The cause of this hypertrophy is systemic hypertension.
(C20.3. *Reproduced by permission of the President and Council of the Royal College of Surgeons of England.*)

cells, but as the process occurs insidiously and sporadically, the actual necrosis is not apparent. A failure to replace lost cells is also a factor in the pathogenesis of atrophy in labile tissues, e.g. the bone marrow. By custom atrophy of the marrow is called *aplasia*, and if not too marked the word *hypoplasia* is used by some authorities. Unfortunately both these terms are used in a different connotation as noted above. It is evident that the nomenclature is illogical and confusing.

## ATROPHY

### Physiological Atrophy

There are numerous examples of structures which are well developed at a certain period of life but which subsequently undergo atrophy or involution. Many *fetal structures*, e.g. the branchial clefts, thyroglossal duct, etc., completely disappear before birth, while others such as the ductus arteriosus atrophy early in postuterine life. From adolescence onwards the lymphoid tissue in the body undergoes atrophy, and is usually replaced by fat. Lymph nodes in the adult are frequently found to be composed of a nodule of fat with a thin surrounding demilune of lymphoid tissue. After the menopause and in old age there is atrophy of the gonads, and as age advances most tissues take part in a generalized atrophy.

## Pathological Atrophy

This may be classified as generalized or local.

### Generalized Atrophy

*Starvation atrophy.* All tissues of the body show atrophy during prolonged starvation. The *cachexia* of malignant disease is in many instances largely dependent upon an inadequate food intake.

Atrophy is most marked in the adipose tissues and in muscle. The brain is least affected. The heart in extreme cases may be reduced to a third of its normal size, and appear brown due to the lipofuscin in its fibres (*brown atrophy of the heart*).

*Senile atrophy.* This is the marked accentuation of the process of physiological atrophy of old age. Brown atrophy of the heart is especially prominent in senility, and other organs, e.g. the liver and spleen, may also show a lipofuscin accumulation in their cells. This substance, also called "wear-and-tear pigment", is produced in the cells by the oxidation of fats.

*Endocrine atrophy.* Hypopituitarism leads to atrophy of the thyroid, adrenal cortex, and gonads. Rarely the whole body becomes stunted, and there is an appearance of premature senility (progeria).

*Atrophy of bone* (osteoporosis) is described on page 448.

### Local Atrophy

*Ischaemic atrophy.* This is a local form of tissue malnutrition in which hypoxia is superimposed. With gradual vascular obstruction the parenchyma of many tissues undergoes atrophy, and this is followed by fibrous replacement. Cerebral atrophy is a feature of cerebral arterial atheroma, and the subsequent neuronal loss with replacement gliosis plays an important part in the atrophy of the cortex and the intellectual impairment of old age.

*Pressure atrophy.* This is a variant of ischaemic atrophy. It follows pressure on a solid organ, the vessels of which are severely occluded. It is the capillaries that suffer the most, and damage is caused both by malnutrition and hypoxia. In this way the capsule around a benign tumour or a cyst is formed (p. 242). Some of the best examples of pressure atrophy are seen in relation to bone (p. 450).

*Disuse atrophy.* The best examples are seen in the locomotor system and in the exocrine glands. The atrophy of bone, ligaments, and muscles that follows joint immobilization must always be borne in mind when limbs are encased in plaster. It also occurs when joints are ankylosed, or if movement is prevented by pain; the atrophy around rheumatoid and tuberculous arthritis is particularly marked. Following the loss of teeth there is atrophy of the supporting alveolar bone.

When the duct of a secreting gland is suddenly and completely blocked, the parenchyma undergoes atrophy, e.g. after total obstruction of a ureter, a salivary duct, or the pancreatic duct. It is interesting to recall that it was this method of producing pancreatic atrophy which was employed by Banting and Best in the isolation of insulin.

*Neuropathic atrophy.* This term is loosely applied to the atrophy of a limb which follows nerve lesions. It has two components. Motor paralysis leads to atrophy of the muscles as well as to a more generalized disuse atrophy. Sensory loss may also prevent use of the limb, and lead to disuse atrophy.

*Idiopathic Atrophy.* There are examples of atrophy in which no cause is evident. In some instances, for example adrenal atrophy causing Addison's disease (p. 475), an autoimmune basis has been suggested. In other cases presenile change or inherited defect is possible.

## ABNORMALITIES OF CELLULAR DIFFERENTIATION

### Metaplasia

*Metaplasia is a condition in which there is a change in one type of differentiated tissue to another type of similarly differentiated tissue.* The importance of the word differentiated should be noted, because its use excludes tumour formation as a form of metaplasia.

## TYPES

### Epithelial Metaplasia

**Squamous Metaplasia.** Many types of epithelium are capable of changing to a stratified squamous variety which may undergo keratinization. It often appears to be the result of chronic inflammation. For instance, squamous metaplasia is common in the gall-bladder and urinary bladder when these organs are chronically inflamed, especially if in addition stones (calculi) are present. It is also seen in the bronchi in chronic bronchitis and bronchiectasis (Fig. 17.4).

While in these examples "chronic irritation" appears to be the cause of the metaplasia, there is one condition in which squamous metaplasia is common, but in which irritation plays no part. This is *hypovitaminosis A*. Squamous epithelia show hyperkeratinization which is manifested in the "toad-skin" appearance of the exposed skin. There is also conjunctival hyperkeratosis, or *xerophthalmia*, and this may be complicated by corneal ulceration and infection leading to loss of sight. Squamous metaplasia is widespread, being found in the nose, bronchi, and urinary tract.

**Columnar Metaplasia.** Squamous epithelium rarely shows metaplasia to a columnar type. It is occasionally seen in the lining of a dental cyst. (p. 297).

Specialized columnar epithelium may change to a more simple type. The conversion of the pseudostratified columnar ciliated respiratory epithelium to a simple mucus-secreting columnar type is commonly seen in chronic bronchitis and bronchiectasis, and may well play an important part in predisposing patients with these conditions to bronchopneumonia.

### Connective Tissue Metaplasia

**Osseous Metaplasia.** The question as to whether fibroblasts can produce osteoid tissue or not is largely a matter of how one defines "fibroblast" and "osteoblast". They certainly exhibit great morphological similarity, and before the appearance of the intercellular substance, whether fibrous tissue or osteoid, they cannot be distinguished. "Fibroblasts" do not normally produce osteoid, but under some conditions they may be regarded as undergoing metaplasia to "osteoblasts". Bone then makes its appearance. An alternative explanation is that the osteoblasts are derived from primitive stem cells.

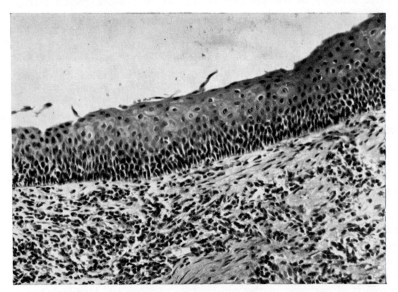

FIG. 17.4. Squamous metaplasia of bronchial epithelium. The normal pseudo-stratified columnar ciliated respiratory epithelium has been replaced by a stratified squamous epithelium. × 200.

Osseous metaplasia is occasionally seen in scars,[11] and also in the fibrous tissue adjacent to any area of dystrophic calcification—cystic goitres, caseous foci in the lung, etc.

**Changes in Mesothelium.** The mesothelial cells lining the pleura and peritoneum may change to an epithelial type, columnar or even squamous.[12-14] This is rare, but is important because such cells cast off into the pleural cavity may be mistaken by the unwary cytologist for cancer cells.

**Tumour Metaplasia.** See p. 267.

### Other Cellular Dystrophies

Dystrophy* may be defined as a disorder, usually congenital, of the structure or function of an organ or tissue due to its perverted nutrition. In its widest sense it includes agenesis, atrophy, hypertrophy, and metaplasia, but in practice the term is usually applied to those disorders which do not readily

* The Greek derivation of this word is as follows: Dys—bad or difficult; Trophe—nourishment.

fit into any of these other categories. The alternative term dysplasia* may also be used for such an abnormal development of tissue, although strictly it should be applied to developmental disorders only. Dyscrasia* literally means a bad mixture (of the four humours), and is now used only by haematologists to describe any blood disorder of uncertain aetiology.

One of the best examples of a dystrophy is the lesion found in pernicious anaemia. Although the abnormal nuclear maturation found in the red-cell precursors in this disease led Ehrlich to describe them as megaloblasts, it was not realized at that time that other cells showed similar changes. Examination of the cells of the gastric, buccal, nasal, vaginal, and other mucosae has revealed certain nuclear abnormalities presumably caused by vitamin-$B_{12}$ deficiency. The changes include pleomorphism, giant nuclei, and large nucleoli.[15] These observations have an important application: the exfoliative cytologist must avoid mistaking these cells for malignant cells in sputum, gastric washings, urine, etc.[16] The premature greying of the hair and the degeneration of the spinal cord indicate that pernicious anaemia is more than merely a haematological disorder.

Many special dystrophies involving muscle, bone, cornea, retina, etc. have been described, but these are outside the scope of this book. It must be reiterated that the term dystrophy has no specific intrinsic meaning, but like dysplasia is used to describe a lesion whose nature is not understood and for which the author can find no other more appropriate name. In recent years dysplasia has acquired a specific meaning when applied to epithelium—most commonly that of the cervix uteri. It is used to describe a type of hyperplasia which is thought to progress to *carcinoma-in-situ* in some cases and later to invasive cancer (p. 281). But dysplasia is also used in other instances, e.g. fibrous dysplasia of bone and mammary dysplasia, in which there is no suggestion of incipient neoplastic change.

In this chapter many different perversions of cell growth have been described. The one thing they all have in common is that they are self-limiting and reversible if the stimulus is removed. In the following chapter neoplasia is considered. Here the perversion of cell growth persists even when the stimulus that produced it is eradicated.

* The Greek derivation of these words is as follows: Dys—bad or difficult; Krasis—a mingling; Plasis—a forming.

## References

1. DONIACH, I. (1960). In "Recent Advances in Pathology", 7th ed., pp. 197–270, ed. by Harrison, C. V. London: Churchill.
2. MacCORMAC, H. and SCARFF, R. W. (1936). *Brit. J. Derm.*, **48**, 624.
3. CALNAN, C. D. and HABER, H. (1955). *J. Path. Bact.*, **69**, 61.
4. WAITE, D. E. (1961). *J. oral Surg.*, **19**, 210.
5. DONOHUE, W. B. (1957). *J. Canad. dent. Ass.*, **23**, 523.
6. LUCAS, R. B. (1972). In "Pathology of Tumours of the Oral Tissues", 2nd ed., p. 121, London: Churchill.
7. LEVER, W. F. (1967). "Histopathology of the Skin", 4th ed., p. 761. Philadelphia and Toronto: Lippincott.
8. HOGAN, M. J. and ZIMMERMAN, L. E. (1962). "Ophthalmic Pathology", 2nd ed., p. 765. Philadelphia and London: Saunders.

9. ANAGNOSTOU, D. and HARRISON, C. V. (1972). *J. clin. Path.*, **25**, 306.
10. ACKERMAN, L. V. and BUTCHER, H. R. (1964). "Surgical Pathology", 3rd ed., p. 960. Saint Louis: Mosby.
11. CLASSEN, K. L., WIEDERANDERS, R. E. and HERRINGTON, J. L. (1960). *Surgery*, **47**, 918.
12. CROME, L. (1950). *J. Path. Bact.*, **62**, 61.
13. DUNNILL, M. S. (1959). *J. Path. Bact.*, **77**, 299.
14. YOUNG, J. S. (1928). *J. Path. Bact.*, **31**, 265.
15. RUBIN, C. E. and MASSEY, B. W. (1953). *J. Lab. clin. Med.*, **42**, 942.
16. BODDINGTON, M. M. and SPRIGGS, A. I. (1959). *J. clin. Path.*, **12**, 228.

*Chapter 18*

# TUMOURS

**Introduction.** The concept that tumour growth is a distinctive clinical and pathological entity has been evolving for many centuries. At first the term "tumour" was applied to any swelling, and the use of the suffix -oma became established to denote such a lesion; even today this relic of the past persists in the use of names like haematoma, hamartoma, tuberculoma, and granuloma. In time the swellings of known aetiology, especially the infective ones, were excluded from the classification of tumours, and there was left a group of swellings of unknown cause apparently produced by the unrestrained growth of the individual's own cells. It appeared that these cells were no longer subject to the normal mechanisms controlling their growth, and had become independent. The trite definition of a tumour as "an autonomous parasite" embodies this concept, but we cannot define a tumour on this basis because we are ignorant about the normal mechanisms of control, and therefore cannot be certain when a cell has escaped from them.

Although the excessive growth of cells is often manifested by the production of a tumour mass, this is not invariable. Sometimes the migration of cells outside the normal confining limits outweighs the bulk of the abnormal proliferation. In this case no "tumour" as such exists—an excellent example is to be seen in the diffuse infiltrating carcinoma of the stomach (p. 418). *Neoplasm*, which literally means new formation or new growth, is a more suitable term. It implies that there is an abnormal type of growth which may be evident not only in the intact animal but also when the cells are grown in culture.

## Types of Tumour

**Classification According to the Tissue of Origin.** Since tumours are formed as a result of the overgrowth of cells, it is logical to name them according to the tissue of origin. The basic subdivision of the body into epithelium and connective tissue is reflected in the recognition of two major groups of tumour: those derived from epithelial cells and those derived from connective tissue. Furthermore within each group there are many subdivisions, just as there are many different types of epithelium and connective tissue.

**Classification According to Behaviour.** An equally important classification is based upon the behaviour of the tumour cells. In some neoplasms the cells always appear to maintain contact with one another, and never wander off into the surrounding tissues nor invade lymphatics or blood vessels. These tumours remain localized, never spread, and are therefore called *innocent*, or *benign*. This contrasts with *malignant* tumours, in which the neoplastic cells invade he surrounding tissues and enter natural tissue spaces such as the lumina of

241

lymphatics and blood vessels. Frequently groups of tumour cells break off, and the resulting tumour emboli become lodged at some distant site, grow, and thereby produce *secondary deposits*, or *metastases*. Between these two extremes of behaviour a third group of *intermediate tumours* is found.

## Benign or Innocent Tumours

### General Considerations and Effects

The cells which constitute this type of tumour show no tendency to invade the surrounding tissues. Instead, the excessive accumulation of cells produces an expanding mass which causes two local effects:

*Pressure atrophy*. Adjacent parenchyma undergoes pressure atrophy while the more resistant connective tissue survives to form a fibrous *capsule*. The tumour is therefore *well-circumscribed*, and is not intimately connected with the surrounding tissue except for those points of entry of the vascular supply. Benign tumours are fairly easy to excise surgically, and provided local removal is complete, they do not recur. A benign tumour within the skull or vertebral column, however, can produce serious effects by pressure.

*Obstruction*. A benign tumour may obstruct a natural passage and cause extensive damage. Obstruction of a bronchus leads to collapse of the lung and bronchopneumonia. A tumour of the intestine may produce intestinal obstruction.

### Gross Characteristics

**Encapsulation.** This is a characteristic feature when the tumour is situated in a solid organ or tissue (see above).

**Shape.** Benign tumours are usually round, but the shape may be moulded by the distribution of surrounding structures. A particular arrangement of fascia may make a tumour oval.

**Size.** Although benign tumours are usually smaller than their malignant counterparts, they may at times attain enormous proportions. The largest tumour in the museum of the Royal College of Surgeons of England is a fibroma of the kidney weighing 82 lb.! A malignant tumour would have killed the patient long before reaching this size.

**Ulceration and haemorrhage** are rare except in certain surface growths.

### Rate of Growth

The rate of growth of a benign tumour is generally slow. It is often erratic, and growth may cease after a period. Enormous tumours are therefore uncommon.

### Hormonal Effects

Benign tumours of endocrine tissue may produce excessive quantities of hormone which can have far-reaching and sometimes fatal effects. A tumour of the islet cells of the pancreas may secrete so much insulin that the blood sugar level falls precipitously, and symptoms of hypoglycaemia occur. These are characterized by convulsions and mental disturbances, as the neurones require a constant supply of glucose. Likewise tumours of the adrenal glands parathyroids, and pituitary may be responsible for characteristic syndromes (Chapter 35).

### Microscopic Appearance

The arrangement of the cells of a benign tumour closely resembles that of the parent tissue. The tumours are therefore described as being *well differentiated*. The cells themselves tend to be regular in size, staining, and shape. Mitotic figures are scanty, and when present are of normal type. The tumour cells are supported and nourished by a network of host connective tissue which consists predominantly of blood vessels, fibroblasts, and a varying amount of collagen. It is called the *stroma*, and although an intimate part of the tumour, it is not itself involved in the neoplastic change.

### Benign Epithelial Tumours

These are of two main types. Benign neoplasia of a surface or lining epithelium produces a warty tumour, or *papilloma* (Fig. 18.1). In a compact gland (e.g. breast) the tumour is embedded in the tissue, and is called an *adenoma*.

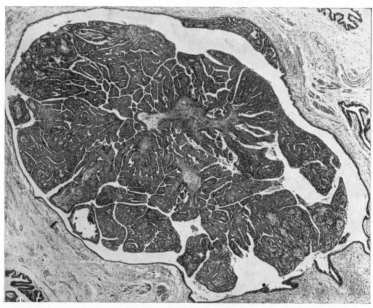

FIG. 18.1. Duct papilloma of breast. There is a large columnar-cell papilloma in the dilated duct. The stalk connecting this polypoid mass to the duct wall has not been included in the section, but the site of thickened epithelium from which it arose is apparent. There is no evidence of invasion. × 26.

### Papillomata

Papillomata may occur on any epithelial surface. Some have a broad base and are described as *sessile*, while others become pedunculated and may be called *polyps*, a morphological term applied to any pedunculated mass attached to a surface and not necessarily neoplastic.

Papillomata are supplied by a core of connective tissue stroma containing blood vessels, lymphatics, and nerves. This is covered by a profuse neoplastic epithelium, composed of either stratified squamous, transitional, or columnar cells, according to that from which it has arisen. The cells show a regular arrangement, and the basement membrane is intact unless there is distortion due to inflammation. The epithelial cells are entirely restricted to the surface, and do not show invasion.

**Stratified Squamous-Cell Papilloma.** Papillomata occur on the skin and other stratified squamous epithelial surfaces, e.g. the tongue and buccal mucosa. There is always *acanthosis*, i.e. a proliferation of the prickle-cell layer, and in the case of cutaneous papillomata there is often excessive keratin formation (*hyperkeratosis*) also. Squamous-cell papilloma is a common tumour of the mouth, and ıs not infrequent in the larynx.

**Transitional-Cell Papilloma.** This occurs throughout the urinary passages, and has characteristic delicate finger-like processes, or fronds, which give it the appearance of a sea anemone. Bleeding is quite common and leads to haematuria. Malignant change is very common.

**Columnar-Cell Papilloma.** This tumour occurs on any surface covered by columnar epithelium, for example in the colon. Papillomata are also to be found in cystic adenomata (see below).

### Adenomata

Adenomata are composed of dense masses of acini lined by exuberant epithelium which may be columnar or cuboidal in shape. They occur in the salivary glands, pancreas, kidney, ovary, and the endocrine glands. They may also arise in the small glands which open on to epithelial surfaces; thus adenomata originate in sweat and sebaceous glands in the skin and the mucous glands of the mouth and respiratory tract.

Intestinal adenomata tend to become polypoid, and in the hereditary condition of *polyposis coli* thousands of tumours are present.[1] Malignant change is almost inevitable, and the patient dies of cancer of the colon. In a related condition, *Gardner's syndrome*, colonic polyposis is found in association with sebaceous cysts, osteomata of the face and skull, and multiple fibromata. This too is inherited as a dominant trait and terminates in colonic cancer.[2]

A rather similar condition is the *Peutz-Jeghers syndrome*,[3-5] in which multiple polyposis of the stomach and intestine (small and large) is associated with a brownish pigmentation peppered around the lips and mouth and sometimes in the skin elsewhere (Fig. 18.2). The polyps are not prone to become malignant, unlike those of polyposis coli; indeed, they are probably hamartomatous rather than neoplastic.

**Cystadenoma.** Sometimes adenomata form elaborate spaces into which papillary ingrowths of neoplastic epithelium occur. These *papillary cystadenomata* are most common in the ovary, but may also be found in the salivary glands and kidneys.

**Fibro-Adenoma.** The common tumour in the breast of young women is the fibro-adenoma. It consists of epithelial and connective tissue elements, both of which are considered to be neoplastic.

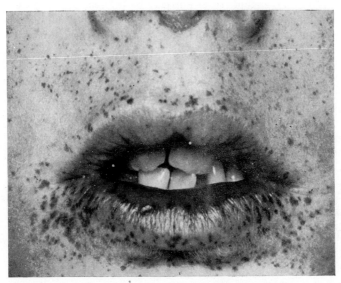

Fig. 18.2. Peutz-Jeghers syndrome. The multiple, circumoral, brown macules are well show. The pigmentation is due to melanin. (*Sheward, J. D.* (1962). Brit. Med. J., **1,** 921.)

### Benign Connective Tissue Tumours

Benign tumours of connective tissue are usually composed of cells which closely resemble the parent tissue. They are supported by an excellent stroma from the adjacent connective tissues, and there is a characteristic tendency to merge with this stroma. The neoplastic cells are not nearly so well demarcated from the stroma as are those of epithelial tumours. The tumours are named according to the cell of origin, e.g. fibroma from fibroblast, osteoma from osteoblast, myoma from muscle, etc.

**Fibroma.** Fibromata are not very common tumours. They consist of circumscribed collections of fibroblasts between which there is a variable amount of collagen. Hard fibromata have much collagen, whereas the softer variety is predominantly cellular. They are found in many sites, e.g. skin, stomach, ovary, gingiva, etc. Fibromata also occur in bones (p. 458). Myxomatous change may be found in some fibromata. Such a tumour is called a *myxofibroma*, or if the change is marked a *myxoma*.

**Myoma.** Tumours of muscle are of two types: from smooth muscle (leiomyoma) and striated muscle (rhabdomyoma).

*Leiomyoma.* This is the commonest of all tumours, being found in the uteri of about 20 per cent of women over 30 years of age. Leiomyomata of the skin, stomach, and intestine are also not uncommon. Usually they are small and often multiple. A leiomyoma is composed of whorls of smooth muscle cells interspersed among which there is a variable amount of fibrous tissue (Fig. 18.3). In due course the muscle element may be replaced by fibrous tissue, and the *fibroleiomyoma* (or fibroid) is produced. Such a tumour may undergo cystic change, or else it may be the seat of dense calcification. On section the whorled interlacing pattern of glistening white fibres resembling watered-silk is characteristic.

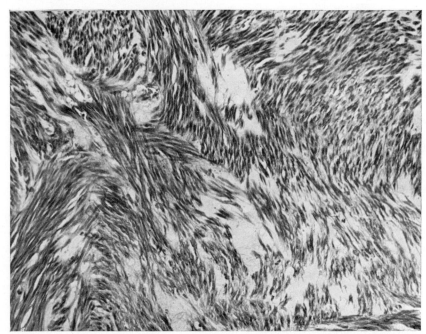

Fig. 18.3. Leiomyoma. There are sheaves of spindle-shaped smooth muscle cells and also areas of replacement by hyaline fibrous tissue. × 200.

*Rhabdomyoma.* Benign rhabdomyomata are exceedingly uncommon.

**Neurofibroma.** The neurofibroma is a tumour derived from the nerve sheath cells of Schwann. Alternative names are neurilemmoma and Schwannoma. These tumours are usually solitary, and are found on the nerves of the limbs, but they may occur in many other sites including the bones and mouth. In gross appearance they closely resemble leiomyomata, and microscopically are composed of spindle cells which have a palisaded, or regimented, appearance, all the nuclei being aligned in one strip and the clear cytoplasm of the cells in an adjacent strip. Many neurofibromata produce collagen, and a stage may be reached in which they are indistinguishable from an ordinary fibroma. (See also neurofibromatosis, p. 294).

**Lipoma.** This common tumour is composed of adult adipose tissue. It is usually subcutaneous, but may be retroperitoneal or subserosal. Oral lipomata are uncommon.

**Chondroma** and **osteoma** are considered in Chapter 33.

## Malignant Tumours

### General Considerations

The cells of a malignant tumour infiltrate and erode the surrounding tissue. Normal cells are enveloped and destroyed, and the tumour edge is therefore ill-defined. Complete excision by surgery is correspondingly difficult, and even if the tumour is removed with much surrounding normal tissue, malignant cells often remain behind, and their continued growth results in a *local recurrence*. In malignant tumours the invading cells spread in the planes of least resistance: finger-like processes extend outwards from the main tumour mass, and this growth produces a fanciful resemblance to the silhouette of a crab. Hence the term *cancer*, which is derived from the Latin word meaning a crab. It is generally applied to all malignant tumours. *A carcinoma is a malignant tumour of epithelial cells, while a sarcoma is one derived from connective tissue.*

Embolic spread of tumour cells is responsible for the production of distant metastases. *Local invasion and embolic spread are the two characteristics of malignant tumours.* Both are probably related to the reduced cell adhesiveness which is a fundamental characteristic of cancer cells, and is evident not only *in vivo* but also in tissue culture—the cells growing out of the explant do not resist mechanical separation as well as do those of normal tissue. The power to invade and spread combined with the capacity for progressive growth make the term malignant particularly suitable for this type of tumour. Death is inevitable in untreated cases, except for those very rare, though well-documented, cases of *spontaneous regression*, in which proven cancers have disappeared of their own accord.[6-10]

### Gross Characteristics

**Lack of Encapsulation.** Malignant tumours have no limiting capsule, because the cells actively infiltrate the adjacent tissues. In certain rapidly growing tumours (e.g. metastases in the liver) cell division exceeds infiltration, and the tumour by its expansive growth may give a false impression of encapsulation. Microscopy, however, always reveals infiltration.

**Shape.** This is irregular in outline and diffuse in definition.

**Size.** Malignant tumours are usually larger than their benign counterparts.

**Ulceration and Haemorrhage.** As would be expected from the destructive property of cancer, these are common features. *Any ulcer which fails to heal within a few weeks should always be regarded as malignant until proved otherwise.* In the mouth exfoliative cytology may be used to aid in the diagnosis of suspicious lesions[11] (p. 280).

### Rate of Growth

Malignant tumours usually undergo a rapid and steady increase in size. This can be of diagnostic importance; for example, if a shadow on a lung or bone radiograph is known to have remained stationary in size for many months, it is unlikely to be due to a malignant tumour.

## Microscopic Features

Microscopically several important features should be noted. The tumour tissue may resemble the parent tissue to a considerable extent, but the similarity is not as great as with benign tumours. Differentiation is not so well developed, and recognition of the tissue of origin is often difficult or even impossible; tumours which show little or no differentiation are called *undifferentiated*. At one time it was thought that normal differentiated cells could become neoplastic and revert to a more primitive state and appearance. This process of "dedifferentiation" is nowadays discredited. Primitive cell-forms are ascribed to a basically primitive cell origin with a subsequent failure of normal differentiation. Neoplastic cells do differentiate, but frequently the differentiation is abnormal and does not conform to that found normally in the tissue. To describe a tumour as poorly differentiated is probably inaccurate, but it is a common practice and means that to the observer the neoplastic cells are making little attempt to resemble the structure of those found normally in the tissue.

Malignant tumours usually show much mitotic activity. The build-up of DNA prior to division results in nuclear enlargement and hyperchromatism. This together with the formation of cells with abnormal numbers of chromosomes accounts for the irregularity in size and shape (*pleomorphism*), and staining which is so characteristic of malignant tumours. Mitoses are not only numerous, but sometimes also abnormal, and the number of chromosomes may diverge from the normal 46. Triradiate mitoses with the formation of three daughter cells are particularly characteristic of malignancy.

*Anaplasia* is a term which was introduced to describe new cells which deviated from the normal and resembled those of embryonic tissue. It is now generally restricted to those cellular changes which are found in malignant tumours. Thus a tumour which shows a high degree of anaplasia is poorly differentiated, and has frequent and bizarre mitoses and cells that are pleomorphic (see Fig. 18.8).

## Effects of Malignant Tumours

Malignant tumours produce their ill-effects in a large number of ways:

**Mechanical Pressure and Obstruction.** Like benign tumours, malignant growths press on adjacent structures and cause obstruction to natural passages. A carcinoma of the colon soon leads to intestinal obstruction. Collapse of a lung and bronchopneumonia are often the features which first call attention to a carcinoma of the bronchus.

**Destruction of Tissue.** In addition, malignant tumours both primary and secondary, infiltrate and destroy tissue. This is well illustrated in bone where destruction may be so marked that pathological fractures occur, and replacement of the marrow results in anaemia.

**Haemorrhage.** Malignant tumours which involve any surface usually ulcerate and bleed. Repeated bleeding causes anaemia, and occasionally the erosion of a large artery leads to a massive fatal haemorrhage. This may happen when a carcinoma of the tongue involves the lingual artery. *Clinically unexplained bleeding from any site should be treated seriously, as it is a common symptom* *of cancer.* Haemoptysis is common in lung cancer, haematuria in urinary cancer, and vaginal bleeding, especially after intercourse, in cervical cancer.

**Infection.** All ulcerative cancers are bound to undergo secondary bacterial infection, and this aggravates the clinical condition. Infection also follows obstruction to the urinary or respiratory passages, e.g. bronchopneumonia occurs in lung cancer, and cystitis and pyelonephritis in cancer of the prostate. Cancer of the mouth interferes so much with swallowing that in due course there is inhalation of food and saliva into the respiratory passages. It is not surprising that suppurative bronchopneumonia is the commonest cause of death in this condition.

**Starvation.** In cancers of the mouth, oesophagus, and stomach there may be a direct nutritional effect due to the failure of food intake.

**Pain.** In advanced malignancy pain may be severe. It occasions anxiety and leads to insomnia.

**Anaemia.** Anaemia is common and may be due to chronic blood loss, mal-absorption of essential dietary components, or bone marrow replacement. Often, however, the cause is obscure.

**Cachexia.** The emaciated appearance of patients with advanced cancer is characteristic, but it is not uncommon for patients to remain obese. The cause of the loss of weight and the generalized body atrophy in cancer has given rise to much speculation. At one time a toxic product of necrotic tissue was postulated, but this has never been substantiated. The present tendency is to attribute cachexia to secondary factors, e.g. starvation, haemorrhage, infection, liver damage, etc.

In advanced malignancy there is usually *pyrexia*, a raised ESR, and a neutrophil leucocytosis, quite apart from any secondary infection. The pathogenesis is obscure.

**Hormonal Effects.** Malignant tumours of the endocrine glands occasionally produce effects due to an excessive production of hormones. This is less common than with benign tumours.

**Carcinomatous Syndromes.**[12] A variety of syndromes have been reported in association with neoplasms which are not explicable in terms of infiltration either by the primary tumour or its metastases. *Muscle weakness* and *skin eruptions*[13,14] are two such examples. Sometimes a patient exhibits signs and symptoms referable to the *nervous system*[15] (weakness, signs of intracranial tumour, etc.) and yet at necropsy no nervous involvement is found. *Venous thrombosis*[16] sometimes leading to fatal pulmonary embolism, is an inexplicable complication of some neoplasms, especially carcinoma of the pancreas. Another curious phenomenon is the *hormonal effects* produced by tumours of non-endocrine origin.[17,18] Thus *hypoglycaemia* is seen in some mesotheliomata, and *Cushing's syndrome* may occur in cancer of the lung. The latter tumour may also produce *clubbing of the fingers*, and sometimes the joints are so swollen that rheumatoid arthritis is closely simulated. The explanation of all these intriguing effects of malignant tumours is not known, but the atypical cells can sometimes produce and secrete hormones or hormone-like substances into the circulation. This is an instance of abnormal differentiation of a malignant tumour.

## Spread of Malignant Tumours

Direct invasion and embolization are the two methods of spread and must be examined in detail.

### Direct Spread

The direct infiltration of the surrounding tissues means that the microscopic edge of the tumour extends beyond what is macroscopically apparent. Infiltration along tissue planes and septa is well shown in cancer of the breast, and in this way the tumour becomes *attached to the skin and deep fascia*

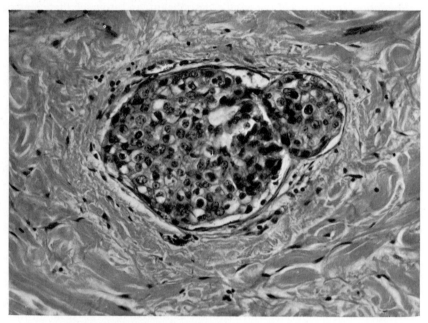

Fig. 18.4. Lymphatic permeation. A lymphatic channel has been completely occluded by a solid cord of cancer cells. The tumour was a spheroidal-cell carcinoma of the breast. × 200.

(Fig. 18.11). Evidence of local invasion of a tumour is an important clinical sign, for it is tantamount to a diagnosis of malignancy.

**Invasion of Lymphatics.** Carcinoma, but not sarcoma, shows a particular tendency to invade lymphatic vessels at an early stage, and the cells may grow as a long, ever-extending cord (Fig. 18.4). The process is called *lymphatic permeation*, and the lymphatic obstruction which it produces can cause lymphatic oedema.

**Invasion of Arteries and Veins.** This is a common event, and may lead to thrombosis and obstruction. It is frequent in lung cancer because so many large vessels are readily accessible to the tumour.[19]

### Spread by Metastases

Groups of cells may become detached, travel in some natural passage to a distant site, become implanted, and finally grow to produce secondary deposits, or *metastases*. Spread *via* the lymphatics, blood vessels, and serous cavities are the most important examples.

**Lymphatic Spread.** Detached groups of tumour cells in an invaded lymphatic are swept into the draining regional lymph nodes. If the cells survive and grow, the node soon becomes replaced by the tumour, and further spread occurs to the next group of nodes by way of the efferent channel. This is a familiar event in the course of carcinoma and melanoma, but is rare in sarcoma. A blockage of lymphatics results in a reversal of lymph flow in other vessels, and metastases may appear in unexpected lymph nodes. This is known as *retrograde embolism*, and the best-known example is the involvement of the left cervical nodes in gastric cancer. This is due to obstruction of the thoracic duct near its entry into the left subclavian vein, so that lymph is diverted up to the neck.

**Blood Spread.** The occurrence of blood-borne metastases is the feature of malignant disease which is responsible for death in most cases. It is also the factor which limits the surgical and radiotherapeutic treatment of cancer.

At first sight the mode of production of secondary tumours is easy to understand. Malignant cells invade small venules, become detached, and are then carried by the blood stream to some distant site where they reach a capillary network. There the emboli become impacted, and the cells proliferate and develop into secondary tumours. A second method of blood-borne metastasis is by way of the lymphatics, for all the lymph eventually drains into the venous circulation.

As would be expected, one of the commonest sites of metastasis for most tumours is the lung. Likewise, primary tumours arising from an area drained by the portal vein regularly metastasize to the liver. Purely mechanical factors would appear to account for this distribution, but closer examination makes such an explanation inadequate.

Many tumours, e.g. of the breast and kidney, give rise to metastases not only in the lungs, but also in the liver, bones, and other organs, and such systemic metastases sometimes occur in the absence of apparent lung deposits. It is possible that these are really present, but have been missed because of an inadequate *post-mortem* examination by the pathologist. Alternatively the cells may have been able to pass through the lung capillaries and become arrested elsewhere, or else there may be a direct venous communication between the primary and secondary sites, e.g. prostate and pelvic bones.

The distribution of secondary tumours might be expected to be related to the blood supply, but this is not the case. Cardiac and skeletal muscle have an abundant blood supply, and yet are rarely the site of metastases. The spleen likewise is not commonly involved. The liver, on the other hand, is frequently studded with secondary tumours regardless of the site of the primary.

There is considerable evidence that malignant cells often reach the blood stream but that most of them die. Only a selected few are able to take root to grow into secondary deposits. What factors govern this are not known. The "seed" may be widespread, but only where the "soil" is suitable does growth occur. Some examples of this *selective metastasis* must now be examined.

(*a*) *Liver*. The commonest organ in which blood-borne metastases occur is the liver, for this organ appears to afford an excellent environment for the growth of tumour cells.

(*b*) *Lung*. This is the next most common site for metastases (Fig. 18.5).

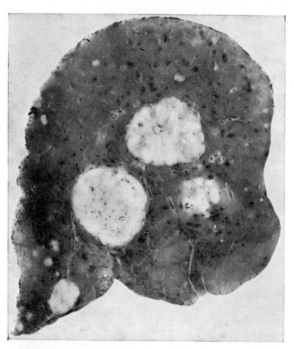

FIG. 18.5. Metastatic carcinoma of lung. Note the circumscribed white deposits. Primary lung cancer infiltrates the surrounding tissue much more obviously. The primary tumour in this case arose from the breast.

(R47.3. *Reproduced by permission of the President and Council of the Royal College of Surgeons of England.*)

(*c*) *Bone*.[20] Carcinomata of the breast, lung, prostate, kidney, and thyroid quite frequently produce bony metastases.

(*d*) *Brain*. Carcinoma of the lung is notorious for the frequency with which it metastasizes to the brain. Indeed, this is the commonest malignant intracranial tumour.

(*e*) *Adrenal glands*. These are frequently the site of secondary deposits of cancer of the lung and breast.

**Transcoelomic Spread.** When a malignant tumour invades the serosal layer of a viscus it causes a local acute inflammatory response. This results in the formation of a serous exudate into the cavity. Haemorrhage into the fluid is common, and therefore *the presence of a blood-stained effusion into a serous cavity should always raise the possibility of malignancy.* Tumour cells may break off and float *free* in the fluid, where they can be detected by the cytologist. They may alight on to other sites in the cavity and form the basis of secondary seedling growths. Such transcoelomic spread is seen in the pleural cavity with cancer of the lung, and in the peritoneum with cancer of the stomach and ovaries.

**Staging of Tumours.** The extent to which an individual tumour has spread can be depicted by assigning it to a particular stage.[21, 22] The criteria used for staging cancers of various organs differ, but a typical example is as follows:

Stage 1. Tumour confined to the organ of origin.

Stage 2. The growth involves the local lymphatic nodes.

Stage 3. Tumour extends to distant lymphatic nodes.

Stage 4. Blood-borne metastases present.

The assessment of the stage is done on clinical grounds aided by histological examination of any available tissue (e.g. lymph nodes if the tumour has been excised), radiology, and other specialized techniques for the detection of tumour in the liver, brain, etc. The method is necessarily inaccurate, but nevertheless this is a useful classification because it is related to the prognosis. Thus with carcinoma of the tongue stage 1 tumours have an average 5-year survival-rate of over 40 per cent, while tumours of stages 2 to 4 have a 5 per cent 5-year survival-rate.[23]

**Dormant Cancer.**[24] A difficulty about staging is the tendency for some metastases to appear many years after the primary tumour has been successfully removed. Such patients may remain well for 10 to 25 years, and then suddenly develop multiple secondary deposits, despite the absence of a local recurrence. It is assumed that the tumour cells were present in the body during the entire period, but for unknown reasons remained dormant. Factors that predispose to the phase of renewed growth after a period of dormancy are intercurrent illness, psychological trauma, and physical injuries. Carcinoma of the breast and kidney and melanoma of the eye are tumours notorious for this tendency towards dormant metastases.

### Malignant Epithelial Tumours

These are called carcinomata, and are the commonest of all malignant tumours. This is probably because epithelium is a much more labile tissue than connective tissue (p. 229). Three types of carcinoma may be recognized:

1. *Squamous-cell carcinoma.*
2. *Carcinoma of glandular epithelium.*
3. *Transitional-cell carcinoma.*

### Squamous-Cell Carcinoma

These tumours arise at any site normally covered by stratified squamous epithelium—skin, mouth, oesophagus, etc. They account for 90 per cent of all malignant oral tumours. At other sites they may occur as a result of tumour metaplasia, or possibly neoplasia in an area of squamous metaplasia, e.g. salivary gland, lung, and urinary tract.

**Macroscopic Types.** Two are usually described:

*The papillary carcinoma* appears as a warty outgrowth with an infiltrating base; this type may arise in a papilloma.

*The nodular type* produces a hard, nodular mass beneath the surface, and shows more rapid infiltration and dissemination. Both types usually ulcerate to form a typical *carcinomatous ulcer*. This has a raised, craggy, rolled edge which is fixed to surrounding skin and deeper structures. The base is composed of white necrotic tissue, which is usually friable and bleeds easily.

**Histological Type.** In considering the histological structure of a squamous-cell carcinoma it is necessary first to understand its formation (Fig. 18.6).

*Formation.* When epithelium shows malignant propensities, there is a progressive proliferation of the prickle-cell layer. This is sometimes so irregular that, even before it actually breaks through the basement membrane, it may give the microscopical impression of malignancy. To this condition the name *carcinoma-in-situ* is applied (p. 280).

The criterion of truly invasive carcinoma is the destruction of the basement membrane by masses of malignant cells, which then stream down into the deeper connective tissue and muscle. As they proceed they tend to break up into separate groups or columns. These clumps may comprise hundreds of cancer cells, or else only a few. In the most anaplastic tumours there may be no attempt at any splitting up, and the tumour mass proceeds in one diffuse sheet.

As the tumour infiltrates it destroys the tissue with which it comes in contact, and this is replaced by a fibrous stroma.

Nearly all malignant tumours excite an inflammatory reaction around them; lymphocytes are particularly numerous. It has been suggested that they play a part in restricting invasion. Once ulceration of the surface occurs, there is a more acute type of response due to secondary bacterial infection.

In those carcinomata which break up into discrete columns, each individual clump may then differentiate partly or completely to resemble the normal epithelium from which it has arisen.

*Differentiation.* Squamous-cell carcinomata vary considerably in the degree of differentiation which they show. When differentiation is good, *epithelial pearls* (also called *keratin*, or *horn*, *pearls*), or *cell nests*, are formed: these are groups of cells, which by differentiating produce a central whorl of keratin (Fig. 18.7.) Surrounding this there are prickle cells, and sometimes a stratum granulosum is recognizable. A basal-cell layer is not well formed. In this way there is a fairly accurate reproduction of the upper layers of normal keratinizing stratified squamous epithelium. The cells are usually fairly uniform in size and shape, their nuclei are evenly staining, and mitoses are scanty. On the whole spread is slow. The skin is the commonest site, but sometimes the oral cavity and bronchus are also the seat of well-differentiated cancers.

The more undifferentiated tumours contain no keratin, although groups of prickle cells may still be recognizable.

Highly undifferentiated, or anaplastic, tumours show no attempt at prickle-cell formation. There is a diffuse sheet of neoplastic cells supported by a scanty, vascular stroma. No attempt at forming groups of cells is recognizable. The cells themselves show great pleomorphism, and mitotic figures abound—some of these are bizarre. Tumour giant cells may be present (Fig. 18.8). It may be impossible to distinguish the tumour from a sarcoma. This type of tumour is usually found in the mouth, bronchus, and cervix.

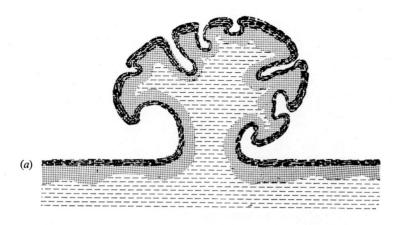

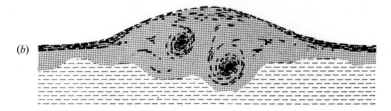

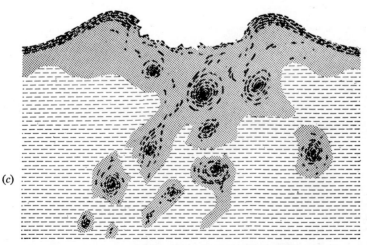

FIG. 18.6. Three types of neoplasia of a keratinizing stratified squamous epithelium.

(a) Benign neoplasia results in an excessive production of regular epithelium, which in order to be accommodated is thrown into a complicated folded structure. This is a papilloma.

(b) In *carcinoma-in-situ* the epithelial overgrowth is irregular; the cells are bizarre, and they lose their polarity. The epithelium is thickened and contains areas of keratinization in its depths. The basement membrane is intact, and there is no invasion.

(c) In carcinoma the basement membrane is destroyed, and atypical cells invade the underlying tissues.

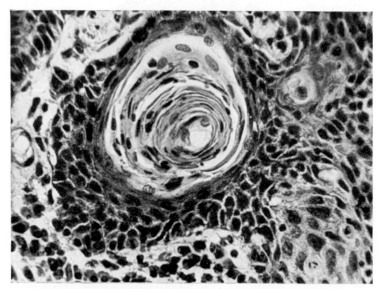

FIG. 18.7. A cell nest, or epithelial pearl. This group of cells was found in a very well-differentiated squamous-cell carcinoma. In the centre differentiation has proceeded to keratin formation, so as to mimic normal stratum corneum. × 380.

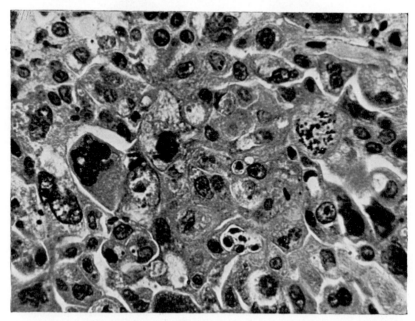

FIG. 18.8. An anaplastic tumour. This section shows the main features of malignant cells—pleomorphism, irregularity in size and staining capacity of the nuclei, giant forms, and an abnormal mitotic figure. × 570.

## Variations of Squamous-Cell Carcinoma

*Transitional-Cell Papillary Carcinoma.* Some squamous-cell carcinomata of the pharynx and lung have a papillary structure, and are composed of a transitional type of epithelium similar to that of the urinary passages. It is better not to call this type of tumour transitional-celled, as it simply causes confusion.

*Verrucous Carcinoma.*[23] This papillomatous well-differentiated tumour occurs in the mouth, larynx, and genital region. It is noteworthy for having a very good prognosis.

*Lymphoepithelioma.* Anaplastic tumours of epithelium overlying lymphoid tissue sometimes contain sheets of undifferentiated cells copiously inter-mingled with lymphocytes. This type of neoplasm usually occurs in the pharynx, especially in connexion with the tonsils. It is of high-grade malignancy, and often the first sign of disease is the appearance of large metastases in the cervical lymph nodes.

**Grading.** Histological grading as described by Broders is of some help in assessing prognosis.[25] Four grades are recognized, according to the degree of differentiation.

Grade 1. More than 75 per cent cell-differentiation.

Grade 2. 50–75 per cent cell-differentiation.

Grade 3. 25–50 per cent cell-differentiation.

Grade 4. Less than 25 per cent cell-differentiation.

Grading on a numerical basis is seldom used because it is time-consuming, and in any case the assessment is subjective.

It is more helpful to define three grades—well-differentiated, poorly-differentiated, and undifferentiated. Although many exceptions are found, the higher the grade the worse is the prognosis, but the more radiosensitive is the tumour.

Some authorities are not convinced that grading is of any great help in the individual case. Certainly the site of the tumour is of great importance. A grade 1 squamous-cell carcinoma of the skin has an excellent prognosis, while in the lung the outlook is poor. Similarly, a grade 4 tumour of the cervix has a much better prognosis than a similar tumour of the lung or pharynx.

## Carcinoma of Glandular Epithelium

These tumours arise from surface, secreting epithelia as well as from under-lying glands. They may arise from columnar-cell papillomata and adenomata.

The pattern of invasion of neoplastic epithelium beneath the basement membrane into the deeper tissue is similar to that already described; in this case the groups of cancer cells, instead of producing keratin, tend to arrange themselves into acinous structures containing a central lumen into which secretion pours. The cells surrounding this lumen may be columnar, cuboidal, polygonal, or spheroidal (Fig. 18.9).

The well-differentiated cancers show excellent acinus formation, which mimics normal glandular structure. These tumours are called *adenocarcinomata* (Fig. 18.10).

In less well-differentiated tumours there are merely clumps of cells surrounded by a stroma, and no attempt at central cavitation to produce

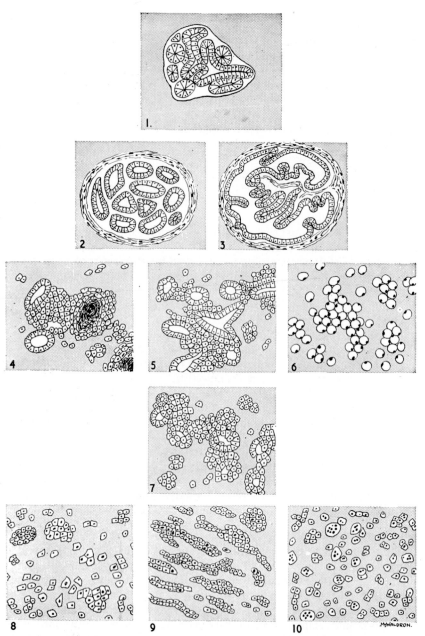

Fig. 18.9. Tumours derived from glandular epithelium. The normal gland (1) is contained in a sheath of connective tissue. Benign neoplasia results in the formation of an adenoma (2) with well-differentiated structure and encapsulation. Cystic dilatation of acini and complicated infolding of the epithelium produce a cystadenoma (3). The remainder of the tumours are malignant. The adenocarcinomata show some tubular differentiation which may be good (5) or poor (7). Lack of differentiation results in a carcinoma simplex (9). The most anaplastic tumours form a sheet of loosely attached cells (8). Giant-cell forms may predominate (10). These anaplastic tumours may be very similar to sarcomata, melanomata, and tumours of squamous epithelial origin. Abnormal differentiation results in squamous metaplasia (4) or the formation of signet-ring cell carcinoma (6).

acini. To this type of cancer the names *carcinoma simplex*, spheroidal-cell, or polygonal-cell carcinoma are applied. It is seen most commonly in the breast, where the cancer clumps are often surrounded by a dense fibrous stroma. Often there is acinus formation elsewhere in the tumour.

The most undifferentiated tumors have diffuse, sheet-like arrangements typical of anaplasia. Distinction from squamous-cell cancers or even sarcomata is sometimes very difficult.

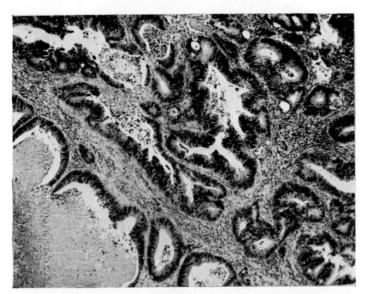

FIG. 18.10. Columnar-cell adenocarcinoma. It consists of large, well-formed acini containing secretion, and is lined by exuberant columnar cells. This well-differentiated tumour arose from the colon. × 80.

**Mucoid Cancer.** The cells of a carcinoma derived from glandular epithelium may contain demonstrable mucus. Sometimes there is so large an accumulation of mucus in the cytoplasm that the nucleus is compressed on to the cell wall. This type of cell is called a *signet-ring cell*. If mucus secretion is marked, the tumour is called a mucoid cancer. Often the stroma contains large lakes of mucus in which there are disintegrating malignant cells. It is a mistake to regard these tumours as degenerate, for they are often highly malignant despite their acellular appearance.

### Transitional-Cell Carcinoma

These tumours occur in the renal pelvis, ureter, and bladder. They are often papillomatous in appearance, but differ from papillomata in having a broader base and showing invasion.

### Stromal Reaction in Carcinoma

The reaction of the invaded tissue to carcinoma cells varies; its growth may be so stimulated that a hard, fibrotic (*scirrhous*) type of tumour is produced. Most breast cancers are of this type (Fig. 18.11). The dense fibrosis appears to be associated with a contracting tendency, which is ill understood. In the breast there is an accompanying retraction of the nipple and dimpling of the skin. Eventually a stony fixation to the chest wall ensues.

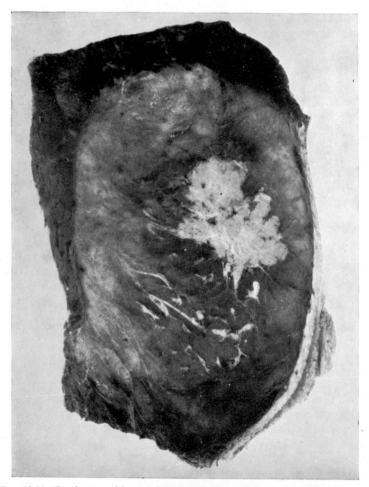

FIG. 18.11. Carcinoma of breast. This is a typical scirrhous carcinoma. Its outline is irregular and badly defined, for it extends sinuously into the surrounding fibro-fatty tissue.

(EB10.1. *Reproduced by permission of the President and Council of the Royal College of Surgeons of England.*)

Scirrhous tumours are also commonly found in the stomach and colon. The contraction causes a "purse-string" deformity, and obstruction of the lumen follows.

When a tumour has little stroma in relation to cell bulk it is soft or brain-like, and is described as *medullary*, or *encephaloid*. Some cancers of the stomach and colon are of this type, and ulceration and bleeding occur rather than early intestinal obstruction.

## Malignant Tumours of Connective Tissue

These are called *sarcomata*. They are much less common than carcinomata, and unlike them, they occur at all ages. While carcinomata tend to be arranged in discrete cellular clumps surrounded by a variable amount of stroma, sarcomata are always disposed in diffuse sheets, in which the neoplastic cells merge inseparably into the stroma.

On the whole sarcomata spread more rapidly than carcinomata, and the prognosis is correspondingly more grave. Early blood-borne metastases are the rule, and the lungs are often riddled with secondary deposits. Lymphatic involvement is very much less common than with carcinoma.

**Fibrosarcoma.** Fibrosarcomata are not encapsulated, and the cells show the cytological features of malignancy—pleomorphism and mitotic activity. Nevertheless, a well-differentiated fibrosarcoma shows considerable cellular regularity and collagen formation, and in practice the distinction from fibroma can be very difficult. Poorly-differentiated tumours show little or no collagen formation, and are then called *spindle-cell sarcomata*. They may be indistinguishable from other anaplastic sarcomata (e.g. leiomyosarcoma, neurofibrosarcoma, liposarcoma, etc.) or even anaplastic carcinomata.

Haemorrhage and necrosis are common features of most sarcomata, because the stroma is delicate and the vascular supply inadequate to meet the demands of the tumour.

**Osteosarcoma.** This is one of the commonest forms of sarcoma, and is described in connexion with the section on bone (p. 459).

**Malignant Tumours of Blood Vessels.** *Angiosarcoma* is a rare tumour which usually arises in the soft tissues including those of the oral cavity, and consists microscopically of poorly-formed vascular channels lined by atypical endothelial cells. *Kaposi's sarcoma* is quite common in certain areas, particularly Eastern Europe and Eastern and Southern Africa. It commences as red or purple nodules on the skin of the legs, but after some years new lesions develop elsewhere, and may also affect the oral cavity and internal organs. Microscopically, the early nodules closely resemble granulation tissue, but later the lesions become more solid as atypical spindle-shaped cells proliferate and produce a more obviously sarcomatous picture.

## Tumours of the Stem Cell and its Derivatives[26]

The neoplastic lesions of these cells are the *lymphomata* and the tumours of the *haematopoietic tissues*.

*Lymphomata.* These are all malignant, and since they vary considerably in their clinical course, many attempts have been made to classify them so that behaviour might be related to histological type. There is no agreed classification and the nomenclature is confusing. Hence it is often impossible to compare the results of treatment in one centre with those of another. The lymphomata are the most common form of malignant tumour after the carcinomata. They arise from the cellular elements of the lymph nodes and bone marrow, and unlike other types of sarcoma, they spread rapidly to other lymph-nodes, eventually becoming systematized. The spleen, liver, and bone marrow are extensively infiltrated, and deposits are also present in the lungs and other organs. Another difference from other types of sarcoma is their extreme radiosensitivity; dramatic remissions follow radiotherapy. Sometimes a localized lesion may be cured, but unfortunately recurrence and systematization are the rule.

The recommended classification is based on two features. The first is the type of cell involved in the neoplastic process, whether lymphocytic or reticulum cell. Hodgkin's disease is given a separate status because of special features which will be described later. The second important feature is whether the neoplastic cells are arranged in distinct nodules or whether they are arranged in a diffuse manner.[27] The *nodular lymphomata* have a better prognosis than their diffuse counterparts, and were at one time grouped together as *giant follicular lymphomata*, or Brill-Symmers's disease, terms which are not now in use. The nodular lymphomata may become diffuse as the disease progresses, but the diffuse ones never become nodular. The lesions therefore always tend to change to a more malignant type.

The following lymphomata are described:

*Reticulum-cell Sarcoma*—nodular or diffuse.

*Lymphocytic Lymphoma*—nodular or diffuse. Each may be poorly, moderately, or well differentiated.

*Lymphoma, mixed cell type*—nodular or diffuse.

*Hodgkin's Disease.* The subdivisions are described later.

**Reticulum-cell Sarcoma (Reticulosarcoma).** This arises from the primitive reticulum cells scattered throughout the lymph node. These cells lay down reticulin fibres, and may assume a fibroblastic activity, laying down collagen also. In reticulum-cell sarcoma the normal architecture of the node is obliterated by a massive infiltration of large neoplastic reticulum cells, some of which may be of giant proportions. It is sometimes difficult to distinguish reticulum-cell sarcoma from an anaplastic carcinoma, and poorly-differentiated tumours are called *stem-cell sarcomata*.

Reticulum-cell sarcoma usually starts in a group of lymph nodes (or more rarely in a tonsil or the small intestine), and soon implicates the spleen and liver which become palpable. It is a disease of later life.

**Lymphocytic Lymphoma.** This tumour is commonly called a *lymphosarcoma*, a term which is deprecated by many experts in the field but which may retain its place by virtue of common usage. The neoplastic cells can vary in differentiation and resemble mature lymphocytes (*lymphocytic lymphosarcoma*) or immature lymphoblasts (*lymphoblastic lymphosarcoma*). An intermediate group can also be recognized. Lymphocytic lymphoma is about twice as common as reticulum-cell sarcoma and affects a similar age group. Clinically the two are indistinguishable. Histologically the architecture of the lymph node is destroyed by sheets or nodules of uniform neoplastic lymphocytes. Indeed, destruction of the normal structures is an important diagnostic feature in helping to decide whether a particular lymph node is affected by a lymphoma or merely a reactive inflammatory process. With one exception lymphomata are uncommon tumours of the oral cavity. The exception is the *Burkitt tumour* (Fig. 18.12), a lymphoma occurring extensively in low-lying, moist regions of Central and West Africa.[28] It is peculiar in being almost exclusively confined to children between the ages of 2 and 14 years, and affecting the jaws (especially the maxilla), ovaries, retroperitoneal lymph nodes, and kidneys. The usual mode of presentation is as an enormous facial swelling with loosening of the neighbouring teeth.

**Lymphoma, Mixed-cell Type.** The lymph-node architecture is destroyed by neoplastic lymphoblasts and reticulum cells. It differs from Hodgkin's disease in that there are no Sternberg-Reed cells.

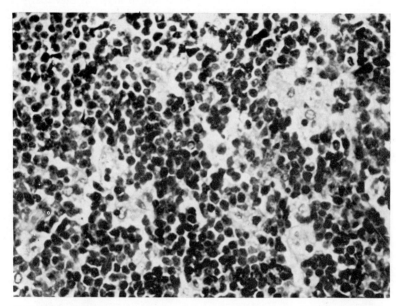

FIG. 18.12. Burkitt's tumour. Note the uniform lymphocytes, interspersed among which are large histiocytes. This is the "starry-sky appearance" stressed in Burkitt's tumour, though seen in other lymphocytic lymphomata also. × 400.

**Hodgkin's Disease.**[29-31] This is the commonest lymphoma, and attacks young and middle-aged adults predominantly. The affected lymph nodes are replaced by a characteristically pleomorphic mass of cells, the most important of which are neoplastic reticulum cells. These vary in size and shape, and include in their number giant cells with double, mirror-image nuclei (*Sternberg-Reed giant cells*, Fig. 18.13). The other cells present comprise lymphocytes, plasma cells, neutrophils, and often many eosinophils. There is a tendency to fibrosis, and sometimes to necrosis. Hodgkin's disease usually manifests with a localized enlargement of lymph nodes, but sometimes constitutional symptoms such as intermittent fever (Pel-Ebstein fever), wasting, and itching of the skin predominate. This is liable to occur especially when the abdominal nodes are primarily involved.

The prognosis of Hodgkin's disease has been related to histological appearances: four types are recognized. In the *lymphocytic predominant type*, previously called paragranuloma (a term now obsolete) Sternberg-Reed cells are scanty and lymphocytes are plentiful. The disease is much less malignant than the pleomorphic type described above, now described as the *mixed cellularity type*. It remains localized for a long time, and is amenable to local treatment such as radiotherapy. A nodular variant (*nodular sclerosing Hodgkin's disease*) also has a relatively good prognosis. The end stage of Hodgkin's disease, and therefore one that has the worst prognosis, is the *lymphocytic depletion type*, which is characterized by a paucity of lymphocytes with either diffuse fibrosis or else a proliferation of atypical Sternberg-Reed cells, this latter variant being previously called Hodgkin's sarcoma.

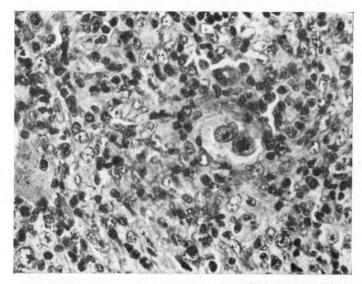

FIG. 18.13. Hodgkin's disease. In the centre of the field there is a binucleate Sternberg-Reed cell. It is surrounded by reticulum cells and lymphocytes. × 350.

The prognosis of Hodgkin's disease is also related to the extent of the disease and a system of staging has been evolved. It ranges from stage I, where there is involvement of the lymph nodes of one region, to stage IV, in which there is widespread disease.

**Other Generalized Lymphomata.** Although the majority of conditions in which there is a malignant proliferation of the stem cell and its derivatives can be placed in one of the categories already described, there are a number of rare diseases which appear to be separate entities. For these the concept of *malignant reticulosis* can be retained. Waldenström's macroglobulinaemia may be cited as an example, for there is a widespread proliferation of cells which are "plasmacytoid"—cells which are neither lymphocytes nor plasma cells.

**Malignant Conditions of the Haematopoietic Tissues.** The most important are the *leukaemias*, in which the malignant cells are found circulating in the peripheral blood, and *multiple myeloma*, in which the marrow is replaced by a plasma-cell tumour. These conditions are discussed in Chapters 26 and 33 respectively.

### Intermediate Tumours

In their behaviour this group of tumours lies between the benign and the malignant groups. Local invasion occurs, therefore the tumours cannot be regarded as benign. Nevertheless they do not show the steady inexorable growth pattern of true malignant tumours. The victims do not inevitably die of the disease if left untreated.

Several types of tumour may be considered under this somewhat controversial group of intermediate tumours, a term coined by Morehead.[32]

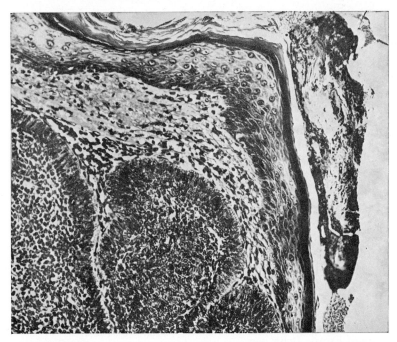

FIG. 18.14. Basal-cell carcinoma. Beneath the epidermis there is a solid mass of basal-cell carcinoma. The cells adjacent to the dermal stroma are arranged at right angles to it in the form of a palisade. × 200.

### Locally Malignant Tumours

The *rodent ulcer*, or *basal-cell carcinoma*, is a typical example of this group. Local invasion is prominent, but metastasis is so rare that it can for practical purposes be ignored.

The tumour is found most frequently on the skin of the face, and appears as an indurated ulcer with a hard, rolled, pearly border. Microscopically the dermis is infiltrated by groups of small round or fusiform cells with prominent darkly-staining nuclei. The layer of cells at the edge of each clump is usually arranged in the form of a palisade, and resembles the germinative layer of the normal epidermis (Fig. 18.14). Indeed, this tumour probably arises from these basal epidermal cells. It differs from squamous-cell carcinoma in that if the cells tend to show differentiation, it is into adnexal structures—hair follicles, sweat glands, or sebaceous glands—but not into cells of the surface epithelium.

The basal-cell carcinoma shows progressive local invasion and destruction of tissue. In its relentless course it may destroy the nose and eye, and finally it can penetrate the skull and lead to meningitis. Nevertheless, growth can sometimes be very slow, and it is common to find small tumours in patients who claim that the lesion has been present for several years.

The ameloblastoma is also a locally malignant tumour (p. 296).

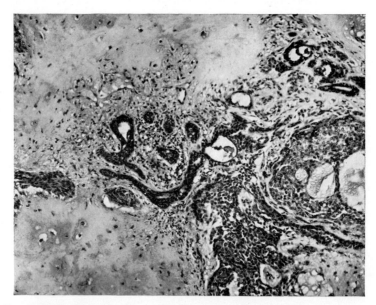

FIG. 18.15. Pleomorphic salivary gland tumour ("adenoma"). There are columns of epithelial cells, some arranged in ductules, surrounded by a dense, rather acellular stroma which resembles hyaline cartilage.  × 110.

### Tumours of Erratic Behaviour

Other tumours are known in which local invasion occurs, and occasionally distant metastases are produced. Usually, however, the distant metastases are small and do not shorten life. These tumours are of erratic behaviour, and a good example is the *pleomorphic salivary gland tumour*.

These tumours are found most commonly in the parotid gland, but may arise from other salivary glands and also the mucous glands of the oral mucosa, trachea, and bronchi. They consist of acini, cords, and thin strands of epithelial cells suspended in a stroma which often has a myxomatous appearance (Fig. 18.15). This was at one time regarded as true cartilage, and the tumour was called a "mixed parotid tumour". It is now realized that the mucoid appearance is due to a sero-mucinous secretion from the tumour cells into the stroma. True cartilage is very rarely found, and when it is present it is due to chondral metaplasia of the stroma.

The tumour may appear well encapsulated, but the capsule is often infiltrated by lateral extensions of growth. Simple enucleation is likely to be followed by recurrence. Furthermore, obvious local invasion may sometimes occur. Occasionally distant blood-borne metastases are encountered, even in tumours which appear "benign" microscopically.

There are a number of other tumours which show a similar erratic behaviour (e.g. "adenoma" of bronchus and carcinoid tumours of the intestine), but they are rare and will not be described. It will, however, be appreciated that as regards behaviour there exist tumours which range from those which may be called completely benign, which never invade and never metastasize, to those which are called malignant and which always invade and always metastasize.

## Difficulties in Tumour Classification

The difficulties encountered in the classification of neoplasms are those which are inherent in the classification of any condition of unknown aetiology. No single classification is wholly satisfactory. By examining tumours from different aspects various subdivisions are possible. While some classifications are more useful than others, none is more correct than the other. Histogenetic and behavioural characteristics form the basis of our present classification, but nevertheless certain difficulties are encountered. Those connected with behaviour have been considered. Difficulties encountered with histogenesis may be considered under five headings:

*Endothelium and Mesothelium.* The flattened lining cells of the serous spaces, like the pleural cavity, and the endothelial cells of blood vessels are sometimes regarded as epithelial, but in fact the tumours which are derived from them usually behave as connective tissue tumours, and are commonly classified as such.

*Undifferentiated Tumours.* A second difficulty in the histogenetic classification is the occurrence of tumours so poorly differentiated that their cell of origin defies recognition. Such anaplastic tumours are given names which are descriptive of the appearance of the cells. Large-cell, small-cell, pleomorphic-cell, giant-cell, spindle-cell, and oat-cell, are all self-explanatory terms when applied to tumours.

*Tumour Metaplasia.* A further difficulty arises when tumour cells differentiate in a direction other than that of the parent tissue; thus sometimes a tumour of glandular epithelium shows differentiation towards a keratinizing squamous-cell type. Such a tumour would be called a squamous-cell carcinoma, although it is of glandular origin (see carcinoma of lung, p. 413).

*Melanoma.* A fourth difficulty is the histogenetic classification of tumours arising from cells whose precise origin is disputed. The best example of this is the *melanoma* of the skin (p. 291).

*Placental and Embryonic Tumours.* Finally certain tumours arise from cells which are not normally present in the adult body. Two groups can be recognized:

(1) *Those of placental origin*, e.g. choriocarcinoma.

(2) *Tumours of Embryonic Origin.* These tumours arise from cells which,

TABLE 18.1

CLASSIFICATION OF TUMOURS

| Tissue of Origin | Behaviour | | |
|---|---|---|---|
| | Benign | Intermediate | Malignant |
| **Epithelium** | | | |
| 1. *Covering and Protective Epithelium* | | | |
| (*a*) Squamous | Squamous-cell papilloma | | Squamous-cell carcinoma |
| (*b*) Transitional | Transitional-cell papilloma | | Transitional-cell carcinoma |
| (*c*) Columnar | Columnar-cell papilloma | | Adenocarcinoma |
| 2. *Compact Secreting Epithelium* | Adenoma. If cystic, cyst-adenoma or papillary cyst-adenoma | | Adenocarcinoma. If cystic, cystadeno-carcinoma |
| 3. *Other Specialized Epithelium* | | Basal-cell carcinoma | |
| | Adenoma | Pleomorphic salivary and mucous gland tumours Carcinoid tumour (argentaffinoma) | Carcinoma |
| **Connective Tissue** | | | |
| Fibrous tissue | Fibroma | | Fibrosarcoma |
| Nerve sheath | Neurofibroma | | Neurofibrosarcoma |
| Fat | Lipoma | | Liposarcoma |
| Smooth muscle | Leiomyoma | | Leiomyosarcoma |
| Striated muscle | Rhabdomyoma | | Rhabdomyosarcoma |
| Synovium | Synovioma | | Malignant synovioma |
| Cartilage | Chondroma | | Chondrosarcoma |
| Bone Osteoblast | Osteoma | Giant-cell tumour | Osteosarcoma |
| Blood vessels and lymphatics | Benign haemangioma and lymphangioma | | Angiosarcoma Kaposi's sarcoma |
| Meninges | Meningioma | | Malignant meningioma |

## CLASSIFICATION OF TUMOURS—*continued*

| *Tissue of Origin* | Behaviour | | |
|---|---|---|---|
| | *Benign* | *Intermediate* | *Malignant* |
| Neuroglia | Astrocytoma, Oligodendroglioma, and Ependymoma* | | |
| Lymphoid and Reticulum cell | Benign lymphoma | | Lymphocytic lymphoma Reticulum-cell sarcoma Hodgkin's disease |
| Haematopoietic tissue | | | Multiple myeloma Leukaemias and polycythaemia vera |
| **Fetal Trophoblast** | Hydatidiform mole | | Choriocarcinoma |
| **Embryonic Tissue** | | | |
| *Totipotential cell* | Benign teratoma | | Malignant teratoma |
| *Pluripotential cell* | | | |
| Kidney | | | Nephroblastoma |
| Liver | | | Hepatoblastoma |
| *Unipotential cell* | | | |
| Retina | | | Retinoblastoma |
| Hind-brain | | | Medulloblastoma |
| Sympathetic ganglia and adrenal medulla | Ganglio-neuroma | | Neuroblastoma |
| **Embryonic Vestiges** | | | |
| Enamel organ | | Ameloblastoma | |
| Parapituitary residues | | Craniopharyngioma | |
| Branchial cyst | | | Branchiogenic carcinoma |
| **Hamartoma** | | | |
| Melanotic | | | Malignant melanoma |
| Angiomatous | ? Benign angioma | | Angiosarcoma |
| "Exostoses" and "Ecchondroses" | | | Chondrosarcoma |
| Neurofibromatosis | Neurofibroma | | Neurofibrosarcoma |

NOTE. Any malignant tumour may be so undifferentiated that it must be classified on a histological basis, e.g. carcinoma simplex, spindle-cell sarcoma, etc.

---

* These tumours are difficult to classify. The common types are locally malignant, but some also metastasize within the central nervous system. Rarely, they appear to be benign in children.

although present in the developing embryo, should normally have disappeared by the time of birth. They are considered in Chapter 20.

An outline of the present classification of tumours is shown in Table 18.I. It is evident that it is far from satisfactory, but since we have little useful basic knowledge regarding the nature of neoplasia this is hardly surprising. There is not even a satisfactory definition of a neoplasm, although that given by Willis is useful:[33] "*A tumour is an abnormal mass of tissue, the growth of which exceeds and is uncoordinated with that of the normal tissue, and persists in the same excessive manner after cessation of the stimuli which evoked the change.*"

It seems certain that the continued growth of tumours is quite useless, and the neoplastic response to a stimulus has no survival value in the evolutionary process. When it is remembered that most tumours occur during the postreproductive years this is not altogether surprising.

## References

1. DUKES, C. E. (1952). *Ann. Eugen. (Lond.)*, **17**, 1.
2. LOCKHART-MUMMERY, H. E. (1967). *Proc. roy. Soc. Med.*, **60**, 381.
3. DORMANDY, T. L. (1957). *New Engl. J. Med.*, **256**, 1093, 1141 and 1186.
4. SHEWARD, J. D. (1962). *Brit. med. J.*, **1**, 921.
5. BURDICK, D., PRIOR, J. T. and SCANLON, G. T. (1963). *Cancer*, **16**, 854.
6. EVERSON, T. C. and COLE, W. H. (1956). *Ann. Surg.*, **144**, 366.
7. BRUNSCHWIG, A. (1963). *Surgery*, **53**, 423.
8. BOYD, W. (1966). "The Spontaneous Regression of Cancer". 99 pp. Springfield, Ill.: Thomas.
9. EVERSON, T. C. (1964). *Ann. N. Y. Acad. Sci.*, **114**, 721.
10. SMITH, R. A. (1971). *Brit. med. J.*, **2**, 563.
11. CAHN, L. R. (1965). *Brit. J. oral Surg.*, **2**, 166.
12. AZZOPARDI, J. G. (1966). In "Recent Advances in Pathology", p. 98, 8th ed., ed. by Harrison, C. V. London: Churchill.
13. SNEDDON, I. B. (1963). *Brit. med. J.*, **2**, 405.
14. WHEELER, C. E., ABELE, D. C. and BRIGGAMAN, R. A. (1967). *Postgrad. Med.*, **41**, 494.
15. BRAIN, R. (1963). *Lancet*, **1**, 179.
16. LIEBERMAN, J. S. *et al.* (1961). *J. Amer. med. Ass.*, **177**, 542.
17. HOBBS, C. B. and MILLER, A. L. (1966). *J. clin. Path.*, **19**, 119.
18. Leading Article (1968). *Brit. med. J.*, **4**, 5.
19. PRYCE, D. M. and WALTER, J. B. (1960). *J. Path. Bact.*, **79**, 141.
20. DRURY, R. A. B., PALMER, P. H. and HIGHMAN, W. J. (1964). *J. clin. Path.*, **17**, 448.
21. GREENOUGH, R. B. (1925). *J. Cancer Res.*, **9**, 453.
22. BLOOM, H. J. G. (1950). *Brit. J. Cancer*, **4**, 259.
23. LUCAS, R. B. (1972). In "Pathology of Tumours of the Oral Tissues", 2nd ed. p. 132 *et seq.*, London: Churchill.
24. HADFIELD, G. (1954). *Brit. med. J.*, **2**, 607.
25. BRODERS, A. C. (1921). *Ann. Surg.*, **73**, 141.
26. ANDERSON, W. A. D. (1971). edr, "Pathology", Vol 2, p. 1336 *et seq.*, St. Louis: Mosby.
27. RAPPAPORT, H., WINTER, W. J. and HICKS, E. B. (1956). *Cancer (Philad.)*, **9**, 792.
28. HARRIS, R. J. C. (1964). *Brit. med. Bull.*, **20**, 149.
29. LUKES, R. J. and BUTLER, J. J. (1966). *Cancer Res.*, **26**, 1063.
30. LUKES, R. J., BUTLER, J. J. and HICKS, E. B. (1966). *Cancer (Philad.)*, **19**, 317.

31. SMITHERS, D. (1972). *Proc. roy. Soc. Med.*, **65**, 61.
32. MOREHEAD, R. P. (1965). In "Human Pathology", p. 63. New York: McGraw-Hill.
33. WILLIS, R. A. (1967). In "Pathology of Tumours", 4th ed., p. 1. London: Butterworths.

*Chapter 19*

# THE AETIOLOGY AND INCIDENCE OF TUMOURS

## Introduction

In spite of a vast amount of research into the cause of cancer, the essential difference between the neoplastic and the normal cell is unknown. Insofar as man is concerned, much is known about the incidence of particular tumours. Careful observations have established that some types of malignancy are particularly common in groups who are subjected to abnormal *occupational* or *environmental* factors. This has led to the recognition of various chemical and physical agents which are responsible, and which are called *carcinogenic agents*. A large number of these is now known.

On a more intimate level hereditary factors have been studied by observing certain families which are known to bear the trait of neoplastic diseases.

The experimental side of cancer research concerns the artificial production of tumours in animals. As in man, *chemical, physical*, and *hereditary factors* have been investigated, and in addition it is possible to study tumours by transplanting them from one animal to another. This work has led to the recognition that cell-free extracts can on occasion induce tumour formation, and that *viruses* appear to be responsible.

Although there are many known causes of cancer in animals, most tumours in man arise spontaneously in response to an unknown stimulus. In a few instances human neoplasms can be attributed to some tangible preceding cause.

The three factors generally recognized as causes of human neoplasia are:
*External chemical and physical agents.*
*Hereditary predisposition.*
*Chronic disease,* usually of an inflammatory nature.
Two additional factors have to be considered, *hormones* and *viruses*.

## External Carcinogenic Agents[1, 2]

### Chemical Carcinogens

It has been known since the eighteenth century that those people whose occupation brings them into contact with coal tar or mineral oil are liable to develop carcinoma of the skin. The chemicals concerned are *aromatic polycyclic hydrocarbons*, and credit is due to the Japanese workers Yamagiwa and Ichikawa, who were the first to produce skin cancers in rabbits by painting their ears with tar. The next step was the isolation of the actual chemical substances in tar which were responsible for carcinogenesis. The first to be discovered, by Kennaway, was the hydrocarbon *1:2:5:6-dibenzanthracene*.[3] Subsequently *methylcholanthrene, 3:4-benzpyrene*, and many others have been isolated. The important agent in human cancer of this type is 3:4-benzpyrene.

Another group of chemicals, the *aromatic amines,* are also carcinogenic.[4, 5] Their importance stems from the fact that workers in the aniline-dye industry are particularly liable to develop bladder cancer. The carcinogen concerned is *2-amino-1-naphthol,* a substance which is excreted in the urine, being formed in the body from aromatic amines, chief among them being $\beta$-naphthylamine, used in the dye, rubber, and cable industries. This is an example of *remote carcinogenesis,* since the agent though taken by mouth, produces its effects in the urinary passages.

Certain *natural foodstuffs* carry a carcinogenic hazard. The mould *Aspergillus flaveus,* which contaminates ground-nut meal, produces a toxin, *aflatoxin,* which is a powerful liver carcinogen. This may well explain why this type of cancer is so prevalent in Africa.

**Genetic Influence in Chemical Carcinogenesis.** An important feature of experimental carcinogenesis is that animals react specifically. Many fruitless years were spent trying to induce coal-tar cancers in rats and dogs, animals which are almost completely resistant. Furthermore, dissimilar strains of animals respond differently. Thus the administration of a particular carcinogenic substance to different strains of animals will produce differing effects. In some there may be no tumour formation at all, while others may show tumours of various organs.

## Physical Carcinogenic Agents

The important relationship between ionizing radiation and cancer is considered in detail in Chapter 21. Ultraviolet radiation exerts its harmful effect in the form of strong sunlight continually acting on the exposed skin of fair-complexioned people. Farmers in Australia and South Africa, sailors, and others habitually exposed to the elements, tend in later life to develop multiple lesions on their faces and hands (*senile,* or *solar, keratoses*), and these sometimes develop into squamous-cell carcinomata. *Basal-cell carcinoma* is also more common in this group of people, as is *carcinoma of the lip.*

## The Latent Period in Carcinogenesis

An important factor notable in all occupational and environmental cancers is the long latent period which elapses from the time of application of the agent to the time of the first appearance of the tumour. This may vary from 5 to over 20 years, and it is evident that there is ample time for the initiating stimulus to be completely forgotten by the patient. The same latent period is also evident in experimental work on animals, although here it is measured in weeks or months rather than years.

## The Precancerous State: Initiation and Promotion[6-8]

During the early years of experimental coal tar carcinogenesis it was noticed that the skin of an animal which had been painted with tar was particularly liable to develop tumours at the site of any wound subsequently inflicted on the painted area. The concept arose that carcinogenesis was a two-stage phenomenon. The application of a carcinogen to the skin produced a change which was called *initiation,* such that when any part of the area was subsequently wounded or damaged by a second agent, which was called a *promoter*, a tumour developed at the site of injury. In addition to trauma itself, non-specific irritants such as croton oil, chloroform, etc. were found to be efficient promoting agents.

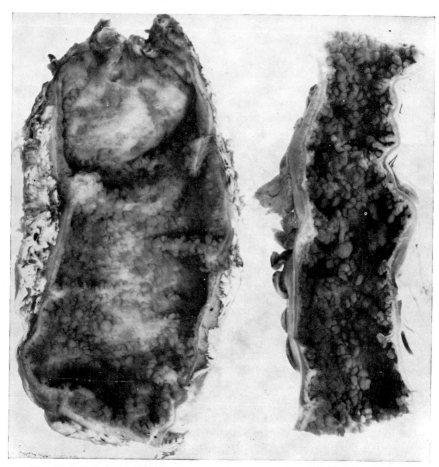

FIG. 19.1. Polyposis coli. The mucosa of the descending colon and rectum is studded with polyps, some of which are pedunculated and others sessile. The bowel wall and the intervening mucosa are normal. None of the polyps shows macroscopic evidence of malignancy.

(A74.4. *Reproduced by permission of the president and Council of the Royal College of Surgeons of England.*)

Skin which had been initiated frequently showed no histological evidence of the change. Initiation could be demonstrated only by the subsequent development of tumours following the application of a promoting agent. Experimental evidence indicated that initiated skin could remain in this state of precancer for long periods. When this concept is applied to occupational cancer, the long latent period between leaving employment and the development of the tumour becomes more readily understandable.

### Hereditary Predisposition

It is doubtful whether there is any significant hereditary predisposition to most of the common types of cancer, for statistical surveys among relatives of cancer patients have not yielded convincing evidence of an increased incidence of tumours in them. Cancer of the breast is possibly somewhat more common in the relatives of affected women than in the population at large.

There are, however, a number of uncommon neoplastic diseases which are inherited.

The trait of *polyposis coli* is transmitted as an autosomal dominant.[9] Multiple adenomata of the colon usually first manifest themselves at puberty (Fig. 19.1). They are not present at birth. By the time the patient reaches the age of 30 years, multiple colonic cancers appear. Life is seldom prolonged over the age of 40 years. Gardner's syndrome is a variant (see p. 244).

*Xeroderma pigmentosum* is inherited as an autosomal recessive trait.[10] The skin is abnormally susceptible to the effects of sunlight, and multiple squamous-cell and basal-cell carcinomata develop on the exposed parts. Death usually occurs within the first decade.

The inherited susceptibility to the action of carcinogen in experimental work has been mentioned above.

### Chronic Disease as a Cause of Cancer

#### Chronic Irritation

Although commonly cited as a cause of cancer, a concept of chronic irritation is too vague to have much meaning nowadays. It is extremely doubtful whether physical irritation acting alone can ever produce cancer, though it may certainly promote a tumour in a field already initiated by a carcinogenic substance. There are, however, a number of chronic diseases which may from time to time be complicated by malignancy. These are called precancerous lesions.

#### Precancerous Lesions

A precancerous lesion is any condition in which cancer is more liable to develop than in the normal tissue. The following examples should be noted:

*Chronic ulcers.* The sinuses of chronic osteomyelitis, and old burn scars occasionally give rise to squamous-cell carcinoma.[11]

*Syphilitic glossitis* was regarded as an important precursor of oral cancer. It was often associated with leukoplakia on the tongue and elsewhere in the mouth, and this condition often proceeds to malignancy. But whether the leukoplakia was due to syphilis, or whether the syphilis was merely a coincidental lesion is not certain.

*Ulcerative colitis.* About 4 per cent of all cases eventually develop carcinoma.[12]

*Cirrhosis.* Primary liver-cell cancer is usually superimposed on a previous cirrhosis. Liver cancer is extremely prevalent in African races and also among the Chinese and Japanese. This is undoubtedly due to the high incidence of nutritional cirrhosis, and is not dependent upon racial factors.

*The Plummer-Vinson syndrome* is associated with post-cricoid carcinoma[13] (pp. 343–344).

*Paget's disease of bone* is occasionally complicated by osteosarcoma.

*Malformations.* There are a number of *hamartomatous lesions* which occasionally become malignant, for example neurofibromatosis.

A *congenitally abnormal organ*, e.g. an imperfectly descended testis, is more liable to malignancy than is a normal one.

### Hormones and Neoplasia[14, 15]

The early observations that oestrogens were a factor in the causation of cancer of the breast in mice led to widespread speculation that such a mechanism was applicable to man. However, it soon became evident that in mice other more important factors are operative, namely *genetic predisposition* and the *Bittner virus*. So far as man is concerned, there is little evidence that hormonal imbalance is responsible for the production of any tumour, except under very unusual circumstances. Thus enormous doses of oestrogen (as secreted by granulosa-cell tumours of the ovary) may lead to endometrial and breast cancer. Vaginal cancer has been reported in young girls whose mothers were given oestrogen during the pregnancy in which they were fetuses.[16, 36]

**Hormone-Dependent Tumours.** If hormones cannot be directly incriminated in the aetiology of human cancer, they are undoubtedly of great importance in maintaining the growth of some tumours. These are called the *hormone-dependent tumours*, and the best example is *carcinoma of the prostate*.

Both the normal prostatic epithelium and the carcinomata derived from it are dependent for their integrity upon a supply of testosterone. If patients with carcinoma of the prostate are castrated, there is often a dramatic relief of symptoms and regression of the tumour and its metastases. Nowadays large doses of stilboestrol are given, and surgical castration is unnecessary. The relief may last for at least five years, and, as many of the patients are over 70 years of age, some succumb to intercurrent illness before the cancer loses its hormone dependency and once more pursues its progressive course.

*Carcinoma of the breast* is another tumour which manifests hormone dependence in some patients. The picture is, however, complicated, because the tumour may depend upon ovarian, adrenal, or pituitary hormones. Nevertheless, in some patients the removal of the ovaries, adrenals, or pituitary produces a marked but temporary remission. In other cases the administration of oestrogens or testosterone may have an ameliorative effect.

### Viruses and Neoplasia[17–19]

Tumour-producing (oncogenic) viruses are arousing much interest, for an increasing number of animal tumours are proving to have a virus aetiology. The first such tumour was fowl leukaemia (Ellerman and Bang, 1908) and it was followed by fowl sarcoma (Rous 1911), rabbit papilloma (Shope, 1932), renal adenocarcinoma in frogs (Lucké, 1934), and mammary carcinoma in mice (Bittner, 1936). The last agent is transmitted from the mother to its offspring in the milk, but the tumour does not occur until the female mice attain maturity, since oestrogens must first act to produce breast development.

Gross (1951) isolated the virus of mouse leukaemia, and in 1953 a second unrelated virus was found in his material. This was remarkable in that it produced tumours in many species of mice, rats, hamsters, and other animals. Furthermore many types of tumour were produced. The salivary glands were especially vulnerable, but tumours of the connective tissues, breasts, and kidneys were also encountered. This agent is now called the *polyoma virus*, and is widely distributed in nature, apparently lying latent in many mice. Certain human and simian *adenoviruses* are oncogenic in baby hamsters, as is also a virus that can be cultivated from the monkey-kidney tissue used in the preparation of poliomyelitis vaccines.

In order to establish the virus aetiology of a tumour it is necessary to transmit the lesion by bacteriologically sterile, cell-free filtrates to other animals. It has also been found that some oncogenic viruses, notably polyoma virus, induce changes in cells grown in tissue culture. This phenomenon, *cell transformation*, is indicated by a rapid proliferation of the cells with copious irregular mitotic activity, and when they are transplanted into animals they exhibit malignant propensities.[20,21] Some tumour viruses contain DNA and others RNA, and both can transform normal cells into genetically stable cancer cells. In the DNA-containing virus, the nucleic acid is integrated into the chromosomes of the host cell. In RNA-containing viruses, the RNA is transcribed into a DNA provirus, which is integrated as above. This process is called *reverse transcription*, because normally it is chromosomal DNA which is transcribed into messenger RNA (p. 16). This reverse phenomenon is an exceptional state of affairs, and is brought about by RNA-dependent DNA polymerase, or reverse transcriptase.[22]

It is important to realize that the mere presence of a virus in a cancer is no indication of its causal role. Cancers frequently harbour *passenger viruses*, which lie latent and play no part in the neoplastic growth.

It is not certain whether oncogenic viruses merely initiate cells which then pursue an independent course of neoplasia (as with chemical agents), or whether the presence of the virus (perhaps in an unrecognized form) is necessary for the continued propagation of the tumour.

At present much research is being done in investigating a virus aetiology for certain human tumours. The essential criterion, the inoculation of suspected viruses into human beings, is clearly impracticable. So far the neoplasm in man which seems most likely to have a virus origin is the Burkitt tumour (p. 263). The *Epstein-Barr virus* is closely associated with it (p. 349), for patients always have a high titre of antibodies to this herpesvirus, which is also associated with infectious mononucleosis. Perhaps a combination of chronic lymphoreticular hyperplasia due to recurrent malarial infection and an assault by this virus produces the Burkitt tumour. This suggestion would help to explain the sharp geographical distribution of the tumour.[23]

### The Origin of Tumours

Two major theories have been put forward:

## Cell Rests

Cohnheim originally suggested that all tumours arose from *cell rests* which had become sequestrated during embryonic development. Neoplastic change in these cells was thought to form the basis of tumours in later life. This explanation is possible in regard to certain teratomata and tumours arising in infancy, but it is no longer acceptable that cell rests give rise to the common tumours in adult life. The postulated rests have never been found, and the evidence is strongly in favour of the concept that tumours are derived from cells which were at one time normal.

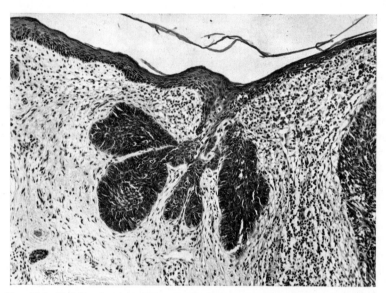

Fig. 19.2. Multifocal origin of basal-cell carcinoma. The epidermis around the small tumour is normal, but at the edge of the section there is part of a much larger basal-cell carcinoma. × 100.

## Origin from Previously Normal Cells

**Fields of Growth.** The modern theory of tumour formation is that in most cases* a whole area of tissue becomes predisposed to neoplasia.[24] Such an area constitutes a *field of growth*. The concept is vital for understanding the current views on carcinogenesis, for in experimental work an area of tissue of the test animal treated with the particular agent becomes an artificially induced field of growth, analogous to that of the human subject exposed to a similar stimulus in the course of his occupation. Clinical substantiation of this theory depends on two observations:

(1) The tendency for *multiple tumours* to arise in a restricted area of tissue (Fig. 19.2).

* It is probable that in some tumours a single cell or cell type becomes malignant, proliferates, and replaces the surrounding normal cells. The monoclonal gammopathies are good examples, and the neoplastic cells produce a single M protein (p. 330).

(2) The frequency of *recurrences* appearing near the area where a primary tumour has been completely removed.

**Multiple Primary Tumours.** There are many examples:

*Multiple squamous-cell and basal-cell carcinomata* of the face.

*Multiple papillomata* of the ureter and bladder.

*Oral cancer.* Multiple primary tumours appear in about 10 per cent of patients with oral cancer. Carcinoma of the mouth is also associated with primary squamous-cell carcinoma elsewhere, for instance in the larynx, oesophagus, or lung.

*Polyposis coli* (Fig. 19.1).

*Cancer of the liver* supervening on cirrhosis is often multicentric.

*Leiomyomata of the uterus.*

**Recurrences of Tumour.** The origin of a recurrent tumour following in the wake of an excised one is sometimes difficult to decide. Malignant tumours infiltrate so insidiously that a group of cells may be left behind to form the origin of a new tumour mass. Nevertheless, there are many good examples of recurrent tumour occurring in an adjacent area of the field of growth. Such recurrences may be seen following the removal of a carcinoma of the tongue in leukoplakia. Thus the field of growth concept of tumour formation has important surgical consequences. Only complete excision of the entire field can ensure that no further tumours develop.

## Multiple Factors as a Cause of Neoplasia

Although the simple two-stage mechanism in the formation of tumours (see initiation and promotion, p. 273) is now less clear in the light of more recent evidence, it is nevertheless true that the production of tumours involves several different factors. This is called *cocarcinogenesis.*

Oestrogens will promote cancer in mouse breast which has been initiated either by application of hydrocarbons or by infection with the Bittner virus. Radiation will induce leukaemia in mice due to the fact that a leukaemia-producing virus is apparently lying latent in the animals.[18] The disease is then transmissible by the virus. The Shope papilloma virus will produce malignant tumours in rabbits when the skin has been tarred beforehand. There is a similar two-stage mode of carcinogenesis in respect of remotely acting agents. Croton oil produces cancer in the skin initiated by the oral administration of the powerful carcinogenic compound 2-acetylaminofluorene.[25] It is no wonder, what with the long latent periods involved and the multiplicity of agents which may be concerned, that the cause of many human cancers remains unknown.

## Early Malignant Lesions

In man the question of early malignant change is of great importance, for it is at this stage that complete eradication of the disease is easiest. In recent years a number of interesting lesions involving epithelial surfaces has been recognized. In these areas there is a typical epithelial proliferation with the cells showing the microscopical changes usually associated with malignancy. They vary in size and shape, have large, darkly-stained nuclei, and show an increased amount of mitotic activity. The cells tend to lose their polarity, and lie haphazardly in relationship to one another. In stratified squamous epithelium there may be foci of abnormal keratinization within the area of cell proliferation, and this is called *malignant dyskeratosis*. However, there is no invasion, and the lesion cannot truly be called malignant. The name *carcinoma-in-situ*, or *intraepithelial carcinoma*, is usually applied.

Carcinoma-in-situ has been described in most epithelia, and is encountered most typically in the skin, where it is called *Bowen's disease* (see Fig. 19.3). It is seen also in the oral cavity either as an isolated lesion or in association with leukoplakia. Carcinoma-in-situ has, however, been most extensively studied in the cervix uteri by means of the technique of exfoliative cytology.

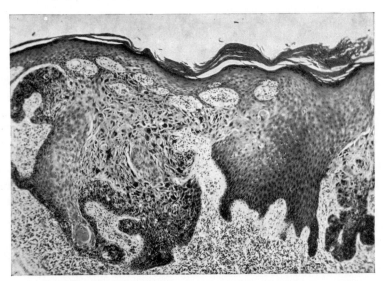

F\ıG. 19.3. Malignant dyskeratosis. The typical pleomorphic appearance of *carcinoma-in-situ* is seen in the proliferating epithelial mass, and in its advancing edge there is a focus of keratinization. Although in places there is a suggestion of invasion, serial sections of the block did not confirm this. × 83.

## Exfoliative Cytology[26–28]

When cancer involves a lining epithelium, some of the neoplastic cells are shed on to the surrounding surface. If the surface is internal these cells are trapped in the secretions of the part, and are ultimately discharged to the exterior. Bronchial carcinoma cells may be coughed up in the sputum, gastric carcinoma cells may be aspirated in the gastric juice, and cervical carcinoma cells may be shed into the vaginal secretions. In recent years much progress has been made in recognizing clumps of cancer cells in such secretions, and sometimes this allows the early diagnosis of malignant disease. The technique was pioneered by Papanicolaou, and has been applied especially to the study of cervical cancer ("Pap smear").

It is often assumed that the onset of malignant change is a sudden event, but exfoliative cytology has shown that in the case of the cervix uteri this is certainly not so. There is considerable evidence that the first change in the epithelium involves certain cellular abnormalities which have been called *dysplasia*. The nuclei are enlarged, show variation in size and shape, and are hyperchromatic (*dyskaryosis*). The epithelium is not as abnormal as has been described in *carcinoma-in-situ*. Nevertheless, a dysplastic epithelium is thought to progress to a state of *carcinoma-in-situ* and finally to one of true invasive squamous-cell carcinoma. The whole process is apparently drawn out over a long period, probably in the order of 10 years. Routine cytological examinations will detect early lesions, which although not cancerous themselves, are thought to progress to invasive, killing cancer. The same situation applies in the mouth. All suggestive or atypical lesions should be smeared to detect the presence of abnormal cells. If these are found, biopsy should be carried out. Dysplastic epithelium may be watched and treated, but if *carcinoma-in-situ* is present, excision of the whole lesion is indicated.

## Incidence of Certain Tumours

### Cancers of the Skin

**Geographical Factors.** The incidence of basal-cell and squamous-cell cancers of the exposed parts of fair-skinned people living in the tropics has already been noted. A more localized example of a geographical incidence of skin cancer is encountered in the *Kangri cancer of Kashmir*. The Kangri, a charcoal-heated basket, is carried close to the skin of the abdomen, and its continued use is often accompanied by carcinoma of the abdominal skin. It is probable that the carcinogenic agents in the fumes initiate the tumour, and the heat of the basket acts as a promoting agent.

**Occupational Factors.** The industrial hazards of exposure to ionizing radiations and polycyclic hydrocarbons are now largely of historic interest, since strict public health regulations have been introduced.

**Hereditary Predisposition.** Xeroderma pigmentosum has already been noted.

**Chronic Skin Lesions** have already been described as precursors of squamous-cell cancer. The prolonged ingestion of arsenic compounds sometimes leads to basal-cell and squamous-cell cancers.

### Cancer of the Lip

This is commonest in elderly, pipe-smoking, agricultural workers; sunlight probably initiates the tumour and the heat of the pipe promotes it to activity.

### Cancer of the Mouth

**Geographical Factors.** Oral cancer is very common among some communities in South-East Asia who indulge in the habit of *betel chewing*.[29] The quid which is kept in the mouth for long periods of time consists of betel nut, spices, tobacco, lime, and buyo leaves. It is probably the betel that is the carcinogenic agent.[30] Cancer of the buccal aspects of the cheek and lower jaw is the usual site, but the tongue may also be involved. Another peculiar habit associated with oral cancer is *reverse cigar smoking* which is practised in parts of India, Sardinia, and Latin America.[31] The lighted end of the cigar is held in the mouth, which is burned in consequence. Cancer of the palate and tongue may ensue.

**Chronic Disease.** Oral cancer has been attributed to hot foods, alcohol, and chronic dental disease, but there is no convincing evidence that this is true. Tertiary syphilis with leukoplakia was said to be an important pre-disposing factor in the past. Women with the Plummer-Vinson syndrome show an increased incidence of oral cancer.

### Cancer of the Lung

The alarming increase in incidence of bronchial cancer in recent years has focussed much attention on the problem. There can be little doubt that *heavy tobacco smoking* predisposes to lung cancer, and that the danger is greater in cigarette users than in pipe smokers.[32] Another factor of undetermined importance is atmospheric pollution with soot and smoke. It probably acts together with tobacco smoking in producing lung cancer.

In certain *industries* cancer of the lung can be attributed to the inhalation of radioactive substances, nickel, chromium, or asbestos. This last produces pleural mesothelioma as well as squamous-cell lung cancer.

There is no evidence that chronic inflammatory diseases such as tuberculosis and bronchiectasis are precancerous.

### Nature of the Cancer Cell

**Changes in Appearance.** The pleomorphism and bizarre appearance of cancer cells have already been described in detail. There is, however, no constant variation characteristic of all malignant cells.

**Changes in Chemical Content.** No definite change in the DNA or RNA composition of malignant cells has yet been described. Extensive investigation of the enzyme contents of malignant cells has shown that tumour cells tend to contain the same enzymes as do the parent tissue, but that the quantity is usually reduced. So far no specific change has been found.

**Antigens.**[33] There is considerable evidence that some tumours are deficient in antigens. Tumours tend to grow as allogeneic homografts and heterografts under conditions where normal tissues would not. It is tempting to think that this lack of antigenicity might be a factor in allowing malignant cells to permeate freely into tissues where normal cells are not allowed to proceed.

On the other hand, some tumours induced by hydrocarbons and viruses develop new transplantation antigens. Tumours introduced by hydrocarbons are capable of manifesting antigenicity in the strain of origin, so that the host becomes resistant to a challenge of the same tumour. The antigens are indi-vidual for the particular tumour. With virus-induced tumours the new trans-plantation antigen is tumour-specific, and is the same for all tumours pro-duced by the particular virus. Anti-viral antibodies are also produced. Some tumours produce new antigens which are not transplantation antigens and their detection can be used as an aid to diagnosis. Thus some carcinomata of the colon produce an antigen normally only found in the fetus (called *carcino-embryonic antigen*), and this antigen together with its antibody can be detected in the plasma.[35] It is interesting that carcinogens, both chemical and virus, are more potent in immunologically inadequate hosts, e.g. the newborn mouse. It seems that immunity to cancer lies primarily in the lymphocytes, and a heavy lymphocyte response around a malignant tumour is of good prognostic import. Immunoglobulins may be of some importance, both in activating complement which lyses some tumour cells and in protecting the tumour cells from the onslaught of lymphocytes (enhancement). These two effects would tend to neutralize each other.[34]

**Changes in Behaviour.** *In vivo.* Progressive growth is characteristic of neoplasia. Malignant tumours invade and metastasize. Even so the phenomena of dormancy and regression indicate that some tumours undergo phases of retrenchment.

*In vitro.* Malignant cells do not on the whole grow as readily in tissue culture as do normal cells. Those that do grow tend to lack the alignment that is seen with normal cells, and there is less adherence to one another and to the glass than is normally seen.

This brief survey of the properties of cancer cells is sufficient to indicate that although there are often many points of difference from the normal, there is no single characteristic by which they can be recognized. Perhaps it is wrong to expect that this should be so. The well-documented morphological features of cancer cells are of great importance to the cytologist and diagnostic histologist, but researches into cell metabolism have been essentially sterile both as regards a reliable cancer test and the elaboration of an effective chemotherapeutic agent. Studies of the antigenic composition and the *in-vitro* behaviour of tumour cells may perhaps yield more fruitful results.

It is humiliating to reflect that the vast majority of tumours in man arise with no apparent cause and appear to develop spontaneously. While some geographical factors are suggestive and a few occupational hazards have been successfully unmasked and controlled, there is still no indication as to the fundamental abnormality in cancer or the nature of its progressive growth.

## Control of Cancer

The most successful approach to the control of cancer at the present time lies in its prevention. The many known physical and chemical carcinogenic agents have already been described, and their avoidance can appreciably reduce the incidence of cancer. A second method of cancer prophylaxis is the treatment of known precancerous lesions. In the previous chapter a point of view has been expressed that cancer must be defined and diagnosed in terms of its invasive behaviour. The observations on the development of uterine cancer have led us to believe that the invasive tumour is the final development of a sequence of precancerous lesions. These lesions are sometimes reflected in the abnormal appearance of the cells, and, in the cervix, they can be detected and treated with relative ease. Cancer of the cervix uteri is therefore a preventable disease, and the same almost certainly applies to cancer of the oral cavity and tongue. Unfortunately in other organs the outlook is less bright. There is as yet no means of detecting the early stages of cancer of the breast, stomach, or colon. All three are extremely common tumours.

It is to be hoped that future discoveries will throw fresh light on the nature of neoplastic growth, so that more efficacious and less mutilating procedures may be developed to deal with the disease. At the present time there is much information regarding animal tumours but remarkably little concerning cancer in humans.

## References

1. HUEPER, W. C. (1954). *Arch. Path.*, **58**, 360, 475 and 645.
2. GOLDBLATT, M. W. (1958). *Brit. med. Bull.*, **14**, 136.
3. KENNAWAY, E. L. (1930). *Biochem. J.*, **24**, 497.
4. BOYLAND, E. (1958). *Brit. med. Bull.*, **14**, 153.
5. WEISBURGER, E. K. and WEISBURGER, J. H. (1958). *Advanc. Cancer Res.*, **5**, 331. New York: Academic Press.
6. BONSER, G. M. and JULL, J. W. (1960). In "Recent Advances in Pathology", 7th ed., p. 384, ed. by Harrison, C. V. London: Churchill.
7. BERENBLUM, I. and SHUBIK, P. (1947). *Brit. J. Cancer*, **1**, 379 and 383.
8. SALAMAN, M. H. and ROE, F. J. C. (1964). *Brit. med. Bull.*, **20**, 139.
9. DUKES, C. E. (1952). *Ann. Eugen. (Lond.)*, **17**, 1.
10. COPELAND, M. M. and MARTIN, H. E. (1932). *Amer. J. Cancer*, **16**, 1337.
11. CRUICKSHANK, A. H., McCONNELL, E. M. and MILLER, D. G. (1963). *J. clin. Path.*, **16**, 573.
12. Leading Article (1967). *Brit. med. J.*, **1**, 322.
13. WYNDER, E. L. and FRYER, J. H. (1958). *Ann. intern. Med.*, **49**, 1106.
14. BIELSCHOWSKY, F. and HORNING, E. S. (1958). *Brit. med. Bull.*, **14**, 106.
15. BONSER, G. M. and JULL, J. W. (1960). In "Recent Advances in Pathology", p. 415, *loc. cit.*
16. Leading Article (1971). *Lancet*, **1**, 1111.
17. ANDREWES, C. (1964). *Brit. med. J.*, **1**, 653.
18. FURTH, J., YOROKO, K. and TAKEMOTO, H. (1962). In "Ciba Foundation Symposium on Tumour Viruses of Murine Origin", p. 138. London: Churchill.
19. LEVY, B. M. (1966). *J. dent. Res.*, **45**, 528.
20. KOPROWSKI, H. *et al.* (1962). *J. cell. comp. Physiol.*, **59**, 281.
21. HABEL, K. (1961). *Proc. Soc. exp. Biol. (N.Y.)*, **106**, 722.
22. Editorial (1970). *Nature*, **226**, 1198.
23. WEDDERBURN, N. (1970). *Lancet*, **2**, 1114.
24. WILLIS, R. A. (1944 and 1945). *Cancer Res.*, **4**, 630 and **5**, 469.
25. RITCHIE, A. C. and SAFFIOTTI, U. (1955). *Cancer Res.*, **15**, 84.
26. WAY, S. (1963). "The Diagnosis of Early Carcinoma of the Cervix." London: Churchill.
27. KOSS, L. G. (1968). "Diagnostic Cytology", 2nd ed. Philadelphia: Lippincott.
28. BAMFORTH, J. (1966). "Cytology in Medical Practice." London: Churchill.
29. ORR, I. M. (1933). *Lancet*, **2**, 575.
30. SURI, K., GOLDMAN, H. M. and WELLS, H. (1971). *Nature*, **230**, 383.
31. KINI, M. G. (1944). *Indian med. Gaz.*, **79**, 572.
32. DOLL, R. and HILL, A. B. (1964). *Brit. med. J.*, **1**, 1399 and 1460.
33. HUMPHREY, J. H. and WHITE, R. G. (1970). "Immunology for Students of Medicine", 3rd ed., p. 580. Oxford: Blackwell.
34. Leading Article (1971). *Lancet*, **2**, 753.
35. ZAMCHECK, N. *et al.* (1972). *New Engl. J. Med.*, **286**, 83.
36. HERBST, A. L. *et al.* (1972). *New Engl. J. Med.*, **287**, 1259.

*Chapter 20*

# DEVELOPMENTAL ANOMALIES: DEVELOPMENTAL TUMOURS AND TUMOUR-LIKE CONDITIONS

**Introduction.** It is incredible that in the course of a few months, a single cell, the fertilized ovum, can proliferate and differentiate into the complex system of organs and tissues that constitute the mature organism. Minor variations are so common that the differences which result are regarded as normal. More serious errors in development result in the production of various malformations which are usually apparent at birth, but which may develop at any time during the growing period of childhood and adolescence. Gross abnormalities may be incompatible with life, and these result in abortion, stillbirth, or neonatal death.

## Causes of Developmental Anomalies

Developmental anomalies may occur either as a result of genetic errors or be due to environmental factors.

**Genetic Errors.** These have been described in Chapter 3. Chromosomal abnormalities should always be looked for when developmental anomalies are present.

**Environmental Factors.** It is becoming increasingly obvious that many external agents are capable of causing serious developmental anomalies. Those that act *in utero* have the most severe effect.

*Infection.*[1] Transmission of infection from the mother to the fetus may cause severe damage. The first trimester of pregnancy is the most dangerous time, as it is during this period that rapid division and differentiation occur. Rubella has acquired a particularly evil reputation: deformities occur in as many as 25 per cent of babies born to mothers who have had this infection during pregnancy.

*Drugs.*[2] A notorious tragedy occurred around the period of 1960, when pregnant women who had taken the sedative thalidomide gave birth to grossly deformed babies. The most common anomalies were absence of limbs or parts of limbs, haemangiomatosis of the upper lips and nose, and malformations of the alimentary tract, heart, and genito-urinary system.

*Cytotoxic agents* also produce malformations, and the use of large doses of *progesterone* can produce genital deformities in female infants. *Lysergic acid diethylamide* (*LSD*) can cause chromosomal damage, abortion, and malformations in rats, and may well do so in humans also. It is obviously wise to avoid the use of all drugs during pregnancy, especially during the first three months.

*Ionizing radiations* (p. 304).

*Rhesus incompatibility*, i.e. erythroblastosis fetalis (p. 347).

It is to be hoped that abnormalities due to external agents will become less frequent as knowledge about the factors involved is acquired.

## Types of Malformation

Although it is a somewhat artificial subdivision, it is convenient to consider the types of malformation under separate headings:

### Failure of Development

There may be complete failure of development of a part (*agenesis*), or the part may remain rudimentary (*hypoplasia*) and never attain a full mature size. In the rare condition of anodontia there is agenesis of the dental lamina and complete absence of all the teeth. Congenital absence of a few teeth (partial anodontia) is more common. Both these conditions may be associated with a general defect of ectodermal structures affecting the hair, nails, and sebaceous and sweat glands (ectodermal dysplasia).

### Failure of Fusion

During development many structures normally fuse, and a failure to do so results in an abnormality. A cleft of the lip and palate occurs as a result of failure of fusion of the globular portion of the median nasal process with the lateral nasal and maxillary processes.

### Failure of Separation

A good example of this is the webbing which may persist between the digits (Fig. 20.1).

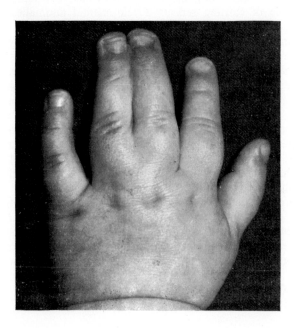

Fig. 20.1. Syndactyly. The third and fourth fingers of the hand are completely fused. (Photograph supplied by Mr. V. S. Brookes.)

### Failure of Canalization (Atresia).

Various channels in the body may fail to canalize, e.g. oesophageal atresia and imperforate anus.

### Ectopia

Sometimes organs and tissues are found in abnormal sites. This is called ectopia, heterotopia, or aberrance. Aberrant adrenal tissue may be found on the surface of the kidney and gonads, and an ectopic testis may be encountered in the abdominal cavity, the perineum, or the pubic area. Ectopic thyroid may be found in the tongue in the region of the foramen caecum, and in some cases no thyroid tissue may be present in its normal situation.

### Heteroplasia

Sometimes there is an anomalous differentiation of a particular tissue in an organ. For instance, small areas of gastric epithelium may be found in the oesophagus. This is called heteroplasia, and must be distinguished from metaplasia, in which the alteration of the tissue occurs after normal differentiation has taken place. Heteroplasia implies that the abnormal differentiation is a primary affair.

### Local Gigantism

Sometimes there is simple overgrowth of an organ or tissue, e.g. an enlarged digit or limb in neurofibromatosis, and this is rather dubiously called "hypertrophy". It is in fact better called local gigantism, because the organ has never been normal in relation to the remainder of the body. In true hyperplasia and hypertrophy the part is initially normal in size and subsequently undergoes enlargement (p. 230).

### Supernumerary Organs

Additional, or supernumerary, teeth may be present; likewise additional digits may occur (polydactyly).

### Hamartomata

A *hamartoma* is a tumour-like malformation in which the tissues of a particular part of the body are arranged haphazardly, usually with an excess of one or more of its components. The term was coined by Albrecht in 1904,[3] and is derived from the Greek word *hamartanein*, to err. The concept it embodies is of great importance, for a large number of common lesions fall into the general category of hamartomata.

A well-known example of hamartoma is the isolated cartilaginous mass not infrequently found in the substance of a lung (Fig. 20.2). This is composed of areas of hyaline cartilage separated by clefts lined by respiratory epithelium. There is no true capsule between the lesion and the surrounding lung. It is evident that this lesion contains several different elements, but that all of these are normally found in the lung. It would appear that it is a malformation derived from a developing bronchus, for all the tissues of a bronchus are present in it, though they are grossly misaligned and there is an excess of cartilage.

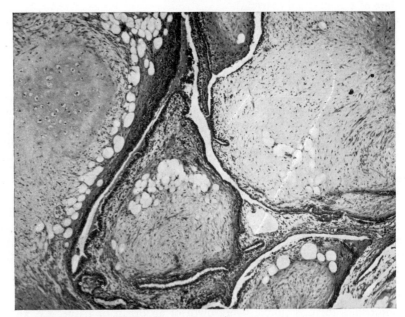

Fig. 20.2. Hamartoma of lung. There are masses of connective tissue intersected by deep clefts lined by respiratory epithelium. In the connective tissue there are areas of adipose tissue, and in the left-hand corner a mass of hyaline cartilage. × 55.

It is very important to distinguish between this type of lesion and a teratoma, which is a true tumour. In a hamartoma: (a) the tissues present are those specific to the part from which it arises, and (b) the lesion has no tendency towards excessive growth. There is no capsule around a hamartoma, as its growth proceeds *pari passu* with that of its surroundings. There is no question of pressure atrophy and therefore no connective-tissue condensation.

It should be noted that many hamartomata are given "tumour-sounding" names. These are so much part and parcel of histopathological nomenclature that they are bound to persist, e.g. angioma, benign melanoma, and chondroma of the lung.

**Vascular Hamartomata.** The very common haemangioma is a hamartomatous malformation and not a true tumour. It is usually present at birth or else appears soon afterwards, and though its growth is sometimes quite active in early childhood, it later becomes quiescent and may even undergo regression as the result of interference with its blood supply. This is particularly true of the strawberry naevus, which starts as an inconspicuous lesion on an infant's face and grows rapidly to giant proportions, but after a few years regresses and finally disappears with scarring. The commonest haemangioma is seen on the skin, where it forms a variety of *naevus*,[4, 5] a word used to describe any type of developmental blemish of the skin. Sometimes vascular naevi are small and spider-like, sometimes raised (strawberry naevi), and sometimes

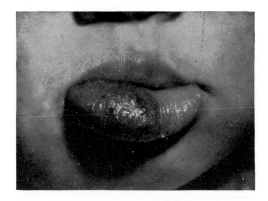

FIG. 20.3. Haemangioma of lower lip. (Photograph supplied by Mr. G. S. Hoggins.)

flattened and extensive (port-wine stain). Characteristically they blanch on pressure due to an emptying of their contained blood. Haemangiomata are also found in the mouth and lips (Fig. 20.3).

Microscopically they consist of poorly-demarcated, non-encapsulated masses and leashes of vascular channels, which are sometimes capacious, and described as *cavernous*, and at other times narrow and well formed (*capillary haemangioma*) (Fig. 20.4).

A noteworthy feature of angiomata is their tendency towards multiplicity. They may occur in several different organs in one patient, and cause characteristic syndromes.[5]

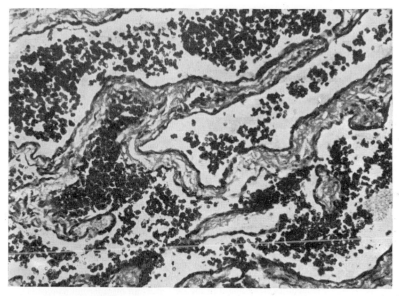

FIG. 20.4. Haemangioma. This is a cavernous haemangioma, and it consists of extensive vascular spaces enclosed in loose strands of endothelial-lined connective tissue. × 200.

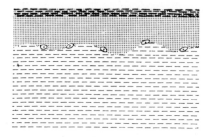

(a) Normal skin.

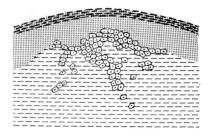

(c) Developing compound naevus.

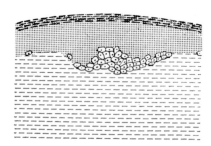

(b) Junctional naevus with activity.

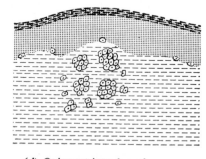

(d) Quiescent intradermal naevus.

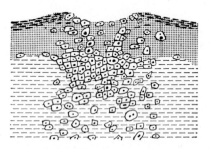

(e) Malignant melanoma.

Fig. 20.5. Diagrammatic representations of the various types of melanotic naevi—only melanocytes and naevus cells are drawn. In the normal skin (a) Melanocytes are present only in the basal layer of the epidermis. A focal proliferation of these cells produces a junctional naevus (b) which may be regarded as a stage in the development of a compound and an intradermal naevus. Such junctional activity is of little importance in a child, but in an adult is much more ominous. (c) Shows the formation of a compound naevus by the invasion of the dermis by melanocytes, or naevus cells. When the junctional activity regresses, the melanocytes remain in the dermis as an intradermal naevus (d). (e) Shows a malignant melanoma which, in addition to junctional activity, shows invasion of the epithelium as well as of the dermis and deeper structures. The cells are atypical, unlike those of the other lesions mentioned.

True tumours of blood vessels—angiosarcomata—are known, but are uncommon (p. 261).

Another type of vascular hamartoma is the lymphangioma. A well-known example is the cystic hygroma of infancy, which forms a characteristic swelling in the neck.[6] It infiltrates the vital surrounding structures so intimately that its complete removal is seldom possible.

**Melanotic Hamartomata.** The common mole, also called a *melanotic naevus* or a *naevocellular naevus*, of the skin is another example of a hamartomatous malformation (Fig. 20.5). The parent cells, the melanocytes, are believed to to originate in the region of the neural crest and to migrate to the epidermis

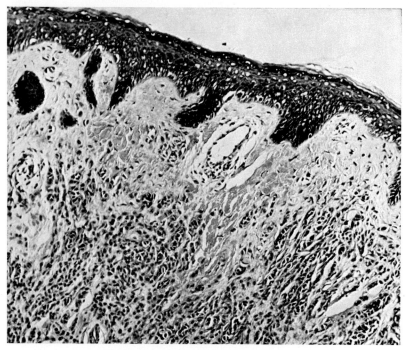

FIG. 20.6. Intradermal naevocellular naevus. Note the extensive collection of naevus cells in the dermis, well separated from the epidermis. × 130.

with the peripheral nerves.[7] Here they become incorporated among the cells of the basal layer. An excessive accumulation of these cells, which are called *naevus cells*, leads to the formation of the melanotic naevus. The cells are shed into the dermis during childhood. Naevus cells remaining in the basal layer of the epidermis are prone to undergo phases of proliferation, called *junctional activity*, but by the age of thirty years all the cells should be embedded in the dermis. Such a naevus is described as *intradermal* (Fig. 20.6). If some of the cells are still attached to the epidermis, the naevus is *compound* (Fig. 20.7), and if there is no dermal migration at all, the naevus is called *junctional*. It is the junctional element of a naevus that is liable to spurts of proliferation (junctional activity), whereas an intradermal

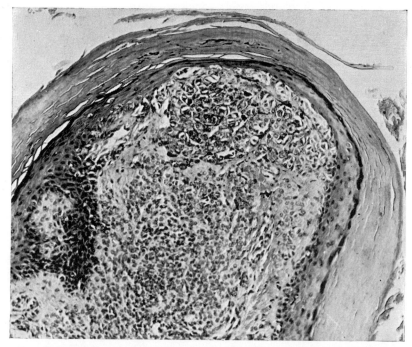

FIG. 20.7. Junctional activity in a naevocellular naevus. The aggregation of naevus cells is not only in contact with the epidermis, but has proliferated sufficiently to cause some thinning. Such an appearance in a child is quite common, but in an adult must be regarded with grave suspicion. × 130.

lesion is inert. Junctional activity is of little significance during childhood,[8] but in adult life any marked degree is to be regarded with suspicion, as it may be the first indication of neoplastic change.

Naevocellular naevi, unlike many other hamartomata, do occasionally become malignant. Lesions on the extremities and genitalia, and especially under the nails are most liable to this change.

*Malignant Melanoma.* If a naevocellular naevus is becoming malignant it increases in size and changes in colour, usually becoming darker, but it may also fade in some areas. It tends to become itchy and may bleed. Microscopically there is marked junctional activity, and the malignant cells are seen to invade not only the dermis but also the superficial layers of the epidermis, which is destroyed, hence the ulceration and bleeding.

The cells of a malignant melanoma show the usual characteristics of tumour cells (Fig. 20.8). They vary in size and shape, and their nuclei are irregular and darkly staining. Mitotic activity is invariable, and tumour giant cells are often present. Usually both the primary tumour and its metastases are well pigmented, but sometimes there is almost complete absence of melanin (amelanotic melanoma).

The commonest site for malignant melanoma is the skin, and it has often been assumed that the majority of tumours arise in pre-existing naevi. This

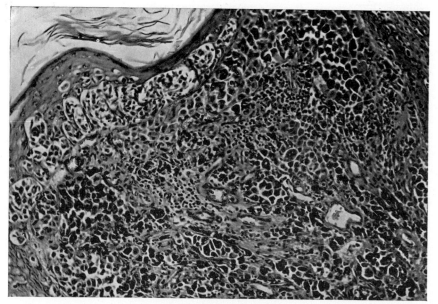

Fig. 20.8. Malignant melanoma. The dermis is infiltrated with pleomorphic tumour cells, some of which are pigmented. The epidermis has been partly destroyed, and elsewhere there was ulceration. × 130.

has been questioned by some investigators[9] who believe that over 90 per cent arise *de novo*, and that the risk of malignancy occurring in a naevus has been greatly exaggerated in the past. This conflict of opinions has not yet been resolved. Three types of melanoma are recognised:[9]

*Nodular Melanoma.* Tumour cells stream into the dermis and invade the epidermis. There is early invasion of local lymphatics, and widespread lymphatic and blood-borne metastases are the rule. Regardless of treatment the prognosis is bad.

*Superficial Spreading Melanoma.* This type is flat and shows irregular pigmentation; in due course nodules may appear. Microscopically the epidermis is invaded and disorganised by melanoma cells, and later the dermis is invaded. The prognosis is better than in the nodular type.

*Lentigo-Maligna Melanoma.* A lentigo maligna, or Hutchinson's freckle, appears as a flat, pigmented macule on the cheek of an elderly person. Microscopically the basal layer of the epidermis contains an increased number of atypical melanocytes, so that the lesion may be regarded as a type of *in-situ* malignancy. After a number of years some patients develop invasive melanoma, which usually leads to the lesion becoming crusted, ulcerated, or nodular. The prognosis is good in this type of melanoma.

Other sites of primary melanoma are the uveal tract of the eye and the juxtacutaneous mucous membranes of the mouth, nose, anus, vulva, and vagina.

**Skeletal Hamartomata.** The common solitary exostosis which grows out from the epiphyseal cartilage of a long bone is a good example of a cartilaginous hamartoma. It stops growing after puberty, when it completely ossifies. The rare condition of multiple exostoses, inherited as an autosomal dominant trait, is a generalized hamartomatous disorder involving many bones. The condition is also called *diaphysial aclasis*.[10]

**Dental Hamartomata.** The *odontome* is a malformation of all the dental tissues. As odontomes are composed of enamel, dentine, and cementum, they are termed composite, and there are several types. The compound composite odontome consists of a number of very small calcified structures which resemble teeth and are called denticles. The complex composite odontome consists of an irregular mass of calcified dental tissues. The odontome may replace a tooth in the arch, or it may be additional to the complete dentition and have arisen from a supernumerary anlage.

**Generalized Hamartomatous Dysplasia.** *Neurofibromatosis* (*von Recklinghausen's disease*) is a well-known condition, inherited as an autosomal dominant trait, in which there is a widespread hamartomatous overgrowth of nerve-sheath tissue. Histologically the lesions closely resemble the tumours described as neurofibromata. The condition may be associated with regional gigantism, which, if the face is affected, produces gross deformity.[11] There may also be café-au-lait spots on the skin. A neurofibromatous lesion may undergo sarcomatous change.

### Persistence of Vestigial Structures

In the course of development many parts which are of immense importance to the embryo undergo obliteration by the time of birth. If this does not happen, these normally vestigial structures persist and may lead to subsequent trouble. The two most important complications are *neoplasia* and *cyst formation*.

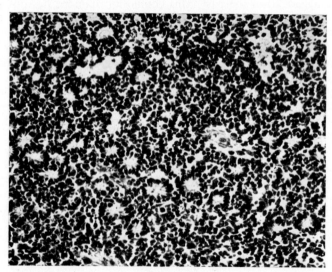

FIG. 20.9. Retinoblastoma. The tumour is composed of small, darkly-staining, fusiform cells arranged in rosette formation. In some of the rosettes there is a central cavity. × 150.

## Neoplasia

Developmental anomalies occasionally form the basis for subsequent tumours. This may occur in a number of ways:

**The Embryonic Tumours of Infancy.** Tumours may arise from primitive undifferentiated cells which are normally present only during embryonic life. The cells may persist into postnatal life and become neoplastic. Such tumours are most common during infancy, although they occasionally occur in later life. The tumours are highly malignant. It would seem that a portion of an organ undergoes a perversion of development to form a neoplasm instead of the normal parenchyma of the part. A good example is the *nephroblastoma* (*Wilms's tumour of the kidney*). Many of these tumours are undifferentiated and are composed of small darkly-staining cells, but sometimes the malignant nephroblasts show differentiation into tubular epithelial structures as well as forming recognizable connective tissue elements. Such tumours are therefore called mixed.

Other tumours of this type arise from the retina (*retinoblastoma*, Fig. 20.9), hind-brain (*medulloblastoma*), and sympathetic ganglion cells and adrenal medulla (*neuroblastoma*). Histologically they resemble each other closely.

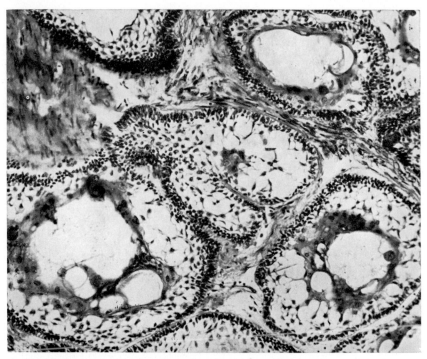

FIG. 20.10. Ameloblastoma. The tumour consists of clumps of fusiform epithelial cells, the outer layers of which form a palisade like that of the basal-cell carcinoma. In the centres of these clumps there is an open meshwork resembling the stellate reticulum of the enamel organ. In some of these aggregations there is cystic change and squamous metaplasia. × 150.

**Tumours Developing in Hamartomata.** This has already been discussed.

**Tumours Arising from Vestigial Remnants.** *Ameloblastoma.* This is a cystic tumour of the jaws which grows slowly and is locally malignant. Both in behaviour and in structure it resembles the common basal-cell carcinoma quite closely. It usually occurs in the mandible, and is seen most often in young adults. It consists of round or angulated clumps of epithelial cells. In the centre of these aggregations there is often an open meshwork resembling the stellate reticulum of the enamel organ. Between the cells there is an accumulation of fluid which gives rise to the cystic appearance typical of this tumour (Fig. 20.10). Other tumours in this group are rare. The *chordoma* arising from the notochord and the *craniopharyngioma* arising from residues of Rathke's pouch may be cited as examples.

**Tumours Arising from Ectopic Organs and Tissues.** Ectopic tissues are particularly liable to neoplastic transformation. Malignancy in ectopic testes is the most important example.

**Teratomata.** These are tumours consisting of multiple tissues foreign to the part from which they arise. The common sites are the ovary and testis. Rarely teratomata are found in the mediastinum, retroperitoneal tissue, and intracranially. Testicular teratomata are composed of cystic spaces lined by a

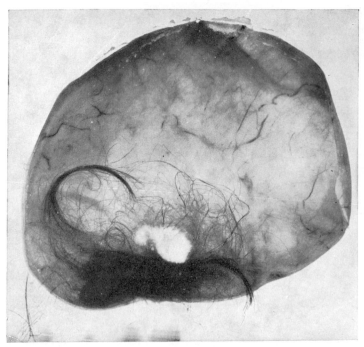

FIG. 20.11. Ovarian teratoma. Note the cystic nature of the tumour. At the base there is a prominent eminence, or umbo, from which a mass of dark hair sprouts.

(EF13.1. *Reproduced by permission of the President and Council of the Royal College of Surgeons of England.*)

variety of different types of epithelium and a connective tissue element which usually contains cartilage, lymphoid tissue, and primitive mesenchyme. The tumour, which affects young men, is highly malignant, and rapidly metastasizes both by the lymphatics and the blood stream. On the other hand, ovarian teratomata are usually well differentiated and benign, and are encountered chiefly in young and middle-aged women. They are usually cystic, and the wall is lined by stratified squamous epithelium and contains sebaceous glands and hair follicles. The cyst is usually filled with a greasy mass of sebaceous material in which there is matted hair. There is often a nodule in the wall, called the umbo, which contains a variety of structures such as bone, teeth, thyroid tissue, brain, etc. The tumour is therefore truly mixed in type (Fig. 20.11).

The origin of teratomata is disputed. One view is that they arise from a totipotent cell which becomes sequestrated from the developing fetus and remains quiescent for a number of years, later to assume independent neoplastic growth. Such a totipotent cell could be expected to produce any type of tissue that is normally present in the body. The curious localization of teratomata to the gonads has, however, given rise to an alternative hypothesis that they occur as a result of the misdirected development of a germ cell.

## CYSTS

It is appropriate to end this chapter with an account of the types of cyst, for many of them have a developmental basis.

The word *cyst*, derived from the Greek *kustis* a bladder, means a *pathological fluid-filled sac bounded by a wall*. The fluid may be secreted by cells lining the wall or it may be derived from the tissue fluid of the area. It is often clear and colourless, but it may be turbid and thick, or contain shimmering crystals of cholesterol. By common usage a cyst does not contain frank pus or blood—in these circumstances the terms abscess or haematoma are employed.

Where the cyst wall is lined by an epithelium, this layer may be derived from developmental residues such as the epithelial rests of Malassez in the periodontal ligament or epithelial residues lying in planes of embryonic fusion. On the other hand it may arise from a normal anatomical structure, such as the cells lining the ducts and acini of an exocrine gland. Often the stimulus which provokes the epithelial proliferation is unknown, as for instance in cysts arising in planes of embryonic fusion like the globulomaxillary cyst. Sometimes chronic inflammation is a factor, as in the development of the *dental cyst*, the commonest of the odontogenic cysts. Here the chronic inflammation in the periapical tissues of a dead tooth stimulates the epithelial rests of Malassez to proliferate and line the liquefied apical granuloma, thus forming a wall of the dental cyst, the contents of which are turbid and characteristically contain cholesterol crystals, which are a product of tissue breakdown.

The classification of cysts is difficult, but the most practical one is based on the pathogenesis of the lesion.

(a) *Developmental.* See below.

(b) *Inflammatory*, e.g. the dental cyst.

(c) *Degenerative*, e.g. cystic changes in goitres, in solid tumours like the uterine myoma (fibroid), and in other pathological lesions like fibrous dysplasia of bone. The basic change is necrosis which is almost always ischaemic in origin. It may occur in vascular disease, as in brain cysts following cerebral infarction, or in a tumour or other lesion with inadequate blood supply. The necrotic debris subsequently becomes liquefied.

(d) *Retention*, e.g. a ranula, which is a cystic dilatation in the submandibular or sublingual gland formed as a result of obstruction of its duct. The name refers to the frog-like swelling produced—*ranula* is Latin for a little frog.

(e) *Implantation*. See epidermoid cyst, page 114.

(f) *Hydatid*, a parasitic cyst, found usually in the liver and lungs, due to the proliferation and expansion of the larval form of the canine tapeworm *Echinococcus granulosus*.

(g) *Hyperplastic*, e.g. mammary dysplasia.

(h) *Neoplastic*, e.g. cystadenoma of the ovary and cystic teratoma.

**Developmental Cysts.** These may arise from ectopic tissues or from the persistence of vestigial remnants.

*Ectopia of Various Tissues.* In ectopia there is a dislocation of tissue into a neighbouring area, where it often becomes cystic. A good example is the *dermoid cyst*, which is due to the sequestration of a piece of skin beneath one of the lines of fusion of the various embryonic body processes. Dermoid cysts occur most commonly in the subcutaneous tissue of the face, usually near the angle of the orbit. Another site is under the tongue (sublingual dermoid). A dermoid cyst is lined by stratified squamous epithelium, and in its wall there are hair follicles, sebaceous glands, and sweat glands. It contains a thick, greasy material consisting of keratin produced by the epithelial lining and sebum secreted by the sebaceous glands. Matted hair is also often present. Unlike a teratoma, it does not include other tissues in its wall.

*Persistence of Vestigial Remnants.* Examples of this type are the branchial and thyroglossal cysts. A branchial cyst develops from a persisting portion of the cervical sinus; it is lined by stratified squamous epithelium and is surrounded by lymphoid tissue.[12] Some odontogenic cysts are also due to the persistence of paradental remnants, e.g. the dentigerous cyst which surrounds the crown of an unerupted tooth, of either the regular or the supernumerary dentition. It is formed by the accumulation of fluid between the layers of the enamel epithelium or between the epithelium and the tooth crown.

## References

1. BROWN, G. C. (1966). *Adv. in Teratology*, **1**, 55.
2. SMITHELLS, R. W. (1966). *Adv. in Teratology*, **1**, 250.
3. ALBRECHT, E. (1904). *Verh. dtsch. path. Ges.*, **7**, 153.
4. MATTHEWS, D. N. (1951). *Proc. roy. Soc. Med.*, **44**, 609.
5. BEAN, W. B. (1958). "Vascular Spiders and Related Lesions of the Skin". Oxford: Blackwell.
6. GOETSCH, E. (1938). *Arch. Surg.*, **36**, 394.
7. MASSON, P. (1951). *Cancer*, **4**, 9.

8. SPITZ, S. (1948). *Amer. J. Path.*, **24,** 591.
9. CLARK, W. H. *et al.* (1969). *Cancer Res.*, **29,** 705.
10. FAIRBANK, H. A. T. (1935). *Proc. roy. Soc. Med.*, **28,** 1611.
11. O'DRISCOLL, P. M. (1966). *Brit. J. oral Surg.*, **3,** 22.
12. WILSON, C. P. (1955). *Ann. roy. Coll. Surg. Engl.*, **17,** 1.

*Chapter 21*

# THE EFFECTS OF IONIZING RADIATION

## Introduction

The ever-increasing use of radioactive substances in both industry and medicine has made the study of radiation damage of great practical importance. On the human body the effects of radiation vary from local tissue necrosis to genetic damage, cancer, and death. With such a perplexing array of effects it is little wonder that the ionizing radiations are regarded with fear and amazement. As their physical nature is so well understood, it might be expected that the mechanisms involved and the damage which they produce would be equally explicable. Such, however, is not the case.

The basic action of ionizing radiations is to produce changes in the structure of the atoms through which they pass. Such changes in turn lead to secondary events in molecules, cells, tissues, and finally in the individual as a whole. These events will be examined in turn, but with so many steps it is not surprising that there are many gaps in our knowledge of the pathogenesis of radiation damage.

## Physical and Chemical Considerations

The energy of the absorbed radiation gives rise to the following changes:
(1) Ions and free radicles are formed.
(2) There is excitation of molecules.
(3) Secondary electrons are generated, and these produce changes similar to (1) and (2) in adjacent areas.

The net effect is that molecules become more reactive and chemical changes ensue. Large biological molecules like DNA and proteins could be affected by two separate processes:

**Direct Action.** Energy absorbed in the molecule itself may lead to chemical change, e.g. denaturation of a protein.

**Indirect Action.** Alternatively chemical change may be induced in a large molecule as a result of the action of an adjacent ion or radicle, e.g. an OH˙ radicle formed from water.

It is generally supposed that ionizing radiations produce a type of biochemical lesion, but if this is so its nature has so far eluded detection.

## Effects on the Cell

Although it would be desirable to explain the cellular damage in terms of the known physico-chemical changes, it must be admitted that this is not yet possible. The effects seen may be summarized:

(1) Immediate death of the cell occurs with very heavy dosage, i.e. 10 000 r or more. This effect occurs regardless of the stage of mitosis and is called

*interphase death.* It is also seen in very sensitive cells, e.g. small lymphocytes, with moderate dosage.

(2) DNA synthesis is inhibited.

(3) Mitosis is delayed, usually due to a prolongation of the $G_2$ phase (see p. 22).

(4) DNA synthesis may occur unrelated to mitosis, so that giant-cell forms are produced. Giant fibroblasts are seen in irradiated skin.

(5) When mitosis does occur in irradiated cells, abnormalities such as chromosome breaks may occur. At this stage the cell may die. Nevertheless, a cell may go through several mitotic cycles before death finally occurs.

(6) The growth rate may be slowed down even in sublethally irradiated cells.

(7) Fractionated doses of radiation do not produce a strictly cumulative effect. Hence there appear to exist intracellular mechanisms whereby radiation damage can be reversed or "repaired".

(8) The sensitivity of cells to damage varies according to the stage in the mitotic cycle when the radiation is given. Maximum sensitivity occurs in most cell-types during mitosis itself. They are relatively resistant during most of the $G_1$ phase, but radiosensitivity returns during the late $G_1$ and early synthetic (S) phases. They are most resistant during the late S and early $G_2$ phases.

Two main theories have been put forward to explain the cellular damage:
*The target theory* supposes that the injury is due to damage in some specific sensitive spot in the cell. Attractive as it may be to visualize a chromosome or an organelle as a target, there is in fact very little to support this theory.

*The poison theory* proposes that the ionization leads to the production of poisonous substances, usually powerful oxidizing agents, which then cause the damage. There is considerable evidence that oxidizing substances are formed in irradiated tissue. Thus chemicals with a reducing action (e.g. cysteine) will give some degree of protection against ionizing radiation. Furthermore, if tissues are irradiated in the absence of oxygen, they show considerably more resistance.[1] This is probably because free oxygen is necessary for the production of oxidizing substances by ionizing radiation. This observation is of some importance in clinical radiotherapy, because many areas of a tumour are relatively hypoxic and might conceivably be protected during irradiation therapy.

### Effects on the Intact Animal

This most important aspect of radiobiology is also the most difficult. A feature which is outstanding is the remarkable *delay* in the appearance of radiation lesions. The actual damage caused by radiation must be almost instantaneous, and yet the effect may not be apparent for days, months, or even years. Experiments with amphibians help to explain this phenomenon. Frogs can be given a dose of radiation which will kill them within six weeks. If the irradiated animals are kept at 5°C, they remain alive for several months, but on being warmed up die within six weeks, like the control animals kept at normal temperature.[2] The experiment indicates that radiation damage manifests itself only when cells are active. This lends strong support to the concept that a biochemical lesion is produced. Such a lesion is not in itself harmful, but produces effects when cellular activity commences. This goes some way in explaining two of the phenomena of radiation damage:

(1) **Relative Sensitivity of Cells.** In the human the germinal cells of the ovary are the most sensitive. Then in sequence follow the seminiferous epithelium of the testis, lymphocytes, the erythropoietic and myeloid marrow cells, and the intestinal epithelium. Least sensitive are nerve cells and muscle cells. This order to some extent parallels the rate of mitosis seen in the various tissues; thus neurones never divide, while epithelial tissue, especially that of the intestine, shows constant mitotic activity.

(2) **The Chronic Nature of Radiation Lesions.** When tissue is irradiated, several phases of damage occur. This is probably because different tissues have different rates of division and metabolic activity, and therefore exhibit damage at different times. Hence an irradiated area shows changes which persist for many weeks or even months and have the characteristics of chronic inflammation, even after a single exposure.

When considering the action of radiation on any tissue, two main effects must be borne in mind.

*The primary effect* of radiation on the tissue concerned.

*The secondary effect*, which is due to damage to adjacent tissues. The most important example of this is the damage to vessels which, by causing thrombosis or endarteritis obliterans, leads to ischaemia. Some authorities attribute much of the beneficial effects of radiotherapy in cancer to this mechanism.

### The Effect of Irradiation on Individual Tissues

**Skin.** Following a single exposure to ionizing radiation, redness (erythema) appears after about 10 days, and the skin shows all the features of acute inflammation. Pigmentation is increased, giving the skin a red dusky colour. With heavy dosage necrosis occurs, and an ulcer is produced. This is very slow to heal, and even when healed the scar may break down after trivial injury. With lower dosage a smouldering chronic inflammation occurs. Fibrosis is evident, and the blood vessels show endarteritis obliterans. The hair follicles and accessory glands are much more sensitive to radiation than is the less active surface epithelium. With a dosage of above 700 r* these structures undergo necrosis, and do not regenerate. The delaying effect on wound healing is described in Chapter 8.

**Gonads.** The ovary and testis are particularly susceptible, and with a dosage of over 500 r the germinal cells are destroyed and permanent sterility results.

**Lungs.** Irradiation of the lungs produces inflammatory changes which culminate in fibrosis.[3] This is sometimes seen as a complication of radiotherapy for lung and breast cancer.

**Bone.** Irradiation of bone produces inflammatory changes which may persist for years, and are punctuated by episodes of painful radionecrosis. If the jaw

---

* The letter r signifies roentgen, a commonly used measurement of radiation. One roentgen is that amount of radiation which under specified conditions produces in 1 ml. of air at NTP, one electrostatic unit of electricity of either charge.

is involved, radionecrosis is often precipitated by the extraction of teeth. Doses of over 1 000 r inhibit growth at the epiphysis, an effect of importance in children. Thus the coincidental irradiation of the mandibular condyle during the ill-advised treatment of an angiomatous hamartoma may lead to cessation of growth with consequent hypoplasia of the mandible.

## Total Body Irradiation[4]

The effects of total body irradiation depend on the dosage, and have been studied in people involved in atomic explosions. It is convenient to describe the effects of total body irradiation under two headings—those occurring during the first two months (immediate), and those occurring later.

## Immediate Effects

Although no hard-and-fast rules can be given, three groups of cases may be recognized:

*Very heavy dosage* (over 5 000 r single exposure) produces severe effects due apparently to direct damage to the brain. Death occurs within a day or two following shock, convulsions, and coma.

*Moderate dosage*, 800–5 000 r single exposure. Loss of appetite, nausea, and vomiting develop soon after irradiation, the reasons for which are not known. The symptoms usually abate, only to recur some 2–3 days later with intractable severity. This latter episode of vomiting is accompanied by severe diarrhoea due to necrosis of the intestinal epithelium. Death usually occurs from dehydration and shock.

*Low dosage*, under 800 r single exposure. Initial nausea and vomiting are less severe, and the subject may then appear to make a complete recovery. Two or three weeks later the results of bone-marrow aplasia become apparent. The serious effects of irradiation at this stage are due to damage to the *haematopoietic* tissues.

## Blood Changes Following Irradiation

*Lymphocytes.* Lymphopenia is the earliest blood change of total body irradiation, and is most marked after a day or two.

*Granulocytes.* The total granulocyte count falls after about a week, and may reach very low levels by the second to sixth weeks. This predisposes to infection, e.g. of the mouth and lungs.

*Platelets.* After a few days the number of platelets drops dramatically, and is very low by 4 weeks. This leads to severe haemorrhage.

*Red cells.* Because the primitive, or erythroblastic, cells are highly radio-sensitive and the mature red cells are resistant, the effect of bone-marrow aplasia on the peripheral count is delayed. The anaemia is of gradual onset and maximal at 6–8 weeks.

## Late Effects of Total Body Irradiation

Those exposed to a sublethal dose may show the following after-effects:

**The Carcinogenic Effect.** It has been realized since the beginning of the century that tumours may develop after the application of ionizing radiation.

The first case, a carcinoma of the skin, was reported in 1902, and subsequently *squamous-cell cancers of the skin* of the hands have been frequently seen in x-ray workers. This also occurred in dental surgeons who held films in position in the mouth. It is important for all those who use x-rays to avoid unnecessary exposure to radiation.

Another danger of exposure to ionizing radiation is the development of *leukaemia*.[5] A high incidence of this disease has been recorded in the survivors of the Nagasaki and Hiroshima atomic explosions[6] and in patients with ankylosing spondylitis treated with radiotherapy.[7] However, the hazard of modern diagnostic radiology is slight.

*Osteosarcoma* has been reported to follow local irradiation years after the treatment of benign or inflammatory bone lesions. The tumour has also followed the injection or ingestion of radioactive substances, such as radium and mesothorium, which are stored in the bones.

**Genetic Effects.** The ability of ionizing radiation to increase the rate of mutation is well established in micro-organisms, plants, and animals. In somatic cells this effect is probably not important, but in the germ cells it is of potential significance, since the new factor is handed down to subsequent generations. It may have a profoundly deleterious effect, since most mutations are harmful.

## Radiotherapy[8]

The destructive effects of ionizing radiations on living cells, particularly those in an active state, have led to their widespread use in the treatment of malignant disease. Nowadays radiotherapy plays an important part in the curative treatment of some primary cancers, as well as in the palliation of those which have already metastasized, and are beyond the scope of surgical excision.

### Factors Influencing Response

Tumours differ widely in their reaction to radiotherapy, and it is only after treatment has been commenced that the response can be assessed. However, some guide to the probable local results of treatment may be given by consideration of the following factors:

**Tissue of Origin.** The relative sensitivities of normal tissues are often reflected in the radiosensitivities of the tumours derived from them. Thus lymphocytic lymphoma, like the parent lymphocyte, is very radiosensitive. Fibrosarcoma, however, like the fibroblasts from which it is derived, is radioresistant.

**Degree of Differentiation and Mitotic Activity.** It is generally taught that within any tumour group the most undifferentiated tumours are also the most radiosensitive. As a generalization this is true, but nevertheless it is found that the histological appearances of an individual tumour are no sure guide to the results obtained in practice. It is found, for instance, that well-differentiated squamous-cell carcinomata of the skin and tongue frequently respond very well.

**The Tumour Bed.** The nature of the stroma supporting a tumour is probably important. If it is avascular as the result of previous irradiation, the tumour is more resistant. This may well be attributable to hypoxia. Some authorities maintain that the connective tissues have a restraining effect on the growth of the tumour. If excessive irradiation is given, the results are said to be much worse than if a modest dose is given, because under these circumstances the tumour bed itself is destroyed.[9] It seems quite certain that all tumour cells are not destroyed by radiotherapy, and that the cure of the patient is related to some other destructive mechanism on the growth of the tumour.

**Nature of the Individual Tumour.** Certain tumours respond extremely well, for example most basal-cell and squamous-cell carcinomata of the skin. On the other hand, squamous-cell carcinoma of the lung generally responds poorly. It is evident that tumours of similar histological appearance in different organs may react very differently to irradiation. The reason for this is not known.

### Cure Rate

The *cure rate* to be expected from radiotherapy must, as with surgical treatment, be considered in relation to the general properties of the tumour. Many malignant conditions, for example lymphoma, cannot be considered as local diseases, and although a tumour mass may respond remarkably well to treatment, the disease progresses sooner or later to its inevitable end. Oat-cell carcinoma of the lung is a similar example.

Radiotherapy is often effective as a palliative treatment. It can reduce the size of a tumour mass and produce relief of symptoms. This is well seen in mediastinal tumours producing obstruction to the great vessels. Radiotherapy may also control haemorrhage from a bleeding tumour, and help to clear up a fungating carcinoma of the breast. Pain from bony metastases may be alleviated. Slowly-growing tumours, like cancer of the breast and Hodgkin's disease, can sometimes be held in check for long periods, and the patient given several years of useful life. It may well be that radiotherapy and surgery are both forms of palliation which allow the body to retard the growth of the tumour. Depending on whether the malignant cells stay dormant for a short or long period, one may speak of a five-year cure, ten-year cure, etc. It is doubtful, however, whether any of our present treatments of cancer can be regarded as producing a cure, if by this is meant the complete eradication of all malignant cells.

### General Reading

ALEXANDER, P. (1957). "Atomic Radiation and Life", 239 pp. Harmondsworth: Penguin Books, Ltd. A simple account of ionizing radiations and their effects.

BACQ, Z. M. and ALEXANDER, P. (1961). "Fundamentals of Radiobiology", 2nd. ed., 555 pp. Oxford: Pergamon Press. Both this and the first edition (1955, London: Butterworths) should be consulted for details on specific aspects of radiobiology.

CRONKITE, E. P. and BOND, V. P. (1960). "Radiation Injury in Man", 200 pp. Springfield, Ill.: Thomas.

GLASSER, O., QUIMBY, E. H., TAYLOR, L. S., WEATHERWAX, J. L. and MORGAN, R. H. (1961). "Physical Foundations of Radiology", 3rd. ed. London: Pitman Medical.

MOLE, R. H. (1960). "The Toxicity of Radiation", in "Recent Advances in Pathology,"
    ed. by Harrison, C. V., 7th. ed., pp. 339–383. London: Churchill.
Various Authors, (1959). *Scientific American*, 201, No. 3. This issue is devoted
    to ionic radiations and their effects.
WARREN, S. (1961). "The Pathology of Ionizing Radiation", 42 pp. Springfield,
    Ill.: Thomas.

## References

1. GRAY, L. H. (1957–58). "Lectures on the Scientific Basis of Medicine", 7, 314.
    London: Athlone Press.
2. PATT, H. M. and SMITH, M. N. (1948). *Amer. J. Physiol.*, 155, 388.
3. SMITH, J. C. (1963). *Amer. Rev. resp. Dis.*, 87, 647.
4. MOLE, R. H. (1959). In "Modern Trends in Pathology", ed. by Collins, D. H.
    p. 91. London: Butterworths.
5. LEWIS, E. B. (1963). *Science*, 142, 1492.
6. HEYSSEL, R. *et al.* (1960). *Blood*, 15, 313.
7. COURT BROWN, W. M. and ABBATT, J. D. (1955). *Lancet*, 1, 1283.
8. RAVEN, R. W. (1959). "Cancer", vol. 5. London: Butterworths.
9. JOLLES, B. (1953). "X-ray Sieve Therapy in Cancer". London: Lewis.

*Chapter 22*

# THE GENERAL RESPONSE TO TRAUMA: HAEMORRHAGE

When the body is injured, there is set in motion a series of events from which scarcely any tissue is exempt. The local events of inflammation and healing have been considered in previous chapters. Here we shall describe the general response to injury. Important changes take place in the *nervous system* and in the *endocrine glands*, but it is in the *cardiovascular system* that the most marked reaction occurs. This is most easily understood by first considering the normal circulation and its reaction to a sudden loss of blood.

## Haemorrhage

Haemorrhage is defined as the escape of blood from the vascular system. The extravasated blood may escape to the exterior or it may remain internal.

### Types of Haemorrhage

**External.** Blood may be coughed up (*haemoptysis*), passed in the urine (*haematuria*), vomited (*haematemesis*), or be passed in the faeces either as fresh blood or, if from higher up in the intestinal tract, as a black, partially digested mass (*melaena*).

**Internal.** Small flat haemorrhages, less than 2 mm. in diameter, are called *petechiae*, or *purpuric spots*; they are usually found in the skin and mucous membranes. A larger, more diffuse, haemorrhagic area is called an *ecchymosis*. A *haematoma* is a discrete pool of blood, usually clotted, in a tissue. Collections of blood in natural spaces are named anatomically, e.g. *haemothorax* (in the pleural cavity), *haemopericardium*, *haemoperitoneum*, *haemarthrosis* (in a joint cavity), etc.

### Effects of Acute Haemorrhage[1]

The vascular system contains about 5 litres of blood, which is kept in motion by the action of the heart so that all the tissues are adequately perfused. The amount of blood reaching any area is determined by two factors—the *calbire of the arterioles supplying it* and the *blood pressure*.

The capacious venous system acts as a reservoir for blood, and therefore when a small quantity is lost, an increase in venous tone reduces the capacity of the circulatory system, so that there is no reduction in the volume of blood reaching the heart (the venous return). Therefore there is no reduction in the cardiac output. When a larger volume of blood is suddenly withdrawn, this reserve mechanism is inadequate. The venous return is diminished, the cardiac output falls, and with it the amount of blood available for perfusing the organs. It is therefore not surprising that the next response to haemorrhage is a series of reactions designed to restore the blood pressure.

### Restoration of Blood Pressure and Redistribution of Blood[2, 3]

*Mechanism.* The fall in blood pressure is detected by the pressure-sensitive carotid sinus and the other baroreceptors, and these reflexly initiate a sympathetic outflow from the central nervous system (Fig. 22.1). The effect is a *vasoconstriction* of the arterioles of the *skin, kidneys,* and *splanchnic area* by direct action, as well as indirectly *via* the adrenal medulla, which is stimulated

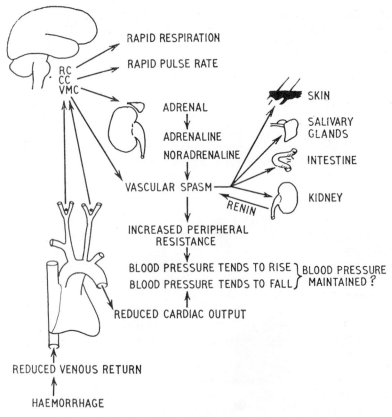

FIG. 22.1. The cardiovascular effects of sudden haemorrhage.

RC (Respiratory Centre)
CC (Cardiac Centre)
VMC (Vasomotor Centre)

to secrete adrenaline and noradrenaline. The lowered blood pressure acts on the juxtaglomerular apparatus and causes the kidney to release renin (p. 365). There is therefore an over-all increase in the peripheral resistance. The blood pressure is restored, and the blood flow to the brain, heart, and respiratory muscles remains almost unaltered. However, the areas affected by arteriolar vasoconstriction tend to suffer; for example the *skin* is cold and pale, the *kidneys* show a reduced urinary output (oliguria), and the *salivary glands* cease to secrete. Thus the vasomotor response to acute haemorrhage causes a *redistribution of blood*, a mechanism which may be regarded as an emergency measure designed to keep the essential organs supplied.

## Restoration of Blood Volume

During the first few hours after a haemorrhage extravascular fluids pass into the blood stream, the volume of which is thereby restored. This is easily demonstrated by following the haemoglobin level. Immediately after a sudden haemorrhage the *haemoglobin level is normal*. During the next 8 hours it falls as dilution occurs, and this process is largely complete by the end of 48 hours.[4] At this stage therefore the haemoglobin level is a good guide to the extent of the previous blood loss. This transfer of extracellular fluid to the blood stream appears to be the result of the reduced capillary hydrostatic pressure which follows the arteriolar vasoconstriction. The osmotic pressure of the plasma due to its protein content is now greater than the hydrostatic pressure, and fluid is drawn into the blood until a balance is achieved (p. 323). Complete restoration of the plasma volume is dependent upon replacement of the lost plasma proteins. These enter the circulation *via* the thoracic duct, and are primarily contributed by the liver.[5]

## Changes in the Blood

Within a few minutes of bleeding the clotting time is considerably decreased, and during the next few hours there is a considerable increase in the level of platelets and neutrophils, which persists for several days. The restoration of the red-cell count is a much slower process, since the body has virtually no reserve store of erythrocytes. New red cells have to be manufactured, and a normal count is not attained until 4–6 weeks later.

The effects of acute haemorrhage depend upon both the volume and the speed with which blood is lost. The normal adult can donate one pint (approx. 500 ml., or 10 per cent of the blood volume) with little discomfort. A sudden loss of 30–50 per cent may well be fatal; however, if spread over a day or so it can be tolerated. If the haemorrhage is so severe that the compensatory mechanisms are inadequate to maintain an adequate blood flow to vital organs, death ensues. This constitutes one variety of *shock*, a subject which will now be considered.

### Shock

Shock is the name given to a clinical state in which the patient has tachycardia (an increased heart rate), and is pale, ashen, and sweating. Two quite separate conditions have been included:

### Vasovagal Attack, also known as Primary Shock, or Syncope[2]

Immediately following injury or loss of blood, a patient may feel nauseated. become giddy, and finally lose consciousness. Convulsions occasionally occur. The attack rarely lasts more than a few minutes, and causes no permanent damage. It is sometimes seen after quite trivial injury, e.g. the insertion of a needle, or even, in nervous individuals, at the suggestion of injury.[6, 7] The attack appears to be mediated by a vasomotor imbalance so that widespread vasodilatation occurs in the skeletal muscles. The blood pressure drops, the heart rate slows, and the cerebral blood flow diminishes so that consciousness is lost. If the patient is laid horizontally, or attains that position spontaneously, he soon recovers. In rare cases death may occur— at least this is one suggestion for the rare cases of sudden death which occur unexpectedly, e.g. when introducing a needle into the pleural cavity or during an attempted abortion. It has been reported that syncope occurring during the induction of anaesthesia may be fatal if the anaesthetic is administered with the patient in the upright position, e.g. in a dental chair.[8]

### Secondary Shock

This is a much more important condition, and it is best to restrict the unqualified term "shock" to it. Shock is seen following many forms of injury; it may occur immediately, or there may be a period of comparative well-being before the characteristic features make their appearance. The patient lies still and apathetic, his temperature is subnormal, his skin cold and clammy, and his face ashen grey. Obvious cyanosis may be present. The blood pressure is low, and the pulse rapid and thready. Little or no urine is passed.

The clinical picture of shock may occur in a variety of conditions, and not surprisingly these have all been assembled under the all-embracing title of "shock". They are:

*Loss of blood* (haemorrhagic shock)
*Post-traumatic*
*Loss of plasma,* e.g. burns
*Loss of fluid and electrolytes*
*Overwhelming infection*
*Cardiogenic shock*
*Anaphylactic shock*

The inclusion of so many divergent syndromes under one heading has tended to obscure our understanding of the condition. They all produce a similar clinical picture which is described as shock, but it is hardly to be expected that the mechanisms involved would be the same in each case. It should also be remembered that a state of shock frequently precedes death regardless of the cause, e.g. electrocution, overdose of drugs, drowning, or following massive total body irradiation (p. 303). To attempt to understand "shock" it is necessary to consider each separately.

**Haemorrhagic Shock.** If following a large haemorrhage the compensatory mechanisms described on p. 308 fail to maintain the blood pressure, either as a result of their own inefficiency, or the excessive load placed upon them by a large haemorrhage, the patient enters into a state of shock. Recovery may occur spontaneously, or as a result of efficient treatment, e.g. transfusion; such shock is therefore said to be *reversible*. It sometimes happens that in spite of vigorous and efficient treatment the blood pressure continues to fall, the patient's clinical condition deteriorates, and death ensues. This is *irreversible shock*.

**Traumatic Shock.** The circulatory changes which follow trauma are very similar to those following haemorrhage. Initial *syncope* may occur, to be followed shortly by secondary shock. The possible causes of the latter are:

*Haemorrhage.*[9] It is often not appreciated that injury, apart from causing external bleeding, leads to an extensive blood loss into the tissues. Thus in a closed fracture of the femur 4 pints of blood may be lost. It is obvious that the swelling of injured parts is produced either by extravasated blood or by inflammatory exudate, i.e. plasma.

In surgical operations it is very important to estimate the amount of blood lost so that it can be replaced. The amount on swabs can be estimated by weighing, or by extracting the haemoglobin and measuring it colorimetrically.

*Toxins* from damaged tissue have been postulated, but their importance has never been substantiated.

*Infection.* There is little doubt that the powerful exotoxins of the pathogenic clostridia exert a profound effect on the circulation. Gas-gangrene even in the absence of substantial traumatic damage causes a shock-like state which may result in death.

*Endotoxic factor.*[10] Since the generalized Shwartzman phenomenon resembles shock, it has been suggested that following trauma the intestinal coliform organisms or their endotoxins enter the blood stream and cause a similar reaction. Nevertheless, this has not been substantiated as an important cause of human traumatic shock, although it is probably important in the severe shock which develops in patients with Gram-negative septicaemia (see below).

In summary, it seems that *blood loss is the most important factor in traumatic shock*.

**Shock Following Burns.**[11,12] The severe shock which follows burning appears to be due to the tremendous loss of plasma in the inflammatory exudate. At a later stage infection with organisms, e.g. *Ps. pyocyanea*, may play a part. An important point of difference from haemorrhagic shock is that there is haemoconcentration rather than haemodilution.

**Shock due to Loss of Fluid and Electrolytes.** Loss of fluid or sodium can lead to such depletion of the extracellular tissue fluids that, unless replacement therapy is instituted, a state of shock develops due to the inadequacy of the circulating plasma volume. This is seen in pyloric stenosis, intestinal obstruction, and cholera, and also in heat-exhaustion due to loss of salt and water in the sweat. As in the shock of burns there is haemoconcentration and the increased viscosity of the blood further impedes the blood flow through the tissues.

In the examples of shock so far considered, it is believed that the capacity of the circulatory system is either normal or reduced. The major factor at fault is a diminished volume of circulating fluid. The term *hypovolaemic shock* is therefore often used. It is evident that a state of shock could also occur if the *capacity* of the circulatory system were to increase without a corresponding increase in blood *volume*. This certainly occurs in the transient vasovagal attack, and is probably the explanation of the shock in severe infections, e.g. septicaemia, and in the Shwartzman phenomenon. This type of shock is often called *peripheral vascular failure*, and is due to peripheral vasodilatation which produces pooling of blood. Often it seems that the blood accumulates in the splanchnic area.

**Shock in Infection.**[13] Shock is seen in a variety of infections. It is prominent in infections with toxic organisms, e.g. diphtheria and gas-gangrene, but it is also a feature of many other severe infections—pneumonia, peritonitis, etc. In recent years a new syndrome, *endotoxic shock* (bacteraemic or Gram-negative shock), has been recognized, and is caused by the sudden entry of Gram-negative organisms into the circulation.[14, 15, 16] It is a complication of any coliform infection, but is usually seen as a sequel to urinary infection. There is a sudden onset of profound shock, and unless treated expeditiously this carries a high mortality. The condition bears some resemblance to the shock seen in the generalized Shwartzman reaction (p. 92).

The shock seen in infection is of complex pathogenesis: at least three factors should be considered:

*Peripheral circulatory failure* due to vasodilatation and pooling of blood, especially in the splanchnic area. This occurs in septicaemic plague,[13] endotoxic shock,[16] and probably in other infections and toxaemias.

*Loss of fluid in the exudate.* In gas-gangrene the profuse loss of protein-rich exudate is responsible for the haemoconcentration and reduction in blood volume.

*Heart failure.* Bacterial toxins, e.g. diphtheria toxin, may damage the myocardium, and an element of heart failure may further embarrass an already failing circulation.

**Cardiogenic Shock.** Myocardial infarction, severe cardiac arrhythmias, and the sudden accumulation of fluid in the pericardium may sometimes lead to a state of shock which resembles that following trauma.[17] A low cardiac output with underperfusion of the tissues is the initial effect, but the resulting metabolic acidosis (see below) causes peripheral vasodilatation and pooling of blood.

**Anaphylactic Shock.** See Chapter 13.

### The Metabolic Upset during Shock[18]

A patient in shock shows a profound *reduction in metabolic rate*, the nature of which is not well understood; it appears that there is a block in carbohydrate utilization.[19] In spite of cutaneous vasoconstriction, and therefore a reduction in heat loss, *the body's temperature falls.* An important effect of shock is that the under-perfusion of tissues results in anaerobic glycolysis with the release of pyruvic and lactic acids into the circulation. There is therefore often a severe *metabolic acidosis*\*.[20] It is evident that an important aspect of shock is that tissues are underperfused with blood. Indeed, it has been stated that "shock is not merely a problem of blood volume, blood pressure, and anaemia, but essentially a problem of flow".[21] A factor to be considered in this respect is sludging.

---

\* The normal pH of the blood is 7·36–7·44. If it falls below 7·36, there is an *acidosis*, and if it rises above 7·44, there is an *alkalosis*. An acidosis due to excess or abnormal acids in the blood is called *metabolic*, whereas one due to carbon dioxide retention in lung disease is called *respiratory*. Metabolic acidosis is present in renal failure (p. 432) and diabetic ketosis (p. 477).

**Sludging**[22, 23]

If the flowing blood of a shocked patient is observed, it will be seen that the red cells are clumped together. This differs from true agglutination in that the masses can be broken up, though with some difficulty. The original description of the phenomenon described the blood as being converted into a "muck-like sludge"—hence the name *sludging*.[23] The *cause* of this is an increase in the level of high-molecular-weight substances (e.g. fibrinogen) in the plasma and a reduction in the low-molecular-weight albumin. The ESR is increased (p. 331). The *effect* is to impede the blood flow through the tissues. Sludging can be prevented or reversed by the infusion of low-molecular-weight substances; for example dextran of MW 40 000 has been used quite extensively.[25]

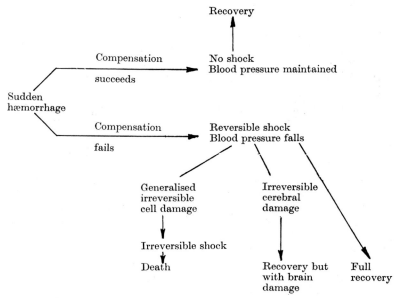

FIG. 22.2. The possible end-results of a sudden haemorrhage.

**Irreversible Shock**

Some patients with shock recover either spontaneously or as a result of treatment. Others steadily deteriorate in spite of all efforts to save them, and there has arisen a concept that there exists a stage from which recovery is impossible. This is called *irreversible shock* (Fig. 22.2).

**The Causes and the Concept.** These must now be examined:

*Prolonged underperfusion of tissue.* Although the selective vasoconstriction and redistribution of blood flow tide the patient over the initial period following injury, they may, if they persist, lead to permanent damage. The *kidney* is particularly vulnerable, and complete anuria may result. However, it is unlikely that this could kill the patient in as short a time as 24–48 hours, the duration of irreversible shock. Superadded *heart failure* and *liver damage* have also been suggested as important factors in making shock irreversible. Also the *metabolic acidosis* may induce vasodilatation and further lower the blood pressure. Whatever the mechanism, there is little doubt that the longer a patient remains in shock, the less likely is he to recover.

*Infection.* The toxaemia of severe infection may damage vital tissues and cause peripheral circulatory failure. This has already been described.

*Inefficient treatment.* It is sometimes not fully appreciated that in hypovolaemic shock the appropriate fluid, whether blood, plasma, or electrolyte-containing fluid, must be poured into the circulation until the blood volume is adequate. The slow drip has no place in the treatment of massive haemorrhage! Large quantities must be given rapidly, and the only limiting factor is the occurrence of an increase in systemic venous pressure, which indicates that the heart is failing to deal with the venous return. A catheter attached to a manometer should therefore be placed in the jugular vein while transfusions are being given.

Patients in shock are very susceptible to the action of depressant drugs like morphine and anaesthetic agents, and may easily be killed by overdosage. Alcohol induces cutaneous vasodilatation, and adds to the hypotension and hypothermia already present. It therefore should not be given to shocked patients.

*Damage to Vital Organs.* An injured patient may have sustained damage to some vital organ, e.g. a laceration of the brain or bleeding into the pericardium. Unless relieved death will ensue—apparently from the mysterious "shock".

**Conclusion.** There are many features about shock which we do not understand. Nevertheless, vigorous, well-designed treatment can save many cases. "Shock" is not a diagnosis which should be accepted unqualified; it indicates that something is wrong—a low blood volume, metabolic acidosis, sludging, arterial desaturation, renal failure, pericardial haemorrhage, etc., all of which may be diagnosed and treated. With severe injury, in old age, and in the chronic sick, death may be inevitable, but the diagnosis of irreversible shock can be made only *post mortem*.

## CONVALESCENCE

Injuries even if too mild to produce shock nevertheless cause considerable metabolic upset. The magnitude of the changes is related to the severity of the injury, and is most marked following severe trauma in those patients who survive the initial period of shock.

Two phases may be recognized: the catabolic and the anabolic.

### The Catabolic Phase

*Protein breakdown.*[26, 27] Body proteins, mostly those of the skeletal muscles, are broken down, and the deaminated portion is used for energy purposes. The nitrogen component is excreted as urea in the urine. There is therefore a *negative nitrogen balance* and *considerable loss of weight*.

*Water and electrolyte metabolism.* During this period water and sodium are retained, and potassium is lost from the body.

The mechanism whereby these changes are brought about is not clear. It is known that trauma stimulates adrenal cortical activity, and that corticosteroids play an important part in the catabolic process. The salt and water retention are related to an increased secretion of aldosterone and antidiuretic hormone which follows trauma.

*Fever, raised ESR, and neutrophil leucocytosis.* These are present, even in the absence of infection.

The catabolic phase lasts only a day or so after minor trauma, for example a simple hernia operation. After a severe burn it may last for 10–14 days, or even longer if infection ensues.

### The Anabolic Phase

Convalescence is completed by a reversal of the changes described in the previous phase. Proteins are rebuilt, and weight and health are restored.

### SUMMARY

The changes that occur in the wounded animal from the time of injury to the return to complete health are highly complex.

During the first few hours the response is concerned largely with circulatory adjustments, the aim of which appears to be the maintenance of an adequate blood supply to vital organs. Energy production is reduced, and the body's temperature falls. Thus the animal needs little food, and is spared the necessity of hunting. During the catabolic phase of convalescence fluid and sodium are retained to help maintain the circulation; in addition, they are needed for the inflammatory exudate around the wound. Energy is now provided by the protein stores, which are also used to build the new tissues during repair and regeneration. As convalescence proceeds and the wounded area heals, the animal becomes fit enough to resume its search for nourishment. Protein catabolism ceases, and energy is produced from ingested food; the depleted stores are replaced, and health is restored.

### References

1. BARCROFT, H. *et al.* (1944). *Lancet*, **1**, 489.
2. DICKINSON, C. J., and PENTECOST, B. L. (1968). In "Clinical Physiology", 3rd ed., p. 63, ed. by Campbell, E. J. M., Dickinson, C. J. and Slater, J. D. H. Oxford: Blackwell.
3. FREEMAN, J. (1963). *Ann. roy. Coll. Surg. Engl.*, **33**, 138.
4. MOORE, F. D. (1959). In "Metabolic Care of the Surgical Patient", p. 162, Philadelphia: Saunders.
5. COPE, O. and LITWIN, S. B., (1962). *Ann. Surg.* **156**, 655.
6. BLAIR, D. A. *et al.* (1959). *J. Physiol. (Lond.)*, **148**, 633.
7. RODDIE, I. C. and SHEPHERD, J. T. (1963). *Brit. med. Bull.*, **19**, 115.
8. Leading Article. (1967). *Brit. med. J.*, **1**, 447.
9. CLARKE, R. *et al.* (1961). *Lancet*, **2**, 381.
10. FINE, J. *et al.* (1960). In "The Biochemical Response to Injury", a C.I.O.M.S. Symposium, Eds. Stoner, H. B. and Threlfall, C. J., p. 377. Oxford: Blackwell.
11. BULL, J. P. (1954). *Brit. med. Bull.*, **10**, 9.
12. BLOCKER, T. G. and BLOCKER, V. (1963). *Progr. Surg. (Basel)*, **3**, 70.
13. SMITH, H. (1960). p. 341 in C.I.O.M.S. Symposium, *loc. cit.*
14. Leading Article (1964). *Brit. Med. J.* **1**, 254.

15. HEALD, R. J. and STRICKLAND, R. L. (1965). *Lancet*, **2**, 242.
16. HOPKINS, R. W. *et al.* (1965). *J. Amer. med. Ass.*, **191**, 731.
17. Leading Article (1966). *Brit. med. J.*, **2**, 481.
18. STONER, H. B. and THRELFALL, C. J. (1960). p. 105 in C.I.O.M.S. Symposium, *loc. cit.*
19. GREEN, H. N. and STONER, H. B. (1954). *Brit. med. Bull.*, **10**, 38.
20. WEIDNER, M. G. and SIMEONE, F. A. (1962). *Ann. Surg.*, **156**, 493.
21. GELIN, L-E. (1963). p. 6 in Proceedings of a Conference on the Evaluation of Low Molecular Weight Dextran in Shock: Pharmacology and Pertinent Rheology, edrs. Eiseman, B. and Bosomworth, P. Washington, D. C. National Research Council, Division of Medical Sciences.
22. KNISELY, M. H., STRATMAN-THOMAS, W. K. and ELIOT, T. S. (1941). *J. Amer. med. Ass.*, **116**, 2430.
23. WELLS, R. E. (1963). *Anesthesiology*, **24**, 828.
24. GELIN, L-E. and SHOEMAKER, W. C. (1961). *Surgery*, **49**, 713.
25. LONG, D. M. *et al.* (1961). *Surgery*, **50**, 12.
26. STONER, H. B. (1961). In "The Scientific Basis of Medicine Annual Reviews", p. 172. London: Athlone Press.
27. JAMIESON, R. A. and KAY, A. W. (1965). In "A Textbook of Surgical Physiology", 2nd ed., p. 71. Edinburgh: Livingstone.

*Chapter 23*

# TEMPERATURE REGULATION: FEVER

## Introduction

One of the most important developments in the higher animals is the evolution of mechanisms whereby a constant environment is maintained for its constituent cells. This fixity of the internal environment has been well recognized since the time of Claude Bernard. Temperature regulation is an important aspect of homeostasis, which in the case of man and other warm-blooded mammals has attained a high degree of efficiency. Cellular activity, involving as it does numerous chemical reactions largely dependent upon enzymatic activity, is very susceptible to changes in temperature. On the other hand, some of the energy released during cell metabolism is emitted as heat. Indeed, the temperature of highly active organs, like the brain and heart, would rise were it not for the cooling effect of the blood stream which carries away the excess heat, and distributes it to those areas where it can be dissipated to the atmosphere, viz. the skin and the mucosa of the upper respiratory tract.

It is probable that the development of a reliable temperature-regulating mechanism has contributed considerably to the biological supremacy of the warm-blooded group of animals.

## The Normal Body Temperature

**Methods of Measuring.** Body temperature is usually measured with the thermometer placed under the tongue, or else in the axilla, groin, or rectum. Of these readings, those obtained from the axilla and groin show the widest variation, and are generally regarded as being least reliable. This is hardly surprising, since the surface skin temperature fluctuates widely, and may approximate to that of the external environment. The rectal temperature is highest, being about 0·3°C (1°F) higher than the arterial temperature.[1, 2] It is said to be the least responsive to changes in the arterial temperature. Thus, if warm saline is infused into a vein, the rise in blood temperature is reflected in an elevation of the sublingual temperature but not that of the rectum. The sublingual temperature taken with the lips closed is therefore held to be the most reliable guide to the arterial temperature.[3]

**Normal Variation.** The normal temperature taken in this way is 36·8°C (98°F), with a range of 36·1°C–37·4°C (97°F–99·3°F). The maximum temperature is generally attained at about 6 p.m., while it is at its lowest at about 3 a.m. In women there is an elevation of the temperature during the middle of the menstrual cycle; its onset is thought to herald ovulation and is probably caused by the action of certain steroid hormones.

## Mechanism of Temperature Regulation[17]

The constancy of the body's temperature is maintained by balancing the amount of heat gained with that lost.

**Sources of Heat.** The major source of heat is from the body's metabolic activity. Heat production under fasting conditions with the individual at complete mental and physical rest is called the *Basal Metabolic Rate* (*BMR*). This ranges from 1 400 to 1 800 calories per day. Under active conditions additional heat is produced by *exercise* and the *ingestion of food*, especially protein.

**Sources of Heat Loss.** Heat is lost from the blood as it perfuses the skin— evaporation of sweat, conduction, and convection all play a part. Since the blood supply to the skin is regulated by the sympathetic nervous system, the latter plays a dominant role in the maintenance of a constant body temperature. Some heat is also lost from the respiratory tract, and in animals this can be increased by panting.

### The Regulating Mechanism

Situated in the hypothalamus is the *heat-regulating centre*, which is sensitive to the temperature of the arterial blood flowing to it.[5] When the temperature falls, cutaneous vasoconstriction is induced *via* the activity of the sympathetic nervous system, and the amount of heat lost is reduced. Furthermore, as the skin becomes cooler the subject feels cold, and may take appropriate voluntary action such as putting on extra clothing. If these mechanisms are inadequate, involuntary *shivering* is induced, and heat production is increased.

When the body's temperature tends to rise, there is a withdrawal of sympathetic vasoconstrictor activity, the skin becomes warm, and heat is lost. The subject feels hot, and may remove clothing, retire to the shade, etc. If these regulating mechanisms do not suffice, heat loss is augmented by sweating.

### Fever

Fever, also called *pyrexia*, may be defined as an elevation of the body's temperature consequent upon a disturbance of the regulating mechanism. When the temperature reaches or exceeds 40·5°C (104°F) the condition is called *hyperpyrexia*. Fever occurs under the following conditions:

**Heat-Stroke.** A rise in body temperature normally occurs during severe exercise when the heat-eliminating mechanisms cannot keep pace with the excessive heat production in the muscles. When the environment is hot and humid, even mild exercise may cause a marked rise in body temperature. Sometimes the heat-regulating mechanism breaks down under these circumstances, and the temperature rises to 41°C (106°F) or more. This is "heat-stroke", or "sunstroke", and unless treated promptly the temperature may continue to rise, reaching 43°C (109°F) or more, a level at which the patient becomes comatose, and permanent brain damage ensues. Death is not uncommon.

**Infection.** Fever is a frequent accompaniment of infection by viruses, bacteria, and larger parasites. The pattern of the pyrexia is often characteristic of particular diseases, e.g. the sudden onset in influenza and the step-ladder rise in typhoid fever (Fig. 7.3).

**Infarction.** Fever is often seen in patients with myocardial infarction.

**Tumours.** Some tumours are particularly liable to produce pyrexia, e.g. Ewing's tumour of bone, renal carcinoma, and Hodgkin's disease.

**Haemorrhage.** This may be followed by fever, especially when it occurs into the gastro-intestinal tract or the pleural or peritoneal cavities.

**Brain Damage.** Cerebral haemorrhage and other intracranial lesions may disturb the central regulating mechanism.

**Injury.** Fever occurs during the catabolic phase of convalescence.

**Fulminating or Malignant Hyperthermia.**[6,7] Although rare, this condition is of importance to practitioners whose patients are given a general anaesthetic. Most of the reported cases have followed the administration of halothane or suxamethonium. The pyrexia develops extremely rapidly, and unless vigorous cooling is employed, the temperature rises to very high levels, e.g. 43°–44°C, and death occurs from cardiac arrest. In most cases the skeletal muscles develop increased tone, and this is presumably the source of the increased heat production. A predisposition to develop malignant hyperpyrexia is inherited in some families, and can be detected by finding an increased blood level of creatine phosphokinase (CPK).

**Miscellaneous Conditions.** Fever is a prominent, but unexplained, feature of many other conditions. Acute rheumatic fever, serum sickness, and gout may be cited as examples.

### Clinical Features

Of all the causes of pyrexia, infection is by far the most important. The development of fever in an acute illness like lobar pneumonia or malaria has been the object of most study. Three stages are described:

**The Cold Stage.** At the onset of illness there is a feeling of intense cold, peripheral vasoconstriction is manifested by pallor, and the patient starts to shiver. Chattering of the teeth completes this picture of the familiar *rigor*. The temperature rises, as does the blood pressure. There is usually a rise in pulse rate of 18 beats per minute for each 1°C rise of temperature (10 per 1°F).

**The Hot Stage.** As the temperature approaches its peak, the peripheral vasoconstriction relaxes and the patient feels dry and warm. Heat loss now balances heat gain, and the temperature remains constant. The "thermostat" of the heat-regulating mechanism is still in control, but is geared to maintain the temperature at a level higher than normal. The extra heat produced is due to the raised metabolic rate caused by the fever. Should hyperpyrexia occur, this regulation may fail. During this phase the blood pressure falls.

**The Sweating Phase.** The temperature begins to fall, and the patient soon experiences a sensation of intense heat. Bedclothes are thrown off, sweating becomes profuse, and the temperature returns to normal. This is described as termination by *crisis*. If the pyrexia subsides slowly, as in typhoid fever, the termination is described as *lysis*.

## The Pathogenesis of Fever

The intravenous injection of Gram-negative organisms produces a sharp rise in temperature. This appears to be due to lipopolysaccharide or polysaccharide substances which are called *bacterial pyrogens*.[8-13] These are thought to act indirectly. They cause the polymorphs to release an *endogenous pyrogen* which acts on the heat-regulating centre. In man there is evidence that a similar pyrogen can be released from monocytes as well as polymorphs. This helps to explain the pyrexia which occurs in infections with organisms that excite a mononuclear response and also fever in patients with agranulocytosis.[14, 15]

The bacterial pyrogens are heat stable, and are of importance because they can produce febrile reactions if present in the fluids used in intravenous therapy, which though sterile, may still cause a sharp rigor. Fluids used for injection purposes must be carefully prepared by distillation to ensure the exclusion of all bacterial products. Such *pyrogen-free fluids* must always be used.

The fact that fever often accompanies necrosis, e.g. in tumours and infarcts, suggests that dead tissue contains pyrogenic substances, and pyrogens similar to those of bacteria have been isolated.[16]

Although recent work has shed some light on the mystery of fever, much has yet to be learned. It would be satisfying to believe that a rise in temperature in infection is a beneficial reaction designed to aid the body's defences. In virus infections this may be so, because fever stimulates the production of interferon (p. 223). However, with most infections there is little evidence that fever is beneficial. For the present we must regard the maintenance of normal temperature as an important homeostatic mechanism for the proper functioning of the body. Any departure from the normal is usually deleterious to well-being and can, if marked, be fatal.

## References

1. EICHNA, L. W. *et al.* (1951). *J. clin. Invest.*, **30**, 353.
2. COOPER, K. E. and KENYON, J. R. (1957). *Brit. J. Surg.*, **44**, 616.
3. CRANSTON, W. I., GERBRANDY, J. and SNELL, E. S. (1954). *J. Physiol. (Lond.)*, **126**, 347.
4. PICKERING, G. W. (1958). *Lancet*, **1**, 1 and 59.
5. BENZINGER, T. H. (1961). *Scientific American*, **204**, No. 1, 134.
6. KALOW, W. *et al.* (1970). *Lancet*, **2**, 895.
7. Leading Article (1971). *Brit. med. J.*, **3**, 441.
8. ATKINS, E. (1960). *Physiol. Rev.*, **40**, 580.
9. WOOD, W. B. (1958). *Lancet*, **2**, 53.
10. WOOD, W. B. (1958). *New Engl. J. Med.*, **258**, 1023.
11. BORNSTEIN, D. L., BREDENBERG, C. and WOOD, W. B. (1963). *J. exp. Med.*, **117**, 349.
12. KAISER, H. K. and WOOD, W. B. (1962). *J. exp. Med.*, **115**, 27.
13. Various Authors (1965). *Proc. roy. Soc. Med.*, **58**, 739.
14. BODEL, P. and ATKINS, E. (1967). *New Engl. J. Med.* **276**, 1002.
15. Editorial (1967). *New Engl. J. Med.*, **276**, 1036.
16. LANDY, M. and SHEAR, M. J. (1957). *J. exp. Med.*, **106**, 77.
17. ATKINS, E. and BODEL, P. (1972). *New. Engl. J. Med.*, **286**, 27.

*Chapter 24*

# DISORDERS OF THE BODY'S FLUIDS: OEDEMA

### The Compartments of Body Fluids[1, 2]

About 70 per cent of the lean body weight consists of water. It amounts to 40–45 litres in the average man, and of this 55–60 per cent (25 litres) is intracellular, and the remaining 40 per cent (15 litres) extracellular. The latter has two components: the extravascular *interstitial fluid* which comprises 12 litres, and the *plasma volume* which is 3 litres.

### Fluid Balance

The total water content of the body is maintained by balancing the fluid output with the intake. This important homeostatic mechanism is not completely understood, and a textbook of physiology should be consulted for the details. It may, however, be noted that fluid balance is controlled by three factors:

1. *Indirectly, by the mechanisms that regulate sodium balance.* Sodium cannot be retained without water.

*Aldosterone* secreted by the adrenal cortex has the effect of increasing sodium reabsorption by the distal tubule of the kidney, and thereby causes water retention. Sodium reabsorption from the proximal tubule is dependent to a large extent on the total glomerular filtrate. When the volume is reduced, as in shock and heart failure, sodium absorption is more complete, and water is therefore also retained.

2. *The mechanisms that regulate the output of water by the kidney.*

The antidiuretic hormone (ADH) from the posterior lobe of the pituitary is important in this connexion. It acts by increasing water reabsorption from the collecting tubules of the kidney.

3. *Regulation of the water intake by the sensation of thirst.*

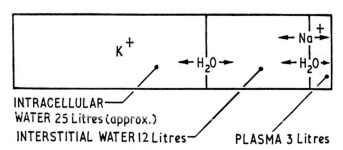

Fig. 24.1. Diagrammatic representation of the three compartments in which the body's water is accommodated. An excess or deficiency of water, which is freely diffusible, produces the greatest effect in the largest compartment, the intracellular one, whereas changes in sodium affect mainly the volume of the interstitial fluid.

321

Water is freely diffusible across the barriers which separate the various compartments (Fig. 24.1). The volume in each is preserved by the osmotic, electrochemical, and hydrostatic forces which are acting upon it. As far as osmosis is concerned potassium, phosphate, and protein are important in the intracellular compartment, while in the interstitial and intravascular spaces sodium, chloride, and bicarbonate have the greatest influence.

Water and sodium metabolism are so closely interrelated that it is convenient to consider them together.

### Disturbances in Water and Sodium Balance[3]

**Pure Water Deficiency.** This follows the deprivation of water, e.g. in people who cannot swallow because of oesophageal obstruction or coma, and during enforced starvation. It is also seen in *diabetes insipidus*, which is due to a lack of ADH. Patients with this disease pass enormous quantities of urine, e.g. 20 litres/day instead of the normal 1–1·5 litres.

*Effects.* Since water can cross the membranes which separate the fluid compartments, they are all depleted. The largest compartment, the intracellular space, is the most severely affected, and the cellular dehydration causes intense thirst and eventually death.

**Pure Water Excess.** The reverse condition, water intoxication, or cellular oedema, occurs when excess water is absorbed and retained. This may be seen in patients to whom too much water is given intravenously (as glucose solution), a situation particularly liable to arise during the postoperative period when water excretion is impaired (p. 314). The effects of water excess are serious. There is vomiting, muscle cramps, headache, convulsions, and sometimes death.

**Combined Salt and Water Deficiency.** Salt, or salt and water, deficiency is seen when there is loss from:

*The gastrointestinal tract,* e.g. severe vomiting or diarrhoea,

*The skin,* due to prolonged excessive sweating (heat-exhaustion),

*The kidney,* e.g. following prolonged administration of diuretics for chronic heart failure.

*Effects.* The effect of salt deficiency is the undermining of the osmotic support of the extracellular fluid. The interstitial fluid volume is reduced in amount, and therefore the patient shows *dehydration.* The eyeballs are sunken, the skin wrinkled, the tongue dry, and the face haggard. Thirst is often absent. Despite a compensatory vasoconstriction, the blood pressure is low and the veins are poorly filled. Little urine is passed, and there is a reduction in the plasma volume, which is evidenced by a rise in the packed cell volume and haemoglobin concentration (haemoconcentration). Unless relieved the condition rapidly terminates in circulatory failure.

**Combined Salt and Water Excess.** This is another artificially induced condition, and is seen in patients with defective renal function who are given excessive amounts of saline solution, e.g. during the early postoperative period, or during the course of acute renal failure.

*Effects.* The fluid is distributed evenly throughout the extracellular compartment which therefore becomes expanded. The manifestations are those of increased venous pressure and oedema, both systemic and pulmonary.

## OEDEMA

*Oedema may be defined as an excessive extravascular accumulation of fluid.* In its usual context it is applied to the morbid accumulation of fluid in the interstitial tissues. It is particularly liable to occur in the various preformed serous sacs, giving rise to *ascites, hydrothorax,* and *hydropericardium,* as effusions into the peritoneal, pleural, and pericardial cavities are specifically called. When generalized, it is called *anasarca,* or *dropsy.* It is, of course, also possible to have intracellular oedema as in hydropic degeneration and in pure water intoxication, but for the remainder of this discussion only the interstitial type will be considered. It is necessary first to understand the normal mechanisms which regulate the distribution of fluid in the body.

### Mechanism of Normal Control in the Systemic Circulation

Starling postulated that the movement of fluid between vessels and the extravascular spaces was determined by the balance of the hydrostatic and osmotic forces acting upon it (Fig. 5.1).[4, 5]

THE FORCES TENDING TO MOVE FLUID OUT OF THE BLOOD VESSELS ARE:

*The hydrostatic pressure in the vessels.* This is generally stated to be 32 mm. Hg at the arterial end of the capillary and 12 mm. Hg at the venous end in the skin of man at heart level.

*The colloidal osmotic pressure of the interstitial fluid.* Since the vascular wall is completely permeable to water and crystalloids, the only effective osmotic forces are those due to the colloids, mainly proteins. The interstitial fluids normally have a low protein content, and this is therefore not an important factor in the formation of the extravascular fluids under normal conditions. Furthermore those proteins which do escape into the tissue spaces are normally removed by the lymphatics.

THE FORCES MOVING FLUID INTO THE BLOOD VESSELS ARE:

*The tissue tension.* This is low (3–4 mm. Hg). Tissue tension is important in relation to the distribution of oedema; for instance lax areas like the face, particularly around the eyelids, ankles, sacrum, and scrotum, tend to accumulate fluid, while tense areas, like the palms and soles, are never the site of marked oedema. A rise in tissue tension is probably an important factor in limiting interstitial-tissue fluid formation in the legs under normal conditions and also in acutely inflamed parts.

*The osmotic pressure of the plasma proteins.* The osmotic pressure of plasma proteins is about 25 mm. Hg, and is due largely to albumin. Since the plasma proteins cannot normally pass through the vessel walls, the vascular permeability is important in regulating the distribution of fluids between the intravascular and the extravascular compartments. In the event of an increase in permeability, an exudate is formed which is rich in protein, e.g. in acute inflammation.

There are indeed two types of oedema:

**An exudate,** the accumulation of fluid due to an increased vascular permeability, such as occurs in inflammation—the fluid contains a high percentage of protein due to the increased vascular permeability.

**A transudate,** the accumulation of fluid due to a hydrostatic imbalance between the intravascular and the extravascular compartments, despite normal vascular permeability. It has a low protein content.

The importance of the lymphatics should not be forgotten. They form an elaborate network in most tissues, and their function is to drain away fluid and protein. The lymph is of considerably higher protein content than is the interstitial fluid itself.

The various factors involved in Starling's hypothesis are depicted in Fig. 5.1 (p. 62). It must be realized, however, that this merely represents an average state of affairs found in many capillaries at the level of the heart. Pressures in individual vessels show considerable variation.

### Types of Oedema

When considering the cause of any type of oedema, it should be realized that the process is usually due to a combination of factors. Starling himself appreciated this, and stated that dropsy was probably never due to a derangement of a single mechanism acting alone.

Oedema can be classified into local and generalized (widespread) types. The local oedemas are the simplest ones to understand because there are usually fewer factors involved in their production.

### Local Oedema

**Acute Inflammatory Oedema** (p. 61).

**Hypersensitivity** (allergic oedema). Oedema is present in all lesions of immediate-type hypersensitivity and in severe delayed-type reactions. It is due to an increase in vascular permeability. The oedema of anaphylaxis is widespread.

**Venous Obstruction.** A rise in venous pressure leads to an increase in capillary pressure, and the result is the formation of a transudate. This is seen in the legs following thrombophlebitis.

**Lymphatic Oedema.** Extensive lymphatic obstruction can produce an oedema of rather high protein content, although not as high as that of an exudate. Chronic lymphatic oedema stimulates an overgrowth of fibrous tissue, and in due course there is fibrous tissue and epithelial hyperplasia so that the affected part becomes grossly enlarged. If marked this is called *elephantiasis*.[6] It is seen in the leg in filariasis due to the obstruction of the lymphatics by a nematode worm. A similar effect is sometimes seen in the arm, when the lymphatics of the axilla are obstructed by cancer of the breast or by the fibrosis which may follow radiotherapy.

*Primary lymphoedema* is a special variety of lymphatic oedema due to a malformation of the lymphatics of the lower limbs. Women are usually the victims. One type of primary lymphoedema is hereditary and congenital, and is called *Milroy's disease*.[7]

### Generalized Oedema

**Cardiac Oedema.** In right-sided and congestive cardiac failure there is a retention of sodium and water by the body as evidenced by an increase in body weight. The distribution of this fluid is influenced by gravity. When the patient is ambulant the legs are affected first, and swelling of the ankles is often the initial symptom. When he is recumbent the oedema appears in the sacral and genital areas. The oedema readily pits on pressure. The pathogenesis of cardiac failure is described in Chapter 28.

**Renal Oedema.** *Acute glomerulonephritis.* Oedema is often the first symptom of this disease. It affects the face and the eyelids predominantly. There is no satisfactory explanation for this facial distribution. At one time it was thought that the oedema was due to damage to the blood vessels, but the more probable explanation is that it is due to heart failure which may follow the sudden rise in blood pressure seen in this condition.

*Nephrotic syndrome.* The outstanding feature of this is proteinuria with hypoproteinaemia. On Starling's hypothesis the diminished osmotic pressure of the plasma proteins can easily explain the generalized oedema, and this is undoubtedly an important factor. However, there are other considerations. A salt-free diet reduces the oedema, especially if combined with diuretics. It seems likely that salt and water retention, perhaps due to an oversecretion of aldosterone, is also important.

*Chronic glomerulonephritis.* The oedema is due to heart failure.

**Famine Oedema (Nutritional Oedema).** [8, 9] The oedema that is seen after prolonged starvation is usually confined to the legs. At first sight it would seem to be explicable in terms of the marked hypoalbuminaemia which is usually present, but there is no close correlation between the level of the plasma proteins and the presence of oedema. The true explanation of famine oedema is not known. An important factor appears to be the loss of compact tissue, mostly fat, and its replacement by a loose connective tissue in which fluid can accumulate without a rise in tissue tension.

Marked oedema is a feature of *kwashiorkor*.[14] This occurs in infants at the time of weaning and is a manifestation of protein deficiency prevalent in Africa, Asia, and Latin America. Failure of growth, anaemia, hypoalbuminaemia, fatty liver, depigmentation of the hair (which may have a reddish hue), and mucocutaneous ulceration are other features of this disease of poverty.

**Hepatitic Oedema and Ascites** are considered in Chapter 31.

**Unexplained Oedema.** Generalized oedema sometimes occurs in the absence of any known cause, and although such cases are uncommon, they indicate that factors other than those already discussed may operate even in the common types of oedema. A well-recognized condition is *cyclical*, or *periodic*, *oedema*, in which there are recurrent attacks of oedema involving skin, mucous membranes, joints, or even internal organs.[10] Usually the area involved is localized, and one type is called *angio-edema*. One patient is recorded as having pain and swelling of the left hand on alternative Wednesdays, lasting one week, for 18 years![11] The immediate cause of the oedema appears to be an increase in vascular permeability, but the cause of this is not known.

One variety of angio-edema is familial and associated with deficiency of the CI-esterase inhibitor of the complement system. How the attacks are precipitated is not clear but activation of the kinin system is probably involved.[12] Apart from skin and gut lesions, acute oedema of the larynx may occur and threaten life.

**Pulmonary Oedema.** This is considered in Chapter 29.

Although dropsy has been recognized as a symptom of disease since the beginning of medical history, it is evident that the mode of its formation is complex. In patients under hypnosis it is sometimes possible by suggestion to produce oedema at the site of previous injury.[13] The mechanism is completely unknown, and it is therefore no surprise to find that the mode of production of oedema in such simple conditions as acute inflammation and heart failure is incompletely understood.

## References

1. SLATER, J. D. H. (1968). In "Clinical Physiology", 3rd. ed. p. 1, ed. by Campbell, E. J. M., Dickinson, C. J. and Slater, J. D. H. Oxford: Blackwell.
2. WILKINSON, A. W. (1969). "Body Fluids in Surgery", 3rd. ed. Edinburgh: Livingstone.
3. MARRIOTT, H. L. (1947). *Brit. med. J.*, **1**, 245, 285 and 328.
4. STARLING, E. H. (1896). *J. Physiol.*, *(Lond.)*, **19**, 312.
5. LANDIS, E. M. (1927). *Amer. J. Physiol.*, **82**, 217.
6. PAUL, M. (1963). *Brit. J. Surg.*, **50**, 897.
7. Leading Article (1963). *Brit. med. J.*, **2**, 1483.
8. PASSMORE, R. and DRAPER, M. H. (1964). In "Biochemical Disorders in Human Disease", 2nd. ed., pp. 24 and 34, ed. by Thompson, R. H. S. and King, E. J. London: Churchill.
9. EALES, L. (1961). In "Recent Advances in Human Nutrition", p. 198, ed. by Brock, J. F. London: Churchill.
10. CLARKSON, B. et al. (1960). *Amer. J. Med.*, **29**, 193.
11. ABBOTT, W. D. (1933). *J. Amer. med. Ass.*, **100**, 1328.
12. EDITORIAL (1969). *New Engl. J. med.*, **280**, 1356.
13. Annotation. (1963). *Brit. med. J.*, **1**, 968.
14. HANSEN, J. D. L. (1961). In "Recent Advances in Human Nutrition", p. 267, ed. by Brock, J. F. London: Churchill.

*Chapter 25*

# SOME ABNORMALITIES OF THE PLASMA PROTEINS

The plasma proteins form a heterogeneous group. They are worthy of study because they not only play an important role in the body's economy, but also, being readily accessible, can be extensively investigated. Changes in their concentration are often of great value diagnostically in clinical medicine.

## Classification of the Plasma Proteins

**Fibrinogen, Globulin, and Albumin.** It should first be appreciated that the plasma proteins have been subdivided according to various physical and chemical characteristics. Their classification is therefore somewhat arbitrary and unsatisfactory. *Fibrinogen* is a protein which during coagulation forms an insoluble fibrin clot. When the remaining serum is half saturated with ammonium sulphate, a precipitate is formed which is composed of *globulin*. The protein which remains in solution is called *albumin*. The normal levels of these proteins are:

| | |
|---|---|
| Albumin | 4·0–5·7 g./100 ml. |
| Globulin | 1·5–3·0 g./100 ml. |
| Fibrinogen | 0·1–0·5 g./100 ml. |
| Total | 6·2–8·2 g./100 ml. |

Other physical characteristics have been used to separate the plasma proteins.

**Electrophoresis.** A more refined separation of the serum proteins is effected by *electrophoresis*. If a mixture of proteins is placed in an electric field at an appropriate pH, there is movement of the individual proteins at different rates, dependent to a great extent on their size and charge. The test can be performed on filter paper, cellulose acetate strip, or starch gel, and after passing an electric current for a suitable time the separated proteins are stained with a simple dye, e.g. light green. Fig. 25. 1 shows a typical electrophoretic separation of serum proteins. If the electrophoresis is performed in a gel, the separated fractions can be detected by adding suitable antibodies. This technique, known as *immunoelectrophoresis*, has revealed a great number of separate fractions which cannot be detected by simple electrophoresis.

**Solubility in Water.** The globulin fraction which is soluble in water is sometimes called the *pseudoglobulin*, while the insoluble portion is the *euglobulin*. Certain proteins precipitate out in the cold. These are called *cryoglobulins*.

**Molecular Size.** Fibrinogen has a molecular weight of 400 000, albumin 65 000, and the globulins range from 45 000 to several million. The ultracentrifuge may be used to separate proteins on a basis of their molecular size (p. 137).

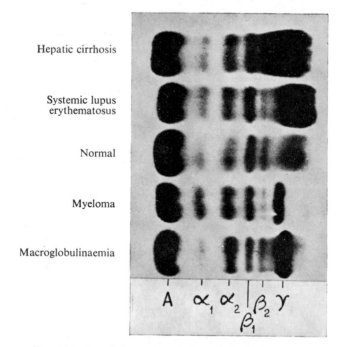

Hepatic cirrhosis

Systemic lupus
erythematosus

Normal

Myeloma

Macroglobulinaemia

FIG. 25.1. Paper electrophoresis in various diseases. In cirrhosis and systemic
lupus erythematosus there is a diffuse increase in the $\gamma$-globulins. This contrasts with the narrow band in myeloma and macroglobulinaemia.

(*From Waldenström, J.* (1958). Triangle, the Sandoz Journal of Medical
Science, 3, 262.)

**Functional Groups.** Another useful method of classifying plasma proteins is
based upon their function. The following groups may be recognized:

(1) *The proteins concerned with clotting,* e.g. fibrinogen, prothrombin, etc.
(2) *The proteins concerned with fibrinolysis,* e.g. plasminogen.
(3) *Hormones,* e.g. of the anterior lobe of the pituitary.
(4) *Enzymes,* for instance alkaline phosphatase.
(5) *Carrier proteins.* Many substances are carried in the blood bound to
specific proteins—thus iron is bound by transferrin. Thyroxine and the
corticosteroids of the adrenals are also bound to specific globulins.
Albumin itself has an important carrier role; for instance it binds
bilirubin. Lipid mobilized from the adipose tissue is transported largely
as unesterified fatty acid bound to albumin.
(6) *The Immunoglobulins.*
(7) *The Components of Complement.*

**Chemical Composition.** Some proteins contain lipid or carbohydrate. The
former are called *lipoproteins,* and the latter *glycoproteins.*

It will be appreciated that any individual protein may be described in a variety of ways. Thus prothrombin is a globulin which is also a glycoprotein. Immunoglobulins are $\gamma$-globulins which may be of small molecular size (150 000) or in the macroglobulin range.

### Source of Plasma Proteins[1]

The principal plasma proteins are all made in the liver, the major exception being the immunoglobulins. This has been elegantly demonstrated by experiments which showed that an isolated perfused rat's liver incorporated radioactive labelled lysine into plasma albumin, $\alpha$-globulin, $\beta$-globulin, and fibrinogen.[2] In the eviscerated rat, however, labelled lysine was incorporated into the $\gamma$-globulins and to a lesser extent into the $\beta$-globulins, but not into albumin.[3]

### Fate of Plasma Proteins

There is a regular turnover of the plasma proteins, but the sites of metabolism are poorly defined. The liver and probably other organs are concerned with the breakdown of $\gamma$-globulin,[4] and there is good evidence that albumin is secreted into the gastrointestinal tract, where it is broken down and its constituent amino acids reabsorbed.[5]

### Abnormalities of Plasma Proteins

There are three types of abnormalities of any protein group. The level may either be raised or lowered, or else an abnormal form of the protein may be present. The term *dysproteinaemia* indicates that there is an imbalance between the proportions of the various plasma proteins. It is generally used to describe the conditions in which the changes are marked, as when an M protein is present or a major component absent.

**Albumin.** The preponderance of albumin together with its low molecular weight make this protein an important factor in the maintenance of the non-crystalloid osmotic pressure in plasma. A low plasma albumin level therefore contributes to oedema formation (Chapter 24).

A low blood albumin level is found whenever there is excessive loss, e.g. in the nephrotic syndrome, with rapidly accumulating exudates, and following haemorrhage, burns, and severe injury. Reduction in the albumin level is also common during acute infection and following trauma. This *acute reaction to stress* is non-specific, and is accompanied by a rise in the $\alpha$-globulin. Hypoalbuminaemia is seen during starvation, particularly if the protein component in the diet is deficient. It also occurs in chronic liver disease following a failure in its manufacture by the damaged liver.

**The Globulins.** The globulins include a wide array of plasma proteins. In some instances there is good evidence that the type of protein which occurs varies in different individuals—thus there are nine different types of transferrin. The type present in any individual is determined by genetic factors in much the same way as are the blood group antigens, and is an example of genetic polymorphism.

In clinical practice the globulin component which is most frequently estimated is the $\gamma$-globulin. This consists mostly of immunoglobulins. The normal level appears to be maintained by constant contact with micro-organisms. Thus, in the germ-free rat* the $\gamma$-globulin level is reduced to about one fifth of normal. When the intestinal flora of such animals is restored the plasma proteins return to normal.[6]

**Agammaglobulinaemia and Hypogammaglobulinaemia.** These are described in Chapter 12, since they are associated with various immunological deficiency states.

**Hypergammaglobulinaemia.** As would be expected, an increased level of $\gamma$-globulin is found in many chronic infections. It is also a feature of certain diseases which have an autoimmune component, e.g. rheumatoid arthritis and systemic lupus erythematosus. The rise in $\gamma$-globulin affects several classes of immunoglobulins, and both K and L types are formed. Presumably many clones of cells are stimulated, and this type of hypergammaglobulin-aemia is called *polyclonal*. It contrasts with the *monoclonal gammopathies*,[7] in which an excess of a homogenous protein is produced. The protein is of one class, and its light chains are either $\kappa$ or $\lambda$, but almost never of both. Such a protein is found most often in *multiple myeloma, Waldenström's macroglobulinaemia*, and sometimes in *malignant lymphomata*. It is therefore called an *M protein*, being named after the first initials of the conditions in which it is found.

Hypergammaglobulinaemia generally presents as a symptomless bio-chemical abnormality which requires further investigation to uncover the primary cause. Sometimes, however, the plasma-protein abnormality may lead directly to secondary effects. In the *hyperviscosity syndrome* the presence of a high concentration of protein, especially a macroglobulin, increases the viscosity of the blood and impedes the peripheral circulation. This produces serious effects when the retina and central nervous system are rendered ischaemic. *Cryoglobulinaemia* (the presence of a globulin in the blood that precipitates in the cold) may occur in hypergammaglobulinaemia, and the precipitation of the protein in the small vessels of the hands leads to ischaemic episodes (Raynaud's syndrome) when the limbs are exposed to cold. Abnor-mal proteins may interact and bind to other plasma components, such as calcium, platelets, and the proteins of the clotting system. A *bleeding tendency* is thereby produced. Although M proteins belong to the immunoglobulins chemically, they have little antibody activity. Indeed, the production of antibody immunoglobulin is often inhibited, and this is manifested as an *increased tendency to infection*. Multiple myeloma often terminates in this manner.

**Multiple Myeloma.**[8-10] The hypergammaglobulinaemia is due to the presence of an M protein which is usually of the IgG class, but may be of the IgA, IgD, or IgE class. The tumour plasma cells manufacture this protein, and in addition often form an excess of the corresponding light chain, either $\kappa$ or $\lambda$. This, being of low molecular weight (22 000), is excreted in the urine as *Bence-Jones protein* (p. 461). The myeloma protein is not itself excreted.

**Macroglobulinaemia of Waldenström.**[11, 12] This rare condition is charac-terized by anaemia, a high ESR, lymphocytosis, and a tendency to haemor-

* A germ-free animal is one that has been specially reared under sterile conditions. Caesarian section is generally employed in the initiation of such a colony.

rhages from the mucous membranes, especially the gingivae, either spontaneously or following dental extraction. The condition runs a prolonged course, and appears to be a disease in which the lymphoreticular system manufactures excessive amounts of a homogeneous M protein belonging to the IgM class. It may lead to the hyperviscosity syndrome.

**Franklin's Disease (Heavy-Chain Disease).**[13,14] This uncommon disease is characterized by painful enlargement of the lymph nodes, fever, splenomegaly, and recurrent bacterial infections. An odd feature is transient, though sometimes severe, oedema and erythema of the soft palate, similar to that seen in infectious mononucleosis. The disease resembles Waldenström's macroglobulinaemia in that it is a type of diffuse lymphoma, lacking the punched-out, tumour-like bony deposits so characteristic of myeloma. The abnormal cells produce a fragment of the heavy-chain molecules resembling the Fc fragment. This abnormal protein is present both in the blood and urine.

### The Lipoproteins[15-17]

The major lipids of the blood are phospholipid, cholesterol and its esters, neutral fat (glyceryl triesters), and free unesterified fatty acid. Apart from the free fatty acid which is bound to albumin, the lipids are carried in the blood as complexes with each other and three carrier proteins. Apoprotein A and apoprotein B combine with lipid to form the $\alpha$- and $\beta$-lipoproteins respectively. Apoproteins A, B, and C combine with lipid to form the pre-$\beta$-lipoproteins and the chylomicrons.

*The hyperlipoproteinaemias* are a group of conditions which may be *primary* and presumably genetic since they tend to be familial, or they may be *secondary* to a wide variety of metabolic abnormalities such as obesity, diabetes mellitus, obstructive jaundice, and an imbalanced diet. Both groups can be subdivided into five types depending on the lipoproteins which are elevated. The hyperlipoproteinaemias are important because some types predispose to the development of atheroma, particularly of the coronary arteries. Lipid can also accumulate in RE cells to form localized deposits of foam cells in the skin and tendons. These are called *xanthomata;* a common example is seen in the eyelids of elderly people. Xanthomata in this situation are called *xanthelasmata*, and they may also occur in the absence of hyperlipoproteinaemia.

### The Erythrocyte Sedimentation Rate (ESR)[18]

When a column of blood mixed with anticoagulant is allowed to stand vertically, the red cells steadily gravitate in a mass due to the fact that their density is greater than that of plasma. The speed at which the sedimentation occurs is dependent upon many complex factors, chief of which are the degree of rouleaux formation and the extent of sludging. Both these phenomena are related to the composition of the plasma rather than to any change in the red cells themselves. Any relative increase in the plasma content of high-molecular-weight substances is found to increase the ESR. Thus an increase in fibrinogen or globulin (especially the $\alpha$ and $\beta$ fractions) has this effect; the 7S $\gamma$-globulins are the least effective. A raised ESR is particularly characteristic of macroglobulinaemia and multiple myeloma. Since albumin inhibits sedimentation, the ESR is increased in hypoalbuminaemia, e.g. in nephrosis. An increased ESR is seen whenever there is tissue necrosis (e.g. myocardial infarction) and following trauma. The factors concerned are poorly understood, but usually there is an increase in the fibrinogen and α-globulin levels, while that of albumin tends to drop. Elevation of the ESR is therefore quite non-specific, but nevertheless the test is a useful investigation. The presence of a raised ESR must always be taken to indicate disease, although the slight rise caused by anaemia, and that normally present during pregnancy, should always be remembered.

The ESR is of value in following the course of a known disease, e.g. tuberculosis and rheumatoid arthritis.

There are several methods of performing the ESR, and a haematology text-book should be consulted for details. The Westergren method is probably the most satisfactory. A column, 200 mm. high, of citrated blood is allowed to stand upright for 1 hour, and the upper level of the red-cell mass is then observed and its height from the top of the plasma recorded. Normally the drop is less than 15 mm. in one hour for men, and less than 20 mm. for women under the age of 50 years, and 20 mm. and 30 mm. respectively for those over that age.[19, 20]

### AMYLOID[21]

Amyloid is an abnormal protein which is found deposited in various organs. When the deposits are extensive the condition is called *amyloidosis*.

**Staining of Amyloid.**[21] In H. & E. sections amyloid appears as a hyaline, eosinophilic, structureless extracellular material. There are three empirical staining reactions by which it may be recognized:

*Iodine.* This may be used either on the specimen itself or on a histological section. Amyloid is coloured mahogany brown, and since in this respect it resembles glycogen, the material was called starch-like, or amyloid, by Virchow. When the iodine is followed by acid, amyloid may turn dark blue.

*Methyl violet.* This is a metachromatic histological stain, for the amyloid changes the methyl violet from a violet to a rose pink colour.

*Congo red.* This is soluble in amyloid, and can therefore be used to stain sections. The amyloid stains an orange colour and when the stained slide is viewed in a polarizing microscope a characteristic green birefringence is imparted. Apart from electron microscopy, this is the most reliable method of identifying amyloid.[21]

The dye is also used in a clinical test for amyloidosis. If a known quantity of Congo red is injected intravenously, its rate of disappearance from the plasma can be measured. When 60 per cent or more disappears within one hour and has not been excreted into the urine, amyloidosis can be diagnosed. Unfortunately, fatal anaphylactic reactions to Congo red have been reported, and the test is generally deprecated.

### Classification of Amyloid Disease

A classification according to associated conditions is the most useful because the amyloidoses are grouped on a clinical basis.

**Secondary amyloidosis,** is the commonest type of amyloid disease. It occurs in chronic infective conditions, especially where there is much necrosis or suppuration, e.g. chronic osteomyelitis, chronic empyema, caseous tuberculosis, and tertiary syphilis. It is also seen in rheumatoid arthritis, Hodgkin's disease, and occasionally in other malignant disease.[22] The distribution of the amyloid is described as *typical*, and is found in the following sites:

*Spleen.* Amyloid is laid down in the walls of the malpighian arterioles, and the cut surface therefore presents a characteristic appearance of *sago spleen* with numerous scattered firm translucent nodules (Fig. 25.2). A diffuse type of amyloid spleen is also recognized, in which the amyloid is laid down in the walls of the sinuses.

*Liver.* The organ is enlarged, heavy, pale, and firm. The amyloid is laid down in the walls of the sinuses between the endothelium and the liver cells (Fig. 25.3).

*Kidney.* The organ is large and pale. The amyloid appears in the glomeruli, which may eventually be converted into hyaline masses. Proteinuria is severe, and the nephrotic syndrome follows.

*Other sites.* Adrenals, lymph nodes, lung, and gut may all be affected. Deposits in the intestine may cause diarrhoea, and biopsy of the rectum is sometimes used as a diagnostic procedure. Amyloid is also laid down in the gingiva, and again biopsy may be employed to facilitate diagnosis.[23]

Generalized amyloidosis is a well-known complication of *multiple myeloma*, and in this it is quite often of atypical distribution as described below.

**Primary Amyloidosis.**[24, 25] This occurs in the absence of any obvious cause. Its distribution may be typical as described in secondary amyloidosis, but more often it is *atypical* and involves the connective tissues of nerves and muscle, e.g. the heart, tongue, and gastrointestinal tract. The staining reaction is often atypical in that the specific stains may not all be positive.

**Senile Amyloid.** Small deposits of amyloid are common in the heart and brain of elderly people and may be regarded as a normal feature of ageing. Occasionally the involvement of the heart may be sufficiently marked for it to cause heart failure.[26]

**Hereditary and Familial Amyloidosis.**[21] Several characteristic syndromes have been described but they are rare. Nevertheless, their existence serves as a reminder that the taking of a family history should never be neglected in a case of amyloidosis.

**Localized Amyloid.** Deposits may occur in the form of localized masses, or "tumours". These are rare, and are generally found in the tongue, larynx, or bronchi.[27] Amyloid may also be found in the stroma of certain true tumours, for example basal-cell carcinoma of the skin, medullary carcinoma of the thyroid,[28] and calcifying epithelial odontogenic tumour.[29–31]

### Effect of Amyloid

The deposition of amyloid generally excites no inflammatory reaction, but there is atrophy of the parenchyma. In an organ with an abundant reserve like the liver this is of little functional significance, but in other situations, for example nerves and kidney, the effects may be severe. Renal failure is a common terminal manifestation of amyloidosis. An affected organ may become rigid and this is important if it has a mechanical function to

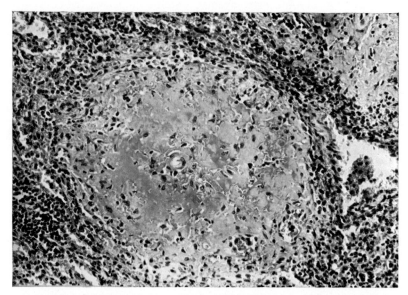

FIG. 25.2. Amyloidosis of spleen. The malpighian body is grossly enlarged, and is replaced by a mass of acellular amyloid. × 160.

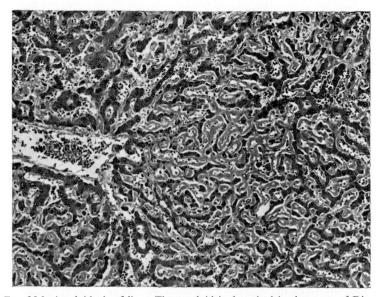

FIG. 25.3. Amyloidosis of liver. The amyloid is deposited in the space of Disse surrounding the sinusoids of the liver lobules. The liver cells adjacent to the amyloid are compressed, and show pronounced atrophy. × 120.

perform, e.g. the heart and tongue. Affected vessels tend to bleed easily, and therefore repeated haemorrhages are to be expected. Since almost any tissue can be involved in amyloidosis, the clinical picture may be extremely varied and the diagnosis should always be kept in mind whenever one is confronted with an unusual case.

### Pathogenesis of Amyloid[21,32]

Electron microscopy reveals that amyloid is a fibrous protein with a characteristic fibrillar appearance (Fig. 25.4).[21,33] The insolubility of these

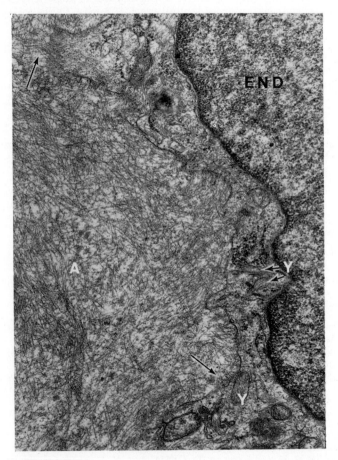

Fig. 25.4. Amyloid-laden rabbit spleen. The amyloid fibrils (A) fill most of the space near the endothelial cell (END), whose plasma membrane bears an intricate relationship to the fibrils, especially in the areas marked by arrows. In several areas (Y) fibrils appear to be intracellular. Osmium-fixed, Epon-embedded tissue, stained with lead citrate. × 24,000.

(*From Cohen, A. S.* (1965), in "International Review of Experimental Pathology" vol. 4, p. 159, eds. Richter, G. W. and Epstein, M.A. New York and London: Academic Press.)

fibrils has delayed their chemical analysis, but recent work has shown that in some cases the amino-acid sequence of the amyloid protein is similar to that of the variable region of the light chains of immunoglobulin.[32,34] Previous investigations had indicated that amyloid did not contain any immunoglobulin determinants.[35,36] Nevertheless, a close relationship between amyloid and immunoglobulin has long been suspected owing to the association of secondary amyloidosis with a prolonged or abnormal immune response such as occurs in chronic infection and multiple myeloma. Either L or K light-chain variable regions can form amyloid, and it is evident that the exact chemical composition of amyloid will vary from one patient to the next. Indeed, there is as yet no proof that all types of amyloid have a similar type of chemical structure, and one example of amyloid has been found in which the amino-acid sequence does not correspond to any known protein sequence.[32] Amyloid as recognized histologically may therefore be less homogeneous than is generally believed, and this may account for the widely differing views which have been put forward concerning its composition and pathogenesis.

If amyloid is a fragment of immunoglobulin, it is possible that it is formed by the digestive activity of macrophages. This would explain the finding that amyloidosis commonly affects organs with a high concentration of RE cells, such as the spleen.[37] An alternative hypothesis is that amyloid, or a precursor, is present in the blood and becomes deposited in a subendothelial or perivascular disposition. It must be concluded that it is still a mystery why amyloid is formed or deposited at certain sites under particular conditions. The stimulus for its formation is not known, but the list of recognized predisposing factors includes inherited abnormality, senility, and a variety of infections, chemical agents, and tumours.

## References

1. HAUROWITZ, F. (1961). In "Functions of the Blood", p. 527, ed. by Macfarlane, R. G. and Robb-Smith, A. H. T. Oxford: Blackwell.
2. MILLER, L. L. and BALE, W. F. (1954). *J. exp. Med.*, **99**, 125.
3. MILLER, L. L., BLY, C. G. and BALE, W. F. (1954). *J. exp. Med.*, **99**, 133.
4. COHEN, S., GORDON, A. H. and MATTHEWS, C. (1962). *Biochem. J.*, **82**, 197.
5. TARVER, H. *et al.* (1961). *Ann. N.Y. Acad. Sci.*, **94**, 23.
6. WAGNER, M. and WOSTMANN, B. S. (1961). *Ann. N.Y. Acad. Sci.*, **94**, 210.
   SELL, S. (1968). *Arch. Path.*, **86**, 95.
   BERGSMA, D. and GOOD, R. A. (1968), edrs. "Immunologic Deficiency Diseases in Man". Birth Defects, Original Articles Series, Vol. IV, No. 1. New York: National Foundation—March of Dimes.
   GOOD, R. A. (1966). In "The Thymus". (A Ciba Foundation Symposium), ed. Wolstenholme, G. E. W. and Porter, R., pp. 470–1. London: Churchill.
7. Leading Article (1968). *Brit. med. J.*, **1**, 460.
8. KORNGOLD, L. (1961), *Ann. N. Y. Acad. Sci.*, **94**, 110.
9. OSSERMAN, E. F. and LAWLOR, D. (1961). *Ann. N. Y. Acad. Sci.*, **94**, 93.
10. OSSERMAN, E. F. (1961). *Amer. J. Med.*, **31**, 671.
11. WALDENSTRÖM, J. (1958). *Triangle*, **3**, 262.
12. MARTIN, N. H. (1960). *Quart. J. Med.*, **29**, 179.
13. FRANKLIN, E. C. *et al.* (1964). *Amer. J. Med.*, **37**, 332.
14. Editorial (1970). *New Engl. J. Med.*, **282**, 1098.
15. STANBURY, J. B., WYNGAARDEN, J. B. and FREDRICKSON, D. S. (1972). *The Metabolic Basis of Inherited Disease*, 3rd ed., 1778 pp. New York: McGraw-Hill.

16. LEHMANN, H. and LINES, J. G. (1972). *Lancet*, **1,** 557.
17. *Bulletin World Health Organisation* (1970). **43,** 891.
18. Leading Article (1960). *Brit. med. J.*, **1,** 1717.
    COHEN, A. S. (1965). In "International Review of Experimental Pathology",
    vol. 4, edrs. Richter, G. W. and Epstein, M. A. New York: Academic
    Press.
19. BOTTINGER, L. E. and SVEDBERG, C. A. (1967). *Brit. med. J.*, **2,** 85.
20. BOYD, R. V. and HOFFBRAND, B. I. (1966). *Brit. med. J.*, **1,** 901.
21. COHEN, A. S. (1967). *New Engl. J. Med.*, **277,** 522, 574 and 628.
22. AZZOPARDI, J. G. and LEHNER, T. (1966). *J. clin. Path.*, **19,** 539.
23. LOVETT, D. W., CROSS, K. R. and VAN ALLEN, M. (1965). *Oral Surg., Oral
    Med., Oral Path.*, **20,** 444.
24. SYMMERS, W. ST. C. (1956). *J. clin. Path.*, **9,** 197.
25. Annotation (1963). *Lancet*, **1,** 1037.
26. POMERANCE, A. (1965). *Brit. Heart J.*, **27,** 711.
27. DOMM, B. M., VASSALLO, C. L. and ADAMS C. L. (1965). *Amer. J. Med.*, **38,** 151.
28. SCHIMKE, R. N. and HARTMANN, W. H. (1965). *Ann. intern. Med.*, **63,** 1027.
29. VICKERS, R. A., DAHLIN, D. C. and GORLIN, R. J. (1965). *Oral Surg.*, **20,** 476.
30. RANLØV, P. and PINDBORG, J. J. (1966). *Acta path. microbiol. scan.*, **68,** 169.
31. GARDNER, D. G., MICHAELS, L. and LIEPA, E. (1968). *Oral Surg.*, **26,** 812.
32. GLENNER, G. G., EIN, D. and TERRY, W. D. (1972). *Amer. J. med.*, **52,** 141.
33. SHIRAHAMA, T. and COHEN, A. S. (1967). *J. Cell Biol.*, **33,** 679.
34. GLENNER, G. G. *et al.* (1971). *Science*, **174,** 712.
35. CATHCART, E. S. and COHEN, A. S. (1966). *J. Biol. Colon.*, **96,** 239.
36. CATHCART, E. S., COMERFORD, F. R. and COHEN, A. S. (1965). *New Engl. J.
    Med.*, **273,** 143.
37. TEILUM, G. (1966). *Lab. Invest.*, **15,** 98.

*Chapter 26*

# DISORDERS OF THE BLOOD

The formed elements of the blood are the red cells (*erythrocytes*), white cells (*leucocytes*), and *platelets*. In the fetus blood formation (*haematopoiesis*) occurs both in the bone marrow and in a few extramedullary sites such as the liver and spleen. After birth haematopoiesis is solely medullary.

## THE RED CELL

### Development

The most primitive blood cell in the marrow is the *haemocytoblast*, a type of stem cell, a large cell with abundant cytoplasm and a nucleus with several nucleoli. If it is directed towards red cell formation it becomes smaller, its nucleus condenses, and its cytoplasm forms increasing amounts of haemoglobin. The first precursor cell is called a *pronormoblast*, which has nucleoli and whose cytoplasm has no haemoglobin. In the next cell type, the *normoblast*, nucleoli have been lost. Three stages are recognized—early, intermediate, and late—depending on the degree of haemoglobinization of the cytoplasm and the pyknosis of the nucleus (Fig. 26.2). Eventually the nucleus is extruded, and a mature red cell is left. These stages of development are indicated in Figure 26.1.

### The Mature Cell

The red cell is a biconcave disc, and in blood films appears as a roughly circular cell. It stains red with the Romanowsky dyes used in haematology*. When young it contains rough endoplasmic reticulum, and this imparts a bluish tint to the cell. This is called *polychromasia*. If such a cell is stained supravitally with brilliant cresyl blue, the RNA stands out as a network, or reticulum, of fine blue strands, and the cell is called a *reticulocyte*. The proportion of reticulocytes to older red cells gives an indication of the activity of erythropoiesis. A *reticulocyte count* should not exceed 2 per cent of the total red cells; if it does it indicates increased red-cell formation. This occurs after:

(*a*) haemorrhage
(*b*) haemolysis
(*c*) successful treatment of an anaemia.

When erythropoiesis is much increased, nucleated forms also appear in the circulation. A good example is haemolytic disease of the newborn (erythroblastosis fetalis—Figure 26.2)†.

---

* These include stains such as Leishman, Jenner, and Giemsa, and consist of a blended mixture of methylene blue and eosin.

† An *erythroblast* is the collective name for any red cell precursor.

THE CELLULAR CONSTITUENTS OF THE NORMAL BONE MARROW

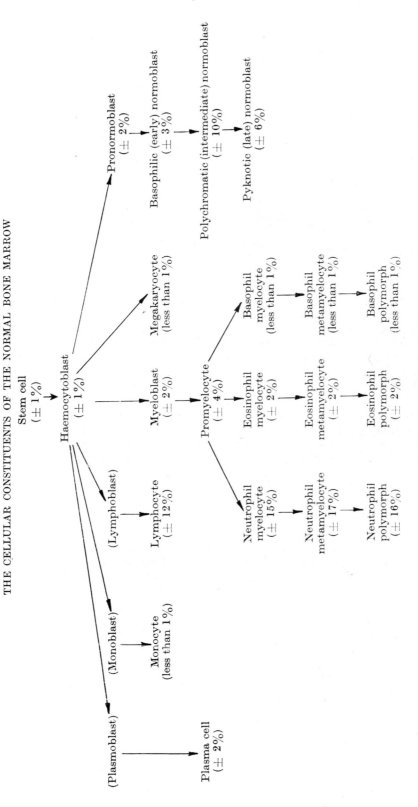

Fig. 26.1. The percentages are a rough average of the normal range of the cells. Plasmoblasts, monoblasts, and lymphoblasts are not normally present.

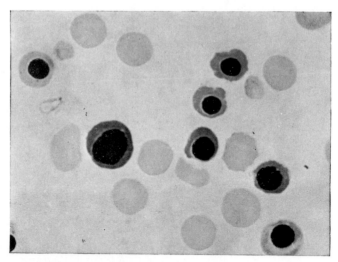

FIG. 26.2. Normoblasts in peripheral blood. The patient was a newborn infant with erythroblastosis fetalis due to Rh-haemolytic disease. One intermediate and six late normoblasts are shown. × 960.

## Examination of the Red Cell

The normal red cell count is 4·6–6·2 million per $\mu$l (or mm$^3$) in males, and the normal haemoglobin content is 14–18 g. per 100 ml. In women the red cell count is half a million cells per $\mu$l less and the haemoglobin level 2 g. per 100 ml. lower. The red cell count is high at birth, but drops precipitously within the first few months.

Unless electronic cell counters are employed red-cell counts are not recommended because of the wide range of error in this investigation. A haemoglobin estimation is simple, and gives adequate quantitative information about the red cells. This can be augmented with a *haematocrit reading*, or *packed cell volume*, if necessary. In this test a thin, cylindrical, graduated tube is filled with blood and centrifuged for half an hour at 3 000 revolutions per minute. In the adult male 40–54 per cent of the volume consists of red cells.

The experienced haematologist derives the most information about the red cell by inspecting a well-made, well-stained blood film. The normal red cell is described as *normocytic* and *normochromic*. If smaller than normal it is *microcytic*, and if larger, *macrocytic*. If poorly haemoglobinized it looks pale and is described as *hypochromic*. A cell cannot be over-haemoglobinized, and so there cannot be hyperchromia. Two other interesting pathological variants are: (*a*) *target cells*, consisting of a central dot and outer rim of haemoglobin, separated by a wide clear area (Fig. 26.5), and (*b*) *spherocytes*, small, perfectly circular cells which are very well coloured.

## Requirements for Red-Cell Formation

Apart from protein, which forms part of haemoglobin, the most important requirements are iron, folic acid, and vitamin B$_{12}$.

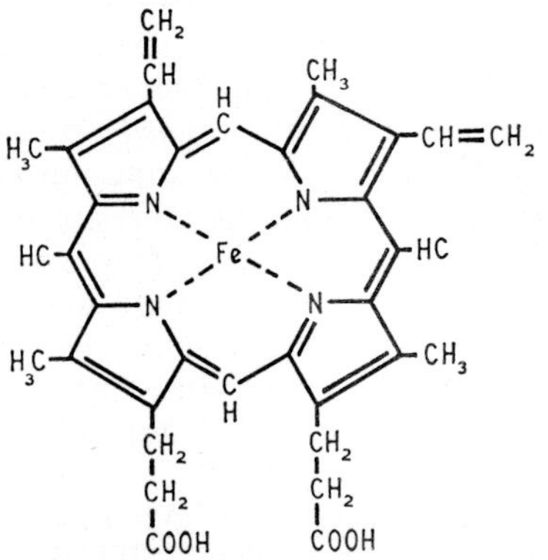

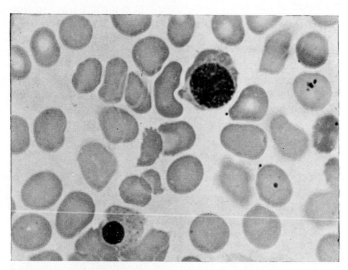

FIG. 26.3. The structural formula of haem. Note the protoporphyrin ring structure which is composed of four pyrrole rings joined by methene ($=CH-$)
bridges. In the centre is a $Fe^{++}$ atom.

**Iron.** In its ferrous form ($Fe^{++}$) iron is an integral part of haemoglobin. As
seen in Fig. 26.3, the iron atom lies in the centre of a porphyrin structure
composed of four pyrrole rings. Iron is absorbed from the food in an ionic
form by the mucosal cells of the duodenum and upper small bowel. Here it
combines, in ferric form ($Fe^{+++}$), with the iron-free protein *apoferritin* to
form *ferritin*, the storage form of iron in the body. Ferric iron is absorbed
as required into the blood stream combined with a plasma globulin called
*transferrin*, or *siderophilin*; it is used for such functions as haemoglobin and
myoglobin synthesis, and the remainder is stored in the RE cells as ferritin.

FIG. 26.4. A megaloblast. Note the large size of the cell and its stippled nuclear
chromatin as compared with the much smaller normoblast and its pyknotic
nucleus. The smear is from the marrow of a patient with pernicious anaemia.
$\times$ 960.

**Vitamins.** The important group belong to the B complex—folic acid and vitamin $B_{12}$. Both are necessary for the proper development of the normoblast; without either (or both) the cell undergoes a perversion of development, remaining large, and retaining a delicate stippled pattern of chromatin instead of showing the nuclear pyknosis of a maturing normoblast. Such a cell is called a *megaloblast* (Fig. 26.4). Both vitamins are present in the diet and absorbed in the small bowel, but whereas folic acid is directly taken up, vitamin $B_{12}$ cannot be absorbed unless bound to a complex mucoprotein secreted by the gastric mucosa. This substance is called *intrinsic factor*. It follows that the gastric secretion is essential for the absorption of vitamin $B_{12}$. Both vitamins are stored in the liver. Vitamin C is also required for red cell production.

**Other substances** required are less well understood. They include copper, cobalt, and hormones, such as thyroxine, adrenal cortical hormones, sex hormones, and *erythropoietin*. The last is probably responsible for the erythropoiesis that occurs after hypoxia. It is formed in the kidneys and possibly in other organs also, and its plasma level is high in most anaemic states.

### Disposal of the Red Cell

The normal life-span of the red cell is about 120 days. The actual manner of destruction is unknown, but the cell material is removed by the RE cells of the liver, spleen, and bone marrow. In these cells the haemoglobin is broken down. The globin portion is released, degraded, and returned to the body's pool of amino acids. The iron portion of the haemoglobin is stored in the RE cells as ferritin, while the porphyrin nucleus is broken down to bilirubin which is excreted by the liver. Normally there is a mere trace of free haemoglobin in the plasma—any that does appear is immediately removed by combination with a globulin component of the plasma proteins called *haptoglobin*, and a large excess is also taken up by the albumin to form *methaemalbumin*. Both the haptoglobin and albumin complexes are removed by the RE cells; none escapes into the urine. It is only when both these proteins are exhausted that free haemoglobin appears in the blood (haemoglobinaemia) and urine (haemoglobinuria).

### THE ANAEMIAS

Anaemia is defined as a condition in which there is a fall in the quantity of either red cells or haemoglobin in a unit volume of blood in the presence of a low or normal total blood volume. The normal blood volume is 5 litres, of which 3 litres is plasma and 2 litres red-cell mass. It might be expected that the blood volume would be reduced in anaemia owing to the decreased number of red cells, but in fact it is little altered as there is a compensatory rise in plasma volume.

The effects of anaemia are attributable to cellular hypoxia. At necropsy there is severe fatty change of the liver, heart, and kidneys, and death is usually attributed to heart failure. The classification of the anaemias is controversial, and the following scheme is recommended:

(1) Acute posthaemorrhagic anaemia, which has been described on page 309.
(2) Iron-deficiency anaemia
(3) Megaloblastic anaemia
(4) Haemolytic anaemia
(5) Anaemia of bone-marrow inadequacy.

### Iron-Deficiency Anaemia

**Causes:** *Chronic blood loss.* This is the most important cause, and is usually due to gastro-intestinal bleeding from a peptic ulcer, tumour, or haemorrhoids. Excessive menstrual loss (menorrhagia) is another factor.

*Defective iron intake.* This may be due to *dietary deficiency*, and is seen quite commonly in infants, pregnant women, and the elderly. It may also be due to defective absorption from the bowel in the *malabsorption syndrome*. This may follow intestinal lesions and also gastrectomy, which is often complicated by intestinal hurry.

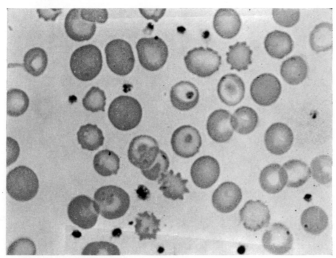

FIG. 26.5. Iron-deficiency anaemia. This film of peripheral blood contains red cells that are hypochromic. Quite a number show a target-like distribution of their haemoglobin. There are numerous platelets present. × 960.

**The pathological findings** are seen in the peripheral blood and bone marrow. There is a moderate anaemia in which the red-cell count is relatively less reduced than the haemoglobin level. *The red cells are markedly microcytic and hypochromic*, and target cells may be present (Fig. 26.5). The reticulocyte count is low unless there has been a recent haemorrhage. The white cells and platelets are normal. The bone marrow shows normoblastic hyperplasia.

Other interesting features seen in some cases of chronic iron-deficiency anaemia are *koilonychia*—spoon-shaped, brittle, lustreless finger nails—and *oral manifestations*—angular stomatitis, denudation of the filiform papillae of the tongue, and dysphagia. These oral features together constitute the

*Plummer-Vinson syndrome\**. Its relationship to iron deficiency is obscure. It is seen especially in anaemic, middle-aged women who have achlorhydria (the absence of hydrochloric acid in the gastric juice), and is sometimes complicated by oral and postcricoid cancer. Atrophic gastritis commonly complicates iron deficiency, and the achlorhydria further impedes iron absorption.

## Megaloblastic Anaemia

The essential feature is the presence of megaloblasts in the marrow, and it is due to a deficiency of folic acid or vitamin $B_{12}$.

**Causes.** *Dietary deficiency.* This is quite common in under-developed countries, and the anaemia is due to a lack of folic acid.

*Pregnancy.* Pregnancy is sometimes complicated by anaemia which is also due to folic-acid deficiency either as a result of a poor diet or because of the extra demands of the fetus.

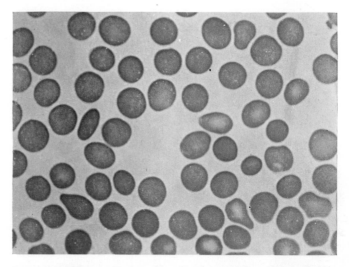

FIG. 26.6. Megaloblastic anaemia. This film of peripheral blood contains well-haemoglobinized red cells which show considerable variation in size and shape. Large forms (macrocytes) predominate. × 800.

*Gastric disease.* The intrinsic factor of the stomach is necessary for vitamin-$B_{12}$ absorption in the bowel, and therefore total resection of the stomach must in time lead to a vitamin-$B_{12}$ deficiency anaemia. However, the most important example is *pernicious anaemia*, an idiopathic condition in which there is progressive atrophy of the gastric mucosa. The stomach fails to secrete pepsin, hydrochloric acid, and finally intrinsic factor itself. Pernicious anaemia is a familial disease, and it is of interest that many patients are of

* This syndrome was first described in 1906 by Paterson, and soon afterwards by Kelly; both were laryngologists. It should rightly be called the Paterson-Kelly syndrome.

blood-group A. Autoantibodies against parietal cells and intrinsic factor are usually present in the patient's serum.

*Intestinal malabsorption* due to intrinsic disease of the small bowel usually affects folic-acid absorption more than it does vitamin-$B_{12}$ absorption.

*Drugs.* Notably the *anticonvulsants* phenytoin sodium and primidone used in epilepsy, and the *antimetabolites* used in the chemotherapy of cancer, antagonize folic acid and can cause a megaloblastic anaemia.

**Pathological Effects.** The *peripheral blood* shows a severe anaemia in which the red-cell count is relatively more reduced than the haemoglobin level. The red cells are conspicuously *macrocytic* and *normochromic*; they show poikilocytosis and anisocytosis, meaning that they vary greatly in size and shape (Fig. 26.6). The reticulocyte count is usually not raised. Both the leucocytes and platelets are reduced in number. *The bone marrow is hyperplastic and contains many megaloblasts* (Fig. 26.4).

There is a mild element of haemolysis in this type of anaemia, and the serum bilirubin is slightly raised. Ineffective erythropoiesis adds to the bilirubin load. The effects are those of a mild haemolytic jaundice (p. 429).

The other effects depend on the cause of the anaemia. Vitamin $B_{12}$ is essential for the proper functioning of the central nervous system, and without it *subacute combined degeneration of the spinal cord* can occur. In this there is demyelination of the posterior and lateral columns of the cord It does not occur in pure folic-acid deficiency.

There is sometimes superficial stomatitis and a smooth tongue denuded of papillae. This is seen characteristically in pernicious anaemia. In the other types of megaloblastic anaemia these changes are inconstant.

### Haemolytic Anaemia

In this condition there is excessive destruction of red cells. This in turn stimulates red-cell formation which is manifested by a reticulocytosis. An increase in reticulocytes that occurs apart from haemorrhage or the treatment of an anaemia is nearly always due to increased haemolysis.

### Causes

The increased haemolysis may be due either to abnormal red cells which are easily destroyed, or to a factor in the plasma which haemolyses normal red cells.

**Corpuscular Defects.** The most important in Northern European races is *hereditary spherocytosis*, or *congenital acholuric jaundice*, in which there is a spherocytic malformation of the red cells. These are very liable to be trapped and destroyed in the spleen. Splenectomy is usually effective in allaying the anaemia while having no effect on the malformed cells.

*The Haemoglobinopathies.* In Negroes the important congenital malformation is *sickle-cell disease*. Here the cells appear normal until deprived o oxygen, when they undergo bizarre sickling. This haemoglobinopathy is considered on page 37. Many other abnormal types of haemoglobin have been found. Thus Hb-C is encountered especially in West-African Negroes, and its presence leads to an anaemia less severe than sickle-cell disease. The haemolytic anaemia characteristic of the Mediterranean races is called *thalassaemia*, or *Cooley's anaemia*. It too is a haemoglobinopathy; no abnormal haemoglobin is formed, but instead there is a failure of synthesis of normal adult haemoglobin and much of the haemoglobin present is of the fetal type. This Hb-F is not normally found in the adult's red cells. The cells are grossly hypochromic, and appear distorted and flattened (*leptocytes*). Cells like these are rapidly destroyed in the body, and a severe haemolytic anaemia ensues.

*Enzyme-deficient Cells.* The observation that certain American Negroes developed an acute haemolytic anaemia when given the antimalarial drugs pamaquin and primaquine, led to the discovery that their cells lacked the enzyme *glucose 6-phosphate dehydrogenase* (*G6PD*). G6PD deficiency is inherited as an incomplete dominant sex-linked trait, and affected individuals usually suffer no ill-effects unless they are given certain drugs. The antimalarials mentioned above are the most important, but the sulphones (used in leprosy), sulphonamides, phenacetin, aspirin, and para-aminosalicylic acid can also precipitate acute haemolytic episodes. Once again the importance of iatrogenic disease is underlined. G6PD deficiency has also been found in Caucasians, especially those from the Mediterranian area, and furthermore other enzyme deficiences have also been found which cause haemolytic anaemia, either spontaneously or under the influence of drugs. The enzymes are those of glucose metabolism, and their normal function is important in maintaining the integrity of the red cell, particularly its haemoglobin content.

## Extracorpuscular Defects

**Autoantibodies.** Amongst the most important plasma factors acting on red cells are *autoantibodies*. Most occur idiopathically, but a few develop in the course of an infection, e.g. mycoplasmal pneumonia, a collagen disease, e.g. systemic lupus erythematosus, or a neoplasm, e.g. reticulum-cell sarcoma and Hodgkin's disease.

*Complete antibodies.* Some antibodies can agglutinate red cells directly in saline suspension, and are called "complete" antibodies. Most of these are not active at body temperature, but become powerful at colder temperatures. They are therefore called "cold" antibodies. Although detected in the laboratory as agglutinins, *in vivo* their action leads to red-cell destruction. They cause a comparatively mild haemolytic anaemia, especially after exposure to the cold.

*Incomplete antibodies.* The more important autoantibodies do not agglutinate red cells in saline suspension. They are, however, adsorbed on to the red cells, which, if washed to remove extraneous protein, and then suspended in an anti-human-γ-globulin serum (obtained by immunizing a rabbit against human globulin), undergo immediate agglutination. The antiglobulin technique described is called the *Coombs test*. Antibodies which coat red cells in saline suspension are termed "incomplete antibodies". *In vitro* they will agglutinate red cells suspended in 20 per cent albumin solution, but in practice the Coombs test is more sensitive. Most "incomplete" antibodies act maximally at 37°C, and are therefore also "warm" antibodies. *In vivo*, incomplete antibodies cause the cells which they coat to be destroyed. They therefore lead to a very severe type of haemolytic anaemia.

**Alloantibodies.**\* The blood-group antibodies can also cause haemolytic anaemia under certain circumstances. A good example is Rh-haemolytic disease of the newborn, in which an Rh-negative mother, married to an Rh-positive man, produces an Rh-positive fetus. During the last part of pregnancy and especially during labour, a leak of fetal cells into the maternal circulation is quite common. The mother is thereby stimulated to produce Rh antibodies. While the first child escapes damage, future Rh-positive fetuses may be attacked by maternal anti-Rh antibodies which cross the placenta. The fetus develops a severe haemolytic anaemia with many nucleated red cells in its circulation (*erythroblastosis fetalis*, Fig. 26.2).

Other important extracorpuscular factors that may lead to haemolytic anaemia are *organisms*, e.g. malarial parasites, *exotoxins*, e.g. the α-toxin of *Cl. welchii*, *drugs*, e.g. lead and sulphonamides, and *severe burns* which damage red cells locally.

**Pathological Effects**

The peripheral blood shows an anaemia in which the red-cell count and haemoglobin level closely correlate. The red cells are normochromic and normocytic. The outstanding feature is a *marked reticulocytosis*, sometimes over 30 per cent. In specific types of haemolytic anaemia malformed red cells may be seen, e.g. target cells, spherocytes, and leptocytes. The red-cell fragility is increased in spherocytosis and decreased in leptocytosis. There is a leucocytosis in acute haemolytic anaemia, but the white-cell count drops to normal in chronic cases. The bone marrow shows marked normoblastic hyperplasia.

There is a moderate to severe haemolytic jaundice in most cases. When intravascular haemolysis occurs, as in some alloantibody and autoantibody reactions, there is also *methaemalbuminaemia* (p. 342) and even *haemoglobinaemia* with *haemoglobinuria*. The presence of free haemoglobin in the plasma may cause renal vasoconstriction and anuria, especially if the haemolysis has occurred as the result of an immunological reaction (p. 363).

Other pathological effects of chronic haemolytic anaemia are *gall-stone (calcium bilirubinate) formation* due to the increased amount of bilirubin in the bile, and a *widening of the marrow cavities* of the bones with absorption of the compact cortex. This is due to the effect of increased, prolonged haematopoiesis. Some congenital haemolytic anaemias, e.g. hereditary spherocytosis and sickle-cell disease, are associated with *chronic leg ulcers*, but the connexion is not understood.

**Anaemia of Bone Marrow Inadequacy**

Anaemia is a complication of many chronic diseases, e.g. rheumatoid arthritis, chronic suppuration, leukaemia, renal disease, and myxoedema.

\* An alloantibody is an antibody present in one member of a species, which is capable of reacting specifically with an antigen present in some other members of the same species (see p. 361). The term isoantibody was previously used in this connexion, but it has been discarded so that the terms will parallel those used in transplantation immunology.

It is normocytic and normochromic, and is not attended by any significant reticulocytosis. It would appear that some deficiency or toxaemia impairs red-cell production, but the mechanism is not known.

Two other important types of anaemia that come into this category are those due to marrow aplasia (*aplastic anaemia*) and marrow replacement (*leucoerythroblastic anaemia*). They are considered later in the chapter.

### Polycythaemia

This is a condition in which the quantity of red cells is raised in a unit volume of blood in the presence of an increased total blood volume. It must be distinguished from haemoconcentration following plasma or fluid loss, in which the blood volume is reduced.

Polycythaemia may be *secondary* to chronic hypoxia, e.g. living at very great altitudes, chronic pulmonary disease, and cyanotic congenital heart disease. It is also seen occasionally in renal carcinoma—the tumour is presumed to secrete erythropoietin—and in Cushing's syndrome.

As a primary condition (*polycythaemia vera*) it is a neoplastic proliferation of the normoblastic element of the marrow. The red cell count may be increased to 10 million cells per mm³. There is often a considerable increase in the white-cell and platelet counts, a change not occurring in secondary polycythaemia. These patients are usually middle-aged or elderly, of florid complexion, with enlarged spleens and livers, and are liable to succumb to thrombotic complications, e.g. mesenteric venous thrombosis, coronary thrombosis, etc. Peptic ulcer is another common complication.

### THE WHITE CELLS

The important white cells are the granulocytes, lymphocytes, and monocytes.

### Development

The precursor cell of the granulocyte series is the *myeloblast*, a cell which resembles the haemocytoblast from which it is derived. As it matures it loses its nucleoli, and is then termed a *promyelocyte*. When specific cytoplasmic granules—neutrophil, eosinophil, or basophil—appear, the cell is called a *myelocyte*. The myelocyte nucleus becomes indented to form a *metamyelocyte*, and is ultimately drawn out into two or three discrete lobes joined by fine chromatin threads. This is the mature granulocyte, often called a *polymorphonuclear* (or polymorph) because of the shape of the nucleus. Most granulocytes are neutrophilic (fine lilac granules), but a few are eosinophilic (large red granules), and an occasional one is basophilic (very large blue granules).

The precursor cells of lymphocytes and monocytes are called *lymphoblasts* and *monoblasts*, but neither is normally present in appreciable numbers in the marrow. A few plasma cells are present in the marrow, but are not normally found in the peripheral blood. Figure 26.1 describes the composition of the bone marrow.

## The Normal White-Cell Count and Its Variations

The total white-cell count in the blood is 4 000–11 000 per c.mm. The range of the differential count is:

| | |
|---|---|
| Neutrophils | 40–75 per cent (2 500–7 500 per $\mu$l, or mm$^3$.) |
| Eosinophils | 1–5 per cent (50–400 per $\mu$l) |
| Basophils | 0–1 per cent (up to 100 per $\mu$l) |
| Lymphocytes | 20–45 per cent (1 500–3 500 per $\mu$l) |
| Monocytes | 3–7 per cent (200–600 per $\mu$l) |

The figures in brackets are the range of "absolute" counts. They are more useful than percentage figures. Thus a drop in neutrophils leads to a rise in the percentage number of lymphocytes—a so-called "relative lymphocytosis" —whereas the actual number of lymphocytes is unchanged. Strenuous exertion, anaesthetics, and emotional stress all produce a transient rise in the number of neutrophils. The main variations in the white-cell count are as follows:*

**Neutrophil Leucocytosis (Neutrophilia).** This common condition is usually due to *infection by pyogenic organisms*, e.g. staphylococcal, pneumococcal, coliform, etc. Some non-pyogenic infections can also lead to a neutrophilia, e.g. plague, diphtheria, and anthrax.

Other important causes are *massive tissue necrosis*, as following a myocardial infarct, *uraemia, acute gout, following severe haemorrhage and haemolysis, rapidly growing malignant tumours*, and *neoplastic disease of the marrow*, e.g. chronic myeloid leukaemia and polycythaemia vera.

**Neutropenia.** This may occur in certain *infections*, such as typhoid fever and brucellosis. It is common during the prodromal period of virus disease and in chronic protozoan infection, e.g. malaria. Overwhelming infection of whatever cause also lowers the neutrophil count.

Other causes of neutropenia are some diseases associated with splenomegaly (*hypersplenism*), and also *pernicious anaemia, bone-marrow aplasia*, and *acute leukaemia*.

**Lymphocytosis.** An absolute lymphocytosis is not common. It is seen in *whooping-cough* and *infectious mononucleosis* (*glandular fever*). In the latter disease the lymphocytes are atypical, and bear a resemblance to monocytes. The disease is an important cause of prolonged fever, and is not uncommon in young adults. Its cause is infective; a herpesvirus called the *Epstein-Barr virus* (*EB virus*) is incriminated, because after the disease there is invariably a high titre of antibodies against this virus in the serum. An interesting feature is the presence in the serum of antibodies which agglutinate sheep red cells to high titre (*Paul-Bunnell test*). There are other types of infectious mononucleosis that are part of cytomegalic inclusion disease and toxoplasmosis, and in these the Paul-Bunnell test is negative.

* The suffix -cytosis implies an excess of cells, e.g. leucocytosis (an increase in white cells), lymphocytosis (increase in lymphocytes), etc. The suffix -penia means a decrease in the relevant cells, e.g. leucopenia, lymphopenia, etc. Neutrophilia is sometimes used as an alternative to neutrophil leucocytosis. Neutropenia denotes a reduction in the number of neutrophil polymorphs, but since this is usually accompanied by a reduction in number of the other granulocytes, the term agranulocytosis is commonly used.

Another important cause of lymphocytosis is *chronic lymphatic leukaemia.*

**Monocytosis.** This is seen typically in *protozoan diseases,* such as malaria, trypanosomiasis, and leishmaniasis. It may occasionally occur in *chronic bacterial infections* also, e.g. tuberculosis and *Strept. viridans* endocarditis. Another cause is *monocytic leukaemia.*

**Eosinophilia.** This is encountered in some *hypersensitivity of atopic type,* e.g. bronchial asthma, hay-fever, and urticaria. *Helminth infections,* especially when the parasites are migrating through the tissues e.g. early schistosomiasis, trichinosis, and hydatid disease, and also filariasis, give rise to a marked eosinophilia. Intestinal worm infestation does not produce such a marked effect.

Eosinophilia is also seen in some skin diseases, e.g. pemphigus vulgaris and exfoliative dermatitis.

## The Leukaemias

Leukaemia is a condition in which there is a widespread proliferation of the leucocytes and their precursors throughout the tissues of the body, with a variable circulating component. The aetiology in man is unknown, and its course invariably fatal. It may follow exposure to ionizing radiations, and is much more common in victims of Down's syndrome than in the general population. In birds and mice the cause is viral (see pp. 276–277).

The classification of leukaemia depends on the rapidity of the disease process and the type of cell involved:

| | | |
|---|---|---|
| Chronic leukaemia | (a) | myeloid (myelocytic) |
| | (b) | lymphatic (lymphocytic) |
| Acute leukaemia | (a) | myeloid (myeloblastic) |
| | (b) | lymphatic (lymphoblastic) |
| | (c) | monocytic (monoblastic) |

The names in brackets allude to the predominant abnormal cell in the blood.

**Chronic Myeloid Leukaemia.** This is a disease usually of middle life. The outstanding haematological finding is an enormous leucocytosis, even up to 800 000 cells per µl. Nearly all of these are neutrophil polymorphs, metamyelocytes, and myelocytes, but there is also a significant increase in the eosinophils and basophils and their precursors. Myeloblasts are not numerous except terminally. If the leucocytes are grown in tissue culture, some show the abnormal Philadelphia chromosome (p. 42).

There is also a slowly progressive normocytic, normochromic anaemia and a gradual fall in platelet count. The bone marrow shows marked proliferation.

Clinically the patient has immense enlargement of the spleen and a lesser enlargement of the liver. Death usually occurs within 3–5 years, and may be heralded by an acute exacerbation in which the blood is flooded with myeloblasts.

**Chronic Lymphatic Leukaemia.** This is usually a disease of later life. There is marked lymphocytosis varying from 20 000 to 250 000 cells per µl. Most of these lymphocytes are mature, and any number of lymphoblasts in the blood is unusual. The polymorph element is reduced. There is a progressive normocytic, normochromic anaemia, and thrombocytopenia. The marrow is less affected than in myeloid leukaemia, and it may show no changes at all initially. Later on it becomes replaced by lymphocytes.

The condition affects the lymph nodes primarily, and the patient usually presents with a generalized lymphadenopathy. Sometimes the tonsils are conspicuously affected, and occasionally there is bilateral salivary-gland enlargement. The spleen and liver are enlarged, but to a lesser extent than in myeloid leukaemia. Death usually occurs in 3–5 years, and is due to anaemia and secondary infection.

**Acute Leukaemia.** The three types of acute leukaemia are best considered together, because it is often very difficult to distinguish between them either haemotologically or clinically. In acute leukaemia the white-cell count can vary from less than 1 000 cells per µl up to over 100 000 per µl. When there is a raised count the blood is flooded with primitive "blast" cells. It is often difficult to be sure whether these are myeloblasts, lymphoblasts, or monoblasts. In some cases the presence of more mature forms helps in the diagnosis, for example, if there are also some myelocytes and polymorphs, the cells are probably myeloblasts, whereas if there are an appreciable number of lymphocytes, the primitive cells are probably lymphoblastic. In any case the number of mature polymorphs is always so small that there is an absolute neutropenia. In cases where the white-cell count is very low, nearly all the circulating leucocytic elements are primitive blast cells, and can be mistaken for lymphocytes by inexperienced workers. This variant of acute leukaemia is sometimes called "aleukaemic leukaemia"; it is an unnecessary category.

In acute leukaemia there is a rapidly progressive normocytic, normo-chromic anaemia and a severe thrombocytopenia. No matter how low the peripheral blood count, the marrow is crowded out with "blast" cells.

Acute leukaemia occurs at all ages. In childhood it is usually lymphatic, but in adult life the myeloid variety is more common. Monocytic leukaemia is the least frequent and occurs most often in middle age. It is not possible to distinguish between them clinically. The onset is usually sudden, though there may have been a period of preceding malaise with obscure anaemia. The main features are high fever, a generalized bleeding tendency due to the thrombocytopenia, progressive anaemia, and necrotic infective lesions which are the result of the poor body resistance accruing from the absence of mature polymorphs (agranulocytosis). Oral and faucial lesions are prominent, and sometimes are the first symptoms which bring the patient for treatment. There is painful confluent ulcerative pharyngitis, stomatitis, and gingivitis. Gross gingival enlargement due to leukaemic infiltration is said to be par-ticularly characteristic of monocytic leukaemia, but it can occur in the other varieties also.

Most patients die within 3 to 6 months, usually as a result of infection or bleeding into vital areas such as the central nervous system. Treatment pro-longs life to about 1 year. It is noteworthy that the lymphatic variety responds well, though only temporarily, to adrenal steroids, whereas the other varieties are unresponsive.

**The Morbid Anatomy of Leukaemia.** There is a monotonous infiltration of leukaemic cells into numerous organs, which are enlarged, soft, and pale in colour. The lymph nodes, spleen, and bone marrow are particularly likely to be crowded out with the responsible cells. The liver is diffusely infiltrated throughout its sinusoids in chronic myeloid leukaemia, while in the lymphatic type it is the portal tracts which are mostly involved (Fig. 26.7). The bone marrow is pinkish-grey in colour, and extends down the shafts of the long bones. No organ is exempt, and massive local infiltrations are characteristic of the acute leukaemias. The other changes are those of diffuse haemorrhage and secondary infection.

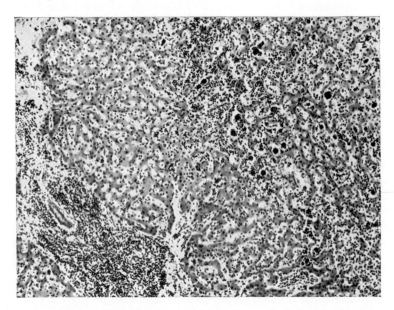

FIG. 26.7. Chronic lymphatic leukaemia. Note the dense infiltration of leukaemic cells especially in the portal tracts. There is a less dense infiltration in the sinusoids. × 100.

### Multiple Myeloma (Myelomatosis).

Multiple myeloma is a condition in which a neoplastic proliferation of plasma-cell series occurs in the marrow. It is considered in Chapter 33.

The blood changes in myelomatosis are non-specific. There is usually a progressive normocytic, normochromic anaemia, but unlike leukaemia, it is exceptional for the abnormal marrow cells to enter the circulation. There is likewise little tendency towards extramedullary collections of these cells.

### BONE-MARROW APLASIA

When the marrow ceases to release mature elements into the circulation, there is a serious drop in the blood count and the condition is described as *aplasia of the bone marrow*. Sometimes the failure of division occurs at the "blast" stage, in which case no mature elements are present, but sometimes the failure in division occurs at the later stage of haematopoiesis. In this case the marrow is crowded with maturing cells, but few enter the peripheral blood. This is called "maturation arrest".

Aplasia of the marrow may involve all three elements, when it leads to diminution of all the cells of the blood (*pancytopenia*), or it may affect only one of the elements. Pure red-cell aplasia is very uncommon, but aplasia of the granulocytes, or *agranulocytosis*, is an important condition. Platelet aplasia occurs in *primary thrombocytopenic purpura*.

**Pancytopenia.** Aplasia affecting all the elements of the marrow (aplastic anaemia) is usually due to an external agent, e.g. *ionizing radiations* or *drugs*, of which the most important are benzene, cytotoxic agents used in cancer chemotherapy, sulphonamides, and chloramphenicol. It is a rare complication of *miliary tuberculosis*, and may be *idiopathic*, in which case it is important to rule out "aleukaemic" leukaemia by a careful study of the bone marrow. An occasional cause is *hypersplenism* (see below).

Haematologically there is a normocytic, normochromic anaemia without any evidence of regeneration in the form of reticulocytes, a leucopenia with neutropenia, and a thrombocytopenia. The marrow is usually severely hypocellular, and those cells present are mostly lymphocytes. The prognosis is bad, and most cases die of infection or intractable haemorrhage. In maturation arrest the cellularity may be normal or even increased, and in these case spontaneous recovery may occur.

**Agranulocytosis.** Aplasia of the white cells is a very serious complication of certain *drugs*, namely amidopyrine (an analgesic), thiouracil, phenylbutazone, chlorpromazine (a tranquillizer), sulphonamides, pyribenzamine (an antihistamine), and dinitrophenol (once used as a weight reducer). It may follow ionizing radiations and cancer chemotherapy also, but is here part of a more widespread aplasia. Some cases are associated with hypersplenism, and some are apparently idiopathic.

There is a profound leucopenia, and nearly all the white cells in the blood are lymphocytes. Red cells and platelets are unaffected. The marrow shows inhibition of white-cell production. The leucopenia leads to a serious deficiency in the body's defence mechanism, and ulcerative, infective lesions occur in the mouth and throat, lungs, gastrointestinal tract, and vagina. Death soon occurs from overwhelming infection, and the lesions all show a virtual absence of polymorphs. The cellular infiltration is lymphocytic and plasma cell.

**Hypersplenism.** The functions of the spleen as regards blood formation are ill-understood. It certainly is active in removing defective red cells from the circulation, and it possibly exerts an inhibitory effect on the formation of white cells and platelets in the marrow. It takes over the function of haematopoiesis when the marrow is destroyed, but normally plays no part in blood formation.

It sometimes happens that conditions leading to gross splenomegaly give rise either to *marrow aplasia* (of all, or of any of the three elements of the blood) or to *haemolytic anaemia*. If the spleen is removed, there may be a cure of the blood disorder even if the primary disease continues unabated. Apparently the enlarged spleen is overactive; it either inhibits marrow function or else has a directly destructive effect on the cells in the circulating blood. When it is associated with aplasia, hypersplenism produces a maturation defect rather than a depression in the earliest stages of haematopoiesis.

Sometimes the splenomegaly is primary, but more often it is secondary to some other condition, e.g. cirrhosis of the liver (when the whole condition is called Banti's syndrome), rheumatoid arthritis, Gaucher's disease, schistosomiasis, or leishmaniasis.

### Bone-marrow Replacement

The normal bone marrow is sometimes crowded out by foreign elements. The commonest is *tumour tissue* from skeletal metastases in cancer of the lung, breast, or prostate, or in cases of multiple myeloma. Sometimes the element is a *lipid-filled macrophage*, as in Gaucher's disease, *fibrous tissue* (myelosclerosis), or even *bone*, as in marble-bone disease of childhood, where there is a failure of replacement of osseous tissue by marrow spaces.

Bone-marrow replacement gives a typical blood picture of *leuco-erythroblastic anaemia*. This consists of a normocytic, normochromic anaemia in which there are many nucleated red cells (normoblasts) in the blood. There is a moderate to considerable polymorph leucocytosis, and many myelocytes and metamyelocytes are also present in the blood. The main feature of this type of blood picture is thus the presence of both immature red and white cells in the circulation. The platelets may be reduced in number, and giant forms are sometimes present.

In longstanding cases the function of the marrow is assumed by the spleen and liver, and in both these organs there may be marked extramedullary haematopoiesis.

### THE PLATELETS AND CLOTTING FACTORS

#### The Normal Platelet

The platelets are small discs, devoid of a nucleus but with fine intracellular granules. They are derived from the large multinucleate *megakaryocytes* by a process of fragmentation of their cytoplasm.

The platelets are important in haemostasis because they readily adhere to damaged vessel walls and thereby prevent haemorrhage. Platelets thus adhere to surfaces and stick to each other, and these properties of *adhesiveness* and *aggregation* have been the subjects of much research because of their possible bearing on the cause of thrombosis (p. 366).

**Platelet Aggregation.** Platelets aggregate immediately in the presence of adenosine diphosphate (ADP). This may be demonstrated *in vitro* by the addition of ADP to a platelet-rich preparation of plasma which is kept agitated. The aggregation can be detected by measuring the ensuing decrease in optical density. Adrenaline, noradrenaline, and 5-HT have a similar effect. *Thrombin* leads to aggregation, but only after a delay of 5–10 seconds. It probably acts by converting platelet adenosine triphosphate (ATP) to ADP.

**Platelet Adhesiveness.** Platelets adhere to a variety of foreign surfaces, and the drop in platelet count when blood is passed through a column of glass beads has been used as an *in-vitro* method of measuring platelet adhesiveness. Platelets will also adhere to vascular endothelium if it is damaged mechanically, and to collagen, but not to pure fibrin.

Adherent platelets swell and release a variety of chemicals (*platelet release reaction*), including lipid (which plays a part in coagulation), 5-HT (which induces vasoconstriction), and ADP. The latter causes platelet aggregation and a small platelet thrombus is built up. This is unstable, and *in vivo* the platelets may break off and be released into the circulation as small emboli. Though clotting is not involved in the mechanism of platelet adhesiveness, the clotting system is soon activated by the lipoprotein surface of the platelets, generally described as platelet factor 3, and by the activation of factor XII. Fibrin is formed, and this is thought to stabilize the platelet thrombus.

Thus following injury, whether extensive or that caused by a pin-prick, the injured vessels are sealed by a mass known as a *haemostatic plug*. At first this consists of platelets, but soon this is consolidated by fibrin formation. Finally the entire aggregate contracts, probably due to the contractile protein in the platelets called *thrombosthenin*. Thrombin released during clotting causes further platelet deposition as well as fibrin formation. Defects in the intrinsic system of blood clotting, such as in haemophilia, do not prevent the formation of a haemostatic plug, and therefore the bleeding time is normal (p. 360). However, the plug is not stable and rebleeding occurs later. Serious bleeding can therefore follow the infliction of a wound such as that caused by dental extraction.

It can be readily understood why a deficiency in platelets or in the clotting mechanism can lead to a bleeding tendency. The normal platelet count is from 150 000 to 400 000 cells per µl. It is raised after injuries and operations (especially splenectomy). A low count is designated *thrombocytopenia*.

### The Clotting Mechanism

Blood clotting itself is a very complex mechanism (Fig. 26.8). In essence it consists of a conversion of *fibrinogen* (*Factor I*) to fibrin by the action of thrombin. This enzyme exists normally as an inert precursor *prothrombin* (*Factor II*), which is activated to thrombin by *thromboplastin* (*Factor III*), in the presence of *ionic calcium* (*Factor IV*). Thromboplastin is a vague, rather unsatisfactory term, and refers to the total activity of the plasma in converting prothrombin into thrombin, but there is no one substance that can be identified as such.

Thromboplastic activity can be generated in two ways. In the *intrinsic* (*blood*) *system*, contact with an abnormal surface leads to the sequential activation of Factors XII, XI, IX, VIII, and X. Activated Factor X, designated Xa, in conjunction with Factor V and platelet factor 3 results in the formation of *blood thromboplastin*, also known as *intrinsic prothrombin activator*, or *prothrombokinase*.

A hypothesis of the activation of these various factors as a serial process is called the *cascade theory of Macfarlane*. It postulates that most of the factors are pro-enzymes, each being activated by the preceding enzyme in a cascade sequence (see Fig. 26.8).

Factor XII is first activated by the contact of blood with a foreign surface, and the product is called Factor XIIa. This activates Factor XI, and Factor

XIa activates Factor IX. Factor IXa in conjunction with Factor VIII and platelet phospholipid, activates Factor X.

In the *extrinsic (tissue) system*, tissue damage results in the release of a tissue factor rich is phospholipid. This in conjunction with Factor VII activates Factor X, which as in the intrinsic system interacts with Factor V and phospholipid, to produce a thrombokinase, called *tissue thromboplastin*, or *extrinsic prothrombin activator*. The tissue factor is found in large amounts

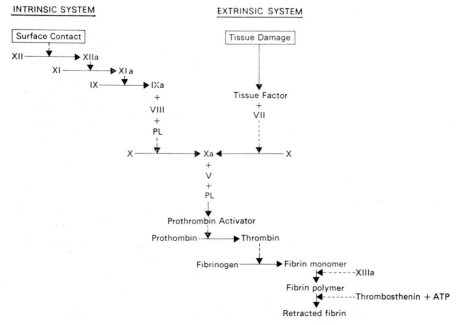

FIG. 26.8. A simplified diagrammatic representation of the blood clotting mechanism. Solid arrows indicate transformation, interrupted arrows denote actions. PL denotes phospholipid which in the formation of prothrombin activator *via* the intrinsic system is derived from the platelets (factor 3). In the extrinsic system, phospholipid is derived from the tissues. There is evidence that platelets in conjunction with Factor XII can form a platelet "tissue-factor" and thereby initiate the extrinsic system. The importance of this *in vivo* is debatable. Not shown in the diagram is the ionic calcium which is required for most of the steps shown.

(After Marcus, A. J. (1969). *New Engl. J. Med.*, **220**, 1213.)

in the brain, extracts of which are used as a source of it in various laboratory tests, such as the prothrombin time. The venom of the Russell viper is also rich in it.

The earliest phase of the intrinsic system is slow, but the extrinsic system is faster because a thromboplastin is readily available. However, once thrombin is formed the process is greatly accelerated—indeed, there is a real cascade, for thrombin potentiates the activity of Factors V and VIII. It also causes platelets to aggregate and so increase the amount of lipid factor 3. This is called the *autocatalytic action of thrombin*. Interestingly, thrombin also destroys Factor VIII after potentiating its reactivity; in this way Factor X activation is stopped when a high concentration of thrombin has been achieved.

The two pathways of blood clotting are both important, for a derangement of either leads to a serious defect in haemostasis. The intrinsic system develops much more slowly than does the extrinsic one, but both are initiated by tissue damage, either by releasing tissue factor or by providing an abnormal surface. In both systems there is activation of Factor X, and from then on there is a final common pathway involving Factor V, phospholipid, prothrombin, and fibrin. Factor XIII stabilizes the fibrin.

It should be noted that the plasma clotting factors (all globulins) are given Roman numerals. They are also given alternative names: Factor V is *labile factor;* Factor VII is *stable factor;* Factor VIII is *antihaemophilic factor;* Factor IX is *Christmas factor;* Factor X is *Stuart-Prower factor;* Factor XI is *plasma thromboplastin antecedent;* Factor XII is *Hageman factor.* The personal names refer to the surnames of the patients in whom a deficiency of the particular factor was first described.

In order to prevent spontaneous intravascular clotting there are also natural anticoagulant mechanisms. The mucopolysaccharide *heparin*, found in the mast cells around small blood vessels, interferes with the action of thrombin. Threads of *fibrin* adsorb thrombin, which is removed from the blood stream.

### Fibrinolysis

In addition there is a specific *fibrinolytic system* (Fig. 26.9) which removes fibrin intravascularly. The lytic agent is plasmin, a plasma protein, normally

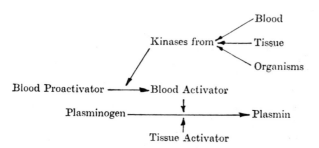

FIG. 26.9. The blood fibrinolytic system.

present as an inert precursor *plasminogen.* This is activated by enzymes called *kinases* present in the tissue and blood and also secreted by some bacteria, e.g. streptokinase from *Strept. pyogenes*. The system is triggered off by such stimuli as exercise, trauma, stress, and anaphylaxis. The actual mechanism of fibrinolysis is not certain, but it seems that the plasmin content of the blood is increased in many conditions, probably as a protection to balance the clotting mechanism.

## Tests of Importance in the Bleeding Diseases

*Platelet count*

*Bleeding time*—the time taken for a small skin puncture to stop bleeding. It varies from 1–9 minutes, and is prolonged when there is a lack of platelets, which, as has been described, are essential for haemostasis.

*Clotting time*—the time taken for a specimen of whole blood to clot. At 37°C this should be from 5–10 minutes. The clotting time is prolonged if there is a deficiency of any of the factors concerned in the *intrinsic clotting system* or in the *common pathway*. The test is insensitive, and a normal result can be obtained even in the presence of a very low level of some clotting factors. The test is not affected by the level of Factor VII (extrinsic system), but is prolonged when a circulating anticoagulant such as heparin is present in excess. The clotting time is widely used to control heparin therapy. Thrombocytopenia does not increase the clotting time, because only a trace of the platelet lipid factor is necessary for the formation of blood thromboplastin.

*Partial thromboplastin time (PTT).* This is the time taken for plasma to clot under the following three conditions:

(a) The test is carried out in a glass tube—the surface activates Factor XII.

(b) A fraction of brain extract called "cephalin" is added. This provides excess phospholipid and makes the test independent of the platelet count.

(c) Calcium chloride is added.

The PTT is a sensitive measure of the factors concerned in the *intrinsic* and *common pathways*.

*Prothrombin time.* In this test equal amounts of brain extract (containing tissue factor), calcium chloride solution, and test plasma are incubated and the time taken for clotting to occur is recorded. A control must be put up at the same time, and this should clot in 10–16 seconds. The prothrombin time is a measure of the factors concerned in the *extrinsic system* (Factor VII) and in the *common pathway* (Factors X, VII, and prothrombin). The intrinsic system is by-passed.

*Capillary fragility test.* This is performed by inflating the cuff of a blood-pressure manometer to a pressure between the diastolic and systolic for five minutes. If positive, the arm and forearm below the cuff show a petechial eruption. This occurs in platelet deficiency, because normally the platelets seal off any defects caused by a sudden rise in blood pressure. The test is also positive if the vessels themselves are abnormal, e.g. in scurvy.

The four tests which can most easily be carried out as an initial investigation of a patient with a bleeding disease are: the *platelet count*, the *bleeding time*, the *partial thromboplastin time (PTT)* and the *prothrombin time (PT)*. If both PTT and PT are normal, the defect is probably in the vessels or the platelets. If either PTT or PT is prolonged, there is probably a defect in the clotting system. If both PTT and PT are abnormal, the defect is most likely in the common pathway. If the PTT is prolonged and the PT is normal, it is the intrinsic system which is most likely at fault. A prolonged PT and a normal PTT is rare, and indicates a deficiency of Factor VII.

In practice, complex defects in haemostasis are best investigated in specialized centres where the activity of each individual factor can be assessed.

## The Bleeding Diseases

These manifest themselves as petechial haemorrhages into the skin, mucous membranes, and viscera (a condition called *purpura*), larger extravasations into muscles, joints, and serous cavities, and by a tendency to prolonged bleeding after injury and operations. There are three factors to be considered in a bleeding disease:

(1) The blood vessels
(2) The platelets
(3) The clotting factors

It must be realized that most bleeding is due to a local vascular lesion or injury. Postoperative bleeding is usually due to a badly-ligated vessel or infection, and epistaxis (nosebleed) is usually due to a vascular disturbance in the nose. Purpura itself may be the result of local factors, e.g. *senile purpura* is due to a loss of connective-tissue support of the smaller vessels, and *orthostatic purpura* may appear on the skin of the legs of people who stand for long periods of time. Generalized purpura is usually a manifestation of a bleeding disease, due either to systemic vascular disease or to thrombocytopenia. It is not usually found in association with defects in the clotting factors. Postoperative bleeding (including that following dental extraction) is due either to thrombocytopenia or a defect in the clotting factors. It is never due to vascular disease acting alone.

## Bleeding due to Vascular Disease

This takes the form of purpura, which may manifest itself internally as haematuria and haematemesis. Bleeding is seldom serious enough to endanger life. Important examples are:

*Anaphylactoid (Henoch-Schönlein) purpura,* is a disease in which small vessels are damaged by immune complexes. It occurs mostly in the young, and is accompanied by skin eruptions, haematemesis, and haematuria.

*Scurvy,* the main bleeding of which occurs from the gingiva, subperiosteally, and into the skin. It is probably due to poor anchorage of the blood vessels following the defective formation of collagen.

*Infections,* such as scarlet fever, haemorrhagic smallpox, and typhus, and also following the administration of *drugs* and *chemical agents* like aspirin and quinine, all of which damage the vascular endothelium usually by the local deposition of immune complexes.

In these conditions there are no specific haematological abnormalities. The capillary fragility test is usually positive.

## Bleeding due to Thrombocytopenia

This is manifested by purpura which may be very marked, severe haematemesis and haematuria, and fatal bleeding into internal viscera, especially the brain. Prolonged post-operative bleeding is another danger, but serious bleeding after relatively minor trauma, such as dental extraction, is uncommon. The bleeding time is prolonged, but the clotting time and PTT are normal. The capillary fragility test is strongly positive and clot retraction is impaired.

Thrombocytopenia may occur as an idiopathic condition (*primary thrombocytopenic purpura*), usually in young people. It appears to be a platelet aplasia—the megakaryocytes, though abundant, are abnormal and do not form platelets. Sometimes the condition remits spontaneously or following splenectomy, but relapses are common and death may occur.

As a secondary condition it occurs in *leukaemia* (especially the acute variety), *marrow aplasia*, *hypersplenism*, and following the administration of certain *drugs*. Here it may be part of a general marrow aplasia, or else the platelet component may be specifically affected. Drugs notorious for their effect on platelets are "Sedormid" (a hypnotic), quinidine, sulphonamides, and organic arsenicals. In some instances these form an antigenic complex with the platelets, which are then lysed by autoantibodies formed against the complex.

### Bleeding due to Defects in the Clotting Mechanism

This is manifested by massive bleeding into the tissues and from the body's orifices. Purpura is unusual, but intractable post-operative haemorrhage is characteristic, and serious, even fatal, bleeding can occur after dental extraction. The partial thromboplastin time is prolonged, and if the defect is severe, so also is the less sensitive clotting time.

The following clotting disorders are important:

**Haemophilia.** This is due to a deficiency of Factor VIII. It affects males only, and is inherited as a sex-linked recessive character (p. 36). The bleeding is very severe, and a special feature is *haemarthrosis*, which is usually recurrent. The organization of the haematoma leads to obliteration of the joint by fibrous adhesions and bony ankylosis. When frozen plasma is warmed to 4°C, a precipitate forms which is rich in Factor VIII. *Cryoprecipitates* prepared in this way are now widely used in the treatment of haemophilia.

**Christmas Disease.** This is due to a deficiency of Factor IX. Its mode of inheritance and clinical manifestations are indistinguishable from those of haemophilia. Only by specialized tests can they be separated.

Although the bleeding time is normal in both haemophilia and Christmas disease, the haemostatic plug which is formed in injured vessels is not stabilized by fibrin, and continued oozing and rebleeding is characteristic. Any fibrin which is formed tends to be removed by the activation of plasmin, and inhibiting this fibrinolytic enzyme might be expected to be of therapeutic value. Epsilon-aminocaproic acid is a plasmin inhibitor, and its administration parenterally before and after dental extraction has been reported to be of value. It can be used in addition to the injection of antihaemophilic globulin.

**Hypoprothrombinaemia.** In this condition there is not only a deficiency of prothrombin, but also of Factor VII, and sometimes of Factors V and X also.

The usual causes are *liver failure* or a *deficiency of vitamin K*. This vitamin is used by the liver for the synthesis of prothrombin and Factors VII and X. Vitamin K is fat-soluble, and is obtained partly from the diet and partly as a result of bacterial synthesis in the intestine. Its absorption is aided by the presence of bile salts, and it is therefore poorly absorbed in *obstructive jaundice*. Vitamin-K deficiency also occurs in the newborn due to an inability of the infant to synthetize it in his bowel. If the mother's intake is also deficient, a serious bleeding state may occur—*haemorrhagic disease of the newborn*. Another cause of hypoprothrombinaemia is the *administration of coumarin anticoagulants*. These inhibit the synthesis of the clotting factors.

**Hypofibrinogenaemia.** A deficiency of fibrinogen is usually acquired as the result of thromboplastic material entering the circulation. This material sets up intravascular clotting, so that the residual blood becomes incoagulable. In addition there is usually an activation of plasminogen, and fibrinolysis and fibrinogen destruction occur together with the clotting. The condition is called *disseminated intravascular coagulation*, or the *defibrination syndrome*, and is characterized by dramatic bleeding. It is met with most commonly as a complication of pregnancy, when amniotic fluid enters the circulation and sets up both clotting and general fibrinolysis. It is also described after *severe trauma, lung operations, incompatible blood transfusions*, in the generalized Schwartzman reaction, and rarely in *widespread cancer*.

### BLOOD GROUPS AND BLOOD TRANSFUSION

The red cells contain many antigens, but for practical purposes those concerned with the ABO and Rhesus blood groups are the most important.

**The ABO System.** The antigens concerned are glycoproteins. The basic antigen is called the H substance. Under the influence of the *A* and *B* genes, it is converted into A and B substances, depending on the presence of either or both genes. At birth there are no corresponding antibodies in the plasma, but within 3–6 months the antibodies corresponding to the antigen *not present* make their appearance. These are called *alloantibodies*, and are capable of agglutinating the red cells of normal people who happen to be of a different blood group, but not those of the same blood group as that of the individual.

The following table describes the distribution of ABO antigens and antibodies:

| Blood group | Antibody normally present in plasma |
|---|---|
| A | anti-B |
| B | anti-A |
| AB | none |
| O | anti-A and anti-B |

Why these antibodies develop is not certain. It is known that many Gram-negative intestinal bacilli have high concentrations of blood-group specific substances, and it is possible that the infant forms antibodies against those to which it is not immunologically tolerant.

To perform a blood grouping it is necessary to treat a suspension of red cells with "anti-A" and "anti-B" serum (derived from a donor with a high titre of these antibodies). If "anti-A" serum causes agglutination of the cells, they are group A; if "anti-B" does it, they are group B. If they are agglutinated by both, they are group AB, and if by neither, they are group O. Although group-O cells contain H substance, anti-H is rarely present in the plasma of group-A and group-B subjects in sufficient strength to cause a significant reaction in the body. It will be noted that the ABO antibodies are "complete", i.e. they agglutinate red cells in saline suspension (p. 346).

**The Rhesus System.** About 85 per cent of the white population of the world have a red-cell antigen which was first noted in Rhesus-monkey red cells. It is called the *Rh antigen*, and cells that contain it are described as Rh-positive. Rh-negative individuals do not normally have Rh antibodies in their plasma (c.f. the ABO system), but if they are immunized by Rh-positive red cells, they form antibodies very easily. Such immunization may follow a mismatched blood transfusion, or occur after the pregnancy of a Rh-negative woman bearing a Rh-positive fetus (p. 347).

Rh-grouping is done by suspending the red cells in serum obtained from a pregnant woman with a high titre of complete Rh antibody. Rh-positive cells undergo agglutination.

### Blood Transfusion

**Indications.** Blood transfusion is an essential procedure in clinical practice. Not only is it mandatory for restoring the blood volume after *severe haemorrhage*, but it is also used extensively in *major operative procedures*. The administration of packed red cells plays a part in the treatment of *severe anaemia* of whatever cause, but if possible this should be treated with the specific agent, e.g. iron, vitamin $B_{12}$, etc., unless the patient's life is in danger. Various blood components are available from transfusion centres, and these are useful in *restoring deficient clotting factors*, such as Factor VIII, prothrombin, and fibrinogen. Blood transfusion plays no part in the therapy of agranulocytosis and severe infection, unless there is concomitant anaemia.

**Storage of Blood.** Blood is collected aseptically from a healthy donor into a glass bottle or plastic bag in which there is an anticoagulant. The one most used is ACD, a mixture of citric *a*cid, trisodium *c*itrate, and *d*extrose. It is stored at 4°C, and must not be allowed to freeze or to exceed 10°C. It can be stored for periods up to 3 weeks. Up to this time most of the red cells survive in the recipient as well as do fresh cells. Leucocytes are eliminated within a day, and platelets too have a very limited survival.

**Cross-matching.** The important elements are the donor's red cells and the recipient's plasma. On the whole the donor's plasma is not important, because, with rare exceptions, the antibodies it contains are so diluted by the recipient's plasma that they are not likely to react with the recipient's cells. It is always preferable to use blood of exactly the same ABO and Rhesus groups as those of the recipient, but group-O blood can be used if necessary, provided it is properly cross-matched. Group O is called the "universal donor", because it is not normally agglutinated by any serum. In extreme emergencies, where delay might lead to death from exsanguination, it is permissible to use uncross-matched group-O Rh-negative blood, but otherwise cross-matching is essential, because (*a*) there may be an error in sample identification, and (*b*) the recipient's serum may contain antibodies other than anti-A, anti-B, and anti-Rhesus.

*Technique of Cross-Matching.* (*a*) Mix a 2 per cent suspension of donor cells and recipient serum at room temperature for 1 hour. Absence of agglutination rules out a "complete" antibody. (*b*) Mix the cells and serum at 37°C for 1 hour. Then centrifuge the cells, wash them three times in saline, and suspend them in an antiglobulin serum (Coombs test). Absence of agglutination rules out an "incomplete" antibody.

**Hazards of Blood Transfusion.** *Incompatibility reactions.* These are usually due to the rapid destruction of the donor red cells by the recipient's plasma. The antigen-antibody reaction leads to the release of vasoconstrictor substances from the red cells, which cause widespread vascular phenomena. There is initial pain along the vein, and this is followed by facial flushing, headache, a sensation of constriction around the chest, and backache. A danger is severe renal arterial spasm with ischaemia of the kidneys. Free haemoglobin in the plasma causes mild renal vasoconstriction, and the presence of vasoconstrictor substances (as well as the original condition that necessitated transfusion) accentuates this markedly. ABO incompatibility leads to much more severe renal effects than does Rh incompatibility, and death from uraemia may occur.

*Bacterial contamination of the blood* due to the adventitious introduction of coliform organisms leads to fatal septicaemia.

*Diseases introduced from the donor,* the most important of which are malaria, syphilis, and virus hepatitis (see HAA, p. 428).

*Febrile reactions* are usually due to the presence of white-cell antibodies formed by the recipient as a result of previous transfusions or pregnancy. Another cause is pyrogens present in the bottles, tubing, or anti-coagulant fluid. The fever is sharp, but usually lasts only a few hours.

*Allergic reactions,* usually urticarial are not uncommon, and are due to some antigen in the donor's plasma to which the recipient is hypersensitive. Life-threatening acute anaphylaxis is rare. Allergic reactions may also be due to the presence of IgE in the plasma of the donor.

*Overloading of the circulation,* leading to heart failure.

*Air embolism* is very rare with modern equipment.

*Thrombophlebitis* following the local irritation of the vein by the needle.

*Transfusional haemosiderosis.* This occurs when repeated transfusions are given frequently over a long period of time. There is a gradual accumulation of iron pigment which is not used in erythropoiesis, and it is deposited in the tissues, where it may set up fibrosis.

*Sensitization.* The transfusion of blood carrying antigens not present in the recipient's cells may stimulate the production of alloantibodies directed against the foreign antigen. These alloantibodies to red-cell, white-cell, platelet, or plasma-protein antigens may complicate future transfusions or pregnancies.

In modern centres blood transfusion is a lifesaving procedure. However, the possible complications are numerous, and except under emergency conditions, transfusion should never be attempted without expert supervision.

## General References

DACIE, J. V. and LEWIS, S. M. (1968). "Practical Haematology", 4th ed. London: Churchill.

DE GRUCHY, G. C. (1970). *Clinical Haematology in Medical Practice*, 3rd ed. 800 pp. Oxford: Blackwell.

WINTROBE, M. M. (1967). "Clinical Hematology", 6th ed., Philadelphia: Lea & Febiger.

## References for Blood Transfusion

BOORMAN, K. E. and DODD, B. E. (1966). "Basic Essentials in Blood Group Theory and Practice", 2nd ed. London: Churchill.

RACE, R. R. and SANGER, R. (1968). " Blood Groups in Man", 5th. ed. 599 pp. Oxford: Blackwell.

GIBLETT, E. R. (1969). "Genetic Markers in Human Blood". Oxford: Blackwell.

MOLLISON, P. L. (1972). "Blood Transfusion in Clinical Medicine", 5th ed., 830 pp. Oxford: Blackwell.

*Chapter 27*

# DISORDERS OF THE CIRCULATION

### The Blood Pressure

The function of the circulatory system is the maintenance of adequate perfusion of blood to all the tissues of the body. Each ventricular contraction ejects a quantity of blood into the arterial system, and in the systemic system the expansion of the elastic arteries prevents an undue rise in pressure. Nevertheless, the arterial pressure rises to a maximum (normally 120–150 mm. Hg), and during the subsequent diastole it falls steadily as blood flows away through the arterioles to the various vascular beds. The lowest pressure (diastolic pressure) reached is generally 60–90 mm. Hg. The major resistance encountered by the blood is in the arterioles, so that by the time the capillaries are reached, the pressure is only about 30 mm. Hg. The blood flow in the major arteries is pulsatile. The elasticity of the major vessels and the high resistance provided by the arterioles reduce this pulsation, so that in the capillaries and veins the blood flow is constant. It follows that whereas blood escapes from capillaries and veins in a constant ooze, it spurts out when an artery is cut.

The physiological mechanisms involved in maintaining the blood pressure will not be described in detail. In the main they involve the regulation of arteriolar tone by the autonomic nervous system in response to stimuli from the aortic and carotid baroreceptors. Low blood pressure (hypotension) is characteristic of shock and Addison's disease. Hypertension will now be considered.

### Systemic Hypertension

A considerable rise in blood pressure is normal in response to emotion, physical exercise, and sexual intercourse.[1] A persistent or recurrent elevation of the blood pressure at rest is abnormal, and is termed *hypertension*. Two types are recognized.

**Primary, or Essential, Hypertension.**[2] This is the common form of high blood pressure, and its cause is unknown. Primary renal or adrenal abnormalities have been postulated but never proven.

**Secondary Hypertension.** Hypertension is characteristic of phaeochromocytoma, where it is due to the effects of adrenaline and noradrenaline produced by the tumour (p. 475). Hypertension is also seen in some adrenal cortical tumours, and is an accompaniment of both Conn's and Cushing's syndromes (p. 476).

The classical experiments of Goldblatt proved that in the dog an obstruction to the renal arterial blood flow could produce hypertension. This is due to the release from the kidney of the proteolytic enzyme *renin*, which acts on

365

a plasma globulin, *angiotensinogen*, converting it into *angiotensin* I. Another plasma enzyme converts this into angiotensin II, an octapeptide which induces vasospasm and produces hypertension.[3]

In man hypertension sometimes, but not always, occurs in acute and chronic glomerulonephritis, pyelonephritis, and other renal diseases. It is not certain whether the mechanism of its production is similar to that of the Goldblatt experiments; present evidence is against such a pathogenesis. Hypertension in unilateral renal lesions is sometimes relieved by nephrectomy, but unfortunately this is not always so.

### Effects and Complications of Hypertension

*Haemorrhage.* Weakened blood vessels tend to rupture more commonly in the hypertensive subject than in the normal; dissecting aneurysm of the aorta, ruptured berry aneurysms of the circle of Willis, and cerebral haemorrhage are all more common in the hypertensive subject.

*Arteriolosclerosis.* The small arteries of many organs show a thickening of their walls, especially the tunica intima, with hyaline material. This is particularly marked in the afferent arterioles of the renal glomeruli, and gradually, as these vessels close down, the glomeruli and tubules which they supply become atrophic and replaced by fibrous tissue.

*Arteriolonecrosis.* Occasionally the blood pressure becomes very high and the arteriolar walls undergo necrosis. This is particularly important in the kidneys, where bleeding occurs and results in haematuria. The affected glomeruli undergo necrosis. This is called *malignant hypertension,* because the patient, if untreated, usually dies within a year or less of renal failure, cerebral haemorrhage, or heart failure, primarily left ventricular in type.

### Thrombosis[4]

In the vascular system it is the platelets and the clotting mechanism which guard against the danger of haemorrhage. The deposition of platelets and fibrin effectively patches any minor defect, and even severed vessels are soon sealed off. The control of platelet deposition and fibrin formation is an excellent example of a homeostatic mechanism designed to steer the body between the two hazards of haemorrhage and thrombosis. Under abnormal conditions an excessive deposit of platelets and fibrin may be formed, and this endangers the circulation by causing obstruction. This is *thrombosis.*

*The coagulation mechanism.* Coagulation, or clotting, may be defined as the conversion of fibrinogen to a solid mass of fibrin. The mechanism is described in Chapter 26 and here it will suffice to note that clotting can be initiated by thromboplastin derived from either the blood (intrinsic) or tissues (extrinsic). The activation of the intrinsic system has two components:

(*a*) Platelets which have become adherent to a surface liberate a lipid factor, and
(*b*) an abnormal surface activates Factor XII (Hageman factor).

Minor degrees of injury are constantly being sustained by blood vessels, and a layer of platelets is soon laid down to prevent haemorrhage. Endothelial cells cover this platelet deposit so that the smooth lining of the vessel is restored, further deposition ceases, and the process is brought to an end. The presence of naturally occurring anticoagulant substances, like heparin, and the constant bathing by the stream of blood, tend to prevent clotting. Nevertheless, small quantities of fibrin are probably formed even under normal conditions, and there exists a *fibrinolytic mechanism* for its removal (p. 357). The active agent *plasmin* is formed on the fibrin threads and leads to their dissolution. Thus, two mechanisms normally prevent the intravascular accumulation of fibrin:

(*a*) Endothelialization of both platelet deposits and areas of damage.

(*b*) The fibrinolytic system.

Under abnormal circumstances these mechanisms are inadequate, and intravascular coagulation becomes excessive.

*Platelet aggregation and adhesion* are described on page 354.

## Pathogenesis of Thrombus Formation

*Thrombosis* may be defined as the formation of a solid mass in the circulation from the constituents of the streaming blood. The mass itself is called a *thrombus*. Thrombosis involves two distinct processes:

(1) *The deposition of platelets on a vascular surface.* This occurs under three circumstances:

    (*a*) When the endothelial lining is damaged or removed.

    (*b*) With vascular stasis, when the platelets fall out of the axial stream and impinge on the wall.

    (*c*) In association with eddy currents, which deflect the platelets to an area on the wall.

Whenever any of these three factors operates to an excessive extent, an abnormal mass of platelets is formed. This is a *pale*, or *platelet, thrombus*.

(2) *The formation of a clot of fibrin in which the blood cells are trapped.*

If the platelet thrombus is not speedily endothelialized, or if there is stasis, blood clot is formed, and in its meshes are trapped the red and white cells. Thrombin is potent in causing platelets to adhere to each other, and its liberation during the process of coagulation readily leads to a further deposition of platelets. In this way a large mass is built up. When blood clot is the major component, it is called a *red*, or *coagulation, thrombus*. Frequently the thrombosis is made up of both red clot and pale platelet components, and is then called a *mixed thrombus*.

The crucial feature of thrombosis is the deposition of platelets on a vascular surface. This can occur only in the presence of a flowing stream, and is therefore produced spontaneously only in the living animal. The clotting is a secondary phenomenon. It follows that the terms "clot" and "thrombus" are quite distinct; a thrombus contains a variable amount of clot, but the important feature is a platelet scaffold which is lacking in a clot; it can be formed only *in vivo*.* Clotting, on the other hand, may occur as part of thrombosis, and is also seen in a column of static blood *in vivo* or *in vitro*.

---

* Highly artificial experimental procedures can, of course, provide an exception to this rule.

Since the cardinal process in thrombosis is the deposition of platelets on an intimal surface, it is evident that the integrity of the vascular system is all-important in preventing it. The two factors are:

(a) The smooth endothelial lining which diminishes frictional resistance between the wall and the circulating blood, and

(b) the streamline of blood along the complex circulatory pathways, which results in the formed elements moving in a central axial stream (p. 61).

The speed of flow prevents local stasis, and the absence of irregularities

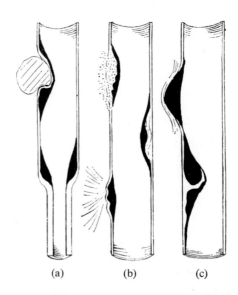

(a)          (b)          (c)

Fig. 27.1. This diagram shows seven different causes of a disruption of the normal streamlining of the blood flow, and the manner whereby platelets (shown in black) are laid down to restore the architecture.

(a) Bulging due to external pressure and spasm.

(b) Endothelial swelling and roughening due to inflammation, a plaque of thickening, e.g. atheroma, and corrugation due to adjacent cicatrization.

(c) Aneurysm, and a hard sclerotic valve.

(*From Hadfield, G.* (1950). Ann. roy. Coll. Surg. Engl., **6**, 219.)

in the walls does not allow the development of eddy currents. The streamline of blood can be threatened in a variety of ways, which are illustrated in Fig. 27.1. These lesions all lead to local stasis as well as to the formation of eddy currents, and the platelets that cover them are actually performing a remedial function. They serve to smooth out the contours of the wall and restore the streamline of blood in the vessel. The small amount of thromboplastin that they generate is dissipated in the flowing blood, and they themselves are rapidly endothelialized. It is when this process is retarded that the platelet mass grows, thromboplastin accumulates, much fibrin is produced, and thrombosis proceeds even to the extent of obliterating the vessel.

## Causes of Thrombosis

Three factors (*Virchow's triad*) must be considered in regard to the mechanism of thrombosis:

*The vessel wall.* The various types of anatomical changes in the vessel wall which may lead to platelet deposition have already been depicted (Fig. 27.1). In general these abnormalities play an important part in thrombosis involving the heart and arteries. In the veins they are of less importance.

*The flow of blood.* The importance of *eddy currents* has already been noted. These lead to platelet deposition, and the resulting thrombus is pale. This occurs in fast moving streams, e.g. over the heart valves and in arteries. *Stasis* is the most important cause of extensive thrombosis involving veins. It is also a factor in inducing thrombosis in the sac of an aneurysm.

*The constituents of the blood.*[5] An increase in the platelet count,[6] increased platelet adhesiveness,[8] and a decrease in the clotting time,[7] such as occur after trauma and haemorrhage, are sometimes important in inducing thrombosis.

It should be noted that usually more than one factor is implicated in causing thrombosis. For instance, there is regional stasis and a high platelet count after an operation, and atheromatous plaques act both by causing a loss of the endothelium and inducing eddy currents.

## Venous Thrombosis

Although disease of the vessel walls is uncommon, stasis is particularly evident in the veins, especially in those of the legs. Thrombosis with a large element of clotting is therefore common. Two distinct entities should be recognized: phlebothrombosis and thrombophlebitis.

## Phlebothrombosis[4]

In this important condition there is extensive thrombosis and clot formation in the veins of the calf. It is due essentially to stasis, and is seen whenever the circulation in the legs is impaired. This occurs whenever the cardiac output is reduced, e.g. in heart failure, shock, and when the metabolic rate is reduced as when a patient is put to rest in bed. The venous return from the legs is greatly facilitated by the squeezing action of the surrounding muscles, and this important mechanism is in abeyance in the bedridden patient. The arms are much less likely to be affected, since they are in constant use in all conscious patients. Following trauma the increased platelet count, increased platelet adhesiveness, and decreased clotting time are further factors favouring thrombosis. Direct damage to the veins, e.g. by a fractured bone, or even the pressure of a pillow on the calf muscles, may be additional precipitating factors. It follows therefore that phlebothrombosis is common in the leg veins whenever a patient is put to bed, especially if he is elderly, if the heart is failing, or if he is in shock or has suffered severe trauma, such as a major operation or haemorrhage.

### Pathogenesis of Phlebothrombosis[4]

Five stages can be recognized (Fig. 27.2).

**Primary Platelet Thrombus.** Following some trivial intimal damage, platelets adhere to the vein walls and form a mass of pale thrombus. This has been likened to the formation of a snow-drift during a snow-storm. Under normal circumstances this would produce no ill-effect, but if stasis is super-added, fibrin formation ensues and a large coralline thrombus is produced.

**Coralline Thrombus.** As fibrin formation occurs and further platelets accumulate, the latter take the form of upstanding laminae growing across

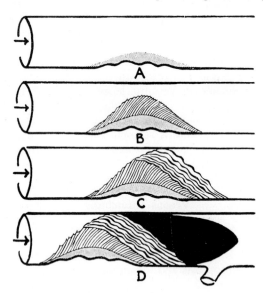

FIG. 27.2. The pathogenesis of phlebothrombosis.
  A. Primary platelet thrombus.
  B. Coralline thrombus.
  C. Occluding thrombus.
  D. Consecutive clot to the next venous tributary.
  (*From Hadfield, G.* (1950). Ann. roy. Coll. Surg. Engl., **6**, 219.)

the stream. Between the laminae there is complete stasis, and fibrin is deposited; in it numerous red and white cells are trapped. This is an example of a mixed thrombus, and on section the alternating layers are seen (Fig. 27.3). The retraction of the fibrin layers leads to the characteristic ribbed or rippled appearance seen when the surface of the thrombus is examined. The elevated platelet ridges are called the *lines of Zahn*, and are a characteristic feature of a thrombus formed in a fairly rapid stream of blood. Their presence is a useful indication that a structure found in a vessel is a thrombus formed during life and not a post-mortem clot (p. 376).

**Occluding Thrombus.** The growth of the coralline thrombus progressively occludes the lumen of the vein, and the ensuing stasis rapidly leads to the formation of an occluding thrombus.

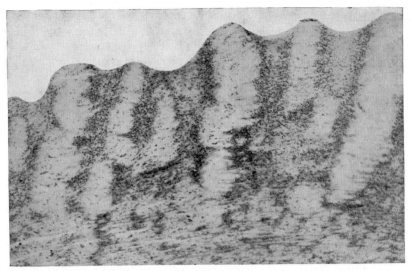

FIG. 27.3. Coralline thrombus. Photomicrograph of vertical section including free surface of a coralline thrombus adjacent to the wall of a large artery. Pale platelet laminae are seen projecting from the surface. Coagulated plasma containing leucocytes lies between them. Many leucocytes are adherent to the platelet laminae.

(*From Hadfield, G.* (1950). Ann. roy. Coll. Surg. Engl., **6,** 219.)

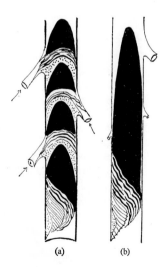

FIG. 27.4. Methods of propagation in phlebothrombosis.

(a) With thrombus formation at each entering tributary.

(b) Clotting *en masse* in an extensive ength of vein.

(*From Hadfield, G.* (1950). Ann. roy. Coll. Surg. Engl., **6,** 219.)

(a)        (b)

**Consecutive Clot.** Once the vein is occluded, blood flow stops and with it stops the thrombosis. The stationary column of blood beyond the thrombus extending to the next entering tributary undergoes coagulation. This is called the consecutive clot (Fig. 27.4), and its free end, or tail, points like a dagger towards the heart.

**Propagated Clot.** When stasis is marked, the clotting process extends up a considerable length of the vein past the entering tributaries to produce a long propagated clot (Fig. 27.4). As this retracts, it lies free in the lumen, and is attached only at the point of original thrombosis. This long, loose structure frequently becomes detached, and is carried to the right side of the heart as an embolus.

## Clinical Features

Clinically phlebothrombosis is remarkably silent. There is little pain in the limb, but direct squeezing pressure on the calf muscles may elicit tenderness. Careful measurement may detect slight oedema. Frequently the first indication of phlebothrombosis is the occurrence of pulmonary embolism.

A recently introduced method of detecting phlebothrombosis employs the injection of $^{125}$I-labelled fibrinogen.[9] This becomes incorporated in the thrombus, and the increase in radioactivity over a vein indicates the presence of thrombosis at that site. After major surgery and myocardial infarction it has been found that venous thrombosis occurs in about 35 per cent of cases.

## Complications

Small emboli lodge in the lungs, and may produce infarction. A more serious complication is massive pulmonary embolism which can produce sudden death. This usually occurs from 7–10 days after injury or operation.

### Thrombophlebitis

Inflammation of a vessel wall may follow the injection of irritant chemicals, e.g. anaesthetic agents, or be a complication of an adjacent area of infection, e.g. a staphylococcal abscess. In either event thrombosis occurs in the area of damage, but as stasis is not present, extensive propagation of the clot does not occur. The thrombosis is therefore relatively localized and firmly adherent. The condition is characterized by pain and swelling in the region of the vein, and is therefore clinically very obvious.

Embolism is most uncommon except in thrombophlebitis due to pyogenic infection, when the organisms may invade the thrombus and cause its softening, so that small infected emboli are released into the circulation. The condition is called *pyaemia*, and the numerous infected emboli become impacted in distant organs, e.g. the lung, where they produce metastatic, or pyaemic, abscesses. If thrombophlebitis affects the portal vein, the *pyaemic abscesses* are found primarily in the liver. This is an occasional complication of suppurative appendicitis.

### Thrombosis in the Atria of the Heart

Atrial thrombosis is generally due to stasis, and the condition is analogous to phlebothrombosis. The thrombi commonly occur in the atrial appendages, and are seen whenever there is stasis, e.g. in heart failure, especially if accompanied by atrial fibrillation. The thrombi may become detached as emboli either in the pulmonary or the systemic circulation depending upon which atrium is involved.

## Thrombosis in Arteries

In the high-velocity arterial system the most important cause of thrombosis is disease of the arterial wall itself. This acts in three ways.

(1) Eddy current formation leads to the deposition of platelets.
(2) There is ulceration of the endothelial lining.
(3) Disease of the arterial wall may so weaken it that aneurysmal dilatation occurs. This leads to local stasis.

The causes of arterial thrombosis are those of arterial damage. Arterial spasm may also initiate thrombosis (p. 386).

### Causes of Arterial Damage
**Inflammation.** This may be:

*Traumatic*, as when an artery adjacent to a fracture is injured.

*Infective.* Arteritis is sometimes seen adjacent to a pyogenic infection and in syphilis. It is, however, less common than phlebitis.

*Idiopathic inflammatory conditions.* There are a number of diseases in which inflammation of the arterial wall leads to thrombosis. *Thromboangiitis obliterans (Buerger's disease)* is the best known. It is seen predominantly in young men. It affects the veins and arteries of the legs, and causes ischaemia which leads to intermittent claudication (pain in the calf muscles on exercise) and ultimately gangrene commencing in the toes. *Giant-cell arteritis* is a disease of elderly people; the affected artery shows thrombosis and a chronic inflammatory granulomatous reaction with many giant cells formed around disrupted elastic fibres. The disease can affect any artery, but commonly it is the temporal one and pain in the temple is a marked feature. The ophthalmic artery is sometimes involved and blindness may result. Rarely the lingual artery is occluded, when ischaemia and pain can affect the oral structures, e.g. the tongue. *Polyarteritis* and other forms of vasculitis can also cause thrombosis.

### Neoplastic Infiltration (p. 250).

**Arteriosclerosis.**[10] This term embraces what is loosely called degenerative arterial disease, and is extremely important. It includes the following:

*Mönckeberg's medial sclerosis.* This affects the large muscular arteries especially those of the lower limbs. The tunica media shows hyaline change and *calcification*. It produces dramatic radiological appearances but does not cause any ill-effects, and is therefore unimportant.

*Diffuse hyperplastic sclerosis.* In this condition the small muscular arteries and arterioles become progressively thickened. The lesions are most marked in hypertension and have already been described.

*Atheroma (or atherosclerosis).* This is the most important.

## Atheroma[10]

Atheroma is the commonest killing disease in all highly advanced civilized communities, and its lesions are present to some degree in almost every adult member. The disease characteristically affects the large elastic arteries like the aorta and its main branches. Of the medium-sized vessels the coronary and cerebral arteries are most commonly involved. This is extremely unfortunate in view of the vital nature of the organs they supply, and it accounts for the lethal effects of atheroma. Atheroma may be considered as consisting of two types of condition.

### Lesions of Atheroma

**Type 1. Yellow Plaques in the Intima (Fatty Streaking).** Foam cells accumulate in the subendothelial layer, and later break down to release their fatty content into the tunica intima. In this way there are produced the yellow streaks which are a common *post-mortem* finding in the aorta at all ages. When they occur in smaller arteries, they do not produce appreciable narrowing of the lumen.

**Type 2. The Accumulation of Fatty Material in the Intima with Additional Fibrosis.** This is the common type of lesion seen in middle and old age. It is sometimes referred to as atherosclerosis.

The lesions, or plaques, are intimal, and consist of a central mass of fatty, yellow, porridge-like material (*athere* is Greek for porridge), which consists predominantly of cholesterol and its esters, and is surrounded and covered by dense fibrous tissue. This gives the plaque a white, pearly appearance. In advanced lesions ulceration with superadded *thrombosis* is common. The fatty material often undergoes *dystrophic calcification*.

### Aetiology

It is not known for certain whether the lesions of type-1 atheroma progress to those of type 2, or whether in fact these are independent diseases. Experimentally lesions closely resembling those of type 1 can be produced in animals by feeding with abnormal diets, usually with a high content of cholesterol. Lesions resembling type-2 atheroma can occur after injuring the arterial wall, thereby producing thrombosis. The subsequent degeneration and partial organization of the thrombus lead to an "atheromatous" plaque. Either of these two mechanisms could be involved in the pathogenesis of human atheroma, and they are not mutually exclusive. Initial lesions produced by dietary indiscretions could progress by additional thrombosis. There is, however, much controversy as to the relative importance of these two mechanisms.

### Effects

*Gradual obstruction.* Atherosclerosis of small arteries, e.g. the coronary and cerebral vessels, produces a plaque which steadily occludes the lumen. This leads to ischaemia of the area supplied.

*Thrombosis.* This leads to sudden complete obstruction.

*Dilatation and aneurysm formation.* The presence of an atheromatous plaque causes atrophy of the adjacent media. The wall therefore weakens, and the artery involved may show either diffuse enlargement (*ectasia*) or a localized dilatation (*aneurysm*). These effects are seen most often in the abdominal aorta, and rupture of such an aneurysm is a not uncommon cause of death.

*Embolism.* Rarely atheromatous material or overlying thrombus becomes detached and embolizes distally.

### Aneurysms[10]

An aneurysm is a local dilatation of an artery or a chamber of the heart due to a weakening of its walls. It may be localized and saccular or diffuse and fusiform.

**Causes.** The weakening of the wall may be due to:
(1) Congenital deficiency, e.g. berry aneurysms of the circle of Willis (p. 468).
(2) Trauma.
(3) Inflammation, e.g. syphilitic aortitis may cause an aneurysm of the thoracic aorta. The condition is now rare.
(4) Degeneration, e.g. atheromatous. This is by far the most common type of aortic aneurysm.

**Effects.** Aneurysms produce harmful effects in a number of ways:
*Pressure.* An aneurysm of the thoracic aorta may press on the oesophagus

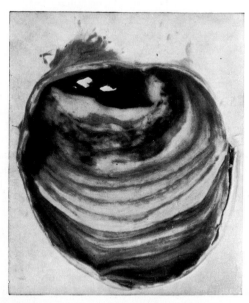

Fig. 27.5. Laminated thrombus in an aneurysmal sac. In this cross-section the sac is seen to be almost completely occluded with laminated thrombus.

(C31b.4. *Reproduced by permission of the President and Council of the Royal College of Surgeons of England.*)

and cause difficulty in swallowing, or on the recurrent laryngeal nerve and lead to changes in the voice.

*Haemorrhage.* Aneurysms may leak for a while, and then suddenly burst.

*Thrombosis.* The sac of an aneurysm soon becomes filled by laminated thrombus (Fig. 27.5). This is due in part to the damage to the endothelial lining and in part to the local stasis.

*Ischaemia* due to blockage of branches of the artery at the site of the aneurysm either by pressure or by occlusion of their ostia with thrombus.

### Dissecting Aneurysm of Aorta

The basic defect is degeneration in the media of the aorta (medionecrosis), the aetiology of which is unknown. If there is rupture of one of the small vessels supplying the wall of the aorta (vasa vasorum), bleeding occurs into the media. This steadily splits the arterial wall into two layers, and eventually a tear extends into the main lumen. This usually occurs in the ascending aorta. Blood is then forced in considerable quantity through this tear, and it produces an extensive stripping of the arterial wall, even down into the abdominal aorta. The disease is quite common, and is usually heralded by the sudden onset of severe chest pain. The effects are serious because the dissection causes blockage of the ostia of important branches of the aorta, e.g. the coronary or renal arteries. Finally the sac of the aneurysm usually ruptures to the exterior, and leads to fatal haemorrhage into the pericardium, the mediastinum, or the peritoneal cavity.

### Thrombosis in the Heart

**Thrombosis in the Atrium** (p. 372).

**Thrombosis in the Ventricles.** Thrombosis is usually seen in the left ventricle overlying an area of infarction.

Coiled thrombi are found in the pulmonary trunk and right ventricle in massive pulmonary embolism. These should not be confused with *post-mortem* clots. The latter are formed after death, and their shape conforms to that of the cavity in which they are formed. They are shiny and elastic, and never exhibit the lines of Zahn which are characteristic of thrombi. Furthermore, in conditions accompanied by a high ESR the blood may separate before it clots, so that there is an upper portion consisting largely of coagulated plasma. This is pale yellow, and is usually called the "chicken-fat clot", while the clot underneath contains sedimented red cells. This is the so-called "red-currant jelly clot".

**Thrombosis on the Valves** pp. 395–398.

### Fate of Thrombi

Fig. 27.6 summarizes the possible fate of a thrombus.

(*a*) Many thrombi undergo lysis, and leave no trace of their previous existence. Plasmin is probably of importance.

(*b*) If an occluding thrombus in an artery or vein contains much clot, it retracts sufficiently for blood to pass by. In this way a new channel is formed. Endothelium quickly lines this passage, and recanalization occurs. In the

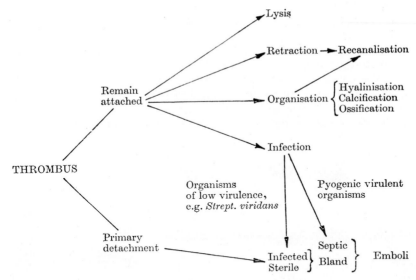

FIG. 27.6. The possible fate of a thrombus.

pulmonary arteries a thin web of connective tissue may be all that remains of a previous life-threatening thrombo-embolism.

(c) A thrombus which is not removed may become organized. In veins the granulation tissue invades it from the mural aspect, and endothelium grows over the thrombus from the adjacent intima. In large, elastic arteries the vasa vasorum from the adventitia do not penetrate as far as the intima, and organization is therefore impaired. Some occurs from the adjacent endothelium, but it is possible that thrombi in arteries undergo degeneration, and are converted into atheromatous plaques.

(d) Organized thrombi may become hyalinized and calcified. This is common in the pelvic veins, and the *phleboliths* so produced may be seen on radiographic examination.

(e) Thrombi may become detached to form emboli.

### Embolism

An *embolus* is an abnormal mass of undissolved material which is transported from one part of the circulation to another. The most satisfactory classification is based upon its composition.

**Types.** Five categories may be recognized.

*Thrombi and clot.* This may be bland or infected.
*Gas*—air and nitrogen.
*Fat.*
*Tumour.*
*Miscellaneous.*

### (1) Emboli Composed of Thrombus or Clot

**Pulmonary Embolism.** The source of the thrombo-emboli is generally one of the veins, most often in the legs. Small emboli block branches of the pulmonary arteries and produce either no effects or else infarction (p. 385). Large quantities of thrombus and propagated clot, however, produce the syndrome of massive pulmonary embolism. In this the main pulmonary artery and its branches are plugged by a mass of coiled thrombus (Fig. 27.7). The clinical effects are dramatic. The patient experiences sudden dyspnoea and chest pain. The obstruction of the right ventricular outflow results in a dramatic fall in

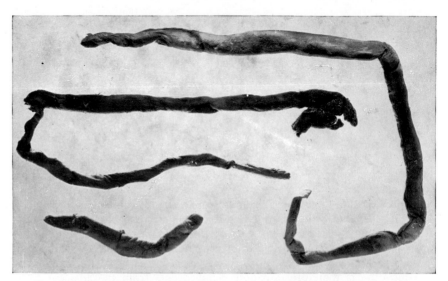

FIG. 27.7. Massive pulmonary embolism. These thrombi were removed from the pulmonary arteries of a man who died suddenly a week after an abdominal operation. There was extensive phlebothrombosis in both calves. Note that the calibre of the thrombi corresponds with the lumina of the leg veins.

(C40.5. *Reproduced by permission of the President and Council of the Royal College of Surgeons of England.*)

left ventricular output; hypotension occurs and consciousness is lost. Death frequently follows. The prevention of massive pulmonary embolism is the prevention of phlebothrombosis. Patients confined to bed must be given leg exercises to increase the venous circulation. Postoperative physiotherapy and early ambulation have done much to reduce this complication of trauma and surgery.

**Systemic Embolism.** The emboli usually arise in the heart, commonly from the left atrium in mitral stenosis or heart failure. Systemic embolism is also a feature of infective endocarditis (pp. 396–398), and it may arise from the mural thrombus formed over a myocardial infarct.

### (2) Gaseous Emboli

**Air.**[11] Air may inadvertently be introduced into a systemic vein, e.g. during a mismanaged blood transfusion. If in considerable quantity, it travels to the heart where it produces foaming in the right ventricle. The right ventricle compresses this foam but cannot expel it. Death therefore occurs rapidly.

During pleural aspirations air may inadvertently be introduced into the pulmonary venous circulation and reach the left side of the heart. From here it may travel to the coronary and cerebral vessels and occlude them. The blockage often has a fatal result.

**Nitrogen: The Decompression Syndrome.**[12, 13] Bubbles of nitrogen appear in the circulation in those who, having been exposed to a high atmospheric pressure, are suddenly decompressed. This occurs in divers, tunnellers, and pilots. Nitrogen, being soluble in lipids, also appears as bubbles in the central nervous system. This effect may result in considerable damage to the spinal cord. Severe pain is produced ("the bends"), and permanent damage or death may ensue. This traditional theory of the pathogenesis of the decompression syndrome is now under doubt, for gas bubbles are often not found in decompressed organs.[14] The possibility of fat embolism (from altered lipoproteins) and platelet thrombus around the fat is suggested by some workers.[15].

### (3) Fat Emboli[16, 17]

Globules of fatty marrow may enter the small veins after a fracture of a long bone; with multiple injuries this embolization may be quite extensive. Usually the emboli are trapped in the lungs and have no harmful effects because of the enormous capacity of the vascular bed. Occasionally, however, emboli pass through the pulmonary capillaries and enter the systemic circulation, where they produce the syndrome of *systemic fat embolism*. Multiple emboli lodge in the kidneys causing haematuria, the brain, where they lead to severe neurological changes, and the skin, where they cause small petechial haemorrhages.

### (4) Tumour Emboli

It is probable that all malignant tumours invade the local blood vessels at an early stage of the disease, and that isolated malignant cells are of frequent occurrence in the circulation. The majority of these emboli are destroyed; only a small percentage develop into metastatic deposits. Occasionally, for instance in carcinoma of the lung, a large mass of tumour becomes detached, and a massive embolus blocks a major artery, e.g. the femoral.

### Miscellaneous Emboli

*Foreign bodies.* A large number of foreign bodies have been reported to undergo embolism, e.g. a polyethylene tube may become detached in a vein and travel to the right side of the heart.

*Parasites.* Various parasites and their ova are carried in the blood stream.

*Red cells.* The blockage of small vessels by sludged aggregates of red cells is commonly seen in infections and following trauma (p. 313).

*Amniotic fluid.*[18] An occasional complication of pregnancy is the sudden introduction of amniotic fluid into the veins of the uterus. This produces a syndrome characterized by shock and a generalized bleeding tendency. This is not attributable to the phenomenon of embolism, but to the initiation of diffuse intravascular clotting and fibrinolysis.

## Hypoxia

Hypoxia is a state of impaired oxygenation of the tissues.

**Types.** Four are commonly described:

*Hypoxic*, due to a low oxygen tension ($Po_2$) in the arterial blood. This is a feature of central cyanosis (p. 393).

*Anaemic*, due to an inadequate level of haemoglobin, which carries the oxygen in the blood.

*Stagnant*, or *ischaemic*, due to an inadequate supply of blood to the tissues. This, as will be seen, is due either to heart failure or some local vascular obstruction, and is a feature of peripheral cyanosis.

*Histotoxic*, due to cellular intoxication which prevents the uptake of oxygen, e.g. cyanide poisoning.

## Ischaemia

Ischaemia is defined as a condition of inadequate blood supply to an area of tissue. It produces harmful effects in three ways:

*Hypoxia*. Oxygen deprivation is undoubtedly the most important factor producing damage in ischaemic tissue, especially in respect of very active cells, e.g. muscle. On the other hand, it plays no part in the lesions produced by pulmonary arterial obstruction, because the alveolar walls derive their oxygen supply directly from the alveolar air.

*Malnutrition*. This is probably of little importance, because the blood contains much more glucose and amino acids than could be metabolized by the amount of oxygen which it contains.

*Failure to remove waste products*. The accumulation of metabolites is the most probable explanation of pain in ischaemic muscles. The presence of waste products or the failure to maintain important electrolyte or other balances is probably a factor in pulmonary infarction.

### Causes of Ischaemia

**General.** Ischaemia may be caused by an inadequate cardiac output; not all tissues are equally affected because of the redistribution of the available blood. The extremities (e.g. finger-tips) tend to be most severely affected, but the ischaemia is rarely sufficiently severe to cause structural damage. Not so, however, with the ischaemia that follows the sudden cessation of the heart's action. Sudden cardiac arrest may occur during the induction of anaesthesia or as a result of coronary thrombosis. The blood supply to the whole body is stopped, but manifestations are in fact confined to a single organ, the brain, which is particularly sensitive to hypoxia. If the arrest continues for 15 seconds, consciousness is lost, and if the condition lasts for more than three minutes, irreparable damage is done.[19] The neurones degenerate and are replaced by glial tissue. If cardiac arrest lasts for more than about eight minutes, death is inevitable. It follows that *all who deal with patients should be capable of diagnosing cardiac arrest (absent heart sounds) and dealing with it by the manoeuvre of external cardiac massage.*

**Local.** By far the most important cause of ischaemia is obstruction to the arterial flow. It should not, however, be forgotten that extensive venous and capillary damage can also produce ischaemia.

**Arterial Obstruction.** Most of the causes of obstruction have already been described. They will therefore be summarized:

*Thrombosis.*

*Embolism.* The effects of an embolus are potentiated by the reflex spasm of the arterial wall, and completed by the rapid development of thrombus over the embolus.

*Spasm* (p. 386).

*Atheroma.* This produces partial obstruction in medium-sized vessels, e.g. cerebral, coronary, and renal arteries.

*Occlusive pressure from without,* e.g. tourniquets and ill-fitting plasters.

**Venous Disease.** Extensive venous obstruction leads to engorgement of the areas drained by the affected veins. This may reach such an intensity that blood flow is impeded and ischaemia results. Mesenteric vein thrombosis is a good example of this; it leads to intestinal infarction. Venous stasis secondary to varicose veins of the legs leads to ischaemic changes of the skin (stasis dermatitis). Ultimately chronic ulceration occurs, often precipitated by local injury.

**Capillary Damage.** In considerations of vascular disease the capillaries are usually forgotten. There are nevertheless many conditions in which so many capillaries in an area are occluded that ischaemia results. An additional effect is bleeding, so that petechial haemorrhages are a common feature of capillary damage even though the extent of the vascular occlusion is insufficient to lead to ischaemia of the area supplied.

*Frost-bite.* The harmful effect of cold on exposed parts is due in large measure to damage to small blood vessels. In mild cases the exudation from the damaged vessels produces large blisters, while if the damage is severe the vessels become completely occluded by thrombus.

*Occlusion of capillaries by red cells.* This occurs when there is severe sludging.

*Occlusion of capillaries by white cells.* This is seen in chronic myeloid leukaemia.

*Occlusion by fibrin.* This occurs in the syndrome of disseminated intravascular coagulation (p. 361). It is a feature of the generalised Schwartzman phenomenon.

*Occlusion by antigen-antibody interaction.* In immune-complex reactions the vessel walls are damaged, and the formation of fibrin and the accumulation of polymorphs occludes the vessels. This is a feature of the Arthus reaction (p. 163). The petechial haemorrhages of infective endocarditis are probably produced by this mechanism (p. 398).

*Occlusion by precipitated cryoglobulins.* In cryoglobulinaemia, the exposure of the extremities to cold causes occlusion of small vessels, and leads to focal ischaemic lesions of the skin with petechial haemorrhages, and sometimes the Raynaud phenomenon.* (p. 330).

*Fat embolism* (p. 379).

*Decompression syndrome* (p. 379).

*External pressure*, e.g. bedsores (p. 111).

## The Effects of Arterial and Capillary Obstruction

The effects depend largely upon the degree of ischaemia produced, and may range from sudden death to virtually no damage at all. The following are the possibilities:

*No effects* occur if the affected area is well supplied by blood vessels which form collateral anastomoses.

*Functional disturbances.* Sufficient blood may reach the area to supply its needs under resting conditions but not under those of activity. This is the cause of the pain in the chest (angina pectoris) in patients with coronary artery disease, and the intermittent claudication in those with peripheral vascular disease (p. 373).

*Cellular degeneration* may affect the parenchyma of an organ and culminate in necrosis. This may be a patchy affair leading to atrophy; it is generally accompanied by replacement fibrosis or, in the central nervous system, gliosis. This type of lesion is seen under two conditions:

(*a*) Sudden complete arterial obstruction of short duration.

(*b*) Partial arterial obstruction of gradual onset.

*Infarction.* See below.

*Sudden death* This occurs in massive pulmonary embolism and coronary occlusion.

## Factors Determining the Extent of Ischaemia in Arterial Obstruction

There are three crucial factors:

**Speed of Onset.** If it is sudden the effects are more severe than if it is gradual, because there is less time for an effective collateral circulation to develop.

**Degree of Obstruction.** A complete obstruction is obviously much more serious than a partial one.

**Anatomy of the Collateral Circulation.** Some arteries have no anastomotic channels; these are called *end arteries.* The central artery of the retina is a classical example; if obstructed there is complete ischaemia of the area supplied. With most arteries there is sufficient anastomosis to ensure that the blood reaches the affected area even when a main branch is occluded. If the anastomotic vessels are well developed, ischaemia is an uncommon phenomenon. The stomach illustrates this well, for it is supplied by three separate arteries which anastomose freely.

**Subsidiary Factors.** There are four subsidiary factors modifying the effects of arterial blockage.

* *Raynaud's disease* is an idiopathic condition in which the digital arteries are unduly sensitive to cold. When cooled, the hands or feet become pale and later cyanosed due to spasm of the digital arteries. In Raynaud's phenomenon, or syndrome, similar attacks occur, but the condition appears to be a complication of some other disease, e.g. cryoglobulinaemia, scleroderma, or lupus erythematosus.

*The pathology of the collateral circulation.* It stands to reason that if the collateral vessels are severely affected with spasm or atheroma they are not likely to assist in maintaining a good alternative blood supply.

*The oxygenation of the arterial blood.*

*The efficiency of the heart.*

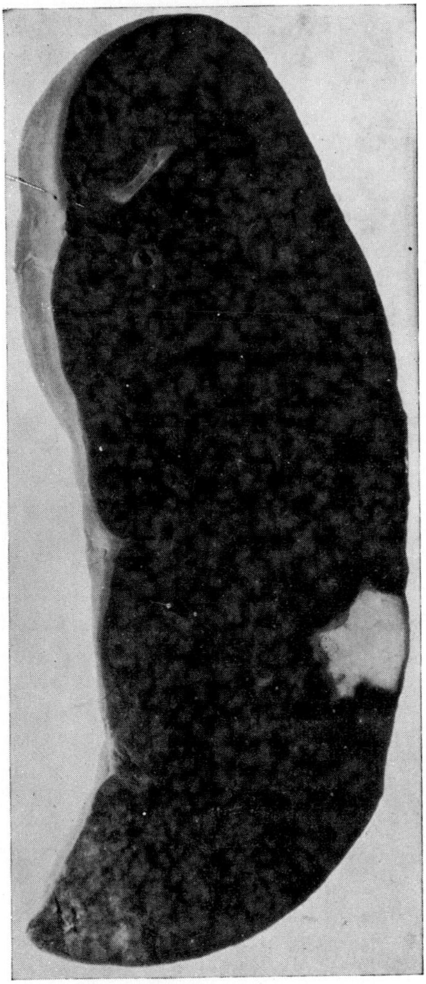

FIG. 27.8. Infarct of spleen. Note the pale, wedge-shaped infarct under the capsule. The lymphoid follicles are unduly prominent. The patient had *Strept. viridans* endocarditis.

(H26.1. *Reproduced by permission of the President and Council of the Royal College of Surgeons of England.*)

*The nature of the affected tissue.* Brain and heart are much more vulnerable to ischaemia than are any other organs. Connective tissue survives much better than does the parenchyma of an organ.

### The Process of Infarction

*Infarction* may be defined as the circumscribed necrosis of tissue due to deprivation of blood supply. It usually leads to a circumscribed area of coagulative necrosis, which is subsequently organized into scar tissue. The process is as follows:

(*a*) There is death of the cells in the area deprived of its blood supply. Blood, either from anastomotic vessels or by venous reflux, continues to seep into the devitalized area for a short time. Thus most infarcts contain a great deal of blood in the early stages, and are swollen and red in colour. The red cells entering the affected area escape from the damaged capillaries and lie free in the dead tissue. Infarcts of lax tissue. e.g. lung and intestine, are much more engorged than are those of compact organs, e.g. kidney and heart.

(*b*) The dead tissue undergoes necrosis. In solid organs the associated swelling of the cells may squeeze the blood out of the infarct. In this way it becomes paler. Infarcts of the spleen and kidneys are characteristically pale, and present a wedge-shaped area of coagulative necrosis, the apex of which is the blocked supplying artery, and the base the capsule of the organ (Fig. 27.8). Infarcts of the heart are also pale, but their shape is more irregular due to the arrangement of the vascular supply.

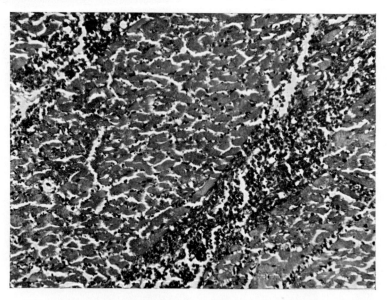

FIG. 27.9. Myocardial infarction. The muscle fibres are necrotic, but their structure is easily recognisable. There is a profuse cellular infiltration, including
many polymorphs, around the necrotic tissue × 150.

(*c*) There is progressive autolysis of the necrotic tissue and haemolysis of the red cells. Microscopically an infarct shows a characteristic structured necrosis with the outlines of the cells being recognizable as ghosts without nuclei. This petrified-forest appearance may persist for many months. (Fig. 27.9).

(*d*) At the same time the surrounding normal tissue undergoes an acute inflammatory reaction. The polymorph infiltration may be so intense as to simulate a pyogenic infection for a while. This is rapidly followed by macrophage activity.

(e) The infarct gradually shrinks and becomes replaced by granulation tissue. Its central portion may, however, take many months to organize, and not infrequently shows dystrophic calcification.

Infarcts in particular organs present certain additional features. In the *lung* the infarct is so filled with blood that it remains red and generally organizes in this stage (Fig. 27.10). In the *intestine* the necrotic bowel wall is soon invaded by putrefactive organisms and becomes gangrenous. In the

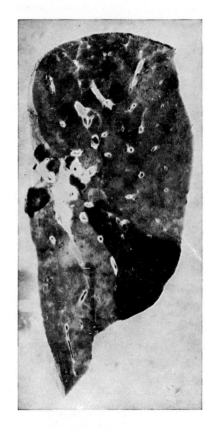

FIG. 27.10. Infarct of lung. Note the dark wedge-shaped infarct in this left upper lobe. It is stuffed with blood.

(R27.3. *Reproduced by permission of the President and Council of the Royal College of Surgeons of England.*)

*limbs* sudden obstruction leads to infarction and wet gangrene, while slow obstruction produces the so-called dry gangrene (p. 55).

In the *central nervous system* the process is somewhat different, because the necrotic tissue undergoes rapid liquefactive necrosis. The end-result is either a glial scar or else, if the infarct is large, a cyst surrounded by a layer of glial tissue.

Infarction of the lung does not occur in healthy people even if a major pulmonary artery is occluded. This is because the bronchial arteries supply well-oxygenated blood. If the bronchial arterial supply is itself impaired, as in heart failure, obstruction to a branch of the pulmonary artery may then lead to infarction. The usual cause of this is an embolus arising from one of the systemic veins. It will be recalled that phlebothrombosis is itself often associated with heart failure.

## Vascular Spasm

Although vascular occlusion is generally caused by an organic lesion, there are a number of conditions in which spasm of the vessel wall plays a most important part. Spasm may occur in either veins or arteries; it is debatable whether the capillaries are capable of independent contraction.

**Venous Spasm.** Trauma applied directly to a vessel wall can cause marked spasm. This is sometimes a source of great difficulty during an inexpert venepuncture. Venous spasm has not been incriminated as a cause of tissue ischaemia.

**Arterial Spasm.** Trauma to arteries frequently produces local spasm, a function which may be of life-saving importance. Cases of avulsion of a limb are on record in which, due to spasm of the main artery, the patient did not die of massive haemorrhage.

This ability of arteries to contract can be utilized by the surgeon who is faced with severe bleeding during the course of an operation. It is a wise policy to pack the wound and await the onset of spasm rather than make heroic though blind efforts with a pair of haemostats. Although this response of the arterial wall to trauma may be of benefit, its effects are sometimes detrimental. Trauma to an artery, e.g. by the close proximity of a bullet path, or the pressure of a plaster, or the application of a tourniquet, may at times produce such persistent and widespread spasm that the area involved becomes ischaemic and infarcted. Absence of the pulse of a limb beyond an area of trauma must be regarded seriously, and efforts should be made to relieve the spasm, lest permanent damage be caused.

Spasm of small arteries is a feature of ergot poisoning and Raynaud's phenomenon. It may lead to gangrene of the extremities. Widespread arteriolar spasm is a feature of shock (p. 312), and has also been incriminated in primary hypertension (p. 365).

## References

1. MASTERS, W. H. and JOHNSON, V. E. (1966). "Human Sexual Response". Boston: Little Brown.
2. HEPTINSTALL, R. H. (1966). In "Pathology of the Kidney", p. 119 and 151. Boston: Little Brown.
3. Leading Article (1963). *Lancet*, **2**, 180.
4. HADFIELD, G. (1950). *Ann. roy. Coll. Surg. Engl.*, **6**, 219.
5. WESSLER, S. and DEYKIN, D. (1958). *Circulation*, **18**, 1190.
6. SHARNOFF, J. G. (1959). *J. Amer. med. Ass.*, **169**, 688.
7. INNES, D. and SEVITT, S. (1964). *J. clin. Path.*, **17**, 1.
8. HAM, J. M. and SLACK, W. W. (1967). *Brit. J. Surg.*, **54**, 385.
9. Leading Article (1971). *Brit. med. J.*, **1**, 305.
10. HUDSON, R. E. B. (1965 and 1970). "Cardiovascular Pathology", A useful reference book for most aspects of vascular and cardiac pathology. In three volumes. London: Arnold.
11. Annotation (1963). *Lancet*, **1**, 96.
12. Annotation (1961). *Brit. med. J.*, **1**, 45.
13. DEWEY, A. W. (1962). *New Engl. J. Med.*, **267**, 759 and 812.

14. FRYER, D. I. (1969). "Subatmospheric Decompression Sickness in Man". Slough: Technivision Services.
15. SAUMAREZ, R. C., BOLT, L. F. and GREGORY, R. J. (1973). *Brit. med. J.*, **1,** 151.
16. LOVE, J. and STRYKER, W. S. (1957). *Ann. intern. Med.*, **46,** 342.
17. SEVITT, S. (1962). "Fat embolism". London: Butterworths.
18. AGUILLON, A. *et al.* (1962). *Obstet. Gynec. Survey*, **17,** 619.
19. DICKINSON, C. J. and PENTECOST, B. L. (1968). In "Clinical Physiology," 3rd ed. p. 64, ed. by Campbell, E. J. M., Dickinson, C. J. and Slater, J. D. H. Oxford: Blackwell.

*Chapter 28*

# DISEASES OF THE HEART

Before commencing dental treatment it is particularly important to ascertain that the heart is normal, because unless precautions are taken, dental treatment may give rise to serious consequences in a patient with a damaged heart. Congenital lesions and valvular abnormalities predispose to infective endocarditis, and myocardial disease may lead to sudden death during anaesthesia.

The types and causes of heart disease are many and various; the effects, ·however, are few in number and stereotyped in nature. Since the heart is a pump, it follows that the diseased and failing heart often pumps inefficiently. The consequences of this are circulatory disturbances which together constitute the syndrome of heart failure. The main features of this will first be described, and the diseases of the heart itself will then be outlined.

## HEART FAILURE

The most important chambers of the heart are the two ventricles. These fill during diastole from the low-pressured venous reservoirs, an effect aided to some extent by atrial contraction. Normally the heart is able to expel all the blood which flows into it. If the venous return is increased in volume, the increased filling of the heart stretches its muscle fibres and the force of the next contraction is increased. This is *Starling's Law of the Heart*. The cardiac output is thus gauged to the venous return, and the heart can satisfy the needs of the body under all normal circumstances.

Under resting conditions the ventricles do not empty completely with each systole, but with exercise their contraction results in more complete emptying. This is mediated by an increase in sympathetic tone, and acting with the greater filling due to the increased venous return, it results in a larger volume (the stroke volume) of blood being ejected with each heart beat. In addition, the heart rate increases. Therefore the heart has a considerable *functional reserve*, and can increase its output from the resting level of 5 litres/min. to 25–30 litres/min.

Prolonged overwork of any chamber causes hypertrophy of the muscle of its walls. This is an additional cardiac reserve, but it should be remembered that the hypertrophied myocardium usually fails unless the strain on it is removed. A large heart is a diseased heart.

When, in the presence of an adequate venous return, the heart fails to supply blood to meet the needs of the body the condition is known as *heart failure*. At first the effects of this are to be seen on exercise, but as the failure increases so the effects are apparent even at rest. Either the left or the right ventricle may fail separately. More usually the heart fails as a whole, and the condition is called *congestive heart failure*.

388

## Effects of Right Ventricular Failure

**Rise in Central Venous Pressure.*** A failure of the right ventricle to eject all the blood which it receives leads to distension of the right atrium by a back-pressure effect. The pressure in the great veins rises, and the *jugular veins are seen to be distended with blood* when the patient sits up in bed. To some extent this *aids* heart function, because the raised pressure causes increased filling of the heart. This by stretching the myocardium *increases* the force of contraction. However, a point can be reached beyond which increased stretching causes a *decrease* in cardiac contraction. Exercise, by increasing the venous return, further reduces the cardiac output; the patient is therefore bedridden. Once past this critical point, therapeutic bleeding increases the cardiac output by reducing the venous pressure. This is the basis for the time-honoured practice of bleeding as a treatment for heart failure. In right-sided heart failure all the organs of the body are congested. This is particularly well seen in the liver, where the centres of the lobules are deeply congested and red (see nutmeg liver, p. 390). Congestion is evident in the skin, especially of the face.

**Cyanosis.** The sluggish circulation allows a more complete deoxygenation of the blood as it passes through the tissues. In the skin this may be detected by the bluish coloration known as *cyanosis*. Cyanosis is evident when the capillary blood contains more than 5 g. reduced haemoglobin per 100 ml. It should be noted that cyanosis due to stasis (*peripheral cyanosis*) is not necessarily due to heart disease. It is seen whenever the circulation is sluggish, e.g. in polycythaemia (where the blood is very viscous), in an area affected by venous obstruction, and in shock. Some people are so sensitive to cold that their ears, nose, and finger-tips become cyanosed even on exposure to a cool atmosphere.

**Polycythaemia.** An increased red-cell count occurs as a result of bone marrow hypoxia.

**Oedema.** Oedema of the dependent parts is a prominent sign of heart failure. It accumulates around the legs and genitalia, and, during recumbency, the sacral region. The pathogenesis of the oedema is complex. In part it is due to the chronic passive venous congestion of the tissues, but a more important factor is the reduced cardiac output. The reduced output of the right ventricle leads to a corresponding fall in that of the left ventricle, for the quantity of blood entering this chamber is the same as the right ventricular output. This reduced cardiac output acts on the kidneys and causes salt and water retention (see below).

## Effects of Left Ventricular Failure

**Rise in Pulmonary Venous Pressure.** The venous distension affects the lungs which become congested and tense. The effort of breathing is increased, and this causes distress (*dyspnoea*). *Pulmonary oedema* is an ever-present danger, and may come on with dramatic suddenness. Rupture of capillaries leads to *haemoptysis*, and the blood which remains in the lungs is converted

* This is the pressure in the right atrium minus the negative intrathoracic pressure.

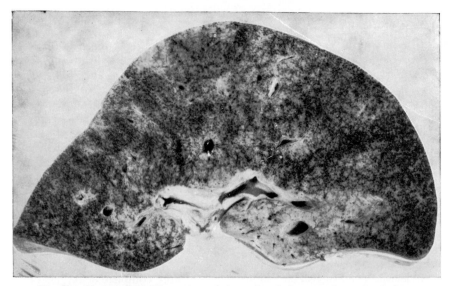

FIG. 28.1. Nutmeg liver. The pattern of alternating dark congestion and pale fatty change is apparent.

(A 95.2. *Reproduced by permission of the President and Council of the Royal College of Surgeons of England.*)

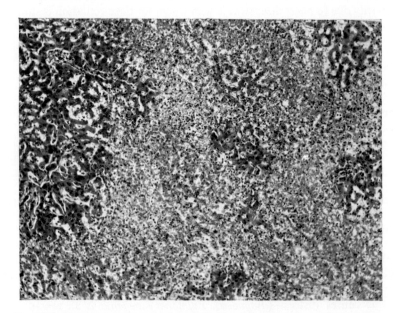

FIG. 28.2. Chronic venous congestion of the liver. There is a virtual disappearance of the liver cells in the central zones of the lobules, and their replacement with engorged, dilated sinusoids. The peripheral cells show fatty change. × 90.

into haemosiderin. This produces a brown pigmentation of the lungs and stimulates fine fibrosis, a condition called *brown induration of the lung*. It is the result of long-standing chronic venous congestion.

It should be noted that in primary left ventricular failure the output of the two ventricles is the same, but the left is functioning with the aid of an increased venous filling pressure. The right ventricle, on the other hand, is working normally. This leads to a redistribution of blood, more being retained in the pulmonary circuit than is normal. In addition to producing pulmonary congestion and oedema, the rise in pulmonary pressure (*pulmonary hypertension*) ultimately causes the right ventricle to fail, and *congestive heart failure* ensues.

**Congestive Heart Failure.** The inadequate cardiac output causes ischaemia. Selective vasoconstriction, e.g. of the skin vessels, causes sufficient redistribution of blood so that the important organs do not suffer damage in the initial stages. Cutaneous arteriolar constriction is an important factor in the pathogenesis of *peripheral cyanosis*. The two organs in which the effect of ischaemia is most marked are the liver and the kidneys.

*In the liver* the ischaemia leads to necrosis of the cells in the centres of the lobules, while the less severely affected peripheral cells show fatty change. The result is the characteristic *nutmeg liver* of congestive heart failure—the centres of the lobules are red and the peripheries yellow (Fig. 28.1 and 28.2).

*In the kidneys* no morphological changes other than congestion are evident, but the impaired renal blood flow leads to *salt and water retention*. This is a very important factor in the causation of cardiac oedema. Venous distension plays its part in determining the location of the oedema rather than in causing its formation.

In the terminal stages of left-sided heart failure *the brain* receives an inadequate blood supply, and this causes an impairment of consciousness and sometimes dementia.

### The Causes of Heart Failure

As previously described, the heart can easily increase its output during exercise. It cannot, however, maintain the high output for long, nor can it continue to function in the face of a high-output pressure. Any condition which imposes a sustained burden on the heart will eventually lead to its failure. It may also fail because of myocardial damage. The causes of heart failure may be considered under three headings:

**Overburdening due to a Sustained Increase in Ventricular Pressure.** This occurs in systemic and pulmonary *hypertension* and also in *aortic and pulmonary valvular disease*. If the semilunar cusps fuse together to produce a narrowing, or *stenosis*, of the valve orifice, the chamber behind the diseased valve, the ventricle, has to generate a high pressure to force blood through the stenosed valve. Hypertrophy of the ventricle occurs, but in time failure ensues. It should be noted that when the mitral valve is diseased, the over-distension of the left atrium causes pulmonary hypertension such that *right ventricular failure soon follows*.

**Myocardial Disease.** Myocardial disease is by far the most important cause of heart failure. It is generally due to ischaemia secondary to atheroma of the coronary arteries (p. 374). Other causes of myocardial failure are myocarditis (e.g. rheumatic and diphtheritic), amyloidosis, and myxoedema. Sometimes a large heart in a normotensive individual fails without obvious myocardial, coronary, or valvular damage. In a few cases this has been attributed to alcoholism,[1] beri-beri, or the excessive ingestion of beer to which cobalt salts have been added during its manufacture.[2] In the remainder no cause is found and the cases are placed in a group called the *cardiomyopathies*.[3] The diagnosis is one of exclusion of known causes.

### Overburdening due to a Sustained Increase in Cardiac Output

**Valvular Defects.** When the aortic valve becomes rigid and *incompetent*, blood flows back into the left ventricle during diastole. An increased volume of blood must therefore be ejected in systole. The actual output of the ventricle is increased, but the effective output is unaltered. A similar result is seen in *mitral regurgitation*, but here the wasted ventricular output is diverted to the left atrium. In both aortic regurgitation and mitral regurgitation left ventricular failure ensues. Pulmonary and tricuspid disease produce comparable effects on the right side.

**High-output Failure.** There are a number of conditions in which there is a sustained increase in the true cardiac output; the most easily understood is thyrotoxicosis, where the increased metabolic rate demands an increased output from the heart. Anaemia and a large arteriovenous shunt have a similar effect. Eventually the overworked heart fails to supply an adequate amount of blood to the tissues even though its output is greater than that of a normal person. This is therefore called *high-output failure* in contrast to the other types described in which the output is low. In both there is an inadequate supply of blood for the needs of the body. The difference lies in the fact that in high-output failure the needs of the body are much greater than normal.

Two types of heart disease may be recognized. There is the group of malformations which are due to faulty development and are therefore congenital, and there are those disorders occurring in a normally developed heart.

### DEVELOPMENTAL ANOMALIES

A large number of developmental anomalies are known, and until recently their differential diagnosis was largely a matter of academic interest. Since cardiac surgeons are now able to offer a chance of cure, this is no longer true, and many techniques have been developed to assist in accurate diagnosis. Only a few of the common anomalies will be described.

**Septal Defects.** The heart develops from a single tube, and a failure in the formation of the septa dividing the left and right chambers is not uncommon. The defects may be between the atria, the ventricles, or both.

**Pulmonary Stenosis.** An unequal division of the truncus arteriosus may result in the development of a large aorta and a correspondingly small pulmonary artery and valve (pulmonary stenosis).

**Multiple Defects.** Developmental anomalies are often multiple. Not only may malformations be found in other organs, but several lesions may be present in the heart itself. A common combination is the *tetralogy of Fallot*. This comprises:

1. *Pulmonary stenosis.*
2. *Ventricular septal defect.*
3. *Overriding of the septum by the aorta, so that blood from the right and left ventricles enters the aorta.*
4. *Hypertrophy of the right ventricle—this is compensatory.*

The effects of Fallot's tetralogy illustrate many of the features of developmental heart disease, and will be considered in some detail.

### EFFECTS

*Murmurs*, often loud, may be heard over the precordium.

*Central cyanosis.* Since blood from the right ventricle enters the aorta directly, there is a considerable *right-to-left shunt*. The arterial blood is therefore not fully oxygenated, and this causes central cyanosis. Patients with Fallot's tetralogy are born as "blue babies". *Central cyanosis* affects all tissues—skin, mucous membranes, tongue, etc. Peripheral cyanosis is due to stagnation; it is seen in the skin when the temperature is reduced and there is vasoconstriction, but not in the mucous membranes, which have a good blood supply. Central cyanosis is found in severe lung disease (p. 400) as well as in direct vascular shunts.

*Polycythaemia*, due to hypoxia of erythropoietic tissue.

*Clubbing of the fingers and toes* is generally marked when the cyanosis is present and of long duration. The pathogenesis is obscure. Clubbing is also found as an idiopathic congenital anomaly of little consequence, in chronic suppurative lung disease (e.g. bronchiectasis and lung abscess), lung cancer, and in *Strept. viridans* endocarditis.

*Underdevelopment.* Unless the defects are corrected the child shows poor development. Early death from infection or heart failure is usual.

**Patent Ductus Arteriosus.** Before birth the ductus transmits blood from the pulmonary artery to the aorta. After birth, as the pulmonary circulation opens up, the ductus should become obliterated, but occasionally this fails to happen. This is an important site for bacterial infection (p. 397).

**Coarctation of the Aorta.** The process of obliteration which affects the ductus may extend to involve the aorta, and lead to the formation of a stricture. Blood then reaches the lower half of the body *via* collateral vessels. The importance of this condition is two-fold. Firstly the area of stenosis may become infected (infective endarteritis), and secondly there is systemic hypertension confined to the upper part of the body. This leads to left ventricular hypertrophy and failure, and sometimes to cerebral haemorrhage. Unless treated, life is seldom prolonged over the age of 40 years.

## ACQUIRED HEART DISEASE

### Arteriosclerotic Heart Disease

The myocardium is supplied by blood through the two coronary arteries.

These vessels are particularly liable to be affected by atheroma, which causes a narrowing of their lumina and subsequent myocardial ischaemia.

**Gradual Coronary Occlusion.** To begin with this has no effect on the resting heart, but on exercise the ischaemia of the muscle causes pain (*angina pectoris*). Characteristically this is felt in the precordium, and spreads to the neck and down the left arm. It comes on with exercise and is relieved by rest. Not every patient with myocardial ischaemia has angina pectoris, and the reason why some escape is not clear. Nor is the mechanism of pain production known. Structurally the myocardium which is rendered ischaemic shows patchy necrosis and subsequent replacement by fibrous tissue. The result is *myocardial fibrosis*. Both coronary arteries may be affected by atheroma. The left ventricle is damaged whichever vessel is affected, and ultimately left ventricular failure ensues.

**Sudden Coronary Occlusion.** Coronary atheroma is particularly liable to be complicated by thrombosis, which leads to a sudden complete occlusion of the lumen. This is the common type of "heart attack"—it comes on suddenly, and is characterized by severe chest pain which is not relieved by rest. The end-results vary considerably:

*Acute functional derangement.* Acute ischaemia may cause sudden death. The left ventricle fibrillates in some cases, while in others ischaemia of the conducting system causes heart block. Sudden death is most common during the first 24 hours, and the value of acute coronary care units is that immediate external cardiac massage or defibrillation can save the lives of a number of these patients.

*Infarction.* If the patient survives, the ischaemic muscle undergoes necrosis. The infarct appears as a firm yellow area of coagulative necrosis with some surrounding haemorrhage and later inflammation. Necrotic muscle releases its enzymes into the blood, and a rise in the levels of SGOT, LDH, CPK, and HBD is a useful indication of myocardial infarction (see p. 53).

Three early complications of myocardial infarction should be noted:

*Pericarditis.* This occurs if the infarct involves the pericardial surface.

*Mural thrombosis* is seen if the infarct involves the endocardium. Portions of thrombus may break off and embolize to systemic organs like the brain and kidney, producing serious and sometimes fatal results.

*Rupture.* Occasionally the necrotic muscle ruptures and this causes haemopericardium and sudden death. Both this complication and systemic embolism are likely to occur at the end of the first week.

About 70 per cent of patients with coronary thrombosis survive their first attack. The infarct is organized to produce a fibrous scar which may later bulge. The aneurysm of the left ventricle so formed may ultimately rupture, but this is an uncommon event. Usually the patient is left with some degree of heart damage, and may have further episodes of coronary thrombosis.

Although myocardial infarction is generally regarded as a consequence of coronary thrombosis, it is by no means the only cause. In *shock* the coronary circulation may be so impaired that infarction occurs. Likewise, *cardiac arrhythmias* causing tachycardia can lead to ischaemia and infarction. In both instances pre-existing coronary atheroma may be a contributory cause. Nevertheless, there are cases recorded of myocardial infarction in patients with widely patent coronary vessels and the possibility of other mechanisms must be considered.[4] Perhaps multiple small platelet emboli impede the small coronary vessels in these cases. Experimentally it can be shown that this is possible, for ADP infused into the coronary artery of a pig leads to the formation of platelet emboli and to infarction.[5] It has even been proposed that a similar mechanism is responsible for many cases of myocardial infarction, and that the coronary artery thrombosis found at necropsy is a secondary event.[6] Whatever the mechanism, there is little doubt that infarction can occur in man without large occlusive arterial thrombi.

## Hypertensive Heart Disease

In systemic hypertension the left ventricle is subjected to a continuous strain. It responds by hypertrophy of its muscle fibres, and for a time bears the strain without failing, but eventually the enormously thick ventricular wall does fail. The chronic left ventricular failure is followed by congestive heart failure. In addition, some patients develop sudden nocturnal attacks of pulmonary oedema. The victim is seized by an ominous sense of suffocation, and the condition is called paroxysmal (nocturnal) dyspnoea (p. 409).

### Rheumatic Heart Disease

Acute rheumatic fever usually attacks children between the ages of 5 and 15 years. It often occurs 2–3 weeks after a streptococcal sore throat, and is believed to be a type of hypersensitivity reaction. However, the relationship to streptococcal infection is not understood; certainly the organisms have not been detected in the lesions of rheumatic fever.

The disease is characterized by fever, flitting pain and swelling of the joints, subcutaneous nodules particularly over bony prominences, and most important of all, involvement of the heart. The pericardium is inflamed, and lesions are found in the myocardium. These take the form of *Aschoff nodes*. They consist of a central area of necrotic collagen surrounded by a zone of inflammatory cells—polymorphs, macrophages, and giant cells. These have up to four vesicular nuclei (with prominent nucleoli) and a basophilic cytoplasm, and are called Aschoff giant cells. Fibroblasts are also present, and the Aschoff node ultimately undergoes fibrosis. Occasionally death from myocardial failure occurs during the acute stage of rheumatic fever, but the microscopic Aschoff nodes seem quite inadequate as an explanation. Dilatation of the valve ring leads to *mitral regurgitation* and this contributes to the heart failure.

The most important lesion of acute rheumatic fever is that which involves the valves. Inflammation (valvulitis) leads to swelling and deposition of small thrombi (called *vegetations*) on the cusps, especially along the line of their closure (Fig. 28.3). While most other lesions of acute rheumatic fever undergo resolution, those of the valves do not. They tend to progress to a state of chronic inflammation, and the cusps become thickened, fibrosed, and contracted. Adjacent cusps adhere to each other rendering the orifice *stenotic*, while the rigid leaflets and thickened, contracted chordae tendineae lead to *regurgitation*. If the aortic valve is affected, it is usually rendered both stenosed and incompetent.

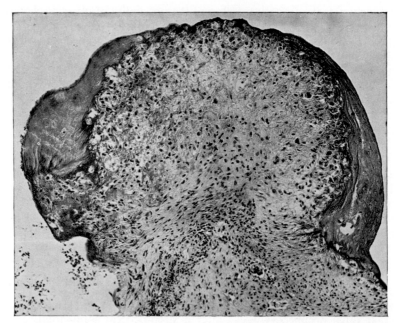

Fig. 28.3. Organizing rheumatic vegetation. The base of the thrombus has been invaded by granulation tissue, while a layer of fibrin (in which there are doubtless aggregations of platelets) still remains on the surface. × 110.

*Mitral stenosis* is the commonest valvular lesion of chronic rheumatic heart disease. Blood is dammed back in the left atrium, and pulmonary venous congestion follows. In mitral stenosis the left ventricle is under no strain and is therefore small, but should there be additional regurgitation or an aortic lesion, the left ventricle becomes enlarged and may subsequently fail.

### Non-Bacterial Thrombotic Endocarditis[7]

Small warty or friable vegetations along the line of closure of the mitral or aortic valves are not uncommon as a *post-mortem* finding. The vegetations are sterile and may be formed on normal or deformed valves. They are of importance in two respects. Occasionally they become detached and embolize to the brain. About 10 per cent of cerebral embolism has been attributed to this mechanism. Secondly the vegetations may form a nidus for the development of infective endocarditis. Usually however, the vegetations of non-bacterial thrombotic endocarditis are of no significance and are removed, probably by lysis.

### Infective Endocarditis

In this condition the valve cusps are invaded by organisms which are usually bacteria, hence the usual name "bacterial endocarditis". But nowadays fungous infections of the valves are seen, and also *Ĉox. burneti* infection in Q-fever, and the condition is better called "infective endocarditis".

**Acute Infective Endocarditis.** During the course of septicaemia, organisms may invade the heart valve and produce an endocarditis which is characterized by the deposition of large friable thrombi (vegetations) on the valve surfaces. The valves themselves may undergo ulceration and rupture. Unless treated, the condition is terminal and leads to *pyaemia*, as fragments of infected thrombus become detached and enter the arterial circulation—usually the systemic. The usual infecting organisms are *Staph. pyogenes* and pneumococci.

**Subacute Infective Endocarditis (and Endarteritis).** The adjective "subacute", hallowed by tradition, is meaningless; the course of the disease is chronic. It is much more helpful to describe the condition in terms of the causative organism than its course. The usual organism is *Strept. viridans*, but sometimes other bacteria, e.g. *Staph. albus*, *Strept. faecalis*, anaerobic streptococci, *H. influenzae*, and coliform organisms, are responsible. A special type may occur in Q-fever. The organism involved is one of relatively low virulence.

The disease occurs typically on vascular endothelium which has been previously abnormal, usually as the result of rheumatic fever. Sometimes a congenital lesion, e.g. a bicuspid aortic valve, coarctation of the aorta, or patent ductus arteriosus, is the seat of trouble, indicating that the condition need not always be an endocarditis. The disease is being encountered more frequently in the elderly than it was previously, and usually there is no obvious preceding valvular disease to account for its localisation. Perhaps minor degenerative lesions are present in the affected valve. The mitral and aortic valves are most commonly affected. The attachment area of ball-valve prostheses (usually aortic) is also liable to infection.

*Prevention.* The organisms reach the heart by the blood stream. *Strept. viridans* is a commensal organism in the mouth. A transient bacteraemia is a frequent event during dental extraction, and may even occur with vigorous mastication. In a healthy individual this is rarely of any consequence, but in a patient with an organic valvular lesion there is a distinct danger that the organisms will localize in damaged areas of the heart and set up endocarditis. Possibly the coincidental formation of non-bacterial thrombotic vegetations causes the organisms to become trapped and set up the infection.

As a prophylactic measure any patient known to have a valvular or congenital heart lesion should be given adequate antibiotic cover before being subjected to dental extraction. It should be given half an hour before the extraction—if given too early, there will be the possibility of the development of more resistant organisms. Long-term chemotherapy is likewise contraindicated, because it merely results in the development of drug-resistant organisms, and, should endocarditis then occur, the infection might be with organisms that are resistant.

In patients who have recovered from infective endocarditis, a recurrence of infection can occur either with the same organism or with a different one. *Strept. viridans* infection can recur even in edentulous patients, and the extraction of sound teeth is not recommended for the prophylaxis of subacute infective endocarditis.[8,9]

*Clinical Features.* The disease runs a chronic course, and unless early, prolonged, and efficient treatment is instituted, the patient dies within one year—usually of heart failure due to valvular destruction or cicatrization, or of a progressive glomerulonephritis, probably of immune-complex allergic aetiology. *Pyrexia* of an irregular type, loss of weight, and *anaemia* are constant features, and the last is in part responsible for the *café-au-lait colour of the skin*. The chronic bacteraemia is responsible for RE hyperplasia which accounts for the *splenomegaly*. *Clubbing of the fingers* is often present, and multiple *embolic phenomena* are characteristic. Large emboli may cause infarction of the brain, intestine, kidney, or spleen; smaller ones have been presumed to be responsible for the *haematuria*, the *splinter haemorrhages* under the nails, and the *petechial haemorrhages of the skin*. However, it seems more likely that these small lesions are due to antigen-antibody complexes causing local vascular damage. *It is important to note that the emboli behave as if they were sterile.* The organisms which they contain are exposed to the bactericidal action of the blood when once they break off from the valves. It is known that the patient's blood contains a high content of antibodies against the causative organisms.

*Pathological Features.* The vegetations are large, red, and friable, and are liable to break off and embolize. Histologically they consist of thrombus containing numerous bacterial colonies which are well protected from the blood stream. The vegetations are attached to the valve by means of granulation tissue, but this is neither profuse nor does it penetrate far into the vegetation. The organisms are once more beyond the reach of the blood. The poor vascularity of the valve cusps is probably the explanation of this inadequate organisation. It is a good example of frustrated repair, and as such typical chronic inflammation.

One of the curious features of this disease is that organisms of relatively low virulence are able to survive in the presence of a high degree of immunity. Their inaccessibility in the thrombus appears to be the explanation.

*Diagnosis.* This depends on a *positive blood culture*. But the disease is so serious that if the clinical picture suggests endocarditis, treatment should be instituted without waiting for pathological confirmation.

Prior to the days of antibiotics the disease was invariably fatal. With modern treatment cure is possible, but the healed valves are often grossly distorted and show calcification.

## Calcareous Aortic Stenosis

This condition, probably arising in a congenitally abnormal valve, usually affects elderly men. The aortic ring and later the valve cusps become calcified, and fuse together producing a tight stenosis. The left ventricle is hypertrophied, but in spite of the overaction of this chamber an inadequate amount of blood is pumped into the aorta. In particular the blood supply to the coronary vessels is impaired, and these patients are in constant danger of sudden death. Surgical replacement of diseased valves by a homograft or a plastic prosthesis is therefore indicated.

A great deal is known about the anatomical features of heart disease, but we are remarkably ignorant about its functional aspects. The action of the myocardium is clearly all-important, but it is just this function which cannot be assessed directly at necropsy. It is humiliating to admit that a failing myocardium cannot be distinguished histologically from a normal one. Perhaps more refined methods of examination will remedy this situation in the future.

## General Reading

HUDSON, R. E. B. (1965 and 1970). "Cardiovascular Pathology", 3 Volumes. London: Arnold.
WOOD, P. (1968). "Diseases of the Heart and Circulation", 3rd ed. London: Eyre and Spottiswoode.
HARRIS, P. and HEATH, D. (1962). "The Human Pulmonary Circulation". Edinburgh: Livingstone.

## References

1. Leading Article (1967). *Lancet*, **2,** 457.
2. HALL, J. L. and SMITH, E. B. (1968). *Arch. Path.*, **86,** 403.
3. CIBA FOUNDATION SYMPOSIUM ON CARDIOMYOPATHIES (1964). Ed. by WOLSTEN-HOLME, G. E. W. and O'CONNOR, M. London: Churchill.
4. SIDD, J. J., KEMP, H. G. and GORLIN, R. (1970). *New Engl. J. Med.*, **282,** 1306.
5. JØRGENSEN, L. *et al.* (1967). *Lab. Invest.*, **17,** 616.
6. SPAIN, D. M. and BRADESS, V. A. (1960). *Amer. J. med. Sci.*, **240,** 701.
7. Leading Article (1967). *Brit. med. J.*, **3,** 812.
8. CROXSON, M. S., ALTMANN, M. M. and O'BRIEN, K. P. (1971). *Lancet*, **1,** 1205.
9. SIMON, D. S. and GOODWIN, J. F. (1971). *Lancet*, **1,** 1207.

*Chapter 29*

# DISEASES OF THE RESPIRATORY SYSTEM

## Normal Function[1, 2]

T' e function of the respiratory system is to enable gaseous exchange to take place between the blood and the atmosphere. Air is inhaled, and as it passes through the nose, nasopharynx, larynx, and trachea it is filtered and humidified. It eventually reaches the small air sacs, or alveoli, of the lung where it comes into close contact with blood in the capillaries, and conditions for gaseous exchange are ideal. Oxygen is added to the blood, and the carbon dioxide which is removed is exhaled. The gas in the alveoli is maintained at a fairly constant composition by the act of breathing. This has two components— ventilation and distribution.

**Ventilation.** This is the bellows-like action of the chest, by which fresh air is drawn in and stale air expired. The volume is approximately 7·5 litres/min. in the adult at rest.

**Distribution.** The inspired air is so distributed in relation to the volume of blood perfusing the lung that the composition of the alveolar gas is maintained at a constant level. Since the arterial blood, as it leaves the lung, is in equilibrium with the alveolar gas, it follows that the gaseous tensions of oxygen and carbon dioxide in the arterial blood are also maintained at this same constant level.

## Respiratory Failure[3, 4]

If through the dysfunction of the lungs there is oxygen lack or $CO_2$ retention, the condition is called *respiratory failure*. In the arterial blood under normal conditions the partial pressure of oxygen, usually written $Po_2$, is about 100 mm. Hg, and the partial pressure of carbon dioxide ($Pco_2$) about 40 mm. Hg. In respiratory failure the $Po_2$ is under 60 mm. Hg and the $Pco_2$ over 49 mm. Hg.

**Lack of Oxygen** (hypoxia). The arterial blood is normally saturated with oxygen, but in respiratory failure both the tension and quantity of oxygen in the blood are reduced. As the blood passes through the tissues it becomes increasingly desaturated, and cyanosis of the exposed parts occurs. The hypoxia stimulates red-cell production in the bone marrow, and leads to polycythaemia. This increases the viscosity of the blood, and by causing stagnation in the tissues contributes to the cyanosis. In addition there is an added strain to the heart, and *heart failure* may occur. Usually the right ventricle is affected, because in most lung diseases causing respiratory failure there is considerable destruction of lung tissue and obliteration of pulmonary vasculature. This causes pulmonary hypertension and strain on the right ventricle.

**Retention of Carbon Dioxide.** An increased tension of $CO_2$ in the arterial blood (hypercapnia) produces vasodilatation of the vessels of the skin and brain. The skin is hot and flushed, and the brain becomes hyperaemic and oedematous.[5] Clinically the latter is manifest as confusion, drowsiness, tremor, and finally coma and death.

## Dyspnoea

In a healthy person the rate and depth of respiration are so regulated that the individual is unaware of the movements involved in breathing. *Tachypnoea* is an increased rate of respiration, and is seen when pain restricts respiratory movement, as in pleurisy, or when the lungs become increasingly rigid, as in congestion or fibrosis. Tachypnoea is sometimes accompanied by an increase in depth of breathing, and the term *hyperpnoea* embraces both conditions. *Dyspnoea* is a condition in which the act of breathing causes distress. It occurs under two main circumstances:

(1) *when tachypnoea or hyperpnoea are of marked degree;*
(2) *when the ventilatory effect produced on inspiration is small in comparison with the muscular effort needed to produce it.* This occurs in any disease interfering with the respiratory excursions of the lung, for instance, fibrosis or congestion. Obstruction to the major air passages, whether due to pulmonary disease like chronic bronchitis or to strangulation, has a similar effect, and produces intense dyspnoea. Psychological factors also play a part. Thus the sudden blockage of a tube through which a person is breathing occasions intense dyspnoea. However, if the subject is asked to block the tube himself the manoeuvre causes no immediate discomfort.

### Bronchial Obstruction[6]

**Causes**

The common causes of bronchial obstruction are:

(1) Tenacious mucus which is not expelled from the respiratory passages, e.g. in asthma.
(2) Chronic bronchitis.
(3) Inhaled foreign bodies, e.g. roots of teeth, peas, etc.
(4) Tumours.

**Effects**

The effects of obstruction depend on whether the obstruction is partial or complete.

**Partial Obstruction.** The partial obstruction of a bronchus impedes the ventilation of the lung distal to the obstruction. It follows therefore that the blood perfusing that part of the lung is inadequately oxygenated, and that in effect a quantity of venous blood is shunted directly into the pulmonary veins and thence to the left side of the heart. Since the blood leaving the lungs is normally fully saturated with oxygen, it follows that no amount of over-ventilation of the unaffected lung can compensate for this shunt effect. The arterial $Po_2$ is therefore lowered. A very important example of partial obstruction of the bronchi occurs in chronic bronchitis, especially after surgical operation[7] (p. 410).

**Complete Obstruction.** Where there is complete obstruction of a large bronchus, the lung distal shows a progressive absorption of its gas content until it becomes completely airless or *collapsed*.

**Infection.** Infection commonly follows bronchial obstruction. Organisms that are inhaled into the affected lung segment become trapped in the mucus, their expulsion is impaired, and bronchopneumonia follows. The infection also involves the bronchial wall, and if long-continued will produce destruction of its muscle and cartilaginous component, so that the bronchus is

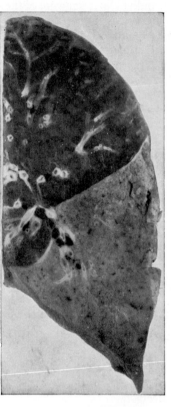

FIG. 29.1. Lobar pneumonia. The left lower lobe is consolidated in the stage of grey hepatization, while the upper lobe is unaffected.

(R30.2. *Reproduced by permission of the President and Council of the Royal College of Surgeons of England.*)

weakened and tends to dilate (*bronchiectasis*). This is frequently seen distal to the obstruction caused by a carcinoma or a foreign body. Quite often bronchiectasis occurs in several parts of the lung as an idiopathic condition, and it is thought to be the result of obstruction by mucus during some previous infection such as measles or whooping-cough.

## Pneumonia

Pneumonia is defined as an inflammation in the alveolar parenchyma of the lung. Exudate usually fills the alveoli which are thereby rendered airless and solid. This is called *consolidation*. Sometimes, however, the inflammatory exudate is restricted to the alveolar wall. This is often called *interstitial pneumonia*, but the term *pneumonitis* is also used.

Two main types of pneumonia are recognized, depending upon the gross appearance of the lesions which result.

## Lobar Pneumonia[8, 9]

This is a disease especially of healthy young adults. The organism concerned is a pneumococcus of high virulence, and is acquired by inhalation from another victim or a convalescent carrier. The disease has a sudden onset with rigors, fever, and pain in the chest. The organisms which reach the lung produce a rapidly spreading inflammatory oedema which soon implicates a whole lobe, and sometimes several lobes (Fig. 29.1).

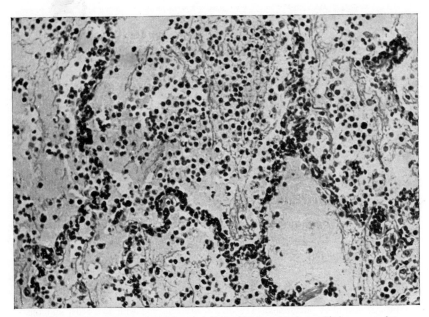

FIG. 29.2. Lobar pneumonia. The alveoli are filled with a loose fibrinous exudate in which there are many pus cells. The alveolar capillaries are engorged with blood. This corresponds to the stage of red hepatization. × 220.

**Pathogenesis.** The fact that infection spreads so rapidly in a gigantic wave of oedematous exudate suggests that allergy is involved in the process. Perhaps the patient has already had a minor pneumococcal infection sufficient to produce an immune response. When now attacked a second time, the reaction of hypersensitivity accompanies the inflammatory response and renders it more intense. An alternative explanation is that lobar pneumonia is a primary infection. When the organisms reach the lungs, they pass on rapidly to the blood stream, where they proliferate in the RE system, and then escape into the blood to produce a septicaemia. When they reach the lungs again, an allergic response occurs due to their reaction with recently formed local antibodies. This mechanism would be analogous to that described in typhoid fever and in syphilis.

**Stages.** Whatever the mechanism, there is no doubt that during the acute stage of the disease there is a septicaemia, and sometimes the pneumococci may localize themselves not only in the lungs but also in the meninges, peritoneum, joints, etc. During the first few days of illness the patient is desperately ill and may die; the lobe of lung affected is *congested* and shows *inflammatory oedema*. It is teeming with pneumococci.

The second stage of the disease is called *red hepatization*, because the congested, consolidated lung has the appearance of liver. Microscopically the alveolar capillaries are dilated, and the alveoli are filled with inflammatory exudate containing oedema fluid, fibrin, and many polymorphs (Fig. 29.2).

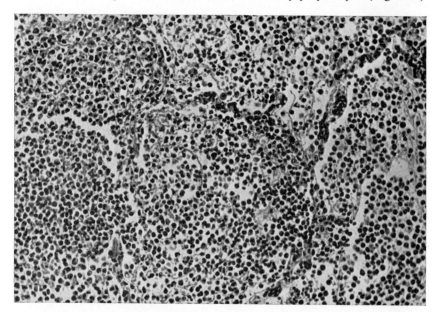

Fig. 29.3. Lobar pneumonia. The alveoli are crowded with pus cells, and the fibrinous exudate is condensed into thick strands. The alveolar capillaries are much less engorged than in Fig. 29.2. This corresponds to the stage of grey hepatization. × 220.

A number of red cells are present also. Gradually the hyperaemia of the lung diminishes, the capillaries shut down, and the lung assumes a grey colour. This is the classical stage of *grey hepatization*. The alveoli are still filled with inflammatory exudate, but the polymorphs show disintegration and fibrin threads appear clumped (Fig. 29.3). The fourth and final stage is that of *resolution*, in which demolition is accomplished by macrophages. The fibrin is removed with great rapidity, and all the debris is cleared away. Fluid exudate and macrophages leave the alveoli mainly by way of the lymphatics. With the removal of all the inflammatory exudate the lung returns to normal, and this is therefore an excellent example of complete resolution. Rarely the exudate in the alveoli is not demolished but persists and is organized into fibrous tissue.

During the acute stage of lobar pneumonia the overlying pleura shows acute inflammation, and is covered with a fibrinous exudate. This is responsible for the creaking pleural rub which may be heard clinically, and for the pain which occurs on inspiration.

### Bronchopneumonia[9]

In bronchopneumonia, unlike lobar pneumonia, there are discrete foci of inflammation round terminal bronchioles. Patches of consolidation are scattered throughout several lobes of the lung, and the condition is usually bilateral (Fig. 29.4). The wildfire spread seen in lobar pneumonia is not present.

There are many varieties of bronchopneumonia. They are best considered under two headings:

(1) *Endogenous bronchopneumonia.*
(2) *Exogenous bronchopneumonia.*

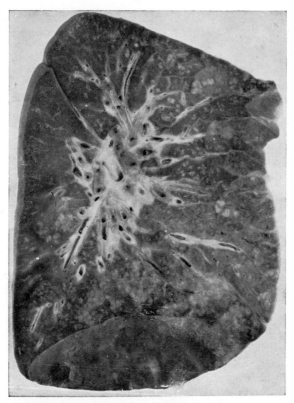

Fig. 29.4. Staphylococcal bronchopneumonia. There are discrete foci of consolidation scattered throughout the lung, and some have formed tiny abscesses.

(R29.3. *Reproduced by permission of the President and Council of the Royal College of Surgeons of England.*)

### Endogenous Bronchopneumonia

This is due to infection with commensal organisms normally resident in the upper respiratory passages. Of these the commensal pneumococci of low-grade virulence are by far the most important. They cause infection whenever the defence mechanisms of the host are impaired. The antagonists are therefore a weakly virulent endogenous organism and an enfeebled host. This contrasts with lobar pneumonia in which the contending parties are a highly virulent organism and a healthy host.

**Causes.**

The conditions leading to endogenous bronchopneumonia may be considered under two headings:

**General Factors.** *Extremes of age.* It is commonest in infancy and old age.

*General debilitating illness.* It is a common terminal event in cancer, cerebrovascular accidents, and uraemia.

*Impaired immune response.* It may occur following total body irradiation, in agammaglobulinaemia, etc.

**Local Factors.** Any local condition interfering with ciliary action and the upward movement of mucus is liable to be followed by bronchopneumonia. The causes may be listed.

*Pre-existing acute respiratory disease.* Bronchopneumonia often complicates influenza, measles, and whooping-cough. In these infections the ciliated bronchial epithelium is shed, and organisms which gain access to the lung cannot be removed.

*Local obstruction.* The trapped secretions form an admirable medium for bacterial growth, and bronchopneumonia is localized to the segment distal to the obstruction. Foreign bodies and tumours of the bronchi are well-known examples.

*Chronic bronchitis and bronchiectasis.* These are important predisposing causes of bronchopneumonia. Two factors are involved. In the first place the ciliated epithelium may be replaced by goblet cells or squamous cells, and this impedes the upward flow of mucus. Secondly the mucus itself is often of viscid consistency, and cannot easily be removed. An excessive amount of mucus appears in the *chronic venous congestion* of heart failure due to the additional fluid contributed by transudation.

*Pulmonary oedema.* In oedematous lung tissue it seems likely that the macrophages are unable to perform their normal function. Infection is therefore quite a common sequel to oedema from whatever cause. The basal oedema which occurs in debilitated, bedridden patients, in those who are unconscious, and following operations often progresses to pneumonia, and is called *hypostatic pneumonia.*

Bronchopneumonia is of much longer duration than lobar pneumonia. If the primary condition is incurable, the pneumonia is merely a welcome terminal event, and there will obviously be little attempt at healing. Even in the childhood bronchopneumonias that follow measles and whooping-cough, a prolonged course is the rule, and is often punctuated by relapses and remissions depending upon whether the organism or the host is gaining the upper hand. Both the onset and the end of the disease are gradual.

### Lesions of Bronchopneumonia

The disease is usually basal and posterior in distribution and is bilateral. If an area of bronchopneumonia is examined microscopically, it is found to consist of acutely inflamed bronchioles full of pus. Some of the surrounding alveoli contain oedema fluid in which there are macrophages and polymorphs, while others are filled with a dense fibrinous exudate in which there are innumerable polymorphs. Some are collapsed as the result of the absorption of air distal to the blocked bronchioles, whereas neighbouring alveoli are empty and distended due to compensatory dilatation. In contrast to lobar pneumonia, where all alveoli in a lobe are at about the same stage of the inflammatory process, in bronchopneumonia there is a very varied picture.

### Sequelae of Bronchopneumonia

*Resolution.* This is much less frequent than in lobar pneumonia.

*Progressive fibrosis of the lung.* This is correspondingly more frequent. It is due to organization of the inflammatory exudate in the alveoli. In addition there is often a continuance of the inflammatory process, so that more and more lung tissue is destroyed and converted into fibrous tissue. This is, of course, the condition of chronic inflammation, and bronchopneumonia often becomes chronic. In due course the infection spreads, and the muscle and elastic tissue of the adjacent bronchi are destroyed and replaced by granulation tissue. In consequence the lumina widen, and eventually the dilatation becomes so extensive that secretion accumulates forming the nidus of further infection and inflammatory destruction. This is the pathogenesis of *bronchiectasis*, which is both a sequel of bronchopneumonia and a predisposing cause of further attacks.

*Suppuration.* Abscess formation is not uncommon, particularly when the host's resistance is exceptionally poor and the causal organism is *Staph. pyogenes.*

### Exogenous Bronchopneumonia

A variety of virulent organisms when inhaled may lead to severe bronchopneumonia. The host may be a healthy adult, or he may be enfeebled as a result of a previous disease. Examples of virulent organisms causing exogenous bronchopneumonia are:

*Staph. pyogenes,* as a result of hospital cross-infection.

*Strept. pyogenes.* This was particularly common in the 1918 influenza pandemic.

*Yersinia (Pasteurella) pestis*—pneumonic plague.

*Mycobacterium tuberculosis* and the deep-seated fungous diseases. This type of disease is quite distinct, as the lesions produced are characteristically chronic. They are described in Chapter 15.

*Mycoplasma pneumoniae* causes an acute pneumonia characterized by a severe cough and widespread lesions in the lungs demonstrable radiologically. The appearance of cold haemagglutinins in the blood and a tendency for the disease to occur in epidemics are other features of this disease, which has a very low mortality rate.

Pneumonia may be due to a variety of *viruses*. Coxsackie viruses, ECHO viruses, and myxoviruses have commonly been incriminated in acute pneumonia especially in children. *Respiratory syncytial virus* is a common offender.[10] The name "virus pneumonia" may be applied to this group of pneumonias, but the term, and also "primary atypical pneumonia", have both been used in the past to describe outbreaks of non-bacterial pneumonia which were in fact caused by *Mycoplasma pneumoniae*. It is best therefore to describe pneumonia in terms of the causative agent.

The histology of this group of pneumonias is poorly defined, since death from the uncomplicated disease is rare. There is usually a lymphocytic and macrophage infiltrate in the alveolar walls so that the lesion may be described as an *interstitial pneumonia*. There is a variable amount of exudate in the alveoli themselves, and the fibrin component often becomes compressed against the alveolar walls as an eosinophilic lining, or *hyaline membrane*.

## OEDEMA OF THE LUNGS

The systolic pressure in the pulmonary artery is 15–25 mm. Hg, and being much lower than that in the systemic vessels, it follows that there is less tendency to oedema formation. The osmotic effect of the plasma proteins is relatively unopposed. Nevertheless, when oedema does occur, two factors tend to ensure that it persists and even spreads.

(1) The loose nature of the lung prevents any appreciable rise in tissue tension, a factor which in other tissues limits the extent of oedema formation.
(2) When once the lungs become oedematous, ventilation ceases, the vessels become hypoxic, and they tend to leak. It follows that in all examples of pulmonary oedema the fluid has a high protein content. It is not possible to distinguish between transudates and exudates as in other tissues.

### Causes of Pulmonary Oedema

**Acute Inflammation.** Oedema occurs in the early stages of pneumonia. It is particularly marked in acute lobar pneumonia, and was seen in the broncho-pneumonia which complicated influenza in the 1918 pandemic. The lungs were described as showing acute haemorrhagic oedema rather than broncho-pneumonia of the classical type. Such a picture is also seen in poisoning with certain gases, e.g. phosgene, chlorine, and nitrogen peroxide. Acute pulmonary oedema also follows the inhalation of gastric juice such as may occur if a patient vomits during the inexpert administration of a general anaesthetic.

**Heart Failure.** Acute pulmonary oedema is a frequent complication of left ventricular failure and is also common in mitral stenosis. Although increased pulmonary venous pressure is the classical explanation, it is unlikely that this is the major cause of pulmonary oedema in heart failure. More important is the effect of a *redistribution of the blood volume*: attacks of acute pulmonary oedema occur quite suddenly, sometimes at night, and they are probably initiated by peripheral vasoconstriction. The amount of blood in the peripheral circulation is thus diminished, and the excess volume is displaced into the pulmonary circulation where it appears as oedema fluid. Support for this contention is the fact that acute pulmonary oedema is a well-known hazard of adrenaline administration. This drug causes peripheral vasoconstriction. It must never be given to patients with acute pulmonary oedema of cardiac origin. In bronchial asthma this drug is beneficial, but in cardiac asthma it can be lethal.

The terms *cardiac asthma* and *paroxysmal nocturnal dyspnoea* are often applied to these attacks of acute pulmonary oedema. The patient wakes up breathless with a sense of oppression in the chest. He sits up, but the dyspnoea increases. Mounting restlessness drives him out of bed to seek the fresh air at the window. The sense of suffocation becomes intense, and with it there is profound distress. The skin has an ashen cyanosis, and there is profuse sweating. The patient may cough up blood-stained sputum, and in severe cases a rapidly spreading pulmonary oedema results in death.

**Overloading the Circulation.** If an excessive volume of fluid is administered intravenously, some of the excess is accommodated in the great veins, but the remainder is diverted to the pulmonary circulation and leads to oedema formation. It is obvious that patients already in heart failure are particularly liable to this complication. Transfusion must be carried out very slowly, and packed red cells should be used instead of whole blood if anaemia is to be corrected.

**Cerebral Damage.** Acute pulmonary oedema is sometimes seen following damage to the brain, e.g. after trauma or cerebral haemorrhage. The most likely explanation is that there occurs considerable sympathetic activity, which by leading to peripheral vasoconstriction causes diversion of the circulating fluid to the lungs, as described above.

## The Pneumoconioses

This group of diseases, produced by the *inhalation of dust*, are mostly occupational in origin. The most important is *silicosis*, which is seen in miners and those who work with finely divided silica. Following the inhalation of this dust there results a chronic inflammatory condition which eventually leads to extensive fibrosis (p. 131). *Asbestosis* produces a similar effect, but, unlike silicosis, is also important in predisposing to cancer of the lung and mesothelioma of the pleura.

## Chronic Non-Specific Lung Disease[11, 12, 13]

This collective title includes chronic bronchitis, emphysema, and asthma, so frequently diagnosed together though often in fact found separately. Their aetiology is unknown, and it is advisable to consider each as a separate entity.

## Chronic Bronchitis[14]

*Definition and Lesions.* This is best defined as a condition in which there is a chronic or recurrent increase in the volume of bronchial mucus, sufficient to cause expectoration, and which is not due to localized bronchopulmonary disease.[12, 15] It is much commoner in tobacco-smokers than in non-smokers, and is very prevalent in England but less so in North America. The bronchial mucosa is thickened by hyperplasia of the mucous glands, and there is an increase in the number of goblet cells in the lining epithelium. True chronic inflammation is not a feature, and Laennec's "bronchial catarrh" would be a better name.

Recurrent inflammation is a common complication, and may be due to infection or the effects of irritant chemicals—smog is particularly dangerous in this respect.

*Effects*. The effect of chronic bronchitis is impairment of ventilation due to bronchial narrowing. The mucosa is thickened and there is excess mucus in, and spasm of, the bronchi. Dyspnoea is a prominent symptom, and as the disease progresses respiratory failure develops. The arterial blood is unsaturated and cyanosis occurs. Hypercapnia and right ventricular failure are also common.

The administration of anaesthetics to chronic bronchitics is particularly hazardous, since any further increase in mucous production or spasm of the bronchi is liable to precipitate respiratory failure.

### Emphysema[14]

*Definition*. The word, introduced by Laennec, is derived from the Greek, meaning an inflation. It is defined as a condition in which there is an increase beyond the normal in size of the terminal air passages. Two distinct types occur.

**Dilatatory Emphysema.**[12] Emphysema due to dilatation of the air passages occurs as a compensatory phenomenon following the removal, collapse, or destruction of the adjacent lung. It is of no importance as a cause of respiratory failure.

**Destructive Emphysema.**[11] This is of great importance, and the unqualified term "emphysema" is generally taken to mean this condition. There is destruction of the alveoli in the walls of the terminal air passages, which are therefore widened. Sometimes large air-filled sacs, or *bullae*, are formed and little lung parenchyma remains. The effect of this lung destruction is to impair gaseous exchange. $CO_2$ can escape rather more easily than oxygen can be taken up. A common effect is therefore arterial desaturation and cyanosis. Dyspnoea is often marked.

### Bronchial Asthma

Asthma may be defined as a condition of widespread narrowing of the bronchial airways, which *changes its severity over short periods of time* either spontaneously or under treatment, and is not due to cardiovascular disease.[12] It is characterized by *paroxysms of wheezing dyspnoea*. The bronchial obstruction is caused partly by spasm of the bronchial muscle and partly by the presence of viscid muscus. The disease often has an hereditary basis, and is one of the manifestations of atopy (p. 162). Its pathogenesis is complex; attacks may be the result of hypersensitivity to some inhaled antigen, but psychological and other factors are undoubtedly involved.

## Tumours of the Lung[6]

The vast majority are epithelial in origin.

### Adenomata[19]

This term has been used to include several distinct tumours. The commonest is the carcinoid. The tumours arise in the wall of a large bronchus and cause partial, and finally complete, obstruction. Distal *bronchopneumonia* and *bronchiectasis* are frequent. The tumours are of intermediate type; they

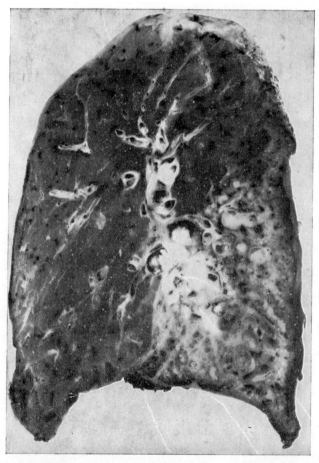

FIG. 29.5. Carcinoma of the lung. This has arisen from the left lower lobe main bronchus and has infiltrated into the lower lobe, which has also undergone fibrosis secondary to collapse, bronchiectasis, and bronchopneumonia. The local hilar lymph nodes are involved. The tumour proved to be a squamous-cell carcinoma.

(R45.1. *Reproduced by permission of the President and Council of the Royal College of Surgeons of England.*)

invade locally but do not commonly metastasize. Hence lobectomy or pneumonectomy is usually curative.

## Carcinoma

Cancer of the lung now ranks as the commonest lethal cancer in males, and is also frequent in females. Cigarette smoking and atmospheric pollution are major factors in its aetiology. Asbestosis is a predisposing cause, and it was also common in the Schneeberg miners who inhaled radioactive substances.

**Gross Appearance.** Two common types of tumour may be recognized:[16]

*Peripheral lung cancers.* These tumours presumably arise in one of the small bronchi or bronchioles, and appear as fairly discrete tumour masses situated in the lung parenchyma. Symptoms are often absent until the pleura and chest wall are invaded, or distant metastases appear.

*Central lung cancers.* These arise in one of the major bronchi, and therefore cause early obstruction with resulting collapse, bronchopneumonia, and bronchiectasis (Fig. 29.5). Frequently the patient presents with fever and symptoms of pneumonia. Haemoptysis is common, the bleeding being either from the tumour itself, or, more often, from the inflamed dilated bronchi beyond.

**Spread.** Lung cancer spreads by all the classical routes:

*Local spread* to involve lung parenchyma, pleura, bronchi, arteries, and veins.

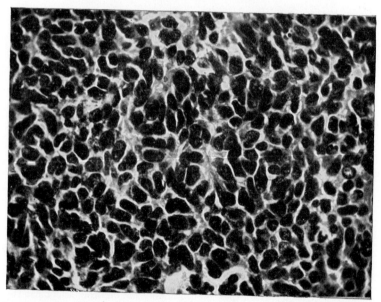

FIG. 29.6. Oat-cell carcinoma of lung. The constituent cells are small, fusiform in shape, and have prominent darkly-staining nuclei. Their shape has given rise to the descriptive term "oat cell". × 500.

*Lymphatic spread* to the hilar and mediastinal nodes. This usually occurs early, and is most marked with the oat-cell tumours.

*Blood-borne metastases.* Secondary tumours are common in the *liver, bones, adrenals,* and *brain.* Even the spleen and bowel, organs not commonly the site of metastases from other tumours, may be involved. It is the frequency of distant spread which makes the prognosis so poor.

**Histological Types.**[17] Although arising from a mucus-secreting epithelium, cancers of the lung are remarkable for their histological variations.

*Squamous-cell carcinoma.* Microscopically this resembles squamous-cell carcinoma arising elsewhere, except that well-differentiated examples are not common. The tumours arise either in areas of squamous metaplasia or by tumour metaplasia in an adenocarcinoma—the latter explanation is the more likely. These tumours may be either central or peripheral, and have the most favourable prognosis.

*Adenocarcinoma.* These tumours are almost always peripheral, and tend to be more frequent in women. Areas of squamous metaplasia are common.

*Anaplastic carcinoma.* These tumours show little or no differentiation; two variants are recognized:

*Large-cell tumours,* which are most probably tumours at the anaplastic end of the scale of squamous-cell carcinoma or adenocarcinoma.

*Small-cell, or oat-cell, carcinoma.* Oat-cell carcinoma of the lung appears to be a distinct tumour, and is probably derived from neurosecretory cells of the bronchial mucosa akin to the argentaffin cells of the intestine.[18] In this respect it shares a common origin with the carcinoid tumour. The tumour is composed of small, darkly-staining cells, may form small rosettes, and may be round or oat-shaped (Fig. 29.6). The tumours are frequently large, and their origin is difficult to determine. They metastasize early and widely. An enormous mediastinal mass may be produced, which impedes the heart's action by directly invading the pericardium and myocardium, and by compressing the great vessels. The tumours are very radiosensitive, but the prognosis is extremely bad.

## References

1. CAMPBELL, E. J. M. (1968). In "Clinical Physiology", 3rd ed., p.93, ed. by Campbell, E. J. M., Dickinson, C. J. and Slater, J. D. H. Oxford: Blackwell.
2. DE REUCK, A. V. S. and O'CONNOR, M. (1962). edrs. "Pulmonary structure and function". A CIBA Foundation Symposium. London: Churchill.
3. Various Authors. (1962). *Proc. roy. Soc. Med.,* **55,** 565.
4. CAMPBELL, E. J. M. (1965). *Brit. med. J.,* **1,** 1451.
5. Annotation (1963). *Brit. med. J.,* **2,** 1486.
6. SPENCER, H. (1968). "The Lung", 2nd ed., New York: Macmillan.
7. HOBSLEY, M. (1963). *Ann. roy. Coll. Surg. Enql.,* **33,** 105.
8. WILSON, G. S. and MILES, A. A. (1964). In Topley and Wilson's "Principles of Bacteriology and Immunity" 5th ed. p. 2018, London: Arnold.
9. REIMANN, H. A. (1962). *Ann. intern. Med.,* **56,** 144.
10. McCLELLAND, L. *et al.* (1971). *New Engl. J. med.,* **264,** 1169 and 1176.
11. SCADDING, J. G. (1959). *Lancet,* **1,** 323.
12. Report of a CIBA Foundation Guest Symposium. (1959). *Thorax,* **14,** 286.
13. HEARD, B. E. (1966). In "Recent Advances in Pathology" ed. Harrison, C. V. p. 348, London: Churchill.

14. HEARD, B. E. (1969). "Pathology of Chronic Bronchitis and Emphysema", 136 pp. London: Churchill.
15. Report of an Expert Committee (1961). *Wld: Hlth. Org. techn. Rep. Ser.*, **213,** 15.
16. WALTER, J. B. and PRYCE, D. M. (1955). *Thorax,* **10,** 107 and 117.
17. KREYBERG, L., LIEBOW, A. A. and UEHLINGER, E. A. (1967). "Histological Typing of Lung Tumours", International Histological Classification of Tumours, No. 1. Geneva: W.H.O.
18. BENSCH, K. G. *et al.* (1968). *Cancer (Philadelphia),* **22,** 1163.
19. Leading Article (1972). *Lancet,* **1,** 1322.

# Chapter 30

# DISEASES OF THE ALIMENTARY TRACT

Although the alimentary tract is usually regarded as being within the body, it is in fact a long tube exposed at each end to the exterior. Its contents, ranging from food in the mouth to faeces in the rectum, are never within the body proper. This is an ideal arrangement, for within the lumen the chemical changes necessary for digestion can occur under conditions which could not be tolerated inside the body itself. One effect of this arrangement is that many litres of digestive fluids are poured into the alimentary tract each day. Normally nearly all of this is reabsorbed, but it can readily be appreciated that if much escaped to the exterior the volume of fluid lost could reach alarming proportions. Vomiting and diarrhoea are potent causes of water and electrolyte depletion, and this is described in Chapter 24. In the present chapter the digestive aspects of the alimentary tract are considered as well as some of its common afflictions.

## The Mouth, Pharynx, and Oesophagus

In the mouth food is masticated and mixed with saliva, which, by virtue of its mucus content, performs a lubricating action in addition to commencing carbohydrate digestion by the enzyme ptyalin.

Swallowing (*deglutition*) is triggered off by the voluntary contraction of the pharyngeal and buccal muscles. This, by raising the larynx and tongue, throws the bolus of food against the posterior pharyngeal wall. Thereafter a wave of peristalsis sweeps the bolus down the muscular oesophagus into the stomach.

**Difficulty in Swallowing (Dysphagia).** This is caused by a great variety of lesions, a few of which will be mentioned.[1]

(1) *Painful conditions* inhibit the voluntary initiation of the act of swallowing, e.g. aphthous ulceration and acute tonsillitis.

(2) *Mechanical interference with deglutition* is seen when the pharynx or tongue is infiltrated with scirrhous carcinoma or amyloid.

(3) *Mechanical obstruction.* This usually occurs in the oesophagus, and is caused by *carcinoma* (Fig. 30.1), either squamous-cell which is usually in the middle third of the oesophagus, or adenocarcinoma arising from the lower portion or the stomach. Less common are *benign strictures*, secondary either to chronic peptic ulcer at the lower end or to the destruction and scarring caused by swallowing corrosive acids and alkalis. The dysphagia of the *Plummer-Vinson syndrome* is associated with obstruction at the upper end of the oesophagus (p. 344; a web is often present in the anterior aspect of the cricopharyngeal area, but whether or not this causes a mechanical obstruction has been debated for years and is still undecided.

(4) *Paralysis of the muscles of deglutition*, e.g. in poliomyelitis affecting the brain-stem and in pseudobulbar palsy (p. 469).

(5) *Neuromuscular incoordination*. In elderly people incoordination of the peristaltic waves and muscular spasm may produce a sensation of obstruction and severe pain. In *achalasia of the cardia* there is a degeneration of the ganglion cells of the lower oesophagus, which results in disturbed peristalsis and a failure of relaxation of the cardiac sphincter. As a result the oesophagus becomes greatly dilated.

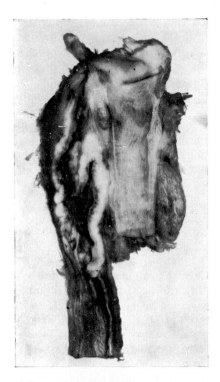

FIG. 30.1. Postcricoid carcinoma of oesophagus. This is a vertical section through the larynx and adjacent oesophagus. The upper part of the oesophagus is surrounded by a polypoid carcinoma which has almost completely occluded the lumen.

(A31.5. *Reproduced by permission of the President and Council of the Royal College of Surgeons of England.*)

(6) *Psychiatric*. Difficulty in swallowing and a sensation of a foreign body in the throat are familiar accompaniments of fear and anxiety.

For clinical purposes dysphagia may be divided into two groups:

*Oropharyngeal dysphagia*, in which attempted swallowing may lead to the inhalation of food or its regurgitation through the nose.

*Oesophageal dysphagia*, in which the common symptom is a sense of obstruction in the chest during swallowing. Carcinoma is the lesion most to be feared, especially if the symptoms are progressive and difficulty in swallowing first affects solids and finally liquids.

### The Stomach

In the stomach the masticated food is softened, moistened, lubricated, and partly digested by the gastric juice. It is kneaded by strong muscular contraction into a semiliquid mass called *chyme*, which is passed steadily into the duodenum.

The gastric juice has four major components:

*Mucus*, which has a lubricating action.

*Intrinsic factor*, without which vitamin $B_{12}$ cannot be absorbed.

*Pepsin*, which commences protein digestion.

*Hydrochloric acid*. This has an important bactericidal action, and also provides the correct pH for the action of pepsin. Its presence is important in the pathogenesis of one of the common disabling afflictions of mankind—*peptic ulceration*.

Wherever acid gastric juice comes into contact with a non-acid-secreting mucosa, peptic ulceration is liable to occur. It is therefore seen at the pylorus, along the lesser curve of the stomach, in the first part of the duodenum, at the lower end of the oesophagus, and at the site of anastomosis between the stomach and small intestine following gastro-enterostomy.

**Acute Ulceration.**[2] *Acute erosions*. Acute shallow ulcers, commonly called erosions, are often seen in the stomach. They are usually multiple, and appear to be caused by dietary indiscretions, alcohol, and the action of irritant drugs, e.g. aspirin. They are shallow and involve little more than the covering epithelium. Healing is rapid and complete. Slight bleeding is common, and may occasionally be severe.

Acute ulceration of the stomach or duodenum is also seen as a complication of burns and severe trauma, and may be related to vagal overactivity. There are usually multiple ulcers and they usually heal rapidly with minimal scarring, but may occasionally erode a large vessel or perforate into the peritoneal cavity, giving rise to severe haemorrhage or peritonitis. Sometimes, after trauma, there is a generalized oozing of blood from the gastric mucosa. In this way much blood is lost without an obvious localized bleeding point.

### Chronic Peptic Ulcer[3]

Chronic ulcers are usually solitary, and present a characteristic appearance. The destructive process penetrates beneath the mucosa to the underlying muscle layers, and this produces a deep, round or oval, punched-out ulcer with straight edges. For reasons which are not known regeneration of the epithelium is inhibited, and chronic inflammation ensues. Healing of the destroyed stomach or duodenal wall is by granulation tissue, and the base of the ulcer consists of inflamed vascular granulation tissue covered by necrotic tissue which forms a slough. Bleeding is therefore common. Deeper in the base of the ulcer the granulation tissue matures to form scar tissue.

**Clinical Features.** Pain in the epigastrium is common and is related to the gastric acidity and spasm of the muscle. It is usually relieved by meals and especially by the administration of alkalis.

**Complications.** *Haemorrhage*. Repeated bleeding is a common cause of iron-deficiency anaemia (p. 343). Sometimes the ulcer becomes attached to an adjacent structure, e.g. the pancreas, and a large artery is eroded. This leads to a massive haematemesis and melaena.

*Perforation*. When the ulcer penetrates to the peritoneal surface it produces a localized fibrinous inflammation which may cause adjacent structures to become adherent to it. If this does not occur the ulcer may perforate, and the gastric or duodenal contents are poured into the peritoneal cavity. The patient immediately experiences excruciating pain, and generalized peritonitis soon develops.

*Cicatrization.* As an ulcer heals, the scar tissue is apt to contract and cause stenosis. Pyloric ulcers are particularly liable to this complication, and the resulting pyloric stenosis causes severe vomiting. This leads to dehydration and metabolic alkalosis.

**Aetiology.** [4, 5] Remarkably little is known about the cause of peptic ulceration. Without the acid content of the gastric juice peptic ulceration cannot occur, but hypersecretion of acid is not constantly related to ulcer formation. Emotional stress and genetic factors probably play a secondary role.

### Cancer of the Stomach

This tumour is not uncommon in Northern European communities, but its incidence is now lower than that of colonic cancer. It is very common in the Japanese. The tumour is either of the fungating, cauliflower type, or else it appears as a typical malignant ulceration. Occasionally the tumour cells invade the stomach wall so diffusely that no definite mass exists. Instead the whole wall is thickened by dense scirrhous tumour (*diffuse infiltrating carcinoma of the stomach*). Histologically the cancer is usually a poorly-differentiated adenocarcinoma. Even with early excision the prognosis is extremely bad.

## The Small Intestine

### The Malabsorption Syndrome[6, 7]

In the small intestine digestion is completed by the action of the digestive juices which are contributed by the liver and pancreas, and the products are absorbed by the intestinal mucosa into the portal vein or the lymphatics. If these functions are impaired, a state of severe undernutrition results, which is called the *malabsorption syndrome.*

**Causes.** The common causes are:

*Lack of bile salts and digestive enzymes,* e.g. in obstructive jaundice and pancreatic disease.

*Lack of absorptive area,* as following massive intestinal resections.

*Intrinsic disease of the intestine itself.* A good example is *idiopathic steatorrhoea,* in which there is a defect of the mucosa which leads to an impaired absorption of fat and many other substances.

**Effects.** The lack of absorption produces some effects which are similar to those of starvation, e.g. following the dysphagia of oesophageal cancer. Thus there is a loss of weight and generalized body atrophy (p. 236).

Fat absorption is usually severely affected, and much fat, some of it undigested, is passed in the faeces, which are pale and bulky. Excess fat in the stools is termed *steatorrhoea.* There is often poor carbohydrate absorption, and the excess carbohydrate is fermented by bacteria in the bowel. The resulting gas formed leads to frothy, offensive faeces.

In addition to the generalized wasting there are the effects of specific dietary deficiencies—in particular of the vitamin B complex, the fat soluble vitamins A and D, and calcium. Calcium is not absorbed because it is bound by the fatty acids in the bowel. This results in a negative calcium balance with mild hypocalcaemia and a tendency to tetany. A deficiency of vitamin D aggravates matters, and the lesions of osteomalacia may occur. A deficiency of vitamin K leads to a low plasma prothrombin level and a bleeding tendency (p. 361). Dermatitis, peripheral neuropathy, and glossitis may all be found, and have been attributed to vitamin A and B deficiencies. The failure of absorption of iron, vitamin $B_{12}$, and folic acid leads to severe anaemia (Chapter 26). The effects of malabsorption from the small intestine are both widespread and serious, and their occurrence is a reflection of the importance of this part of the digestive tract.

## The Large Intestine

The colon has two main functions: the absorption of water and electrolytes and the formation of a convenient receptacle for faeces, so that they may be discharged at the individual's own convenience. Acute inflammation of the colon results in a derangement of its functions, and the diarrhoea that results causes great inconvenience as well as a considerable loss of water and electrolytes. Two severe infections are recognised:

**Bacillary Dysentery.** This is an acute infection of the colon caused by organisms of the genus *Shigella*. The incubation period is short (24–48 hours), and the disease is characterized by fever, abdominal pain, and diarrhoea which can lead to severe dehydration and death.

**Amoebic Dysentery.** This is caused by a protozoon, *Entamoeba histolytica*, which invades the colonic mucosa and produces shallow ulceration. The disease may be acute with severe bloody diarrhoea, but more usually it is chronic, and the patient has several foul-smelling, sometimes blood-stained stools each day. Occasionally the amoebae invade the blood stream and cause *amoebic hepatitis*; a liver abscess may ensue.

Both types of dysentery are most common in the tropics and in those who live under crowded, unhygienic conditions.

Ulcerative colitis is described on page 128.

**Carcinoma of the Large Intestine.** The large bowel ranks with lung and breast as the most common site of fatal malignant disease in Europeans. The rectum and sigmoid colon are most frequently involved. The tumour is usually a well-differentiated adenocarcinoma, and it breaks down to produce a typical carcinomatous ulcer. This tends to encircle the gut and produce obstruction. The passage of blood and mucus in the stools with constipation alternating with diarrhoea are the usual clinical features. The tumour invades locally, metastasizes to the regional lymph nodes, and finally invades the blood stream to give metastases in the liver and elsewhere. Growth is often relatively slow, so that the prognosis following resection is well correlated with the stage of the tumour[8] (see p. 253).

**Carcinoid Tumours of the Intestine.** These are not common but are of great interest. They occur in the appendix, ileum, colon, and occasionally in the stomach and pancreas. They are derived from the argentaffin cells, and are of intermediate malignancy. Tumours of the appendix tend to remain localized, but the ileal ones sometimes produce metastases in the liver. These lead to the

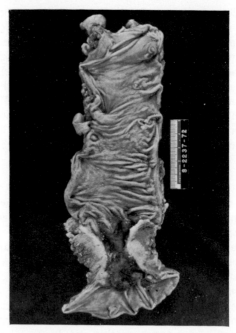

Fig. 30.2. Carcinoma of the colon. The tumour has arisen from the recto-sigmoid junction, and involves the whole circumference of the bowel, producing stenosis. The pericolic fat has been invaded. (*Photograph supplied by Dr. J. B. Cullen.*)

*carcinoid syndrome*—diarrhoea, valvular lesions of the right side of the heart, asthmatic attacks, and periodic flushing of the face. The pathogenesis of this syndrome is not clear, but the release of 5-hydroxytryptamine by the tumour, the activation of the plasma kinins, and the deposition of platelets on the heart valves are all involved.

## Specific Nutritional Deficiencies[9-11]

A detailed description of all the deficiencies which may occur either as a result of inadequate dietary intake or malabsorption is beyond the scope of this book. Deficiencies of vitamins C, D, and K are described elsewhere, and so also are the various factors required for haematopoiesis. Two other vitamin deficiencies will be described, since they produce oral and cutaneous lesions.

### Vitamin A

This fat-soluble vitamin is found together with vitamin D in high concentration in many fish-liver oils. It has two main functions in the human body: it is in part responsible for the maintenance of structure of the mucous membranes, and it plays a vital role in night vision. Since carotene can be converted into vitamin A, this vegetable pigment can replace the vitamin in the diet.

**Effects of Deficiency.** *Night-blindness.* In the retina vitamin A (or carotene) is converted into visual purple (rhodopsin), and utilized by the rods which are responsible for vision in dim light. An early manifestation of vitamin-A deficiency is therefore night-blindness.

*Changes in skin and mucous membranes.* These are mentioned on p. 237. It should be noted that there is no evidence that an excess of this vitamin affords any protection against common virus infections, e.g. the common cold. Indeed, a great excess of the vitamin is harmful, causing neurological and gastrointestinal disturbance.[12] It is for this reason that polar-bear liver is poisonous—a fact well known to Eskimos and Arctic explorers.

### The Vitamin B Group

Many factors are included in this group, and some, if not all, are necessary components of the diet in man. Many of them act as coenzymes in various metabolic processes, and it is not possible to explain the various and specific manifestations which their deficiency occasions. The most important members of the group are vitamin $B_1$, or thiamine, and nicotinic acid.

### Deficiency of Thiamine ($B_1$)

This causes beriberi, which is uncommon in European countries except in association with the malabsorption syndrome. Two forms are recognized.

*Wet beriberi.* This is characterized by high-output cardiac failure and marked peripheral oedema.

*Dry beriberi.* In this condition there is degeneration of the peripheral nerves ("peripheral neuropathy"). Burning pain and loss of sensation in the limbs are characteristic.

### Deficiency of Niacin (Nicotinic Acid)

A deficiency of this vitamin causes *pellagra*, the manifestations of which may be considered under three headings:

*Dermatitis.* A characteristic dusky red dermatitis occurs on the exposed parts, and is aggravated by exposure to sunlight. Oral lesions are a frequent and early manifestation of pellagra. The entire oral mucosa is inflamed (*stomatitis*), and in particular the tongue is swollen, painful, and fiery-red (*glossitis*). The lips are swollen, red, cracked, and painful (*cheilosis*), and this is especially marked at the angles of the mouth (*angular stomatitis*).

*Diarrhoea.* This is common: the stools are watery and offensive.

*Dementia.* Confusion and other manifestations of cerebral dysfunction occur.

### Riboflavine ($B_2$) and Pyridoxine ($B_6$)

A deficiency of these factors has been incriminated as a cause of glossitis, cheilosis, and angular stomatitis in man.

It is evident that there is a considerable overlap in the symptoms caused by deficiencies of members of the vitamin B group. In practice a mixture of them all should be administered if a deficiency of one is suspected.

## General Reading

Bockus, H. L. (1963–65). "Gastroenterology", 2nd ed. in three volumes. Philadelphia: Saunders.

## References

1. Almy, T. P. (1967). In Cecil-Loeb "Textbook of Medicine", 12th ed., ed. by Beeson, P. B. and McDermott, W., p. 838. Philadelphia and London: Saunders.
2. Brooks, F. P. (1966). *Medical Clinics of North America*, **50**, 1447.
3. Illingworth, C. F. W. (1953). "Peptic Ulcer". Edinburgh: Livingstone.
4. Shay, H. (1961). *Amer. J. digest. Dis.*, **6**, 29.
5. Menguy, R. (1964). *Amer. J. digest. Dis.*, **9**, 199.
6. Booth, C. C. (1965). In "Recent Advances in Gastroenterology", ed. by Badenoch, J. and Brooke, B. N., p. 162. London: Churchill.
7. Hourihane, D. O'B. (1966). In "Recent Advances in Pathology", 8th ed., ed. by Harrison, C. V., p. 320. London: Churchill.
8. Dukes, C. E. (1958). In *Cancer*, Vol. 2, p. 136, ed. by R. W. Raven. London: Butterworth.
9. Wohl, M. G. and Goodheart, R. S. (1960). In "Modern Nutrition in Health and Disease", 2nd ed. Philadelphia: Lea and Febiger.
10. Wagner, A. F. and Folkers, K. (1964). "Vitamins and Coenzymes". New York: Interscience Publishers.
11. Spies, T. D. *et al.* (1959). In "Diseases of Metabolism", ed. by Duncan, G. G. Philadelphia: Saunders.
12. Stimson, W. H. (1961). *New Engl. J. Med.*, **265**, 369.

*Chapter 31*

# DISEASES OF THE LIVER

The liver is the largest organ in the body and its functions are manifold. Both anatomically and functionally it occupies a key position in relation to the digestive system, for nearly all the venous blood from the gastrointestinal tract reaches it *via* the *portal vein*. It is therefore not surprising that the liver performs many functions connected with fat, carbohydrate, and protein metabolism. Another activity of the liver is the secretion of bile, which, in addition to having a digestive role, also contains the end-products of haemoglobin metabolism.

## Degenerative Conditions

The liver cells, or *hepatocytes*, are very susceptible to the effects of many poisons. Poisonous mushrooms (*Amanita phalloides*), carbon tetrachloride, chloroform, and many drugs (important among which is the anaesthetic agent halothane) can all cause severe liver damage, either by direct action or by some type of hypersensitivity response. Infections, in particular with the viruses of hepatitis, can also produce liver damage.

The effects of hepatotoxic agents can vary from mild cloudy swelling and fatty change to extensive necrosis.

## Hepatic Necrosis

*Types:* If the liver cells are severely affected, they die and undergo necrosis. This usually has a *zonal distribution*, which means that the cells of a particular zone in every lobule undergo necrosis—*centrilobular necrosis* is the most common (Fig. 31.1 (*b*)). Sometimes the foci of necrosis are erratically distributed; this is termed *focal necrosis*, or spotty necrosis. It is typical of virus hepatitis.

Occasionally the necrosis is more extensive and involves wide tracts of liver. Whole lobules are destroyed, and the name *massive necrosis* is appropriate.

**Results.** The outcome of necrosis depends upon the severity of the lesions: *Zonal and focal necrosis.* The patient may have no symptoms, or suffer from an acute febrile illness with jaundice and gastrointestinal symptoms and then recover. The necrotic liver cells autolyse and are removed. The sinusoidal structure and reticulin framework of the liver lobules remain intact, and as the surviving liver cells divide, the destroyed ones are replaced, and there is complete restoration of the liver to normal (Fig. 31.1 (*a*)).

*Massive necrosis.* The patient may die of liver failure in the acute phase— this is seen after acute poisoning and occasionally in virus hepatitis, but quite often no cause can be found. If the patient survives, the lobular structure of the necrotic liver collapses, and the destroyed areas are replaced by scar

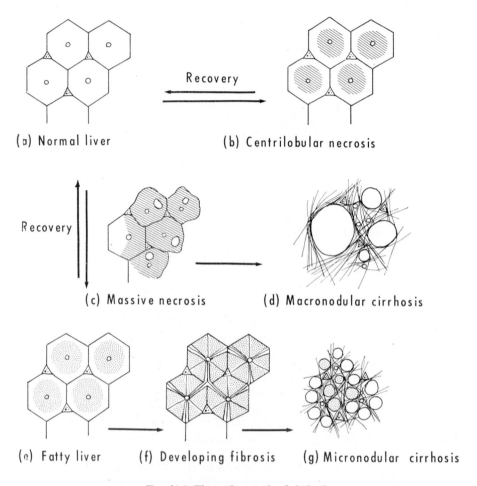

FIG. 31.1. The pathogenesis of cirrhosis

(a) Depicts four normal liver lobules as hexagonal structures each with a central hepatic vein. Between the lobules are the portal triads, each containing branches of the hepatic artery, bile duct, and portal vein. In (b) there is centrilobular necrosis, and when liver cell regeneration occurs there is complete return to normal. (c) Shows massive necrosis with collapse of the affected lobules. When regeneration occurs, a coarsely nodular cirrhotic liver is produced as depicted in (d); in some areas normal lobules will be found. A fatty liver (e) may return to normal. However, if it persists over a long period, fibrous septa form and these divide up the lobules (f). Some liver cells degenerate, and as regeneration occurs a finely nodular cirrhotic liver develops (g). No normal lobules remain.

(*Drawn by Margot Mackay, Department of Art as Applied to Medicine, University of Toronto.*)

tissue. Isolated groups of liver cells show regeneration, but since there is no normal scaffold on which they may disperse, they form irregular nodules called *regeneration nodules*. The final result is a form of *cirrhosis of the liver* (Fig. 31.1 (*c* and *d*)).

### Hepatocellular Degeneration and Fatty Change

The changes are described in detail in Chapter 4. Cloudy swelling, hydropic degeneration, and fatty change may all result from the effects of poisons, hypoxia, or infection. Fatty change is the most important lesion, and is often caused by an inadequate diet. It is also common in *chronic alcoholism*.

If the cause of the fatty liver is removed, complete recovery is usual—not so if the condition is allowed to persist indefinitely. Gradually fibrous tissue forms, and hepatic cells become isolated as the lobules are split up (Fig. 31.1 (*f*)). Some cells undergo necrosis, others regenerate, and there results a finely nodular cirrhotic liver not fundamentally different from that seen after massive necrosis (Fig. 31.1 (*g*)).

### Cirrhosis of the Liver

The term cirrhosis was introduced by Laennec who was impressed by the tawny colour of the liver in this condition, but this is due merely to fatty change of the liver cells. The essential feature is diffuse destruction of the parenchyma and its replacement by fibrous tissue which disrupts the normal lobular architecture of the liver. There is also active regeneration of liver cells occurring at the same time as this fibrous reparative process (Fig. 31.2).

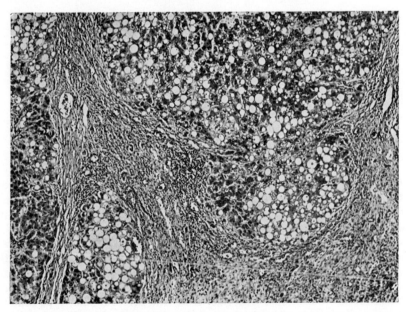

FIG. 31.2. Cirrhosis of the liver. A thick strand of fibrous tissue intersects two nodules, the cells of which show severe fatty change. × 50.

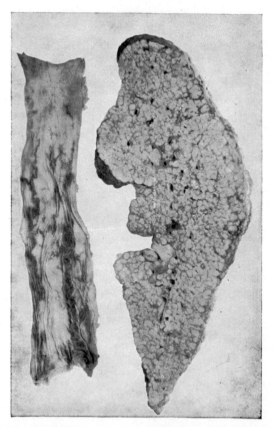

FIG. 31.3. Cirrhosis of the liver. This section of liver shows pale nodules of
regenerating parenchyma, interspersed among which there are bands of
dense scar tissue.
The lower end of the oesophagus has been included—it is opened to show a
length of dilated, tortuous submucosal veins. The patient died of haematemesis consequent on the rupture of one of them.

(EA27.1. *Reproduced by permission of the President and Council of the Royal College
of Surgeons of England.*)

Cirrhosis is best regarded as an *end-stage condition*, as it can be the end-
result of liver damage due to many causes—poisons, alcohol, inadequate diet,
infection, genetic error, etc. Classifications are very unsatisfactory since in
most cases the cause is unknown. A descriptive classification is the most useful
and is based on the liver's nodularity. If the nodules are small and of uniform
size (Fig. 31.3) the term *micronodular cirrhosis* is applied. This contrasts with
*macronodular cirrhosis* (Fig. 31.1 d), in which the nodules are of varying size
and many of them are large. Micronodular cirrhosis may be idiopathic, but
is often found in alcoholics with fatty liver; the macronodular type follows
massive necrosis. It must be emphasized that there is no sharp line of division
between these two types of cirrhosis.

Cirrhosis is a serious condition, and the patient is in constant danger of developing complications which may be fatal.

## Complications of Cirrhosis

**Hepatocellular Failure.** This is described later.

**Porto-Systemic Shunt.** During the development of cirrhosis many branches of the portal and hepatic veins are obliterated. The pressure in the portal radicles rises (*portal hypertension*), and blood from the portal vein is shunted into the systemic veins following the development of anastomoses. This has two serious effects:

*Haemorrhage.* An important group of anastomoses develops at the lower end of the oesophagus. The veins are thin-walled and tend to bleed. Sudden, massive, and often fatal haemorrhage is the result. The blood is usually vomited up (*haematemesis*).

*Intoxication.* Products from the intestine by-pass the liver and reach the remainder of the body. This leads to a *faecal odour* of the breath, and is thought to be the cause of the confused mental state and *coma* which patients dying of cirrhosis often develop.

**Ascites.** Fluid in the peritoneal cavity is common in cirrhosis, and is in part due to the portal hypertension. In addition, the destruction of hepatic venules leads to a greatly increased formation of lymph in the liver. Some of this is drained away by the lymphatics, but these appear to be inadequate and the excess lymph exudes from the liver surface into the peritoneal cavity. Hypoalbuminaemia and hyperaldosteronism are other factors in the pathogenesis of ascites and the generalized oedema which sometimes develops.

## Virus Hepatitis

Two distinct types are known:

**Infective Hepatitis.** Infective hepatitis, due to Virus A, commonly occurs in institutions like schools and military camps. It is contracted following the ingestion of contaminated food, and has an incubation period of about *one month*. The virus causes a patchy focal necrosis from which complete recovery is usual, but occasionally there is massive necrosis which may be fatal. The infective agent persists in the blood and in the faeces for many months. Such *convalescent carriers* do not usually have HAA (p. 428) in their blood, but may transmit the infection by donating blood or by contaminating food.

**Serum Hepatitis.** This infection is caused by Virus B which is present in the blood of carriers for long periods. The usual means of transmission is by the injection of contaminated serum. Minute quantities only are necessary; unless instruments are sterilized between patients, there is a very real danger that the virus will be transmitted from one person to another. Drug addicts who use the intravenous route ("main-liners") are common victims, and it has been described following tattooing. The tattooist often tries the needle on himself, and may not sterilize it between customers. Blood transfusion is the greatest hazard (see p. 363). Serum hepatitis has a very long incubation period, about *three months*, and the source of infection may be forgotten and difficult to trace. The disease resembles infective hepatitis very closely, but tends to be more severe, permanent liver damage may be incurred, and death from massive necrosis is commoner than with the short-incubation virus A hepatitis. Prophylactic passive immunization with $\gamma$-globulin is useful against infective hepatitis, but is of little avail against serum hepatitis. There appears to be no cross-immunity between the two viruses.

Summarizing the differences between the two viruses, it is apparent that virus A is generally transmitted by the ingestion of faecal material and is sometimes responsible for epidemics of hepatitis. It is occasionally transmitted by blood transfusion and it produces a sharper, brisker, less dangerous type of disease in a younger age group than Virus B. Virus B, on the other hand, is commonly transmitted by the parenteral administration of blood or blood products, but it is probable that it too can be transmitted by the oral route and be responsible for some sporadic cases of hepatitis.

Neither Virus A nor Virus B has been grown or isolated for certainty, but the presence of Virus B in the blood can now be detected with some assurance. Symptomless carriers of the virus as well as patients suffering from serum hepatitis have an antigen present in the blood which by chance was first discovered in the blood of an Australian aborigine, and therefore called *Australia antigen*. It is also called *hepatitis associated antigen (HAA)* or *hepatitis B antigen (HB ag)*. Electron microscopy has revealed that the antigen consists of several characteristic particles. These may be virus components but do not seem to be complete virus, and the relationship between the HAA and the infective agent of serum hepatitis remains to be clarified.

Nevertheless about 50 per cent of individuals who receive HAA-positive blood develop hepatitis, and it is now routine practice to screen all blood donors for HAA. Very small quantities of blood are capable of transmitting the disease, and it is therefore mandatory that all needles, instruments, and other equipment which has come into contact with one patient's blood should either be discarded or else adequately sterilized before use on another patient. This is of particular importance to the dentist, since his instruments, needles, scalpels, dental forceps, etc., often enter the gingival tissues and become contaminated. If the patient is a known HAA-carrier, the danger is obvious and the operator himself is at risk should he inadvertently injure himself with an instrument. Outbreaks of hepatitis are notorious in some units whose work entails the use of blood (e.g. in haemodialysis units).

## Bile Formation and Jaundice

Of all the symptoms of liver disease, *jaundice*, or *icterus*, is the most immediately apparent. Nearly all the tissues in the body are coloured a bright yellow. In addition to the skin, the conjunctivae and oral mucous membrane are discoloured, and in the early stages jaundice is sometimes most apparent in these sites, especially in dark-skinned individuals. Jaundice is due to an excessive amount of bilirubin in the plasma and tissues. Its development can be understood only in relation to bilirubin metabolism.

**Bilirubin Metabolism.** When red cells are broken down, the porphyrin moiety of the haemoglobin is converted into *bilirubin* in the cells of the reticulo-endothelial system. Bilirubin is insoluble in water, and following its release from the RE cells it is carried in the blood stream attached to albumin. The liver has three important functions in regard to bilirubin:

It *extracts* it from the blood.

It *conjugates* it with glucuronic acid to form bilirubin diglucuronide.

It *excretes* the conjugated bilirubin into the bile.

Under normal conditions 15–20 per cent of the bilirubin excreted is derived from sources other than red-cell destruction. Some of this originates from the bone marrow during the formation of haemoglobin (*ineffective erythropoiesis.*) The amount formed in this way may be increased in disease, for example pernicious anaemia, and contribute to the jaundice.

## Types of Jaundice

**Obstructive Jaundice.** This occurs when there is an obstruction to the passage of conjugated bilirubin from the liver cells to the intestine. The bilirubin diglucuronide is absorbed back into the blood, and if the obstruction is complete the patient rapidly becomes deeply jaundiced. The conjugated bilirubin is soluble in water, and is easily excreted by the kidneys. Therefore the *urine is dark*, and this contrasts with the *faeces which are clay coloured*. Two major types of obstructive jaundice may be recognized. In one (*extrahepatic cholestasis*) the bile duct is blocked, for instance by a gall-stone in its lumen or by a carcinoma of the head of the pancreas. In the second type the obstruction is assumed to be in the liver itself (*intrahepatic cholestasis*). One important cause of this is the administration of certain drugs, for example chlorpromazine (Largactil) and other phenothiazine derivatives.

**Haemolytic Jaundice.** This is the second type of jaundice to be considered. The excessive destruction of red cells causes an increased rate of bilirubin formation, and the liver is unable to deal with the increased load. The bilirubin in the blood is unconjugated, and is therefore insoluble in water and not excreted in the urine. This type of jaundice is said to be *acholuric*. The faeces contain an excess of bilirubin. Haemolytic jaundice rarely reaches the intensity of the obstructive variety.

**Hepatocellular Jaundice.** This is considered below.

## Hepatocellular Failure

It is convenient to complete this survey of liver disease by summarizing the important features of liver-cell failure. It is often called *cholaemia*, and may occur as a terminal event in many forms of liver disease. Thus it is seen in necrosis, cirrhosis, and occasionally when the organ is involved by tumour.

## Manifestations of Liver-Cell Damage

**Jaundice.** This is due partly to a failure of the liver to take up bilirubin from the blood, and partly to its failure to excrete conjugated bilirubin. This hepatocellular variety of jaundice is therefore of mixed type.

**Neuropsychiatric Manifestations.** These include abnormalities in behaviour, a "flapping" tremor of the arms, confusion, convulsions, and coma.

**Bleeding Tendency.** The liver manufactures most of the plasma clotting factors, e.g. fibrinogen and prothrombin. In liver disease an abnormal bleeding tendency is not uncommon. Surgery, even dental extraction, should be attempted with caution.

**Hypoalbuminaemia.** The liver also manufactures albumin, and it is not surprising that the blood level falls in many chronic liver diseases. Hypoalbuminaemia contributes to the formation of ascites and generalized oedema.

**Failure of Detoxification.** Many drugs, e.g. morphine and barbiturates, are detoxified or excreted by the liver. In patients with liver failure a normal dose of such a drug may precipitate coma and death.

**Fever.** Pyrexia is not uncommon, but its cause is not known.

In the terminal stages, severe electrolyte imbalance occurs. The patient sinks into a state of cholaemic coma with deepening jaundice, and the end is precipitated by renal, cardiac, or peripheral circulatory failure.

## Tumours of the Liver

*Benign tumours* are rare and unimportant. *Primary carcinoma* is an occasional complication of cirrhosis, and is therefore quite common in those countries where this disease is rife. Metastatic deposits of tumour are extremely common in the liver in cases of disseminated malignant disease. The common sites for the primary carcinoma are the breast, lung, and gastrointestinal tract.

A raised level of *alkaline phosphatase* in the serum is characteristic of metastatic tumour and is a useful clinical test. Each nodule of tumour obstructs a number of small bile ducts, and the test is positive before there is significant retention of bilirubin. Jaundice is not common in tumours of the liver unless it is associated with cirrhosis or it occurs as a terminal event. This emphasizes the tremendous reserve capacity of the liver and its ability to regenerate (see also p. 117).

## General Reading

ARIAS, I. M. (1960). *Medical Clinics of North America*, **44**, 601. An account of the metabolism of bilirubin.

FERRIS, A. A. (1972). *Brit. med. Bull.*, **28**, 131. An account of Australian antigen.

POPPER, H. and SCHAFFNER, F. (1957). "Liver: Structure and Function". New York: McGraw-Hill.

POPPER, H. and SCHAFFNER, F. (1961–1972). "Progress in Liver Disease", vols. 1–4, New York and London: Grune and Stratton. These books provide a very complete and detailed account of liver disease.

ROUILLER, C. (1963–64). "The Liver", in two volumes. London and New York: Academic Press. Reference books covering many aspects of liver disease and experimental work.

SCHIFF, L. (1963). Edr. "Diseases of the Liver", 2nd ed. Philadelphia: Lipincott.

SHERLOCK, S. (1968). "Diseases of the Liver and Biliary System", 4th ed., 809 pp. Oxford: Blackwell. A very readable account of liver disease with a strong clinical bias.

THOMPSON, R. P. H. (1970). *Brit. med. J.*, **1**, 223. Physiology of bilirubin in relation to jaundice.

*Chapter 32*

# DISEASES OF THE KIDNEY

## The Function of the Kidneys

The kidneys are essential for life because of the part they play in the excretion of waste products and in the regulation of the extracellular fluid. They control the concentration of its various electrolytes, contribute to acid-base balance, and are intimately concerned in the regulation of water balance. These functions depend on the secretion of urine, which entails two distinct processes:

(*a*) the passive filtration of plasma through the glomeruli, so that the escaping fluid is similar to plasma except that it is virtually free of protein.

(*b*) the passage of this filtrate through a complex system of tubules, where its content of solutes is altered and·its pH is modified. The resulting fluid is urine.

The glomerulus and its tubule together constitute the *nephron*, and this opens into a large collecting tubule which empties into a calyx of the renal pelvis. From here the urine passes down the ureter to the bladder, where it is held until it can be voided by micturition.

Many alterations take place in the composition of the glomerular filtrate as it passes through the tubules:

There is reabsorption of all the glucose, about 80 per cent of the water, and many electrolytes from the *proximal convoluted tubule*.

There is an active secretion of hydrogen and potassium ions by the *distal convoluted tubule*, and this is balanced by a reabsorption of sodium, chloride, and bicarbonate ions.

There is reabsorption of more water in the *distal convoluted tubules and the collecting tubules*—this function is under the control of the pituitary antidiuretic hormone, which makes the tubular cells more permeable to water exchange, while sodium reabsorption from the *distal tubule* is controlled by aldosterone.

## Renal Failure: Uraemia

Renal failure is a state in which the body's metabolism is deranged as the result of dysfunction of the kidneys. Renal insufficiency usually first manifests itself in a disturbance of urine formation and this is followed by various systemic effects which culminate in a clinical syndrome described as *uraemia*. The most conspicuous biochemical feature of uraemia is the retention of nitrogenous substances in the blood. An indication of the extent of dysfunction may be obtained by measuring the blood urea level (normally 15–35 mg. per 100 ml., or 10–20 mg. per 100 ml. if expressed as blood urea nitrogen, BUN). The blood creatinine level rises similarly.

**Clinical Features of Uraemia.** Since the diagnosis of uraemia is largely clinical, it is convenient to describe its main features at this stage:

(*a*) cerebral symptoms, e.g. drowsiness, headache, convulsions, and coma. These are possibly due to disturbances of fluid balance and the retention of ill-defined waste products.

(*b*) deep, sighing respirations, which are due to metabolic acidosis.

(*c*) muscular twitchings, and occasionally muscular spasms, due probably to hypocalcaemia.

(*d*) nausea, vomiting, and diarrhoea. These are possibly due to the excretion of urea into the stomach and intestine, where it is converted into ammonia by the urease secreted by local organisms.

(*e*) hiccup, gastrointestinal bleeding, pruritus (itching of the skin), purpura, and acute fibrinous pericarditis.

Although many of the features of uraemia are unexplained at the present time, it seems certain that electrolyte imbalance and failure in acid-base regulation are more important than is the retention of nitrogenous substances.

Renal insufficiency may either appear acutely, or else develop gradually as a terminal feature of chronic destructive renal disease. These two types will be considered separately.

**Acute Renal Failure.** This manifests itself by a sudden diminution in the urinary output (*oliguria*), and this may be followed by complete cessation (*anuria*). This must not be confused with sudden failure to pass urine due to an obstruction, an event which commonly affects men with prostatic enlargement and is called *retention of urine*.

The condition is a common clinical emergency, and is usually due to *sudden renal ischaemia due to vasoconstriction*. This occurs:

(*a*) whenever there is a sudden decrease in blood volume such as may follow severe haemorrhage, burns, and persistent vomiting or diarrhoea.

(*b*) following the escape of free haemoglobin or myoglobin into the circulation, as after incompatible blood transfusions and crushing injuries to the muscles of the limbs.

(*c*) following certain complications of pregnancy.

If the cause is remedied in time, the change may be reversed without any structural damage to the nephron, but if it persists, necrosis of parts of the tubules follows (*acute tubular necrosis*). This may lead to death, and even if the patient survives it may take many months for renal function to be completely restored.

The manifestations of acute renal failure are severe oliguria—complete anuria occurs in the worst cases—associated with the retention of nitrogenous substances, potassium, phosphate, and other anions in the blood. The pH of the blood falls due to the failure of tubular secretion of hydrogen ions (*metabolic acidosis*), and there is an increase in the volume of extracellular water. The patient may die of overhydration, potassium intoxication, infection, or the retention of unclassified toxic metabolic products.

If he survives, there follows a period when large quantities of urine are passed (*polyuria*), because the kidneys cannot conserve electrolytes and water. Life is then in jeopardy because of dehydration and electrolyte loss. Regeneration of tubular epithelium occurs quite rapidly, but a perfect functional recovery is unusual.

**Chronic Renal Failure.** This too is common in clinical practice, and is usually due to *chronic destructive renal diseases* like chronic pyelonephritis, glomerulonephritis, and bilateral renal tuberculosis. *Vascular disease*, e.g. malignant hypertension, is another cause, and so is *obstruction to the outflow of urine*, as follows prostatic enlargement, urethral stricture, and cancer of the pelvic organs. *Hypercalcaemia* (p. 447) and *diabetes mellitus* (p. 477) also lead to kidney damage and chronic renal failure.

The manifestations of chronic renal failure are complex and diverse. There is usually moderate dehydration, as the diseased kidneys cannot conserve water and sodium properly. Potassium is usually retained, and a metabolic acidosis develops. Phosphate retention is a prominent feature, and it may, if long-standing, lead to a reciprocal lowering of the plasma calcium level and secondary hyperparathyroidism.

Many chronic renal diseases are complicated by *hypertension*. A fall in renal pulse pressure stimulates renin formation (p. 365), but it is uncertain whether this is the means whereby hypertension occurs in renal disease.

Another feature of chronic renal failure is intractable *anaemia*. The kidneys secrete erythropoietin (p. 342), and it may be that the production of this hormone is impaired in chronic renal disease. Both acute and chronic renal failure, if unrelieved, culminate in *uraemia* which is the harbinger of death.

### The Protein-Losing Kidney

Normally only a trace of protein escapes into the glomerular filtrate, and this is reabsorbed by the proximal tubule. There are a number of conditions in which the permeability of the glomerulus is increased, so that large amounts of protein escape into the filtrate and are voided with the urine. Albumin, the smallest of the plasma proteins, is affected the most severely, and hypoalbuminaemia results. The occurrence of proteinuria, hypoalbuminaemia, and oedema is called the *nephrotic syndrome*, and it may be a complication of such chronic diseases as glomerulonephritis, diabetes mellitus, renal amyloidosis, and systemic lupus erythematosus. It may also occur in *nephrosis* as a primary lesion of the glomerulus. Several entities are recognized. In some types, particularly the nephrosis of children, the glomeruli appear normal by light microscopy but abnormalities can be detected electronmicroscopically. In other types, the basement-membrane zone is seen by light microscopy to be thickened, a change which is described as "membranous". The disease is alternatively known as idiopathic membranous glomerulonephritis.

The main features of the nephrotic syndrome are:

(*a*) severe proteinuria

(*b*) hypoproteinaemia, especially affecting the albumin level of the plasma.

(*c*) generalized oedema due in part to the hypoproteinaemia and perhaps also to hyperaldosteronism.

(*d*) susceptibility to infection, due possibly to a loss of immunoglobulins in the urine.

(e) a raised level of lipids in the blood. The blood cholesterol (normally about 250 mg. per 100 ml.) may exceed 1 000 mg. per 100 ml. The cause of this is unknown.

In the early stages renal function is well maintained and the blood pressure is normal, but later renal failure and uraemia may occur.

### Glomerulonephritis

*Acute glomerulonephritis* (*Bright's disease*) usually occurs in childhood and adolescence. It often develops about ten days after a *Strept. pyogenes* tonsillitis or pharyngitis, and can also follow three weeks or more after streptococcal impetigo. Acute glomerulonephritis is more prone to follow

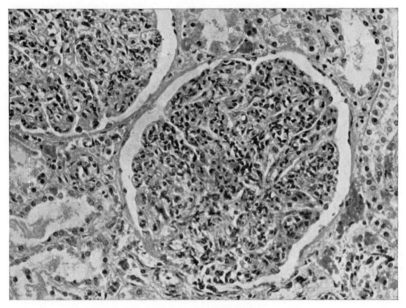

FIG. 32.1. Acute glomerulonephritis. The glomerulus is greatly enlarged, and is hypercellular. The tuft is virtually bloodless due to occlusion of the vascular lumina. × 220.

infection with certain strains of *Strept. pyogenes*, particularly type 12. The pathogenesis is not completely understood, but it appears that streptococcal antigen stimulates the production of specific antibodies and that antigen-antibody complexes are deposited in the glomeruli. These activate the complement system, and this leads to local damage. In the early stages the glomeruli are enlarged, and appear hypercellular due to an infiltration of polymorphs and a proliferation of the glomerular cells (Fig. 32.1). The capillary channels are narrowed, and the reduced flow through the glomeruli is responsible for the oliguria.

Most patients with acute nephritis recover and experience no further renal trouble. However, in a small percentage of cases death occurs in the acute stage from acute renal failure. In other cases there is progression of the disease, and this causes death either within about one year (*rapidly progressive glomerulonephritis*) or after many years (*chronic glomerulonephritis*). In the latter event most of the glomeruli are converted into hyaline masses, the tubules undergo atrophy, and there is fibrous replacement of the renal parenchyma.

Clinically the acute phase is accompanied by oliguria. The urine has a smoky appearance due to the presence of many red cells. Facial oedema is another usual feature. There is moderate hypertension which may lead to heart failure.

Chronic glomerulonephritis may be silent for a long time, apart from moderate proteinuria, but eventually the manifestations of chronic renal failure and uraemia develop. Hypertension and heart failure are common. Some cases develop a nephrotic syndrome.

## Pyogenic Infections of the Kidney

**Acute Pyelonephritis.** Bacterial infection of the kidney is very common. The infecting organisms are usually the Gram-negative intestinal bacilli, including *Ps. pyocyanea* and *Proteus* species. Two routes of infection have been described:

*Haematogenous.* It is believed that most infection is blood-borne from the colon. In healthy individuals the few organisms that escape through the glomerular filter are voided expeditiously in the urine, but if there is obstruction to the outflow of urine, the organisms flourish and set up *acute pyelonephritis*. This is manifested by numerous small cortical abscesses and a streaking of the congested medulla due to pus cells in the tubules. The renal pelvis is also acutely inflamed.

*Ascending infection.* There is a rival hypothesis that infection spreads upwards from the bladder, because in practice the renal lesion is often preceded by acute cystitis. An "ascending infection" following the reflux of urine up the ureters is a possibility, for it is known that such reflux can occur. Nevertheless, even in these cases the renal infection could be blood-borne following a bacteraemia associated with the acute cystitis, perhaps aggravated by catheterization.

It is evident that obstruction to the urinary flow is the most important factor predisposing towards infection. This obstruction may be ureteric or urethral. Ureteric obstruction may be due to stones or a congenital anomaly (Fig. 32.2). The ureter proximal to the obstruction dilates (*hydroureter*), and the pressure of urine is transmitted back to the renal pelvis, which also undergoes dilatation (*hydronephrosis*). If this persists, the kidney itself undergoes progressive atrophy. The hydronephrotic kidney is liable to infection, which may convert it into a pus-filled sac, or *pyonephrosis*.

Urethral obstruction leads to a bilateral hydroureter and hydronephrosis. Prostatic enlargement (p. 232) is a common and most important example, for it causes chronic, partial obstruction of the urethra and this leads to dilatation of the bladder with muscular hypertrophy of its walls, hydroureter, and hydronephrosis with steady destruction of renal parenchyma. It predisposes to infection, and even a mild prostatitis precipitates an attack of acute

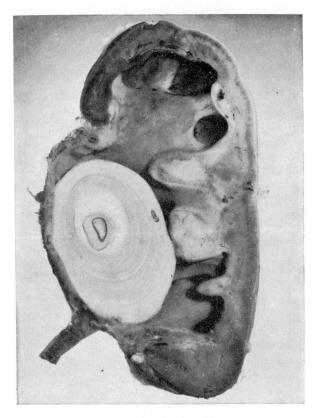

FIG. 32.2. Hydronephrotic kidney. The pelvis is greatly dilated, and it contains a
large calculus which has been sectioned to reveal its laminated structure. The
kidney substance has been severely destroyed.

(U25.3. *Reproduced by permission of the President and Council of the Royal
College of Surgeons of England.*)

obstruction, an emergency which occasions much apprehension and pain
as well as jeopardizing renal function even more.

**Chronic Pyelonephritis.** In many cases of acute urinary infection, there is
recurrence or the development of chronicity. This is *chronic pyelonephritis,*
the commonest cause of chronic renal failure. Its pathogenesis is uncertain,
for there is often no obvious obstruction to or stasis in the urinary passages.
It may be that intrinsic renal lesions, especially the scars of previous infections,
are the predisposing factors for smouldering infection. There is a gradual
destruction of the renal parenchyma, which is heavily infiltrated by lymphocytes, plasma cells, macrophages, and variable numbers of pus cells. The
glomeruli are gradually converted into hyaline masses, the tubules undergo
atrophy and obliteration, and the parenchyma is replaced by fibrous tissue
(Fig. 32.3). At first, the process occurs in wedge-shaped subcapsular foci, but
eventually it becomes diffuse. Surviving tubules undergo dilatation, and are

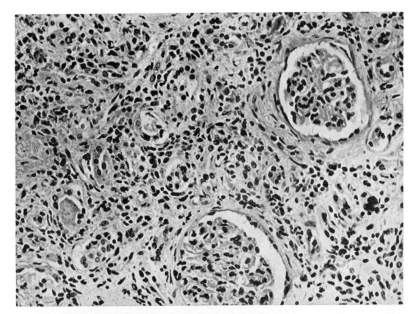

FIG. 32.3. Chronic pyelonephritis. Most of the parenchyma of the kidney has been replaced by fibrous tissue heavily infiltrated with small round cells. A few atrophied tubules can still be recognized, and two glomeruli, one showing early periglomerular fibrosis, are included in the section. × 220.

often filled with eosinophilic protein material which gives them a thyroid-like appearance. Hypertensive vascular changes are often severe. Ultimately the kidney resembles that found in chronic glomerulonephritis. Indeed, the end stages of many renal diseases are barely distinguishable from one another.

Acute pyelonephritis is accompanied by fever and rigors, and the urine is full of polymorphs. As the infection becomes chronic, the symptoms subside and the urine contains fewer pus cells and organisms. Later on chronic renal failure and hypertension develop.

### Tumours of the Kidney

**Adenoma.** The common benign renal tumour is the *adenoma*. It usually appears as a pin's-head-sized, white or yellow nodule situated just beneath the capsule. Its cells are usually arranged in a papillary cystadenomatous pattern, and they sometimes have a clear cytoplasm, thereby closely resembling those of the carcinoma.

**Carcinoma of the Kidney.** This is the malignant counterpart of the adenoma. It presents at a pole of the kidney as a large encephaloid mass, which on section has a variegated appearance: areas of orange are interspersed amid white stroma and red foci of haemorrhage (Fig. 32.4). Microscopically it consists of large spheroidal cells with a clear cytoplasm. These are arranged

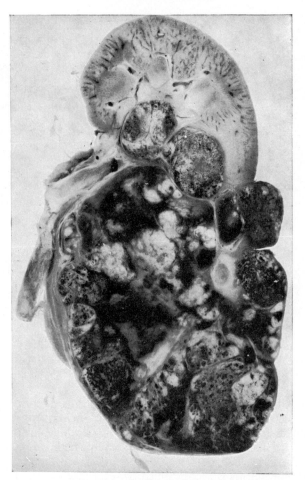

FIG. 32.4. Carcinoma of the kidney. The lower pole has been replaced by a large
encephaloid tumour which is infiltrating into the upper pole and compressing
the ureter. Note the variegated appearance of the tumour.

(EU30.1. *Reproduced by permission of the President and Council of the Royal
College of Surgeons of England.*)

in tubular acini in very well-differentiated tumours (Fig. 32.5). These cells
resemble those of the adrenal cortex, and it was once believed that the tumour
arose from ectopic adrenal rests situated on the surface of the kidney. This
belief was the origin of the name *hypernephroma*, which is still widely used in
connexion with the tumour. It arises in fact from the renal tubular epithelium,
and all grades of transition can be found between it and the tubular adenoma.
The clear appearance of the cells is due to their high content of lipid and
glycogen, both of which tend to be lost during histological processing. The
carotenoids dissolved in the lipid give rise to the orange colour of the
tumour. The best name for this tumour is *clear-cell carcinoma of the kidney.*

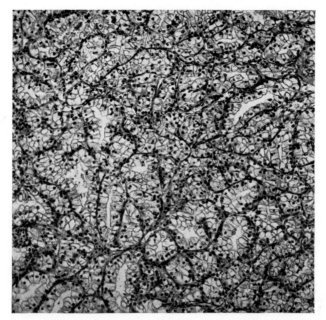

FIG. 32.5. Clear-cell carcinoma of the kidney. It consists of round and polygonal cells with copious clear cytoplasm. This example is quite well differentiated, for many of the cell groups are arranged in acini. × 130.

Clinically carcinoma of the kidney is often silent for a long time. Haematuria and an abdominal mass are two common presenting features. Distant lymphatic and blood-borne metastases are common, the liver, lungs, and bones being especially vulnerable. Indeed, a skeletal metastasis is sometimes the first indication of the tumour.

Another interesting feature is the phenomenon of dormancy (p. 253)—bony deposits may suddenly erupt many years after the successful removal of the affected kidney.

The other important renal tumour is the *nephroblastoma*, or *Wilms's tumour*, an embryonic tumour of infancy discussed in Chapter 20.

### General Reading

BLACK, D. A. K. (1967). "Renal Disease", 2nd ed. Oxford: Blackwell.
DE WARDENER, H. E. (1967). "The Kidney", 3rd ed. London: Churchill.
HEPTINSTALL, R. H. (1966). "Pathology of the Kidney". London: Churchill. This book is devoted largely to the morphological aspects of renal disease.
MERRILL, J. P. and HAMPERS, C. L. (1971). "Uremia", 115 pp., New York and London: Grune and Stratton.

*Chapter 33*

# DISEASES OF BONE AND JOINTS

**Introduction.** In early embryonic life condensations of mesenchyme are laid down at the sites of future bone formation, and by the end of the second month ossification commences. In the development of some bones, notably the cranium and the clavicle, there is a direct conversion of the membranous sheet of mesenchyme to bone. Bones formed in this way are called *membrane bones*. The base of the skull and the long bones develop in a different way: in these the mesenchyme differentiates into cartilage which is subsequently *replaced* by bone. The cartilage cells swell up and die, and the intervening matrix then calcifies. This *calcified cartilage* is eroded by osteoclasts, and at the same time osteoblasts lay down lamellar bone (see below); the process continues at the epiphyseal ends of long bones until adult stature is reached. This type of bone formation is called *endochondral ossification*. Some bones, for example the mandible, are formed by a mixture of the two processes of ossification.

## Structure of Bone[1-5]

Bone is composed of calcified osteoid tissue; the latter consists of collagen fibres embedded in a mucoprotein matrix (osseomucin). It is the special composition of this ground substance which imparts to bone its characteristic properties, and it is here that the bone salts are deposited. The exact composition of these salts is not known, but they are generally considered to have a hydroxyapatite structure.

Depending upon the arrangement of the collagen fibres, two histological types of bone may be recognized.

**Woven, Immature, Fibrillary, or Non-Lamellar Bone.** This shows irregularity in the arrangement of the collagen bundles and in the distribution of the osteocytes. The osseomucin is usually basophilic, and is less abundant than in mature bone. It also contains less calcium.

*Formation.* Woven bone is formed wherever ossification occurs primarily in loose connective tissue. This occurs in three situations:

    (*a*) During the formation of membrane bones.

    (*b*) When bone forms in the midst of the differentiating granulation tissue of a healing fracture.

    (*c*) In certain bone disorders and in osteogenic tumours.

**Lamellar or Mature Bone.** In this type of bone the collagen bundles are arranged in parallel sheets either in the form of concentric Haversian systems or flat plates.

In the outer dense *cortex* of a long bone Haversian systems predominate, while flat plates are seen under the periosteum and endosteum. This type of bone is called *compact bone*.

The central portion of long bones is hollowed out to form the medullary cavity, which contains marrow. Only a few spicules of bone remain. These are constructed of flat bundles of collagen, although in the wider trabeculae Haversian systems may be found. The central trabeculated part of the bone is called *cancellous*, and it should be noted that, like "compact" bone, this is a term related to the gross appearance.

*Formation.* Lamellar bone is formed when bone is laid down on a previously calcified structure. This may be:

(*a*) calcified cartilage, as in normal endochondral ossification and in replacement of the cartilage which forms during the healing of a fracture;

(*b*) woven bone, as during the early growth of membrane bones;

(*c*) lamellar bone itself, as during the circumferential growth of all bones.

In the normal adult the entire skeleton is composed of lamellar bone.

## Metabolic Functions of Bone: Calcium Metabolism[6–8]

Bone serves as a store for calcium and phosphorus, containing 99 per cent of the total body calcium (about 1 Kg.) and 90 per cent of the total body phosphorus. The remaining 1 per cent of the calcium is a vital part, for it is available to the soft tissues and is necessary for neuromuscular activity, cardiac rhythm and enzyme activity.

Calcium in the blood exists in three forms:

*Ionized calcium*, which is diffusible and constitutes 65 per cent of the total plasma calcium.

*Protein-bound calcium*, which is non-diffusible, being attached to albumin.

*Non-ionized, diffusible calcium*, which exists for the most part as citrate, and constitutes the smallest fraction.

The *ionized calcium* is the most important fraction. It is in equilibrium with the calcium salts in bone, and its level is regulated by the hormone of the parathyroid glands (*parathormone*) and possibly also by *calcitonin*, a hormone secreted in man by the parafollicular, or C, cells of the thyroid gland. Vitamin D may also play a minor role. In clinical practice it is the total serum calcium that is usually measured, and if the level of the plasma proteins is unaltered this gives a reliable guide to the level of the ionized fraction. The normal serum calcium is 9·2–10·4 mg. per ml., and is remarkably constant in health due to the efficiency of the regulating mechanisms.

Phosphorus occurs in the blood as an inorganic phosphate, and its level is 2–4 mg. per 100 ml. The range is slightly higher in children, 3–5 mg. per 100 ml.

The serum calcium and phosphate together maintain a reciprocal relationship. Thus, if there is a rise in serum level of one, there is a fall in that of the other. However, if the level of one is low, the other does not necessarily rise.

Alkaline phosphatase is manufactured by osteoblasts, but the precise role of this enzyme in bone formation is not understood. Nevertheless, since some of the enzyme escapes into the blood, the serum level is a good index of the over-all osteoblastic activity within the body. The measurement of the alkaline phosphatase level in the blood is therefore a useful aid in the diagnosis of generalized bone disorders.* The level is normally 1·5–5 units (Bodansky), or 3–13 units (King-Armstrong), in adults and slightly higher in children.*

Although bone appears rigid and inert, it is as susceptible as the soft tissues to adverse circumstances and deleterious agents; indeed, the effects on bone are often more severe and permanent.

There is a continuous process of remodelling throughout life with bone resorption by *osteoclasts* and bone deposition by *osteoblasts*, each keeping pace with the other. If either predominates osteoporosis or osteosclerosis results. *Osteoporosis* is a condition in which osteoid matrix, although reduced in amount, is normally mineralized. The bony trabeculae are greatly thinned, and the bone as a whole is weakened and liable to fracture. The radiographic appearance is therefore one of rarefaction.

Osteoporosis may be brought about by either excessive destruction of bone or defective formation, and may occur in a number of conditions in a localized or generalized form (pp. 450 and 448).

In *osteosclerosis* there is excessive formation of osteoid, which being calcified, makes the bones appear dense on a radiograph.

### Classification of Generalized Bone Disorders

There is no very satisfactory classification of generalized bone disorders, but they may be considered under three headings:

1. *Developmental abnormalities*, of genetic or unknown cause.
2. *Abnormalities due to metabolic disorders.* These include endocrine disturbances and vitamin deficiencies or excesses.
3. *Abnormalities occurring in the adult*, generally of unknown cause.

Although this is a convenient classification, there is an overlap between the groups, and in some examples a localized form of the disease may occur.

### DEVELOPMENTAL ABNORMALITIES

There are a few rare conditions of bone which are due to some failure during the developmental process.

### Cleidocranial Dysostosis[10]

This condition is sometimes inherited as a dominant characteristic, and is characterized by the complete agenesis of a bone or part of a bone. The clavicle is most often affected, but defects have also been reported in the pelvic girdle and long bones. When the clavicles are absent, the subject is able to approximate the shoulders across the chest (Fig. 33.1).

* Very high levels of alkaline phosphatase are found in obstructive jaundice. Liver disease must therefore be considered. The total blood alkaline phosphatase activity consists of the summation of the effect of five isoenzymes. These can be measured separately. Bone alkaline phosphatase is the most unstable and is the one referred to here. Another important alkaline phosphatase is derived from liver and its blood level is raised in bile-duct obstruction.[9] The level is not only raised in obvious jaundice due to main bile-duct obstruction, but also with multiple bile-ductule obstruction when jaundice is absent. A raised level is therefore a useful indication of the presence of multiple secondary carcinoma.

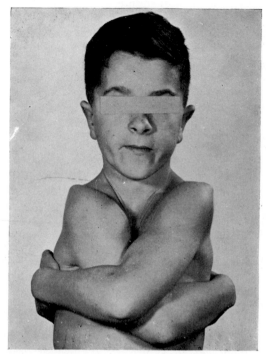

FIG. 33.1. Cleidocranial dysostosis. The two shoulders can be approximated across the chest because of the absence of intervening clavicles.

(Photograph supplied by Mr. T. D. Foster.)

There may also be retardation or failure of closure of the fontanelles, and the two halves of the frontal bone may not fuse. There is also associated a general failure of eruption of the teeth.

### Osteogenesis Imperfecta (Fragilitas ossium)[11]

This condition may be present at birth (*congenital type*) or may develop later (the *tarda form*).

In the congenital type multiple fractures occur *in utero* or during birth, and the prognosis is poor. In the tarda form the condition is less severe, for, if the child survives, the tendency to fracture decreases after puberty.

The bones in osteogenesis imperfecta are generally thin and brittle. The cortex is thin, and there is a decrease in the amount of cancellous bone. The fragility results in the frequent occurrence of fractures which occur either spontaneously or as a result of trivial injuries. Although there is rapid healing of the fractures, the bone is of abnormal consistency. The multiplicity of fractures generally leads to severe deformities.

The disease is inherited as an autosomal dominant character with incomplete penetrance. The pathogenesis is obscure, but it is thought that there is a generalized hypoplasia of mesenchyme. This theory is supported by the fact that affected subjects are of short stature, and have lax ligaments which lead to hypermobility of the joints. In addition the sclera is sometimes thin and semi-translucent, so that it appears blue due to the pigmentation of the underlying choroid.

**Dentinogenesis Imperfecta (Hereditary Opalescent Dentine).** This is a condition affecting that part of the tooth of mesenchymal origin (dentine), and may be seen in association with osteogenesis imperfecta or may occur without any bony involvement.

### Fibrous Dysplasia

The aetiology of this condition is unknown. It is characterized by the appearance of areas of bone resorption and replacement by fibrous tissue in which there are thin trabeculae of woven bone in the shape of Chinese characters. The marrow space is also obliterated in the affected areas. Any bone may be affected, either in its entirety or only focally. Fibrous dysplasia includes a wide variety of conditions which may well be excluded from this group as our knowledge increases. Two main types are described:

**Polyostotic Fibrous Dysplasia.** This manifests itself early in life. There is an insidious onset, and a pathological fracture may be the presenting symptom. The condition usually affects one side of the body only. When the skull and facial bones are involved there is much disfigurement. The disease process usually ceases when growth has ended.

A more severe form of the condition is accompanied by pigmentation of the skin (café-au-lait spots), endocrine dysfunction resulting in sexual precocity in young girls, and disturbances of growth and development (*Albright's syndrome*). The reason for the pigmentation and endocrine disturbance is not known.

**Monostotic Fibrous Dysplasia.** Some authorities believe that this is a reparative reaction following trauma or infection. Despite the histological similarity to the polyostotic form it does not seem to progress to the latter. Monostotic fibrous dysplasia is much more common than the polyostotic form. It occurs in young people, and may affect any bone including the jaw in from 10–15 per cent of cases.[12,13]

### Familial Fibrous Dysplasia ("Cherubism")[14]

This disease, first described by Jones in 1933,[15] resembles monostotic fibrous dysplasia but is inherited as an autosomal dominant trait with incomplete penetrance. The bone is replaced by loose, oedematous fibrous tissue in which there are scattered giant cells. Bony trabeculae like those of fibrous dysplasia are not present.

Characteristically there is enlargement of the jaws and there may be submaxillary lymphadenopathy. Involvement of the orbital floor with upward displacement of the eyes combines with the large jaws to give a cherubic appearance.

Bony expansion of the jaws occurs particularly in the mandibular molar region—it commences in the first two to three years of life, and gradually ceases as growth terminates. There may be a premature loss of primary teeth and some disturbances of the permanent dentition with an absence of teeth and failure of eruption of those present.

Radiographs of the jaws show extensive symmetrical areas of radiolucency which have a multilocular appearance. Involvement of bones other than those of the skull and mandible can occur, but it is rare.

There is some doubt as to the exact nature of the condition. Jones, who coined the named cherubism, considered that it was an anomaly of dental development. Others regard it as a fibrous dysplasia or a bone dysplasia. Others do not commit themselves, and consider the condition a familial osseous dysplasia or fibrous swelling of the jaws.[16]

### Achondroplasia (Chondrodystrophy Fetalis)

This disease is transmitted as an autosomal dominant factor. The essential feature is defective endochondral bone formation, and the long bones of the limbs are therefore short. The trunk and head are of normal size, but the middle third of the face is depressed due to the premature cessation of cartilaginous growth and synostosis of the bones of the cranial base. There is relative or true protrusion of the lower jaw. This type of dwarf, who has normal intelligence, is very muscular and agile, and is frequently seen in the circus ring.

### Osteopetrosis (Albers-Schönberg Disease, Marble-Bone Disease)[15]

There is increased deposition of bone in this condition, so that the bones are hard, heavy, and inelastic. The cortex is greatly thickened, and the marrow cavity is much reduced in size. This disease is inherited as an autosomal recessive trait.

Although the bones are thickened and hard, they are liable to fractures because of their inelasticity. Leuco-erythroblastic anaemia may occur as a result of the reduction of bone-marrow space. Later on blindness, deafness, and facial paralysis develop, because the cranial nerves are constricted as they pass through the bony foramina of the skull.

## ABNORMALITIES DUE TO METABOLIC DISORDERS

### Endocrine Disturbances

Changes may take place in the skeleton as a result of many endocrine dysfunctions; the pituitary and parathyroid glands are most important, and will be considered here. Hyperthyroidism and hypothyroidism are described in Chapter 35.

**Hyperpituitarism.** Hypersecretion of growth hormone in the young, whether due to an adenoma or hyperplasia of the acidophil cells of the anterior lobe of the pituitary, leads to an excessive growth at the epiphyses of the entire skeleton. The result is *gigantism*, and in addition to excessive skeletal growth there is also an increase in the size of the viscera.

If hypersecretion of growth hormone occurs after closure of the epiphyses, the distal, or acral, parts of the body are affected, and *acromegaly* results. There is a generalized increase in thickness of all the bones of the skeleton due to subperiosteal appositional bone growth. The typical acromegalic appearance is one of overgrowth of the mandible (*prognathism*), prominence of the supraorbital ridges and malar bones, and enlarged hands and feet. The prognathism is a result of further growth in the cartilage in the head of the condyle.

**Hypopituitarism.** Pituitary deficiency in childhood results in dwarfism, and is usually due to destruction of the gland by a tumour. The pituitary dwarf is quite different from the achondroplastic dwarf, for the head, body, and limbs are all well proportioned though diminutive. General growth processes are slow, and become arrested at an early age. There is also a delay in the development and eruption of the teeth.

**Hyperparathyroidism.**[18-22] An excessive secretion of parathormone produces rarefaction of the bones which may be generalized, or of more irregular distribution to produce *osteitis fibrosa cystica.* Hyperparathyroidism can be understood only after the properties of parathormone are first appreciated.

The main action of parathormone is to regulate the equilibrium between the calcium in the blood and that in the bones. An increased secretion causes resorption of bone, a rise in the level of the plasma calcium, and increased excretion of calcium in the urine. Parathormone secretion is thought to be regulated by the level of the calcium in the plasma. The view that calcium can be directly removed from bone by a process of diffusion, or *halisteresis,* is not generally accepted. It is thought that osteoclastic activity is always necessary before calcium can be removed—the two views are not in fact irreconcilable. If bone salts are removed by diffusion, the exposed osteoid may be removed by osteoclastic activity. Whatever the mechanism, in hyperparathyroidism there is excessive osteoclastic activity, and as bone is removed it is replaced by fibrous tissue.

Hyperparathyroidism can be divided into two groups:

*Primary hyperparathyroidism,* due to the excessive production of parathormone, as a result of either idiopathic hyperplasia or neoplasia—generally benign. *The level of serum calcium is raised.*

*Secondary hyperparathyroidism,* due to hyperplasia of the glands with hypersecretion induced by a persistently *low level of serum ionized calcium.* This is seen most frequently in two groups of conditions:

(1) rickets and osteomalacia (p. 448),
(2) chronic renal disease.

The relationship between renal disease and parathyroid function is complex. In chronic renal disease the inability to excrete phosphate results in a raised serum phosphate. This in turn causes a depression in the serum calcium level. The low serum calcium stimulates the parathyroids and leads to their hyperplasia. Their hypersecretion increases the mobilization of calcium from the bones, and produces progressive demineralization. The calcium is excreted *via* the kidney, where calcareous deposits may occur in the tubules and cause further renal damage. The effects on the growing skeleton are severe, and may result in dwarfism.

*Osteitis fibrosa cystica (von Recklinghausen's disease of bone).* In the early

* This is a poor name because the condition is not inflammatory, nor is it always cystic.

stages of this disease there is generalized bone involvement which is manifested by bone pains, softening and bending of the bones with resulting
deformity, and spontaneous fractures due to the decreased strength of the
bones.

As there is excretion of calcium *via* the kidneys, renal calculi are not
uncommon, and may sometimes be responsible for the presenting symptoms,
e.g. haematuria, pain, and urinary infection. The deposition of calcium in
other tissues is common (metastatic calcification—see below). In some cases
the bones are enlarged, and contain tumour-like lesions composed of osteoclasts and localized blood-filled cysts. These *brown tumours*, as they are called,
closely resemble giant-cell tumours of bone (p. 458), and are seen typically at
sites which normally contain haematopoietic tissue: the skull, jaw, ribs, and
spine. The brown coloration is due to the content of haemosiderin.

Occasionally the first indication of the condition is a cyst-like lesion of
the jaw. The radiographic description is of a "ground-glass" appearance of
the affected bone. There is resorption of bone, and although the lamina dura
may be lost, the teeth are not usually affected. The diagnosis may be confirmed
by finding a raised serum calcium level and lowered serum phosphate. The
serum alkaline phosphatase is usually considerably raised.

### Metastatic Calcification[23]

*Metastatic calcification* is the deposition of calcium salts in normal tissue
other than osteoid or dentine due to a derangement of calcium or phosphate
metabolism. The most common cause is hypercalcaemia due to hyperparathyroidism or extensive destructive lesions of bone, e.g. multiple osteolytic
tumours. However, it may also occur in hyperphosphataemia, as in chronic
renal disease. The common sites of metastatic calcification are the *lung*,
*gastric mucosa*, and *kidney*, all situations where acidic substances are excreted
—the $CO_2$ of the alveolar gas, the hydrochloric acid of the gastric contents,
and the hydrogen ions of the urine.

The renal lesions are the most serious, for, combined with the effects of
calculi which may also occur with hypercalcaemia, they rapidly lead to renal
failure.

### Inadequate or Excessive Amounts of Vitamins

For normal growth and development to occur, there must be an adequate
intake of protein, carbohydrates, and fat. In addition, certain vitamins and
minerals are essential. Several diseases result from inadequate ingestion,
absorption, and utilization of these substances, and give rise to characteristic
skeletal lesions. The effects of these changes are more severe if they occur
during childhood, when bone is being formed rapidly.

### Vitamin-C Deficiency: Scurvy

Deficiency of ascorbic acid results in the defective formation of collagen
fibrils, and there is an excessive accumulation of ground substance. Osteoid
and dentine, as well as unspecialized connective tissue, are affected. There is
weakness between the epiphyses and shaft of the bones, and complete
separation may occur. There is generalized osteoporosis. The teeth may
become loosened, and there is a tendency to gingival haemorrhage (p. 359).

### Vitamin-D Deficiency: Rickets and Osteomalacia

The body obtains vitamin D from the food and by synthesis in the skin under the influence of ultraviolet light. An inadequate diet (particularly in those countries where there is not much sunlight) and the malabsorption syndrome will therefore lead to its deficiency. Vitamin D appears to aid the absorption of calcium and phosphorus from the intestine, and in addition it also has a slight parathormone-like action: excessive doses lead to hyper-calcaemia and hypercalcuria. The main effect in vitamin-D deficiency is *an impaired calcification of cartilage and osteoid.*

**Rickets.** In vitamin-D deficiency there is a lowering of the levels of calcium and phosphate in the blood, while the alkaline phosphatase level is con-siderably raised. There is a failure of calcification of the epiphyseal cartilage, which is therefore not removed or replaced by osteoid. Continued growth of this cartilage causes a considerable enlargement of the bone ends. Similarly, the costo-chondral junctions are enlarged, producing the clinical deformity called the "rachitic rosary". Growth of bone length is impaired, and the child is dwarfed. Even the osteoid which is formed is poorly calcified, and the weakened bones are liable to deformities and fractures: knock-knees, kyphosis (forward curvature of the spine), and other deformities are common.

In infants there is a thickening of the frontal and parietal eminentia, and flattening and thinning of the occipital region (craniotabes), and there may be delayed eruption of the teeth. Fortunately, this florid picture of rickets is rare in civilized countries.

*Vitamin-D Resistant Rickets.*[24] There are a number of hereditary conditions in which rickets occurs in spite of an adequate vitamin-D intake. Usually this is associated with an abnormal excretion of amino acids in the urine.

**Osteomalacia.** The counterpart of rickets in the adult is osteomalacia. It is more common in women, because pregnancy imposes an additional drain on the supplies of calcium.

In the normal adult, bone is continually being remodelled; it is removed by osteoclasts and replaced by osteoblasts laying down osteoid which promptly calcifies. If this calcification fails, the bones consist largely of osteoid and the result is osteomalacia: there is an abundance of osteoid but poor calcification, in contradistinction to osteoporosis, where the matrix is normally calcified but reduced in quantity.

All bones are affected, but it is the weight-bearing regions where the most severe effects are seen. Severe pelvic distortion may cause complications in subsequent pregnancies, and collapse of the vertebrae gives rise to pain due to compression of the spinal nerves in the intervertebral foramina.

## ABNORMALITIES OF BONE OCCURRING IN THE ADULT

### Generalized Osteoporosis[8, 25, 26]

*Disuse osteoporosis.* Prolonged recumbency produces considerable osteo-porosis in most bones. It would seem that stress and strain are a necessary stimulus for the maintenance of bone structure. Immobilization leads initially to osteoclastic resorption of bone and the mobilization of excessive amounts of calcium, which results in hypercalcuria and sometimes renal-stone formation. This is then followed by a phase of quiescence in which the bone shows little osteoclastic or osteoblastic activity. If movement is resumed, the bones gradually return to normal. The blood levels of calcium, phosphate, and phosphatase are normal in disuse osteoporosis.

*Idiopathic osteoporosis.* Osteoporosis, especially of the pelvis, spine, and ribs, is not uncommon in old age (*senile osteoporosis*), and compression of the vertebral bodies causes backache as well aş a considerable loss of height. The condition is also seen in women who have passed the menopause (*post-menopausal osteoporosis*), and this has been attributed to hormonal imbalance. Occasionally osteoporosis occurs in a younger age-group for no very obvious reason.

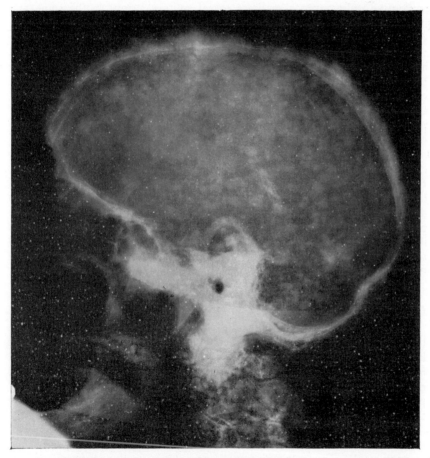

Fig. 33.2. Paget's disease affecting the skull. Note the uneven thickening of the outer table and the blurring of the demarcation between the inner and outer tables.

(Radiograph supplied by Professor H. C. Killey.)

*Other types of osteoporosis.* Osteoporosis is also seen when collagen formation is impaired as in,

(*a*) Scurvy.

(*b*) Excessive glucocorticosteroid levels, e.g. Cushing's disease and with prolonged administration of adrenocortical hormones.

(*c*) Impaired supply of protein, e.g. starvation and the malabsorption syndrome.

### Paget's Disease of Bone (Osteitis Deformans)

Described first by James Paget in 1876, this condition is considered by some to be an inflammatory disease. However, despite much study its aetiology and nature are unknown. It occurs in people over the age of 40 years, predominantly in men. It is perhaps more common than was originally thought, as routine radiographs sometimes reveal solitary lesions in the spine and pelvis without clinical manifestations. The involved bones show much thickening of the cortex due to the dominance of osteoblastic activity.

Initially the bone is softened due to osteoclastic resorption, and the affected area shows increased vascularity. The bending of softened, weight-bearing bones results in deformities, and is adequate reason for the alternative name of osteitis deformans. Later there is irregular subperiosteal deposition, and the bones become hard and thickened (Fig. 33.2). The serum calcium and phosphate levels are within normal limits, but the alkaline phosphatase may be raised as much as fifty times above normal.

The skull is frequently affected, and later it may become obviously enlarged. When the jaws are affected the teeth show marked hypercementosis. Bone pain may be an early feature. Blindness, deafness, headaches, and facial paralysis are complications that may occur as a result of compression due to the increased bone formation. Sarcoma of bone complicates the condition in about 1 per cent of patients. The reason for this is not known; it appears that the excessive proliferative activity of the bone leads eventually to neoplastic growth.

## BONE DISORDERS CAUSED BY PHYSICAL DISTURBANCES

### Localized Osteoporosis

**Due to Immobilization.** The local disuse of a bone causes osteoporosis in the same way as does total recumbency, and the immobilization of a joint leads to marked osteoporosis of the adjacent bones. This occurs after fractures and also in diseases of the joints themselves, e.g. tuberculous and rheumatoid arthritis. It is very pronounced in paralysed limbs; indeed, if paralysis occurs in childhood, as after poliomyelitis, the whole limb including the bones fails to attain adult size.

**Pressure Atrophy.** Expanding lesions which exert pressure on the surrounding bone cause local ischaemia due to compression of the blood vessels, and atrophy results. Thus a benign tumour or cyst may produce a sharply-defined area of rarefaction. In an attempt to offset the weakness that ensues more bone is produced by the periosteum opposite the lesion, so that the mass appears to cause expansion of the bone. This is well seen in the giant-cell tumour and in the ameloblastoma. It should be noted that cartilage, being avascular, does not undergo pressure atrophy. Therefore an aneurysm of the descending aorta pressing on the vertebral column causes atrophy of the vertebrae but spares the intervertebral discs. For the same reason benign tumours and cysts do not destroy the epiphyseal cartilage of a long bone.

## Fractures[2, 27, 28]

**Exciting Causes**

EXCESSIVE MECHANICAL FORCE

*Direct violence*, e.g. depressed fracture of the skull.

*Indirect violence*, e.g. fracture of the condyle of the mandible following a blow on the chin (Fig. 33.3).

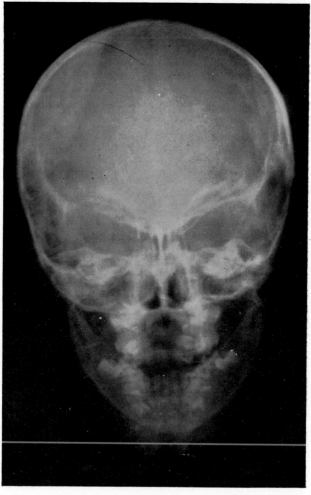

FIG. 33.3. Fractured condyles in a child aged 3 years following a fall on her chin.

452 DISEASES OF BONE AND JOINTS

*Muscular action.* Sudden unexpected strains during violent exercise may cause fractures in normal bones (*spontaneous fractures*). Likewise the violent convulsive movements of tetanus and strychnine poisoning may result in the collapse of a vertebral body, causing wedging.

ABNORMAL BONE

A fracture may occur in a diseased bone subjected to a normal strain (*pathological fracture*). Any lesion which causes weakness may be responsible, e.g. osteitis fibrosa cystica, osteogenesis imperfecta, simple bone cyst, and tumour. Secondary carcinoma must always be borne in mind, and indeed a pathological fracture may be the first indication of a malignant lesion, e.g. carcinoma of lung or breast.

**Stages in Fracture Healing (Bone Regeneration)**

The stages in healing of a fracture are illustrated diagrammatically in Fig. 33.4. It must be remembered that the entire area is not all at the same stage of healing at the same time; while the centre may be at an early stage, the changes adjacent to the bone ends are much more advanced. However, for descriptive purposes it is convenient to divide the healing process into separate stages.

**Stage 1: Haematoma Formation.** Immediately following the injury there is a variable amount of bleeding from torn vessels, and a haematoma is formed.

**Stage 2: Traumatic Inflammation.** The tissue damage excites an acute inflammatory response, with vasodilatation and a polymorphonuclear leucocytic infiltration. The hyperaemia has been held responsible for the decreased density of the adjacent bone ends often noted radiologically. This "decalcification" is presumably a form of osteoporosis due to osteoclastic activity, but the pathogenesis is not clear. The depolymerization of the ground substance which accompanies the inflammatory reaction causes a loosening of the attachment of the periosteum to the bone. The haematoma therefore attains a fusiform shape.

**Stage 3: Demolition.** Macrophages invade the clot and remove the fibrin, red cells, inflammatory exudate, and debris. Any fragments of bone which have become detached from their blood supply undergo necrosis, and are attacked by macrophages and osteoclasts.

**Stage 4: Formation of Granulation Tissue.** Following the demolition there is an ingrowth of capillary loops and mesenchymal cells derived from the periosteum and endosteum. The importance of the periosteum in fracture union has been much disputed in the past. The cells of its deeper layer certainly have osteogenic potentiality, and together with its blood vessels contribute to the granulation tissue.

In fractures of the neck of the femur the head is dependent upon the periosteum for its blood supply. If this is damaged, there is ischaemic necrosis of the head. Hence in this situation the integrity of the periosteum is of great practical importance. In a rib following subperiosteal resection the periosteum alone is capable of effecting complete regeneration. Here it probably acts partly by forming a limiting membrane around the haematoma, and partly by providing cells and blood vessels for the granulation tissue.

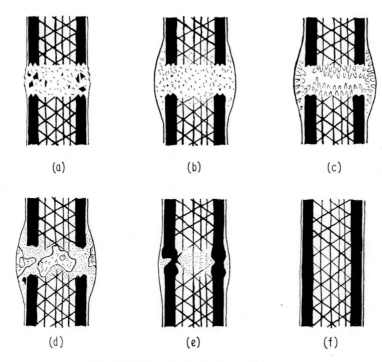

FIG. 33.4. Stages in the healing of a fracture.

(a) Haematoma formation.
(b) Stages 2 and 3. Acute inflammation followed by demolition. Loose fragments of bone are removed, and the bone ends show osteoporosis.
(c) Stage 4. Granulation tissue formation.
(d) Stage 5. The bone ends are now united by woven bone, cartilage, or a
mixture of the two. The hard material is often called callus, and can be divided
into three parts—internal, intermediate, and external. The intermediate callus
is that part which lies in line with the cortex of the bone, while the external
callus produces the fusiform swelling visible on the outside of the bone.
(e) Stage 6. Lamellar bone is laid down, and calcified cartilage and woven
bone are progressively removed.
(f) Stage 7. Final remodelling.

In fractures of the long bones, however, it must not be forgotten that a
very extensive area of cancellous bone is exposed. From this the endosteal
osteoblasts and the medullary blood vessels grow out to form the granulation
tissue. Under these circumstances the periosteum is of much less importance.

During these early phases the pH is low, and this is spoken of as the
*acid tide*.

**Stage 5: Woven Bone and Cartilage Formation.** The mesenchymal
"osteoblasts" next differentiate to form either woven bone or cartilage. The
term "callus", derived from the Latin and meaning hard, is often used to
describe the material uniting the fracture ends regardless of its consistency.
When this is granulation tissue the "callus" is soft, but as bone or cartilage

formation occurs it becomes hard. The word is used loosely by surgeons, radiologists, and pathologists, but exact definition of its various stages is difficult and serves no useful function. If the term is used, it is probably best to apply it to the calcified hard tissue uniting the bone ends.

*Formation of Woven Bone.* The osteoblasts form both the collagen fibres and the osseomucin, in which they are embedded. The osteoid is in this way formed by the maturation of granulation tissue, and as in the repair of ordinary connective tissue progressive devascularization occurs. The collagen bundles are irregularly arranged with no attempt at lamellar structure.

After about ten days the pH of the uniting fracture increases. During this *alkaline tide* the osteoid undergoes calcification, and thereby becomes woven bone. Osteoblasts produce an alkaline phosphatase which may play a part in the calcification, in that it may lead to a local supersaturation of phosphate due to its effect on hexose phosphates. Resorption of bony spicules may at the same time produce a local supersaturation of calcium ions.

The bone ends thus become united by woven bone. It forms a fusiform mass which is arbitrarily divided into internal, intermediate, and external callus (Fig. 33.4).

Woven-bone formation is found whenever the bone ends are adequately immobilized. It normally occurs in human fracture healing, and is a predominant feature in healing of tooth sockets. In experimentally-produced fractures in animals adequate immobilization is difficult to attain, and then the granulation tissue matures not to woven bone, but to hyaline cartilage as described below.

*Formation of Cartilage.* The mesenchymal cells ("osteoblasts") behave as chondroblasts and form cartilage, i.e. the cells actively lead to the formation of a specialized ground substance in which the collagen fibres are embedded. These cartilage cells swell and die, and the intervening matrix undergoes calcification. Cartilage formation is seen in fractures in which movement occurs, not only in experimental animal fractures, but also human fractures where complete immobilization is impractical, e.g. ribs.

In many fractures both cartilage and woven bone are formed. Both are capable of forming a calcified scaffold on which the final adult-type, lamellar bone can later be built. The two embryological methods of bone formation, endochondral and intramembranous ossification, are faithfully repeated in later life during the regeneration of bone.

**Stage 6: Formation of Lamellar Bone.** The dead calcified cartilage or woven bone is next invaded by capillaries headed by osteoclasts. As the initial scaffolding ("provisional callus") is removed, osteoblasts lay down osteoid which calcifies to form bone. This time its collagen bundles are arranged in orderly lamellar fashion. For the most part they are disposed concentrically around the blood vessels, where they form Haversian systems. Adjacent to the periosteum and endosteum the lamellae are parallel to the surface as in the normal bone. This phase of deposition of definitive lamellar bone merges with the last stage.

**Stage 7: Remodelling.** The final remodelling process, involving the continued osteoclastic removal and osteoblastic formation of bone, results in the formation of a bone which differs remarkably little from its previous state.

The *external callus* is slowly removed, the *intermediate callus* becomes converted into compact bone containing Haversian systems, while the *internal callus* is hollowed out into a marrow cavity in which only a few spicules of cancellous bone remain.

The healing of a socket following the extraction of a tooth is similar to that of a fracture. After an extraction the socket fills with blood which forms a clot, which within a few days is replaced by granulation tissue. Woven bone is laid down in the socket and this is later replaced by lamellar bone. There is a covering of compact bone. As the alveolar bone is no longer required to support the tooth, remodelling takes place and results in a reduced ridge in that area. The extraction of a tooth produces an open wound, and the healing process also includes epithelialization over the granulation tissue.

A complication that sometimes occurs is the condition known as a "dry socket"; this is a focal osteomyelitis and may occur if the blood clot disintegrates or is lost. The exposed bone becomes necrotic, and sequestration follows. The condition is extremely painful and healing is slow.

### Abnormalities of Fracture Healing

*Repair, or fibrous union.* Although the cells of the granulation tissue are called osteoblasts, they are capable of differentiation along several lines. They can form bone, but if immobilization is not complete, cartilage may develop. When movement is even more free, the cells behave as fibroblasts, and the bone ends become united by ordinary scar tissue. Whether this can ever undergo ossification is debatable. It is claimed by some authorities that fibrous tissue can become replaced by bone, but that it is a very slow process. From a practical point of view fibrous union is an unsatisfactory end-result of healing, because in many cases it is permanent.

Occasionally with excessive movement the cells differentiate into synovial cells, and a false joint, or *pseudarthrosis*, results. This is a well-recognized sequel of fractures of the tibia.

*Non-union.* Complete lack of union between the fracture ends results from the interposition of soft parts. Muscle or fascia separating the bone ends may prevent the formation of a uniting haematoma. Under these conditions union of any sort is impossible. This phenomenon is utilized in the treatment of some disorders of the temporomandibular joint in order to create a new joint.

*Delayed union.* In the presence of a continuous haematoma any of the causes of delayed healing (p. 111) retard bone regeneration.

**Causes of Impaired Healing.** If the adverse conditions are severe, fibrous union may be the end result. In practice the following are the most important:

*Movement.* Movement of any sort is harmful, because it causes damage to the delicate granulation tissue, and thereby excites an inflammatory reaction. In surgical practice every attempt is made to reduce movement to a minimum. In the case of impacted fractures this is usually easy, but in other instances where the bone ends are mobile, recourse may have to be made to pins, plates, or other forms of internal splinting. The bone ends must not be over-distracted, for this leads to slow healing. Indeed, if on the contrary the bone ends are brought together under high compression, there is rigid immobilization and healing is speeded.[29]

*Infection.* By prolonging the acute inflammatory phase, infection is an important cause of slow union or non-union. Since the tension of exudate in a bone is liable to lead to extensive ischaemic necrosis with sequestrum formation, it is particularly important to avoid infecting previously closed fractures during open reduction. Absolute asepsis must be maintained by employing a no-touch technique.

*Poor blood supply.* While complete loss of blood supply results in necrosis of bone, poor blood supply leads to slow granulation tissue formation and therefore slow union. Certain sites are notorious for this complication, e.g. fractures of neck of femur, shaft of tibia, and the carpal scaphoid. In these situations the avoidance of other possible causes of delayed healing, e.g. movement, is particularly important. The slow healing of fractures in old age is probably due to ischaemia.

**Myositis Ossificans.** If there is an extravasation of the fracture haematoma into the surrounding muscles, its subsequent organization and ossification results in the condition of *traumatic myositis ossificans.*

### Disorders of the Bone Marrow

Disorders of the haematopoietic tissue of the marrow produce obvious effects in the circulating blood, and are considered in Chapter 26. There remain a number of disorders of uncertain nature which affect the reticulo-endothelial system as a whole, but since bone lesions are common it is convenient to consider them here.

### Lipid-Storage Diseases[30]

The lipid-storage diseases are examples of inherited disturbances of lipid metabolism associated with a specific enzyme defect. Excess lipid accumulates in various organs, the RE cells being particularly affected in Gaucher's and Niemann-Pick disease. Several types of each of these diseases are known, and they are inherited as recessive traits.

**Gaucher's Disease.**[31] In this disease there is a massive accumulation of a glucocerebroside due to a deficiency of the enzyme glucocerebrosidase. Glucocerebroside is probably derived from effete white and red cells in the RE system and it is not surprising that here is found the main accumulation of lipid. The swollen RE cells are called Gaucher cells and their presence causes massive enlargement of the spleen and liver. Destructive lesions may occur in the bones, especially the femur, due to collections of Gaucher cells in the marrow eroding the cortex, which is thinned. The marrow replacement may cause a leuco-erythroblastic anaemia.

The adult form of the disease runs a protracted course. In the brain glucocerebroside is derived from gangliosides, which have a rapid turnover in infancy. It follows that central-nervous-sytem involvement with severe mental retardation and death is a feature of the infantile and juvenile neuro-pathic forms of Gaucher's disease.

**Niemann-Pick Disease.**[32] This rare and usually fatal disease occurs pre-dominantly in Jewish children. It is familial, and is due to a defect in the metabolism of a phospholipid, sphingomyelin, which accumulates in the RE system as well as certain parenchymal cells. Not only are the spleen, lymph nodes, and bone marrow involved, but the kidney, lungs, brain, and adrenals may also be affected. There is physical and mental retardation. A generalized rarefaction with circumscribed foci of bone resorption may occur.

## Histiocytosis X[33]

The three conditions in this category, Letterer-Siwe disease, Hand-Schüller-Christian disease, and eosinophilic granuloma of bone, although differing markedly in clinical behaviour, are nevertheless regarded as variants of the same disease process. Their differences are probably due to the age at which they occur—the younger the patient, the more severe is the form. Histologically there is a focal infiltration of large macrophages which may sometimes contain lipid. Interspersed among them there are polymorphs, eosinophils, and other small round cells. The nature of the disease process is unknown.

*Letterer-Siwe disease.* This acute fatal condition occurs in young children. There is enlargement of spleen, liver, and lymph nodes. In fact there is a universal destructive proliferation of the RE cells, and few organs escape.

*Hand-Schüller-Christian disease.* This disease runs a more chronic course, and affected children may survive into adult life. Characteristically there are focal areas of radiolucency in the skull. If the orbit is involved, exophthalmos (protrusion of the eyeballs) results, and if the sella turcica is

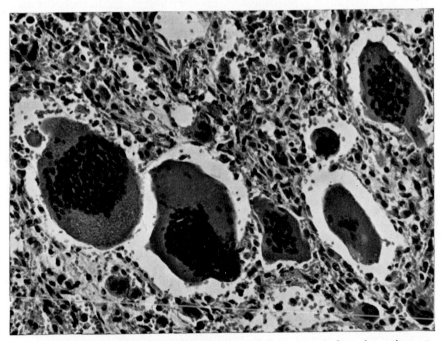

Fig. 33.5. Giant-cell tumour of bone. The tumour is composed of very large giant cells resembling osteoclasts and also a smaller spindle-shaped fibroblastic element. × 200.

implicated, diabetes insipidus may develop as a result of destruction of the posterior lobe of the pituitary. Loosening of the teeth is also quite a common feature if the jaw is affected. The destructive histiocytic lesions may eventually heal by fibrosis.

*Eosinophilic granuloma of bone.* A much older group is affected by this disease, which usually produces a solitary, localized area of bone destruction. Occasionally, however, multiple lesions are present, and when these are widely scattered the disease is not clearly delineated from Hand-Schüller-Christian disease. The affected areas are swollen and painful. The jaws are frequent sites of predeliction, and the lesions present diagnostic difficulties when they are closely related to the teeth.

## TUMOURS[34]

### Tumours of Bone

The tumours of bone form a complex group of neoplasms, for in spite of the apparent simplicity of bone structure, the histogenesis of some of the tumours which arise from it is quite obscure. The occurrence of tumours in the adjacent marrow and the frequency of skeletal metastases add further to the confusion.

Quite often the initial diagnosis of bone tumour is made on radiological grounds, but it must be emphasized that histological confirmation by biopsy is essential before treatment is attempted. The "characteristic" appearances of certain tumours, e.g. osteosarcoma, are often absent, and furthermore may be mimicked by other lesions.

**Benign Tumours.** *Osteoma, chondroma, fibroma,* etc. are all recognized, but are rare, especially in the jaws. Many lesions described as tumours are in fact hamartomata, e.g. angioma, or variants of other non-neoplastic conditions, e.g. fibrous dysplasia, reaction to trauma, etc.

### Intermediate Tumours

**Giant-Cell Tumour of Bone (Osteoclastoma).** This tumour of uncertain histogenesis is usually found in patients between 20 and 40 years of age. It is composed of a mixture of spindle cells and giant cells resembling osteoclasts (Fig. 33.5). The tumour destroys bone locally by pressure atrophy and in some cases by actual invasion. This produces the characteristic soap-bubble appearance seen radiologically. About 15 per cent of giant-cell tumours metastasize to the lungs.

The tumour is usually seen in the long bones, and is very rare in the jaws. In the past it was commonly reported in the jaws, but this was probably due to the misdiagnosis of other non-neoplastic conditions. Some of these should be noted:

*Central giant-cell reparative granuloma.* This appears as a central, expanding lesion in the tooth-bearing portion of the jaw, usually the mandible. It occurs between the ages of 10 and 25 years, and closely resembles a giant-cell tumour histologically. Nevertheless, it is thought to be non-neoplastic; it never metastasizes, and is perhaps a reaction to haemorrhage.

*Brown tumour.* See p. 447.

*Peripheral giant-cell reparative granuloma* (*giant-cell epulis*). This should

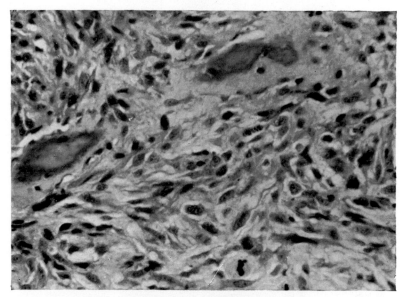

FIG. 33.6. Osteosarcoma. The tumour consists of sheets of spindle-shaped cells intimately connected with the intervening stroma. Two spicules of osteoid are included. Note the mitotic figure at the lower edge on the section. × 350. (Photograph supplied by Dr. A. D. Thomson.)

not be confused with a giant-cell tumour. It arises from the gingivae or periosteum as a result of chronic infection or irritation.

## Malignant Tumours

*Fibrosarcoma, angiosarcoma*, etc. are described, but are rare.

**Chondrosarcoma.** This tumour is composed of atypical cartilage cells, but it is notoriously difficult to distinguish from a benign chondroma histologically. Local invasion and later metastasis to the lungs are the main features.

**Osteosarcoma.** Osteosarcoma is the most common and the most malignant of this rare group of primary bone tumours. It usually occurs in children and young adults, but is found in older persons as a complication of Paget's disease or as a result of the deposition of radioactive substances in the bone. The tumour is composed of malignant osteoblasts which are usually very pleomorphic; giant cells are often abundant. Well-differentiated tumours may produce variable amounts of cartilage and osteoid, which may or may not calcify to form bone (Fig. 33.6). The surrounding normal bone is destroyed, and radiologically a poorly-differentiated tumour appears *osteolytic*, as there is an irregular bony defect. The tumour lifts up the periosteum, and if neoplastic bone is formed, it tends to be laid down around the periosteal vessels as they penetrate the tumour mass. This leads to the characteristic sun-ray appearance of the *osteosclerotic* type of tumour (Fig. 33.7). The out-

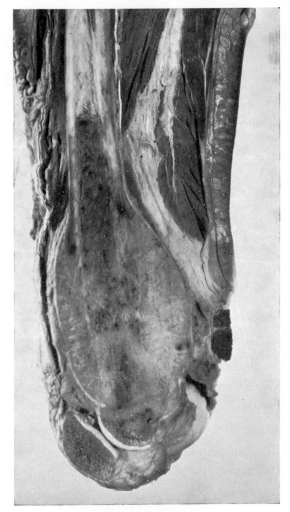

FIG. 33.7. Osteosarcoma. This has arisen from the lower end of the femur and has
spread almost to the knee joint. The tumour has lifted up the periosteum, and
has assumed a fusiform shape. There is a radiating ("sun-ray") disposition of
newly-formed bony spicules in this spindle-shaped mass.

(S72.5. *Reproduced by permission of the President and Council of the Royal
College of Surgeons of England.*)

look for a patient with osteosarcoma is extremely poor, for pulmonary
metastases appear early.

### Tumours of Bone Marrow (Myelogenic Tumours)

These rare tumours arise in the haematopoietic and reticulo-endothelial
cells of the bone marrow. The three included in this group are *Ewing's tumour,
reticulum-cell sarcoma,* and *multiple myeloma.*

**Ewing's tumour.** This tumour occurs in young children, and most often affects the shaft of a long bone. It is composed of sheets of small round cells, and is osteolytic. The raised periosteum may produce layers of new bone around the tumour, leading to an onion-like appearance radiologically. The nature of Ewing's tumour is obscure. It appears to be a distinct entity, but can be closely mimicked by reticulum-cell sarcoma and metastatic neuroblastoma. It is radiosensitive, but the prognosis is bad because it usually metastasizes to other bones and viscera.

**Reticulum-Cell Sarcoma.** This tumour occurs in an older age-group. It is osteolytic, and nearly always appears as an isolated tumour. It is radio-sensitive, and its prognosis is better than that of Ewing's tumour.

**Myeloma.** A tumour composed of neoplastic plasma cells is occasionally encountered as a *solitary myeloma* in the tonsil or nasopharynx. More commonly the tumours are multiple and are found in the bones, especially the vertebrae, ribs, sternum, and skull (*multiple myeloma*). The disease occurs in patients over the age of forty, and the osteolytic tumours produce characteristic punched-out areas on a radiograph. The results of these tumours are serious. Not only do they lead to the destruction of the surrounding cortex and cause spontaneous fractures and collapse of the vertebral column, but they may also produce so much demineralization of the skeleton that hyper-calcaemia and renal failure may follow. Pain is an early symptom.

The tumour cells form large amounts of a homogeneous immunoglobulin called *myeloma protein* (p. 330). Some tumours produce an excess of its component light chain, which has a molecular weight of about 22 000 (*Bence-Jones protein*), and is small enough to pass through the glomeruli into the urine, where it can be recognized by its tendency to precipitate between the temperatures of 60°C and 80°C, and to redissolve on further heating. On cooling a similar phenomenon occurs between 80°C and 60°C. This protein may also precipitate in the tubules of the kidney, causing ob-struction and renal failure.

### Metastatic Tumours

Secondary tumours of bone are much more common than the primary ones. They develop from blood-borne metastases of carcinoma of the prostate, breast, bronchus, kidney, stomach, and thyroid. They are characteristically osteolytic, with the exception of carcinoma of the prostate which is osteo-blastic. Pathological fractures and pain are the usual presenting symptoms.

The jaws are rarely affected, but when secondary deposits do occur it is usually in the mandibular molar area. A deposit in the jaws has been known to give rise to symptoms before the primary growth manifested itself.

### DISEASES OF JOINTS

A joint consists of two or more opposing *cartilage-covered bone ends* united by a sleeve of connective tissue called the *capsule*, the innermost layer of which is modified into a secreting membrane called the *synovium*. This consists of one or more layers of flattened or cubical cells that secrete a clear, pale, viscid fluid (*synovial fluid*) which contains small quantities of albumin and globulin and also a significant amount of mucin. Not only does the synovial fluid lubricate the joint, but it is also the main, if not the only, source of nourishment of the hyaline cartilage covering the bone ends. The amount of synovial fluid in the joint is very small—there is only about 0·5 ml. in the knee joint.

**Arthritis.** This is an inflammation of a joint. There is usually an increased amount of synovial fluid present due to a concomitant inflammation of the synovial membrane (*synovitis*). Arthritis may be traumatic, as after the twisting or the forcible hyperextension or hyperflexion of a joint. This may lead to a minor tear of the capsule, called a sprain, but if more severe the rupture of the capsule may cause a partial or complete displacement of the bone ends. A partial displacement is called a subluxation, and a complete one a dislocation. Simple sprains heal spontaneously, but the weakness of a ruptured capsule may predispose to a recurrent dislocation.

Another type of arthritis is *infective* in aetiology. This may follow a penetrating joint injury, when the infection is introduced from outside, or it may be blood-spread during the course of a systemic illness. The most important type of haematogenous arthritis is the suppurative arthritis that occasionally occurs in the course of such pyogenic diseases as gonorrhoea, lobar pneumonia, and staphylococcal septicaemia. Sometimes the infection may be of a more chronic type, e.g. tuberculosis and syphilis. Suppurative arthritis, unless energetically treated in the early stages with antibiotics, leads to the rapid destruction of the articular cartilages, and the whole cavity is filled with exudate which organizes and obliterates the space. In this way the joint is destroyed, and the bone ends are united by fibrous tissue. This is called an *ankylosis*, and it may undergo ossification later. A bony ankylosis is characteristic of a burnt-out suppurative process, whereas tuberculous arthritis usually terminates in a fibrous ankylosis.

By far the most important types of chronic arthritis are *rheumatoid arthritis* and *osteoarthritis*.

### Rheumatoid Arthritis

This common disease occurs most frequently in young adults, especially women. It is characteristically polyarticular (affecting many joints) and symmetrical. The small joints of the hands and feet are usually worst affected, but the knees also suffer badly. It is a systemic disease, and in the active phases there is mild pyrexia, weight loss, and sweating bouts. A moderate anaemia often develops.

The affected joints are swollen, tender, and painful. In the early stages the synovial membrane is acutely inflamed; it proliferates into villous folds in which there is a heavy infiltration of lymphocytes and plasma cells. Later on the lymphocytic infiltration becomes more copious and lymphoid follicles may also develop. There is a steady encroachment of granulation tissue from the articular margin on to the cartilage. This inflammatory tissue forms a *pannus* over the cartilage and destroys it. The joint space is gradually obliterated by fibrous adhesions, and eventually ankylosis occurs. In this late stage there is severe atrophy of the adjacent bones and muscles, and the overlying skin is smooth and shiny. The results of advanced rheumatoid arthritis are tragic to see. Progressive contractures lead to flexion deformities seen especially in the distorted hands with the characteristic ulnar deviation of the fingers, and the flexed, ankylosed larger joints which render the patient immobile. There may be limited movement in the temporo-mandibular joints, and occasionally ankylosis occurs.

The nature of rheumatoid arthritis is unknown, but the basic lesion seems to be a fibrinoid necrosis of collagen. It is therefore classed among the collagen diseases (p. 172). The systemic nature of the process is evidenced by *subcutaneous nodules* which develop over pressure points; these consist of a

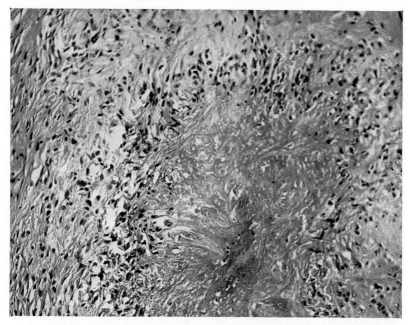

FIG. 33.8. Rheumatoid nodule. There is an extensive central area of necrotic collagen surrounded by a palisade layer of fibroblasts. In the periphery there is a reparative fibrosis and a moderate small round cell infiltration. × 200 approx.

(*From Bywaters, E. G. L. and Scott, F. E. T.* (1960). *"Rheumatism and the connective tissue diseases", in* Recent Advances in Clinical Pathology, *Series III, edited by S. C. Dyke, p. 301, Fig. 6. London: Churchill*).

large area of necrosis surrounded by a palisade of fibroblastic cells and a diffuse zone of lymphocytes and plasma cells (Fig. 33.8). Inflammatory and fibrotic lesions are also encountered in the *heart and pericardium, lungs, arteries,* and *eyes.* Enlargement of the *spleen* and *lymph nodes* is also often present. *Amyloidosis* is an important complication; indeed, it is the only significant fatal lesion in rheumatoid arthritis, which may otherwise smoulder on for many years and produce complete crippling.

The sera of most patients with rheumatoid arthritis contain an auto-antibody which reacts against human immunoglobulin. This antibody is called *rheumatoid factor*, but its significance in the pathogenesis of the disease is not known.

**Ankylosing Spondylitis.** This condition resembles rheumatoid arthritis so much in its histological appearance and pathogenesis that some authorities simply regard it as a variant which attacks the spinal column primarily. But there are differences: (a) young men are usually affected, (b) the vertebral joints and the large peripheral joints are affected, whereas the small distal joints are seldom involved, and (c) there is bony ankylosis of the spinal and peripheral joints, and the spinal ligaments and the margins of the inter-vertebral discs undergo ossification. In due course the spinal column is converted into a composite bony mass, the so-called bamboo spine. Sub-cutaneous nodules are not present, nor is the rheumatoid factor. There may be ocular and cardiovascular complications.

## Osteoarthritis

Osteoarthritis, despite its name, is not an inflammatory disease of joints but rather a degenerative one. It is one of man's commonest afflictions, for it is essentially an accentuation of the normal ageing process of articular cartilage. The nourishment of the hyaline cartilage is normally rather precarious, depending on the synovial fluid. The constant wear and tear on the joints after many years' activity leads to a gradual deterioration of the central part of the articular cartilage. This process is greatly aggravated by concomitant trauma to a joint, especially that sustained during athletics. The aetiology of osteoarthritis is unknown, but genetic and metabolic factors seem to be involved. It is a disease of later life, but it can affect a traumatized joint in a younger person. The spine and the large weight-bearing joints, especially the hips, are most severely affected, but the smaller joints do not escape. Osteoarthritis, unlike the rheumatoid variety, is not a systemic disease. The general health is not affected, and the victims tend to be obese.

The condition commences with a softening and fraying of the articular cartilage. It becomes progressively thinner, and ultimately the underlying bone is exposed. This increases in density, and its surface becomes hard, worn, and polished, a change called *eburnation*. Meanwhile there is an in-explicable proliferation of cartilage cells at the margin of the articular area. The new cartilage that is formed soon ossifies. The result is that the periphery of the articular cartilage is raised and bossed; this is called *lipping*, and is an important radiological finding. The peripheral new bone may become elongated into irregular *marginal osteophytes*. Not only do these interfere with the range of the joint's movement, but they may also become nipped off to form *loose bodies* (also called "joint-mice"). These are a constant nuisance because they tend to be caught between the opposing bone ends during movement; the result is "locking" of the joint, which may be excruciatingly painful if a fringe of synovium is included. A prominent site for osteophytes is the terminal interphalangeal joint of the fingers of elderly people. These produce the painless bony swellings called *Heberden's nodes*.

There is no primary synovial change, but later the membrane is thrown up into vascular villous folds. There is no inflammatory change except after locking, which produces a traumatic synovitis. These joints do not become ankylosed, but the destruction of articular cartilage and the osteophyte formation seriously limit movement, which may be very painful. Fortunately the operation of arthroplasty is now so successful that many people crippled with osteoarthritic hips have been restored to activity with artificial metallic joints (see p. 131).

**Tumours of Joints.** The only significant one is the *synovioma*, and this arises much more often from the synovial membrane of a tendon sheath than from a joint. It is usually a benign tumour with cleft-like spaces and large giant cells.

There is a condition of generalized proliferation of the synovium, which is reddish brown in colour, found most often in the knee joint. Histologically there are giant cells, lipid-filled macrophages, and haemosiderin in the synovial villi, and the condition is called *pigmented villonodular synovitis*. The histological picture resembles that of a synovioma, and it is probable that this is a benign synoviomatous change in a joint. The blood pigment may be the end-result of repeated trauma.

The malignant synovioma resembles other sarcomata in its general behaviour.

## General Reading

COLLINS, D. H. (1966). "Pathology of Bone". London: Butterworths.

## References

1. BLOOM, W. and FAWCETT, D. W. (1962). In "A Text-book of Histology", 8th ed., p. 153. Philadelphia: Saunders.
2. HAM, A. W. (1965). In "Histology", 5th ed., p. 384. Philadelphia and Montreal: Lippincott.
3. McLEAN, F. C. and BUDY, A. M. (1959). *Ann. Rev. Physiol.*, **21**, 69.
4. GOLDHABER, P. (1962). *New Engl. J. Med.*, **266**, 870.
5. BAKER, S. L. (1959). In "A Textbook of X-Ray Diagnosis", 3rd. ed., vol. 4, p. 55, ed. by Shanks, S. C. and Kerley, P. London: Lewis.
6. FOURMAN, P. (1963). In "Bone Metabolism in Relation to Clinical Medicine", p. 12, ed. by Sissons, H. A. London: Pitman.
7. FOURMAN, P. (1960). "Calcium Metabolism and the Bone". Oxford: Blackwell.
8. BALL, J. (1960). In "Recent Advances in Pathology", 7th ed., p. 293, ed. by Harrison, C. V. London: Churchill.
9. WIEME, R. T. and DEMEULENAERE, L. (1970). *J. clin. Path.*, **24**, Suppl. (*Ass. Clin. Path.*), **4**, 51.
10. FORLAND, M. (1962). *Amer. J. Med.*, **33**, 792.
11. McKUSICK, V. A. (1966). "Heritable Disorders of Connective Tissue", 3rd ed. St. Louis: Mosby.
12. HOUSTON, W. O. (1965). *J. oral Surg.*, **23**, 17.
13. ZEGARELLI, E. V. and KUTSCHER, A. H. (1963). *Dent. Radiog. Photog.*, **36**, 27.
14. JONES, W. A. (1965). *Oral Surg., Oral Med., Oral Path.*, **20**, 648.
15. JONES, W. A. (1933). *Amer. J. Cancer*, **17**, 946.
16. LUCAS, R. B. (1972). "Pathology of Tumours of the Oral Tissues", 2nd ed., p. 368. Eiinburgh: Churchill Livingstone.
17. SMITH, N. H. H. (1966). *Oral Surg., Oral Med., Oral Path.*, **22**, 699.
18. LEADING ARTICLE (1961). *Lancet*, **2**, 641.
19. DENT, C. E. (1962). *Brit. med. J.*, **2**, 1419 and 1495.
20. ROTH, S. I. (1962). *Arch. Path.*, **73**, 495.
21. DONIACH, I. (1960). In "Recent Advances in Pathology", 7th ed., p. 258. *loc. cit.*
22. PYRAH, L. N., HODGKINSON, A. and ANDERSON, C. K. (1966). *Brit. J. Surg.*, **59**, 245.

23. MULLIGAN, R. M. (1947). *Arch. Path.*, **43**, 177.
24. BURNETT, C. H. *et al.* (1964). *Amer. J. Med.*, **36**, 222.
25. BARTTER, F. C. (1957). *Amer. J. Med.*, **22**, 797.
26. FRASER, R. (1962). *J. Bone Jt. Surg.*, **44B**, 485.
27. URIST, M. R. (1959). In "Wound Healing and Tissue Repair", p. 65, ed. by Patterson, W. B. Chicago: The University of Chicago Press.
28. PRITCHARD, J. J. (1963). In "The Scientific Basis of Medicine Annual Reviews", p. 286. London: Athlone Press.
29. MÜLLER, M. E. (1969). In "Recent Advances in Orthopedics", p. 79, ed. by Apley, A. G. London: Churchill.
30. STANBURY, J. B., WYNGAARDEN, J. B. and FREDRICKSON, D. S. (1972). Edrs, "The Metabolic Basis of Inherited Disease", p. 730 *et seq.* New York: McGraw-Hill.
31. HSIA, D. Y., NAYLOR, J. and BIGLER, J. A. (1959). *New Engl. J. Med.*, **261**, 164.
32. CROCKER, A. C. and FARBER, S. (1958). *Medicine (Baltimore)*, **37**, 1.
33. JOHNSON, R. P. and MOHNAC, A. M. (1967). *J. oral Surg.*, **25**, 7.
34. LICHTENSTEIN, L. (1966). "Bone Tumors", 3rd ed. St. Louis: Mosby.

*Chapter 34*

# DISEASES OF THE CENTRAL NERVOUS SYSTEM

The brain and spinal cord are of such complexity that only those features of neuropathology which are relevant to dental surgery will be described in this chapter.

## Cellular Components

The important component of the central nervous system is the nerve cell, or *neurone*. The highly specialized neurones with their long axonal processes are held in position and insulated from each other by a specialized connective tissue called *neuroglia*. This has three components:

The *astrocytes* are closely associated with the bodies of the nerve cells and the blood vessels.

The *oligodendroglia* encloses the axons and forms their myelin sheaths, an insulating function which is essential for the conduction of nerve impulses.

The *microglia*, as the name implies, are small cells, and are of mesodermal, reticulo-endothelial origin.

The extreme susceptibility of the neurones to hypoxia has been noted previously (p. 380). Permanent brain damage can easily occur if the brain is rendered ischaemic; this may occur during periods of hypotension in the course of a surgical operation. Inadequate ventilation of the lungs with oxygen is not uncommon during the inexpert administration of nitrous oxide as an anaesthetic, and is another important cause of cerebral hypoxia.

## Meninges

The coverings, or *meninges*, of the central nervous system are three:

The *pia mater* closely envelops the brain and spinal cord.

The *dura mater* is closely adherent to the bony-ligamentous protective housing provided by the skull, vertebral column, and the connecting ligaments.

The thin, translucent *arachnoid* covering lies between the pia and the dura.

The space between the arachnoid and the pia is called the *subarachnoid space* and contains *cerebro-spinal fluid* (*CSF*). This fluid originates in the choroid plexuses, perfuses the ventricles, and finally escapes through the foramina in the roof of the fourth ventricle to reach the subarachnoid space.

## Effects of Increased Intracranial Pressure

Although the rigid bony enclosure of the brain is a necessary protective shield, its presence has some attendant disadvantages. Any lesion which takes up space within the skull (*space occupying lesion*) tends to cause a rise in intracranial pressure, and this increases the pressure in the veins. Initially some CSF and venous blood are displaced, but soon, as venous obstruction is produced, there is a marked rise in CSF pressure, which has very serious effects. If of sudden onset, the blood supply to the brain is so reduced that the cerebral hypoxia causes rapid *loss of consciousness*. When the lesion develops gradually, severe *headaches* are common, and there is also progressive *mental impairment*. The pressure on the venous return from the retina causes oedema which can be seen with an ophthalmoscope as swelling of the optic disc (*papilloedema*). Eventually *blindness* follows. *Haematoma, abscess* with inflammatory oedema, and *tumour* are examples of space occupying lesions.

### Traumatic Lesions of the Central Nervous System

An injury involving the jaws is sometimes accompanied by a much more important injury to the brain. Blows on the head produce damage to the region underlying the injury and to the brain at the opposite pole—this is the so-called *contre-coup injury*. Minor injuries cause petechial haemorrhages and traumatic inflammatory oedema, while more severe ones may actually tear the brain (*laceration*), and haemorrhage may be of sufficient magnitude to cause death. Some degree of haemorrhage into the subarachnoid space is common in all head injuries, and can be detected by examining the cerebro-spinal fluid obtained by lumbar puncture.

**Subdural Haemorrhage.** It sometimes happens that a venous sinus or vein is torn, and blood escapes into the loose subdural space to produce a subdural haematoma. If small, this is of little importance. If large, it organizes at the periphery and its centre remains fluid. The cyst which is formed imbibes fluid, and enlarges to form a *chronic subdural haematoma* which acts as a space occupying lesion. The injury which causes this type of lesion is often relatively mild, and in an elderly or alcoholic patient may be completely overlooked. Weeks later headaches and other signs and symptoms of raised intracranial pressure appear.

**Extradural Haemorrhage.** This occurs when the *middle meningeal artery* is torn, usually in association with a fracture of the skull involving the temporal region. Unconsciousness may occur immediately after the injury, but the patient often recovers and feels well for a few hours. This *lucid interval* is deceptive, for presently, as the bleeding proceeds. increasing signs of raised intracranial pressure appear, and are followed by coma and death. It is evident that all cases of head injury, except the most trivial, should be observed carefully for 24 hours. This applies particularly to persons suspected of being drunk—a state which may be mimicked by the combination of medicinal brandy given by a well-wisher and an extradural haemorrhage.

### Non-Traumatic Vascular Lesions

**Subarachnoid Haemorrhage.** This is not uncommon in the 20–50 year age-group. The haemorrhage stems from a ruptured aneurysm of one of the major cerebral arteries in the neighbourhood of the circle of Willis. The aneurysms lie in the subarachnoid space and are from 0·5 to 1·0 cm. in diameter—because of this size they are often called *berry aneurysms*. They are thought to arise at the site of congenital defects in the elastic coat of the arteries. Sometimes they are multiple.

**Cerebral Haemorrhage and Infarction.** Atheroma and hypertension both predispose to cerebral haemorrhage (sometimes called cerebral apoplexy). The common site is from the lenticulostriate artery, well named the artery of cerebral haemorrhage, and the region of the brain affected is therefore the internal capsule. The immediate effects of haemorrhage tend to be more severe than those produced by thrombosis. In both there is the clinical picture commonly called a "stroke".

*With haemorrhage* there is usually sudden loss of consciousness, and as blood disrupts the substance of the brain, coma deepens and death ensues. This is not, however, inevitable, and the bleeding may stop.

*Thrombosis* often occurs during sleep, and although consciousness may be lost this is not invariable. Thrombosis causes *infarction*, which can itself lead to later haemorrhage in the damaged area.

The infarct is usually pale, and in those patients who survive the area softens (colliquative necrosis). The microglial cells enlarge, become phago-cytic, and appear as large foamy macrophages. The damaged nerve fibres are not replaced to any extent, and the area heals by proliferation of astro-cytes to produce a *glial scar*. The area of brain thus collapses, and sometimes a central cyst remains where once were the long tracts from the motor cortex to the spinal cord. It should be noted that any nerve cells destroyed are not replaced.

In both haemorrhage and thrombosis the neurological picture is commonly that of *hemiplegia*—loss of voluntary movement on the side of the body opposite to that of the lesion.

Quite apart from acute episodes of thrombosis or infarction, cerebral atherosclerosis can lead to multiple, bilateral, ischaemic lesions in the brain. The characteristic mental deterioration of old age is one effect, but if the lesions are extensive there may be severe bilateral damage to the cortico-spinal tracts. Bilaterally innervated muscles such as those of the tongue and pharynx are affected, and the condition is called *pseudobulbar palsy*.

## Infections of the Central Nervous System

**Bacterial Infections.** Pyogenic bacteria may produce a diffuse infection of the subarachnoid space, which is called *meningitis*, or a localized suppuration in the brain substance (*cerebral abscess*).

### Meningitis

**Mode of Infection.** Two routes are common:

*Blood-borne. H. influenzae* and *N. meningitidis* (meningococcus) gain entry to the blood, presumably from an infection in the upper respiratory tract. The route is probably *via* the choroid plexuses, where the organisms are filtered out of the blood. The infection spreads through the ventricular system and reaches the subarachnoid space in the region of the basal cisterns. It is here that the most severe effects are seen. The pia and arachnoid are acutely inflamed, and there is a massive polymorph and fibrinous exudate into the subarachnoid space. With modern chemotherapy the patients often survive, but even then the exudate may undergo organization, and the foramina in the roof of the fourth ventricle become blocked. Cerebrospinal fluid accumulates in the ventricular system which expands accordingly—this is one mechanism whereby *hydrocephalus* develops. In the young child the pressure exerted on the developing bones leads to a tremendous enlargement of the vault in the skull.

Tuberculous meningitis is mentioned on p. 194.

*Local spread.* Meningitis may follow the spread of infection from the middle ear or mastoid air cells—sites of infection that used to be quite common in childhood. It is also a complication of a fractured skull when the wound is exposed to the exterior or the nasal cavity. Fracture of the cribriform plate of the ethmoid is followed by an escape of cerebrospinal fluid into the nose (*cerebrospinal rhinorrhoea*). Meningitis may follow.

## Cerebral Abscess

As with meningitis these are two modes of infection:

*Blood-borne.* Patients with chronic chest infections (empyema, lung abscess, and bronchiectasis) sometimes develop a cerebral abscess. The infection is presumably blood-borne; an alternative explanation is that spread occurs from an infected nasal air sinus—a common accompaniment of chronic chest suppuration.

*Local spread.* As with meningitis this occurs from an infected middle ear or nasal air sinus.

**Virus Infections.** A large number of virus types cause infection of the central nervous system, e.g. the viruses of mumps, rabies, and the various forms of arbovirus encephalitis. Poliomyelitis is described on p. 224.

## Tumours of the Central Nervous System

**Primary.** The tumours are the *gliomata,* and several types are described—the common one being the *astrocytoma.* A curious feature of all gliomata is that, although they are locally invasive and may metastasize within the central nervous system, *none of them ever produces distant metastases.* In spite of this the prognosis is very poor because of the difficulty in surgical removal.

The *meningioma* is a benign tumour arising from the arachnoid granulations of the dura; it is not therefore a tumour of the brain itself. Nevertheless, it is included here because the effects produced are very similar to those of a cerebral tumour. It produces pressure atrophy of the underlying brain, and, unless removed, kills the subject by its local effects or because of an increased intracranial pressure.

**Secondary Tumours.** These are more common than primary growths. Carcinoma of the lung in men and carcinoma of the breast in women are the common primary tumours in these cases.

### General Reading

BLACKWOOD, W., MCMENEMEY, W. H., MEYER, A., NORMAN, R. M. and RUSSELL, D. S. (1963). "Greenfield's Neuropathology", 2nd ed. London: Arnold.

RUSSELL, D. S. and RUBINSTEIN, L. J. (1963). "Pathology of Tumours of the Nervous System", 2nd ed. London: Arnold.

BIGGART, J. H. (1961). "Pathology of the Nervous System", 3rd ed. Edinburgh: Livingstone.

*Chapter 35*

# DISEASES OF THE ENDOCRINE GLANDS

**Introduction.** While the nervous system exerts major control of the activity of higher animals, there is an additional mechanism whereby one group of cells can influence another. This is by their secretion into the blood stream of potent chemicals (hormones), which, being carried by the circulation, can exert influence on some distant part. Secreting cells which perform this endocrine function are being recognized in increasing numbers, for not only are they situated in the well-known endocrine glands, but are also found scattered in other tissues. For instance, when food enters the pylorus, the hormone called *gastrin* is secreted, and this stimulates the fundus of the stomach to produce hydrochloric acid. When acid enters the duodenum, *secretin* is formed, and this causes the pancreas to pour out its alkaline juice.

This chapter deals only with the common disorders of the major endocrine glands.

**Mode of Action of Hormones.** Some insight into the potent and highly specific action of hormones is now being gained. Many protein and peptide hormones appear to act on specific receptor sites on the cell membrane, where they activate the adenyl cyclase enzyme system. This catalyses the conversion of adenosine triphosphate to 3′,5′-cyclic adenosine monophosphate (cyclic AMP), an agent which acts as a messenger within the cell and stimulates it to activity by regulating protein and RNA synthesis. Steroid hormones appear to act directly on specific nuclear receptors.

## The Pituitary Gland

Although small, the pituitary secretes an amazing variety and number of hormones.

**The posterior lobe** and the associated infundibulum and hypothalamus secrete antidiuretic hormone (ADH) and oxytocin, a hormone which causes the pregnant uterus to contract at term. The antidiuretic hormone (vasopressin) renders the distal tubules of the kidney more permeable to water, so that a concentrated urine is produced (p. 321). Destruction of the posterior lobe, e.g. by tumour, causes *diabetes insipidus*, the chief symptoms of which are the passage of huge quantities of very dilute urine and great thirst.

**The anterior lobe** produces seven hormones:

(1) Adrenocorticotrophic hormone—ACTH
(2) Melanocyte stimulating hormone—MSH
(3) Thyroid stimulating hormone—TSH
(4) Growth hormone—GH
(5) Follicle stimulating hormone—FSH

(6) Interstitial-cell stimulating hormone—ICSH; in the female this acts as a luteinizing hormone—LH

(7) Lactogenic hormone, or prolactin

## Disorders of the Pituitary

Hyperplasia or neoplasia of the anterior pituitary may be associated with the hypersecretion of one or several of the pituitary hormones. On the other hand, non-hormone-secreting tumours of the pituitary, or tumours arising in its neighbourhood, may press on and destroy the parenchyma and so lead to a diminished hormonal secretion. This also occurs when the pituitary is destroyed by other lesions, e.g. infarction or inflammation. The clinical picture may therefore be complex, and only the more common types will be outlined. Tumours in the pituitary region give rise to two additional characteristic effects due to their anatomical situation: compression on the optic chiasma causing loss of the temporal visual fields of both eyes (bitemporal hemianopia) and enlargement of the sella turcica which is detectable radiologically.

**Hyperpituitarism.** The acidophil cells are usually involved, and the effects of excessive growth hormone are predominant. If the condition arises in childhood the result is *gigantism*: the individual is well proportioned but huge. Hyperpituitarism after the epiphyses have fused leads to *acromegaly*.

Hyperplasia or an adenoma of the basophil cells may be the primary cause of Cushing's syndrome, which is described on p. 476. The pituitary secretes an excess of ACTH and MSH, and after adrenalectomy this overactivity can be even accentuated, so that generalized hyperpigmentation results, as in Addison's disease (p. 475).

**Hypopituitarism.** In children the effect is largely related to a lack of growth hormone, and well-proportioned dwarfism is the result. Puberty does not occur in these *Lorain-type*, or Peter Pan, individuals. Another less common presentation is that of overweight and somnolence, resembling the fat boy in Dickens's "Pickwick Papers". This is called *Fröhlich's syndrome*.

In adults hypopituitarism usually manifests itself as hypothyroidism with some evidence of adrenal cortical deficiency. It sometimes occurs after parturition, and is thought to be due to infarction of the gland. The condition is then called *Sheehan's syndrome*. The classical type of hypopituitarism, *Simmonds's disease*, in which extreme wasting is the main feature, is in fact very rare.

## The Thyroid Gland

The thyroid gland has the unique property of being able to trap iodine from the blood and incorporate it as thyroglobulin in the colloid of its vesicles. By the action of a proteolytic enzyme the iodine-containing thyroid hormones thyroxine and triiodothyronine are released. This occurs when the gland is stimulated by thyroid stimulating hormone (TSH) from the anterior pituitary. TSH secretion is itself stimulated by a low blood level of thyroid hormone.

The inconspicuous C-cells of the thyroid secrete calcitonin, but so far no syndrome has been described in relation to an excess or deficiency of this hormone.

**Action of the Thyroid Hormones.** In spite of much research the precise mode of action of the thyroid hormones is not known. However, much has been learned by comparing the normal individual (euthyroid) with those who suffer from excessive or diminished secretion (hyperthyroid and hypothyroid).

*A deficiency* causes:

A reduction in metabolic rate.

Impaired mental and physical growth. This is most marked in childhood.

Anaemia—this is less constant.

*Excessive secretion* increases the metabolic rate, and it has been suggested that there is uncoupling of oxidative phosphorylation, i.e. energy produced by oxidative metabolism is dissipated as heat, and is not stored in the high energy bonds of ATP. Since muscular contraction is dependent on ATP, this may explain why muscle weakness is a common symptom, and may at times be extreme.

**Goitre.** Any enlargement of the thyroid is called a goitre, and to a minor extent this occurs at times of stress, e.g. puberty and pregnancy. Indeed, in ancient Egypt the rupture of a thread tied round the neck of a bride was used as an indication of pregnancy. A more potent cause is a diet deficient in iodine, because the thyroid, being unable to manufacture its hormone, cannot check the secretion of TSH which stimulates it to activity. Before iodine was added to table salt, goitres were common in many parts of the world for this reason—in the Great Lakes area of North America, the Andes, the Himalayas, and Derbyshire, England. Repeated phases of hyperplasia followed by involution led to the formation of large nodular goitres containing many colloid-filled areas, some of which showed necrosis and dystrophic calcification (*nodular colloid goitre*).

The goitres associated with hyperthyroidism, Hashimoto's disease, and neoplasia are described later.

**Hypothyroidism.** Hypothyroidism used to be frequent in areas of endemic goitre, but it may also be due to causes other than iodine lack—for instance, a congenital absence of the thyroid gland. The effects in the child differ from those in the adult.

*Cretinism.* An insufficiency of thyroid hormone in the infant leads to cretinism. The child has a bloated face, protruding tongue, and vacant expression, and becomes mentally defective (Fig. 35.1). There is a retardation of growth with delayed ossification and delayed epiphyseal union. There is also delay in dental development.

*Myxoedema.* This is the manifestation of hypothyroidism in the adult. There is a reduction in mental and physical activity, and the patient exhibits a characteristic bloated appearance due to a curious oedema of the skin. There may be an increase in bone density due to a diminution in excretion of calcium and phosphorus.

**Hyperthyroidism.** This is also known as *thyrotoxicosis*, and occurs in two forms.

*Primary hyperthyroidism (Graves's disease).* This disease is characterized by a diffuse enlargement of the thyroid gland (goitre) due to a marked hyperplasia of its epithelial elements. There is a raised metabolic rate which

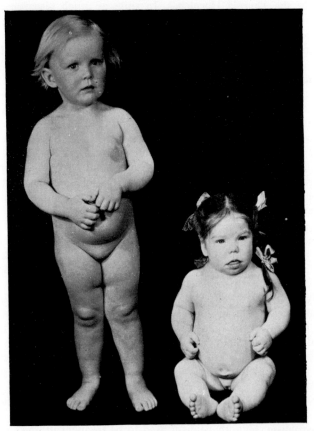

FIG. 35.1. Cretinism. Note the dwarfed appearance of the cretin as compared with a child of like age on her right. Other distinctive features are the torpid expression, round face, eyes set widely apart, enlarged protruding tongue, and the umbilical hernia.

(Photograph supplied by Mr. G. S. Hoggins.)

manifests itself by a persistent increase of the heart rate, and the individual is typically jumpy and nervous. The hands are warm and sweating; they are seldom at rest, and exhibit a fine tremor when the fingers are stretched out. The eyes have a characteristic appearance—the eyelids are retracted, giving the patient a staring expression; in severe cases the globe is actually pushed forwards to produce *exophthalmos*. The cause of thyrotoxicosis is not known. An *exophthalmos-producing factor* has been isolated from the blood, and so also has a thyroid stimulating substance. The latter is not TSH, for its action is slower—hence its name, *long-acting thyroid stimulating factor* (*LATS*). It is not of pituitary origin, and it has been suggested that it is an antibody formed in the lymphoreticular system.

If left untreated, thyrotoxicosis often terminates in heart failure. In long-standing cases osteoporosis may occur. This is due to an increased osteoclastic activity which leads to the excessive excretion of calcium and phosphorus in the urine.

*Secondary hyperthyroidism.* This occurs as a secondary phenomenon in a patient who is already suffering from a goitre from some other cause, e.g. iodine deficiency. The disease is less severe than Graves's disease, and exophthalmos does not occur.

**Hashimoto's Disease.** Like most thyroid disease this is more common in women than men. The gland is diffusely enlarged, showing atrophy of its epithelial elements and a massive infiltration with lymphocytes and plasma cells. There are immunoglobulin antibodies to thyroglobulin present in the blood, and their detection is of value in diagnosis. It seems unlikely that these antibodies are destructive to the thyroid tissue, and if Hashimoto's disease is an autoimmune disease, the antibodies concerned are probably cell-bound (p. 171).

**Tumours.** Benign encapsulated nodules in the thyroid gland are common, but the majority are probably focal areas of hyperplasia. These are usually multiple (nodular colloid goitre).

*Carcinoma* was apparently not uncommon in goitrous districts, but is nowadays distinctly rare.

### The Adrenal Glands

#### The Adrenal Medulla

The cells of the adrenal medulla liberate adrenaline (epinephrine) and noradrenaline (norepinephrine) in response to sympathetic stimulation. These hormones cause a redistribution of blood such that the individual is better adapted for fight or flight. A rare tumour, the *phaeochromocytoma*, derived from the medulla secretes these agents in excess and leads to systemic hypertension.

#### The Adrenal Cortex

Three major groups of hormones (corticosteroids) are secreted:

*Glucocorticoids*, e.g. corticosterone, hydrocortisone (cortisol), and cortisone. In physiological concentrations these accelerate the synthesis of glucose from non-carbohydrate precursors, and inhibit the actions of insulin.

*Mineralocorticoids*, e.g. aldosterone. This primarily affects electrolyte metabolism. It causes sodium retention and increases potassium loss in the urine.

*Sex hormones*, e.g. oestrogen, androgens, and progesterone.

**Adrenal Insufficiency—Addison's Disease.** Idiopathic atrophy, perhaps by an autoimmune process, or destruction, usually by tuberculosis, is the cause of Addison's disease. A low blood pressure, loss of appetite, loss of weight, weakness, and eventual death are the main features. As would be expected there is hypoglycaemia, a fall in serum sodium (*hyponatraemia*), and a rise in serum potassium (*hyperkalaemia*). The skin and mucous membranes, including the oral mucosa, show increased melanin pigmentation. This is because the low plasma hydrocortisone level stimulates the excessive production of pituitary ACTH and MSH. Both these hormones, especially MSH, cause a darkening of the skin by an effect on the melanocytes.

**Adrenal Hypersecretion.** Idiopathic hyperplasia, adenoma, or rarely carcinoma may be associated with hypersecretion of corticosteroids. The clinical pictures are often mixed, but three main patterns may be discerned.

*Adrenogenital syndrome.* In boys puberty may occur prematurely, even as early as four years ("infantile Hercules"). In girls male characteristics may develop. In adult women this masculinization is called *virilism*, e.g. atrophy of breasts, cessation of menstruation, growth of beard, deepening of the voice, etc.

*Conn's syndrome.* Excess aldosterone secretion produces a low serum potassium, sodium and water retention, and hypertension.

*Cushing's syndrome.* The major features are obesity, hyperglycaemia, osteoporosis, hypertension, and increased body hair growth in women. The syndrome, or mild forms of it, is commonly seen when corticosteroids (hydrocortisone, prednisone, etc.) are administered in pharmacological doses. Rounding and swelling of the face (moon face) is particularly characteristic.

**Uses and Complications of Glucocorticosteroid Therapy.** Although the mode of action of corticosteroids is not understood, the following effects and complications should be noted:

*Anti-inflammatory action*—this may be used to advantage when bacterial inflammation might produce serious damage, e.g. in the eye. Antibiotics must also be administered, otherwise the infection may spread.

*Lymphoid atrophy and depression of the immune response.* This may be used to advantage in treating acute lymphatic leukaemia, autoimmune diseases, and hypersensitivity states, e.g. asthma.

*Infection, particularly tuberculosis,* may occur due to the actions above lighting up a quiescent focus.

*Interferon production is inhibited.* Virus infections may therefore be aggravated.

*Wound healing, contraction, granulation tissue formation, and collagen formation* are all inhibited.

*Osteoporosis.* Collapse of vertebrae and other fractures may occur after trivial injury.

*Peptic ulcer and its complications* are more common.

*Diabetes mellitus* may develop.

*Cataract* formation is a further complication.

*Cushing's syndrome.* See above.

## The Islets of Langerhans

### Diabetes Mellitus

This is a disorder of carbohydrate metabolism due to a disturbance of the normal insulin mechanism. *Insulin* is a hormone secreted by the $\beta$ cells of the pancreatic islets of Langerhans. It promotes the entry of glucose into the body's cells, where the glucose is metabolized: most is oxidized to $CO_2$ and water, while the remainder is either converted into neutral fat, stored as glycogen, or used in the formation of amino acids and glycoproteins.

**Effects of Insulin Deficiency.** Glucose metabolism is severely impaired. Its level in the blood—normally 70–100 mg. per cent in the fasting state—rises;

this is called *hyperglycaemia*, and when it exceeds 170–180 mg. per cent, it escapes into the urine (*glycosuria*). Its presence leads to an increased secretion of urine in order to contain it, an effect called *osmotic diuresis*. This leads to a loss of water and electrolytes, and the patient becomes dehydrated.

Furthermore protein is broken down to amino acids, which are metabolized in the liver to form glucose. This process of *gluconeogenesis* is associated with an increased excretion of nitrogenous substances in the urine with resulting bodily wasting. There is also an increased breakdown of fat in the adipose tissue, and the plasma level of free fatty acids rises. Most of these are oxidized to $CO_2$ and water, but where there is a great excess, some of the fatty acids are converted by the liver into *ketone bodies*, e.g. acetone, acetoacetic acid, and $\beta$-hydroxybutyric acid. This condition of *diabetic ketosis* is extremely dangerous, for unless treated at once with insulin, the patient lapses into a state of severe metabolic acidosis and coma, which terminates rapidly in death.

The main symptoms of diabetes mellitus are the passage of large amounts of urine (polyuria) and thirst.

**Types of Diabetes Mellitus.** The tendency to develop diabetes mellitus is inherited, but it seems likely that environmental factors are also important. The disease occurs in two clinical forms.

*Early-onset diabetes.* This affects children and young adults, and appears to be due to an absolute failure of the pancreas to secrete insulin. The disease is severe, wasting is marked, and without treatment the patients die in diabetic coma.

*Maturity-onset diabetes.* This occurs in the middle-aged and elderly. The amount of insulin in the blood is normal or may actually be raised, but for reasons which are not clearly understood it is not fully utilized. This may be due to the presence of insulin antagonists (perhaps antibodies), an abnormality in the type of insulin, or an unresponsiveness of the tissues themselves. Glucose utilization by adipose tissue is not impaired, and fat therefore accumulates. These patients are usually obese, their diabetes is mild, and they can often be treated successfully by diet alone.

## Complications of Diabetes Mellitus

*Diabetic ketosis and coma.*

*Susceptibility to infection*, both pyogenic and tuberculous. Oral sepsis is common.

*Vascular disease.* Diabetics are liable to more severe atheroma than are non-diabetic subjects of like age. In addition there is a characteristic thickening of the intimal layer of small vessels. The combined effect is to produce severe ischaemia affecting particularly the heart, limbs, kidney, nerves, and retina. This causes:

*Coronary thrombosis;*

*Gangrene of the legs,* usually of the true, or "wet", variety;

*Renal disease.* Sometimes the nephrotic syndrome but ultimately chronic renal failure ensues;

*Retinal damage,* leading to blindness.

The balance between insulin and glucose requirement is easily upset by infection and trauma. Any diabetic patient who is subjected to surgery should therefore have skilled medical treatment.

## General Reading

CATT, K. J. (1970). Lancet, **1**, 763, 827, 933, 1097, 1275 and 1383, and **2**, 255 and 353. Series of articles entitled "ABC of Endocrinology".

MARTIN, L. (1964). "Clinical Endocrinology", 4th ed. London: Churchill.

MEANS, J. H., DeGROOT, L. J. and STANBURY, J. B. (1963). "The Thyroid and its Diseases". New York: McGraw-Hill.

WHITE, P. (1965). Edr., A symposium on diabetes, *The Medical Clinics of North America*, **49**, 855 *et seq*. Philadelphia and London: Saunders.

WILLIAMS, R. H. (1962). "Textbook of Endocrinology", 3rd ed. Philadelphia: Saunders.

*Chapter* 36

## DISEASES OF THE SKIN

### Introduction

The number of diseases of the skin which have been described in the literature far exceeds that of any other individual organ. There are many reasons for this: the skin is exposed to the external environment and is a complex, composite organ. It contains hair follicles with associated sebaceous glands, eccrine and apocrine sweat glands, a surface epithelium, and a connective-tissue element with a loose papillary dermis between the epithelial elements and the reticular dermis, itself composed of dense collagenous bundles and coarse elastic fibres. The ease with which the skin can be examined and biopsied and the importance that mankind has given to its appearance have further added to the complexity of dermatology. This chapter describes some common skin reactions, particularly those which may also affect the oral mucosa. Some diseases, e.g. pemphigus vulgaris and lichen planus, can affect the mouth either initially or to a major extent. Biopsy of these mucosal lesions is sometimes difficult, and histological interpretation is frequently unsatisfactory. The finding of more typical lesions on the skin is therefore rewarding, since skin biopsy is easy and pathological interpretation clear-cut.

### Terminology

An area of altered skin, usually red (erythematous), whether pigmented or non-pigmented is, if flat and not palpable, called a *macule* if less than 1·0 cm. in diameter and a *patch* if larger. Similar areas which are palpable (usually they are raised and indurated, but in atrophic conditions may be depressed) are called *papules* if small and *plaques* if over 1·0 cm. in diameter. A lesion containing a visible accumulation of clear fluid is a *vesicle* if small and a *bulla* if large (over 0·5 cm. or 1·0 cm. according to definition). *Pustules* contain pus. If flakes of keratin are seen obviously adherent to the lesion it is called *squamous*, while shallow *erosions*, or *ulcers*, are termed *excoriations* if they are produced by mechanical trauma of scratching. *Crusts* consist of dried serum and other debris.

### Dermatitis

Dermatitis or eczema are synonymous terms used to describe a particular skin-reaction pattern which primarily involves the epidermis. Three stages are recognized, the initial acute reaction passing into the subacute and chronic phases if the cause persists.

**Acute Dermatitis.** The epidermis shows intercellular oedema (*spongiosis*) which terminates in the separation of epidermal cells and the formation of vesicles or bullae. The dermis shows a perivascular infiltrate composed mostly of lymphocytes (Fig. 36.1). The vesicles may rupture, and clinically acute dermatitis presents as palpable erythematous vesicular lesions which may rupture and leave a weeping or crusted surface.

**Subacute Dermatitis.** Spongiosis and vesicle formation are still evident, but the epidermis reacts by increased mitotic activity so that it becomes thicker (*acanthosis*). Keratinization is disturbed with the result that, in places, the granular layer is absent and the overlying mature keratinocytes retain their nuclei (*parakeratosis*).

**Chronic Dermatitis.** Spongiosis is scanty or absent but acanthosis is marked. Excess keratin is formed (*hyperkeratosis*), and in places there is parakeratosis (Fig. 36.2). Clinically, chronic dermatitis appears as indurated scaly papules or plaques, and the skin markings tend to be accentuated. This latter process is known as *lichenification*.

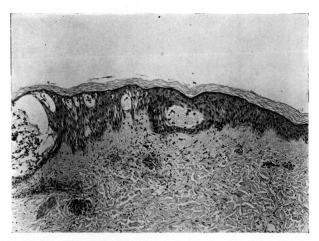

Fig. 36.1. Acute dermatitis. This is an example of acute allergic contact dermatitis due to poison ivy. The epidermis shows spongiosis, and in many places the cells have torn apart to produce intra-epidermal vesicles. The largest of these is on the left-hand side, and contains coagulated exudate and a number of inflammatory cells, mainly lymphocytes. The dermis shows a mild inflammatory reaction, again with a lymphocytic infiltrate. ×120.

The causes and clinical types of dermatitis are many and various. Externally applied chemical irritants are a frequent cause of dermatitis (contact dermatitis); a common example is the chronic lichenified hand eczema seen in housewives whose hands are repeatedly in contact with water, detergents, and other household agents. Alkalis, acids, and many industrial chemicals can act as primary irritants, and if applied over a long period lead to refractory chronic dermatitis. Individuals with a dry skin, and particularly elderly people, may develop dermatitis due to exposure to water, soaps, and detergents which, to a normal person, are harmless. An example of a potent chemical which acts as a primary irritant is mustard gas, a volatile liquid invented specifically for its ability to produce an acute dermatitis.

The development of cell-mediated sensitizing antibodies toward chemicals results in the production of *allergic contact dermatitis*. Iodine, formaldehyde, dyes, plants, and nickel used in jewellery are amongst the many agents which can cause this allergic type of dermatitis. It should be noted that the skin of the face is particularly sensitive and can react to agents which elsewhere cause little trouble. Thus, dermatitis around the eyes can be due to a nail-polish which causes no trouble on the hands. Ultraviolet light may act on chemicals present in the skin (either applied topically or taken systemically) and so alter them as to cause either direct irritant effects (*phototoxic dermatitis*), or the formation of a new antigen and subsequent sensitization (*photoallergic dermatitis*). Agents which are well known to cause this sensitizing effect when applied topically are perfumes, coal-tar derivatives, and halogenated salicylanilides (used in deodorant soap). The face is commonly affected, and

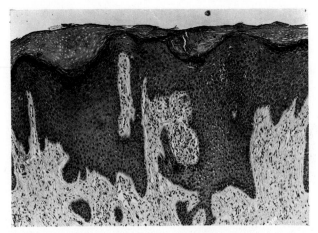

Fig. 36.2. Chronic dermatitis. The epidermis shows marked hyperkeratosis and acanthosis with irregular elongation of the rete ridges. There is a focus of parakeratosis, and the dermis shows a sparse infiltration by lymphocytes. The changes should be compared with normal skin present on the right-hand side of Fig. 36. 1. ×120.

an example of particular interest is the sensitizing effect that the eosin in lipstick has in the production of sun-sensitive cheilitis.

Many drugs taken internally have a similar effect, e.g. chemotherapeutic agents (sulphonamides, tetracycline, and griseofulvin), diuretics (chloro-thiazide), and tranquillizers (phenothiazines and chlorpromazine), to mention some of the main groups. It is evident that with any patient who has a disease of the skin or mucous membrane, the nature of which is not imme-diately apparent, it is of great importance to enquire what drugs have been applied locally or used systemically.

Infantile eczema and atopic dermatitis occur in atopic individuals, but the pathogenesis is obscure, for although the associated respiratory symptoms appear to be caused by a type I hypersensitivity reaction, the skin lesions are more complex and the damage may be cell-mediated (see page 166). A feature of some forms of dermatitis, including the atopic variety, is marked itching (pruritus); this leads to scratching and self-perpetuation due to continued physical trauma. The condition is then referred to as *chronic neurodermatitis*. Localized plaques of neurodermatitis due to scratching—the back of the neck and the front of the ankle are favourite sites—are referred to as *lichen simplex chronicus*.

### Papulosquamous Eruptions

The description of this wide group of dissimilar diseases, which includes secondary syphilis and ringworm, will be restricted to two common examples, both of unknown aetiology.

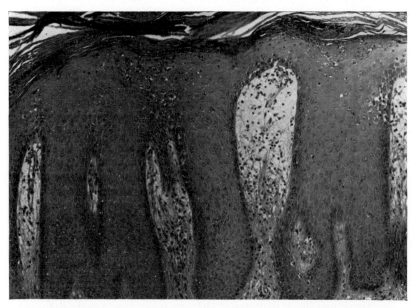

FIG. 36.3. Psoriasis of the skin. The epidermis shows marked hyperkeratosis, parakeratosis, and acanthosis. The elongation of the rete ridges is particularly well shown, and the broad club-shaped processes are seen to anastomose on the left side of the picture. The papillae between the rete ridges exhibit the highly characteristic vasodilatation and oedema. There is a sparse inflammatory infiltrate in this part of the dermis, and cells are seen to be migrating through the epidermis. These cells are for the most part polymorphonuclear leukocytes, and small collections of them appearing in the keratin layer are a characteristic feature of psoriasis. They are called Munro micro-abscesses. ×120.

**Psoriasis** occurs as scaly papules and plaques commonly situated on the elbows, knees, and other extensor surfaces. It frequently affects the scalp and adjacent forehead but the oral cavity is rarely involved. Histologically, it resembles chronic dermatitis, but the acanthosis involves a regular elongation of the rete ridges and the intervening papillary dermis is usually oedematous and vascular (Fig. 36.3).

**Lichen planus** occurs as pruritic, somewhat violaceous, flat-topped papules. Any site may be involved but common areas are around the wrists and

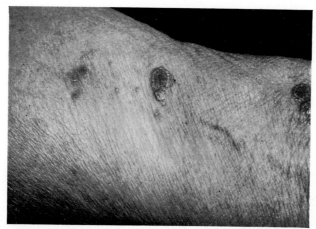

FIG. 36.4. Lichen planus on the anterior aspect of the wrist. The lesions are flat-topped papules and show the diagnostic white lines called Wickham's striae. In this case they are well shown around the periphery of the larger papules. The faint dark circle near the edge of the large central papule indicates the area which was biopsied. It showed the typical appearance of lichen planus, and the changes, particularly the prominent granular layer, were most pronounced in the region of the striae.

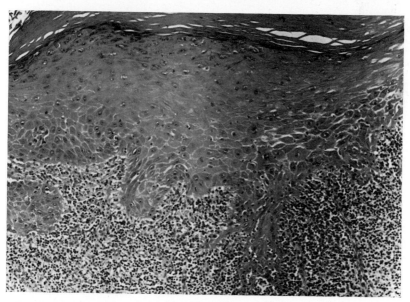

FIG. 36.5. Lichen planus of the skin. The epidermis shows marked hyper-keratosis, but there is complete absence of parakeratotic nuclei. The granular layer is increased in prominence, and the epidermis shows acanthosis with elongation of some rete ridges. The basal layer of the epidermis has been replaced by flattened cells, and the epidermis has a saw-tooth appearance. The characteristic band of lymphocytic infiltrate in the papillary dermis is well shown. × 120.

ankles. The mucous membranes are commonly affected, and in about 15 per cent of cases these are the only areas involved. In the oral mucosa the lesions are white and form a lace-like network on the buccal mucosa. The glans penis which is another common situation. Lichen planus of the oral mucosa is rarely followed by malignancy. (Fig. 36.4.)

Lichen planus of the skin has a very characteristic histological appearance. There is acanthosis and hyperkeratosis, but three features distinguish typical lesions sharply from those of chronic dermatitis and psoriasis:

1. Parakeratosis is absent.

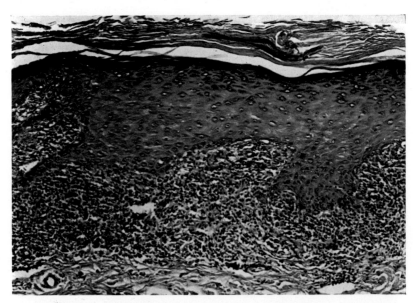

FIG. 36.6. Lichen planus of oral mucosa. The appearances are very similar to those shown in Fig. 36.5. The prominent granular layer is well shown; normally the oral mucosa does not show this. Occasional parakeratotic nuclei are seen in the keratin layer, a feature not seen in lichen planus of the skin. The loss of the basal-cell layer is particularly well shown. The lymphocytic infiltrate is closely applied to the epithelium, and in places cells are migrating between the epithelial cells. × 120.

2. There is hydropic degeneration or loss of the basal-cell layer of the epidermis.

3. The superficial, or papillary, dermis shows a dense well-delineated band of lymphocytic infiltration. (Fig. 36.5.)

The oral lesions are similar in appearance except that, as with the normal mucosa, parakeratosis is present. (Fig. 36.6.)

### Diseases Characterized by a Dermal Inflammatory Reaction

An inflammatory reaction in the dermis is present in many skin diseases including those which appear primarily to affect the epidermis, e.g. dermatitis and psoriasis. A localized area of dermal inflammation is a feature of many infections, e.g. tuberculosis and erysipelas, but there is a group of conditions in which a widespread vascular reaction occurs for no very apparent reason. The most mild example in this group is urticaria.

**Urticaria.** In acute urticaria ("hives"), there is an acute inflammatory reaction in the dermis with vasodilatation, mild polymorph accumulation, and marked oedema. Multiple areas of dermal oedema occur, at first red but later becoming pale. The lesions resemble the changes seen in triple response of Lewis (page 72). Acute urticaria may be a type I hypersensitivity reaction mediated by IgE, but is also seen in immune-complex disease. It follows the ingestion of a particular food or drug, and as with other hypersensitivity reactions, small quantities of the agent can be sufficient to induce an attack. Thus, the menthol in a cigarette or toothpaste can precipitate acute urticaria in a sensitized person. Repeated attacks of urticaria may occur over many years (chronic urticaria), and in these patients the cause is rarely found.

Urticaria affects the dermis. When the subcutaneous tissues are also involved, the condition is termed *angio–oedema*. In both urticaria and angio-oedema the mucous membranes, including that of the tongue, can be involved. In one type of hereditary angio–oedema, there is a deficiency of Cl-esterase inhibitor. This is a serious condition, for lesions occur in the intestine causing colic, and in the larynx causing death from asphyxiation.

**Toxic Erythema.** This general term is applied to many conditions in which the epidermis is normal, at least in the early stages, but there is a dermal inflammatory reaction showing vasodilatation and a perivascular collection of cells, chiefly lymphocytes. As an acute condition toxic erythema accompanies many virus infections (e.g. measles, German measles, and infectious mononucleosis) and the intake of drugs. Damage to blood vessels by immune complexes is the probable pathogenesis.

**Erythema multiforme.** This may be regarded as a severe variant of toxic erythema. The onset is sudden and the patient rapidly develops symmetrical lesions of varying types—urticarial, erythematous macules and papules, and sometimes vesicles. Target, or iris, lesions are characteristic. The dermal oedema is sometimes so marked that it progresses to form a subepidermal vesicle or bulla. The dermal reaction causes secondary degenerative changes in the epidermis. The severity of the dermal inflammatory reaction and the degenerate appearance of the epidermal roof serve to distinguish these lesions from those of bullous pemphigoid (see below). Erythema multiforme is often idiopathic, but it sometimes appears to be precipitated by a variety of factors, e.g. previous herpes simplex of the lips, drug intake, exposure to sunlight, to mention but a few. Erythema multiforme tends to affect the extremities, and can also cause lesions on the mucosal membranes. Severe cases of erythema multiforme which affect the oral mucosa are termed the *Stevens-Johnson syndrome.*

## Vesiculo-bullous Diseases

The formation of vesicles or bullae is the outstanding feature of this group of diseases, and for accurate diagnosis a biopsy of an *early* lesion is often necessary, because the situation of the vesicle is of vital importance in differential diagnosis. Some vesicles are intra–epidermal, while others form beneath the epidermis. It should be noted that a late subepidermal vesicle becomes intra–epidermal as tongues of regenerative epidermis cover the base. This is one of the reasons for biopsying an early lesion.

### Subepidermal Vesicles

**Bullous pemphigoid.** A dermal inflammatory reaction is followed by the formation of a subepidermal vesicle. The disease is not uncommon, and is characterized by the occurrence of crops of *tense* vesicles and bullae appearing on the trunk and sometimes on the mucous membranes. The disease is chronic, tends to occur in elderly people, and is sometimes the first manifestation of a tumour of some internal organ. A disease with similar histology, *benign cicatrizing mucosal pemphigoid*, affects the oral mucosa and the conjunctiva.

**Erythema multiforme.** This has already been described.

**Dermatitis herpetiformis.** In this disease groups of vesicles appear, and are severely pruritic. Histologically, the dermis shows an inflammatory reaction initially restricted to the papillae and characterized by the presence of numerous eosinophils. The mucous membranes are rarely affected.

**Porphyria cutanea tarda** and **epidermolysis bullosa** are rare causes of subepidermal bulla formation.

### Intra-epidermal Vesicles

The superficial subcorneal vesicles and pustules of candidiasis and impetigo can generally be diagnosed clinically without the aid of biopsy. So also can the spongiotic vesicles of acute and subacute dermatitis. The fluid in these vesicles contains inflammatory exudate, but a few detached epidermal cells may be present. This contrasts with an important group of blistering diseases in which the vesicles are formed as a result of a loss of adherence between adjacent epidermal cells. The detached cells become rounded off and lie free in the fluid. This process is called *acantholysis*, and is a dominant feature of two groups of diseases.

1. **The Pemphigus Group.** In pemphigus vulgaris the acantholytic process commences immediately above the basal layer of the epidermis, so that a suprabasal acantholytic cleft is formed. The basal layer remains unaffected and resembles a columnar epithelium covering the dermal papillae (Fig. 36.7). The term papillomatosis is applied to this appearance. Clinically, the patient develops *flaccid* vesicles and bullae which rupture leaving extensive raw areas. The distinction from bullous pemphigoid is important, because pemphigus vulgaris is often fatal and can be kept under control only by heavy immunosuppression. Bullous pemphigoid is chronic and tiresome but rarely fatal. Pemphigus vulgaris often affects the oral mucosa; sometimes this is the predominant and presenting symptom.

2. **The Virus Vesicle Group.** In zoster, varicella, smallpox, vaccina, and herpes simplex, acantholytic intra–epidermal vesicles are formed. Fusion of epidermal cells may produce multinucleate giant cells; some of these are acantholytic and seem to be floating free within the vesicle. There is a marked dermal inflammatory reaction present in most examples. The distinction between the individual members of this group is difficult to make histolo-

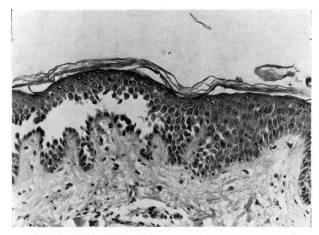

Fig. 36.7. Pemphigus vulgaris. The epidermal cells are seen to lack cohesion, so that an intraepidermal vesicle is formed. Isolated acantholytic cells lie in the cavity. It can readily be appreciated that the vesicle will be flaccid, and that pressure on it will result in lateral extension. This is known as Nikolsky's sign. The papillae of the dermis are covered by a layer of relatively unaffected basal cells which have been likened to a row of tomb-stones. ×200.

cially, but electron microscopy of the vesicle fluid and other virological techniques can be used to identify the cause.

### The Collagen Diseases

Two diseases in this group (see page 172) primarily affect the skin.

**Lupus Erythematosus.** In *systematic lupus erythematosus* many organs are affected—kidney, serous membranes, joints, brain, heart, and skin. The characteristic skin eruption is a diffuse erythema of the malar regions ("butterfly rash"). In *chronic discoid lupus erythematosus* lesions are confined to the skin, generally the face and other sun-exposed areas. Patients frequently complain that sunlight makes the disease worse. The lesions are well defined, erythematous, and scaly, and show evidence of atrophy. When the scalp is involved, there is hair loss (*alopecia*). Indeed, lupus erythematosus is an important cause of alopecia with scarring, and the lesions are very similar to those produced by lichen planus and scleroderma of the scalp. The oral mucosa is affected in about 15 per cent of cases of chronic discoid lupus erythematosus; the lesions are erythematous and hyperkeratotic so that leukoplakia is simulated. The histopathology of both the localized and systemic types of lupus is very similar, but whereas the chronic discoid variety generally shows more scarring and atrophy and remains localized, the systemic type is serious and death is often due to renal involvement or the effect of immunosuppressive therapy. (Fig. 36.8.)

**Scleroderma.** This disease also occurs as a localized form (*morphoea*) involving any area of skin, and a systemic variety (*systemic sclerosis*) which affects large areas of skin as well as internal organs—particularly the oeso-phagus, other parts of the gastro-intestinal tract, and the kidneys. Dysphagia is sometimes a marked feature, and oesophageal reflux may lead to a foul taste in the mouth. A characteristic oral radiological finding in scleroderma is widening of the periodontal membrane. The major cutaneous lesion is an increase in thickness of the dermis by fibrous tissue, so that the skin becomes indurated and bound down. When this affects the face, an immobile mask-like appearance with pinching of the nose is characteristic. Systemic sclerosis is often associated with Raynaud's syndrome (see page 382).

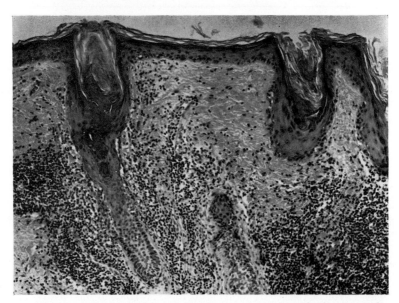

Fig. 36.8. Chronic discoid lupus erythematosus. The epidermis shows atrophy which, in this slide, is particularly marked around the orifices of the hair follicles. There is hyperkeratosis, and the hair follicles are atrophic and their mouths filled with keratinous plugs. The basal layer of the epidermis is poorly seen, and in some areas there is a vacuolated appearance due to hydropic degeneration of the basal cells. In the dermis there is a patchy lymphocytic inflammatory infiltrate which has a tendency to be arranged around hair follicles. In the follicle on the left, the inflammatory infiltrate is closely applied to the epithelial cells so that the junction between the two is poorly seen. ×120.

## Hamartomata

The hamartomata of the skin are termed naevi. The common melanotic and angiomatous varieties are considered elsewhere.

## Tumours of the Skin

**Squamous-cell Papilloma** is generally used as a descriptive term which covers a number of separate entities. One variety is present at birth and is a type of hamartoma termed an *epithelial naevus*. Although non-neoplastic and benign, it often recurs after simple removal by curettage. The common wart (*verruca vulgaris*) is a type of papilloma due to an infection by one of the papovaviruses. In elderly people it is very common to find multiple *seborrhoeic* *keratoses* on the backs of the hands, trunk, and face. They are papillomata often with considerable acanthosis and melanin pigmentation. Clinically they appear to be "stuck on" the surface of the skin either as elevated warty papillomata or as flat, roughened, pigmented plaques. Curettage effects an easy cure. They are not premalignant, but when heavily pigmented are liable to be confused with other pigmented lesions—melanotic naevi, pigmented basal-cell carcinoma, Hutchinson's freckle, or malignant melanoma.

Other benign tumours are not uncommon: fibroma, lipoma, neurofibroma, etc. These will not be further considered.

### Malignant Tumours of the Skin

The most common malignant tumour of the skin in white races is the basal-cell carcinoma (page 265). See Fig. 36.9.

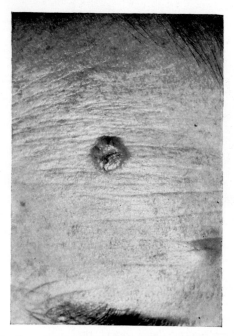

FIG. 36.9. Basal-cell carcinoma on the right side of the forehead of a 56-year-old man. The lesion has the typical appearance with a depressed centre and a raised, rolled edge over which dilated blood vessels can be see traversing. The dome-shaped swelling just above the medial aspect of the eyebrow has the features of an epidermoid cyst, commonly called a sebaceous cyst, or wen.

**Squamous-cell Carcinoma.** This tumour commonly arises on the sun-exposed skin in a pre-existing *actinic keratosis* (Fig. 36.10). Actinic keratoses are areas of epidermal dysplasia caused by prolonged, repeated exposure to sunlight. They appear as scaly erythematous areas on the face or hands, and in contradistinction to seborrhoeic keratoses, they must be regarded as precancerous. Squamous-cell carcinoma arising in an actinic keratosis is invasive, but metastasis is late and the prognosis is good. Squamous-cell carcinoma may also arise in normal skin or in a chronic erythematous lesion called *Bowen's disease*. This is a type of *carcinoma-in-situ*, and can occur on any part of the body. This type of squamous-cell carcinoma is more malignant than that arising in an actinic keratosis. Squamous-cell carcinoma must be differentiated both clinically and pathologically from a keratoacanthoma, which it closely resembles and which also occurs on a sun-exposed area (see page 232).

**Melanoma.** Malignant melanoma of the skin can arise in three ways:

1. In *normal skin*. Some tumours invade the dermis early (*nodular melanoma*), and also metastasize early so that the prognosis is very bad.

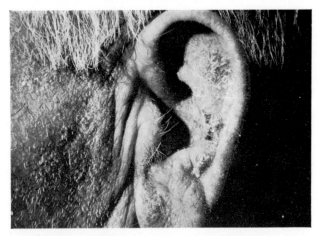

FIG. 36.10. Actinic keratoses on the left ear of an elderly man who had spent much of his working life out of doors. The lesions are erythematous and hyperkeratotic. The epidermal dysplasia is a precursor of carcinoma, and an area of crusting in the centre was regarded as suspicious. Biopsy at this site revealed no evidence of squamous-cell carcinoma.

Other tumours have a much better prognosis, for although they involve the epidermis and papillary dermis over an area, there is no early deep invasion (*superficial spreading melanoma*).

2. In *pre-existing naevocellular naevi* the incidence of malignancy is unknown, but considering the number of naevi in the average person, it must be very uncommon. Danger signals which suggest malignancy are a recent increase in size, ulceration, bleeding, and change in colour.

3. In *Hutchinson's freckle*. Hutchinson's freckle is a pigmented patch or plaque usually on the face, which microscopically shows atypical proliferation of melanocytes in the basal layer of the epidermis. It may be regarded as a *melanoma-in-situ*. After many years the melanocytic cells invade the dermis, and malignant melanoma develops. Even then the prognosis is good, in contradistinction to malignant melanoma which arises on normal skin.

Other malignant tumours of the skin, for example lymphomata (*mycosis fungoides*) and sarcomata, occur but are very uncommon.

The management of skin tumours is beyond the scope of this book, but it should be emphasized that before radical treatment is undertaken a positive biopsy must be obtained. The hypothetical possibility of disseminating tumour by biopsy, even in the case of malignant melanoma, is more than offset by the tragedy of treating a benign lesion by radical means. The study of skin tumours has highlighted several curious pseudomalignant lesions. Thus, keratoacanthoma closely mimics carcinoma, nodular fasciitis resembles sarcoma, and before diagnosing malignant lymphoma of the skin it is necessary to exclude certain pseudolymphomatous lesions which may arise spontaneously (pseudolymphoma of Spiegler-Fendt) or as a result of trauma such as an insect or tick bite.

## References

1. LEVER, F. W. (1967). "The Histopathology of the Skin", 4th edn, 794 pp., Philadelphia: Lippincott.
2. MILNE, J. A. (1972). "An Introduction to the Diagnostic Histopathology of the Skin", 363 pp. London: Arnold.
3. ROOK, A., WILKINSON, D. S. and EBLING, F. J. G. (1972), edit. "Textbook of Dermatology", 2nd edn, 2118 pp. Oxford: Blackwell. An exhaustive standard English text in two volumes.
4. FITZPATRICK, T. B., ARNDT, K. A., CLARK, W. H., EISEN, A. Z., VAN SCOTT, E. J. and VAUGHAN, J. H. (1971) Editors. "Dermatology in Medicine", 2048 pp. New York: McGraw-Hill. An exhaustive standard American text.

# INDEX

Main references are indicated by bold numerals.
Illustrations are referred to by *italic* numerals.